Food *for* Today

Helen Kowtaluk

Now 8 Chapters of GLOBAL FOODS

Ninth Edition

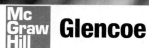 **Glencoe**

New York, New York   Columbus, Ohio   Chicago, Illinois   Peoria, Illinois   Woodland Hills, California

—Dedication—

This ninth edition is dedicated to Helen Kowtaluk, who passed away in late 2004. Throughout her long career in publishing, Helen was committed to providing students with quality educational materials, of which *Food for Today* is the prime example.

Safety Notice

The reader is expressly advised to consider and use all safety precautions described in this textbook or that might also be indicated by undertaking the activities described herein. In addition, common sense should be exercised to help avoid all potential hazards and, in particular, to take relevant safety precautions concerning any known or likely hazards involved in using the procedures described in *Food for Today.*

Publisher and Author assume no responsibility for the activities of the reader or for the subject matter experts who prepared this book. Publisher and Author make no representation or warranties of any kind, including but not limited to the warranties of fitness for particular purpose or merchantability, nor for any implied warranties related thereto, or otherwise. Publisher and Author will not be liable for damages of any type, including any consequential, special or exemplary damages resulting, in whole or in part, from reader's use or reliance upon the information, instructions, warnings or other matter contained in this textbook.

Brand Name Disclaimer

Glencoe/McGraw-Hill does not necessarily recommend or endorse any particular company or brand name product that may be discussed or pictured in this text. Brand name products are used because they are readily available, they are likely to be known to the reader, and their use may aid in the understanding of the text. The publisher recognizes that other brand name or generic products may be substituted and work as well as or better than those featured in the text.

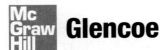

Contents in Brief

Unit 1: FOOD IN YOUR LIFE

Chapter 1: The Amazing World of Food... 22
Chapter 2: Diversity at the Table 34
Chapter 3: The Food Supply...................... 48
Chapter 4: Food Science & Technology 62

Unit 2: NUTRITION BASICS

Chapter 5: Nutrients at Work 76
Chapter 6: Carbohydrates 90
Chapter 7: Proteins & Fats 102
Chapter 8: Vitamins & Minerals............... 116
Chapter 9: Water & Phytochemicals......... 130

Unit 3: HEALTH & WELLNESS

Chapter 10: Nutrition Guidelines............... 142
Chapter 11: Keeping a Healthy Weight 158
Chapter 12: Health Challenges 172
Chapter 13: Life-Span Nutrition 182

Unit 4: FOOD DECISIONS

Chapter 14: Eating Patterns 196
Chapter 15: Vegetarian Food Choices 210
Chapter 16: Meal Planning 220
Chapter 17: Shopping for Food 234
Chapter 18: Serving Food 250
Chapter 19: Etiquette................................. 266

Unit 5: KITCHEN BASICS

Chapter 20: Food Safety & Storage............. 278
Chapter 21: Preventing Kitchen
            Accidents................................ 296
Chapter 22: Equipping the Kitchen............. 306
Chapter 23: Conserving Resources............. 330

Unit 6: THE ART OF COOKING

Chapter 24: Using Recipes 342
Chapter 25: Preparation Techniques 354
Chapter 26: Cooking Methods.................... 366
Chapter 27: Developing a Work Plan 382
Chapter 28: Creative Additions.................. 390
Chapter 29: Preserving Food at Home........ 400

Unit 7: FOOD PREPARATION

Chapter 30: Fruits.................................... 412
Chapter 31: Vegetables 430
Chapter 32: Grain Products 448

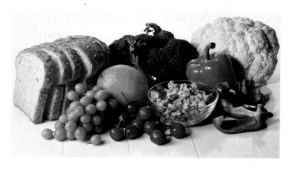

Chapter 33: Legumes, Nuts & Seeds............ 462
Chapter 34: Dairy Foods 476
Chapter 35: Eggs...................................... 490
Chapter 36: Meat 506
Chapter 37: Poultry 520
Chapter 38: Fish & Shellfish 532
Chapter 39: Beverages 544

Unit 8: FOOD COMBINATIONS

Chapter 40: Sandwiches & Pizza................. 558
Chapter 41: Salads & Dressings 570
Chapter 42: Stir-Fries & Casseroles 582
Chapter 43: Soups, Stews & Sauces 592

Unit 9: THE ART OF BAKING

Chapter 44: Baking Basics.......................... 608
Chapter 45: Quick & Yeast Breads 622
Chapter 46: Cakes, Cookies & Candies 634
Chapter 47: Pies & Tarts............................ 648

Unit 10: GLOBAL FOODS

Chapter 48: Foods of the United States
            & Canada 660
Chapter 49: Foods of Latin America &
            the Caribbean 672
Chapter 50: Foods of Western & Northern
            Europe.................................... 682
Chapter 51: Foods of Southern Europe 694
Chapter 52: Foods of Eastern Europe &
            Russia 706
Chapter 53: Foods of Southwest Asia &
            Africa..................................... 716
Chapter 54: Foods of South &
            Eastern Asia 726
Chapter 55: Foods of Australia &
            Oceania 738

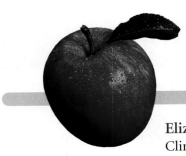

Nutrition Consultant

Elizabeth Shipley Moses, M.S., R.D., C.D.E.
Clinical Nutritionist, Falls Church, Virginia

Teacher Reviewers

Judy Karen Hellums Brown, M.A., NBCT
Department Chair & Culinary Arts Instructor
Madison City Schools, Madison, Alabama

Veronica J. Campbell
Family & Consumer Sciences Educator
Clintonville School District, Clintonville,
    Wisconsin

Renée F. Dickson
Family & Consumer Sciences Teacher
McGuffey School District, Claysville,
    Pennsylvania

Rooney (Lois A.) Dively
Instructor & Gifted Coordinator
Macomb CSU District #185, Macomb, Illinois

**Christine Grovenstein, M.S. Health
Education, CFCS**
Family & Consumer Sciences Teacher
Joe E. Newsome High School, Lithia, Florida

Carole Havelick
Family & Consumer Sciences Teacher
Lakewood High School, Lakewood, Colorado

Eleanor L. Keppler, M.S., CFCS
Family & Consumer Sciences Department Chair
Lawrence Central High School, Indianapolis,
    Indiana

Lana L. Knepp
Family & Consumer Sciences Coordinator
Mifflin County School District, Lewistown,
    Pennsylvania

Teresa Ann Lofty, Ed.S.
Family & Consumer Sciences Teacher
Whitwell High School, Whitwell, Tennessee

Paula Wright Long
Family & Consumer Sciences Teacher
Huntsville City Schools, Huntsville, Alabama

Bonnie Ollinger
Family & Consumer Sciences Teacher
Melbourne High School, Melbourne, Florida

Lynne G. Pritchett
Family & Consumer Sciences Instructor
Gilmer High School, Ellijay, Georgia

Jody Snyder
Family & Consumer Sciences Educator
Steilacoom Historical School District #1
Steilacoom, Washington

Cheryl Swartz
Family & Consumer Sciences Instructor
USD #254, Medicine Lodge, Kansas

Linda Crichlow White, M.S., M.L.S.
Media Specialist
Parkland Middle School, Rockville, Maryland

Anita L. Wilham
Family & Consumer Sciences Teacher
Greenwood Community High School
Greenwood, Indiana

Contents

Unit 1: FOOD IN YOUR LIFE

Chapter 1: The Amazing World of Food 22

• The Power of Food • The Pleasures of Food • The Creative Side of Food • The Career Possibilities of Food • The Global View of Food • Food in Your Future

Career Prep *About the Career Features* 30

Chapter 2: Diversity at the Table 34

• What Is Culture? • Influences on Cuisines and Customs • Similarities in Global Cuisines • Food Customs Today • Food Customs in the U.S.

Career Pathways *Author—Madhur Jaffrey* 45

Chapter 3: The Food Supply 48

• The Food Chain • The Food Supply in the United States • Global Food Problems • Global Water Problems • What Can Be Done?

Career Prep *Career Opportunities* 58

Chapter 4: Food Science & Technology 62

• The Scientific Side of Food • Expanding the Food Supply • Improving Health • Improving Meal Preparation • Food Technology Trade-Offs

Career Pathways *Food Scientist—Craig "Skip" Julius* 71

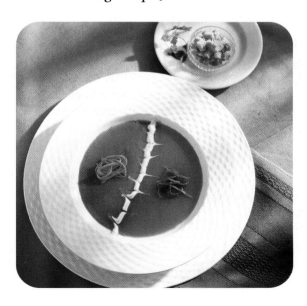

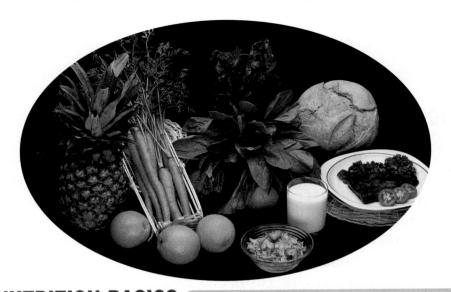

Unit 2: NUTRITION BASICS

Chapter 5: Nutrients at Work 76

• The Nutrients in Foods • The Digestive Process • Absorption of Nutrients
• Nutrient Transportation • Nutrient Storage • Metabolism • An Incredible
Journey

Career Pathways *Nutrition Consultant—Sylvia Meléndez-Klinger*.................................. 87

Chapter 6: Carbohydrates 90

• What Are Carbohydrates? • Making Carbohydrates • Digesting
Carbohydrates • Carbohydrates in Food • The Need for Carbohydrates
• Carbohydrates in the Diet

Career Pathways *Chef—John Rivera Sedlar* 99

Chapter 7: Proteins & Fats 102

• Protein • The Lipid Family

Career Prep *Aspects of Industry* 112

Chapter 8: Vitamins & Minerals 116

• What Are Vitamins? • What Are Minerals?

Career Prep *Using Knowledge and Skills* 126

Chapter 9: Water & Phytochemicals 130

• The Nutrient Water • Phytochemicals

Career Prep *Preparing for the Work World* 136

Unit 3: HEALTH & WELLNESS

Chapter 10: Nutrition Guidelines...................................... 142

• Reliable Resources • Dietary Supplements • Separating Fact from Fiction

Career Pathways *Food Editor—Andria Scott Hurst*.. 155

Chapter 11: Keeping a Healthy Weight 158

• The Ideal Body Myth • The Overweight Epidemic • What Is a Healthy Weight? • Managing Weight • A Healthful Weight-Loss Plan • Commercial Weight-Loss Plans • Gaining Needed Weight • Maintaining a Healthy Weight

Career Pathways *Fitness Consultant—Peter Nielsen*.. 169

Chapter 12: Health Challenges 172

• Stress • Illness and Recovery • Chronic Health Problems • Eating Disorders

Career Prep *FCCLA Opportunities*.. 178

Chapter 13: Life-Span Nutrition 182

• Nutrition for a Lifetime • Pregnancy • Infancy • Childhood • Adolescence • Adulthood

Career Prep *Interests and Aptitudes*.. 190

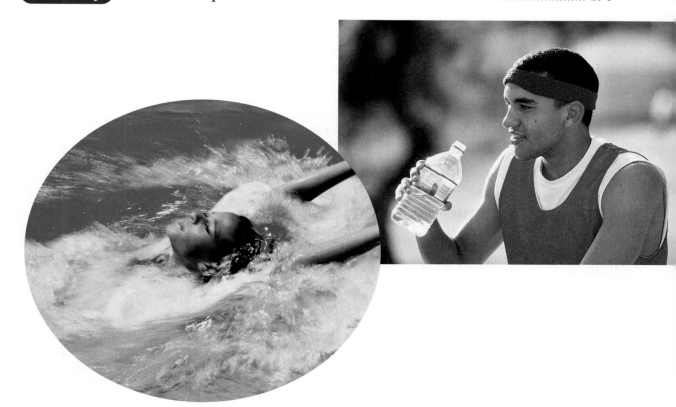

Unit 4: FOOD DECISIONS

Chapter 14: Eating Patterns 196
- What Influences Food Choices? • Eating Patterns • Choices for Eating Out
- Evaluating Your Food Choices • Decision Making

Career Pathways *Publicist—Dick Dace* *207*

Chapter 15: Vegetarian Food Choices 210
- Types of Vegetarians • The Vegetarian Decision • Vegetarian Nutrition
- Daily Food Choices • Exploring Vegetarian Foods

Career Prep *Goal Setting* *216*

Chapter 16: Meal Planning 220
- Meal Planning and Real Life • The Food Budget • Other Resources
- Planning for Convenience • Planning for Appeal • Weekly Meal Planning
- Planning for One

Career Prep *Education and Training* *230*

Chapter 17: Shopping for Food 234
- Where to Shop • Plan Your Shopping • Using Food Labels • Getting Quality
- Getting Your Money's Worth • Checking Out • Responsible Shopping
- Resolving Purchasing Problems

Career Prep *Managing Resources* *246*

Chapter 18: Serving Food 250
- Tableware • Table-Setting Basics • Serving Meals at Home • Service for
Large Groups • Enjoyable Family Meals • Packing a Lunch • Serving Meals
Outdoors • Entertaining

Career Pathways *Professor—Bill Quain* *263*

Chapter 19: Etiquette.. 266
- Table Etiquette Basics • Restaurant Etiquette

Career Prep *Locating Job Opportunities* *272*

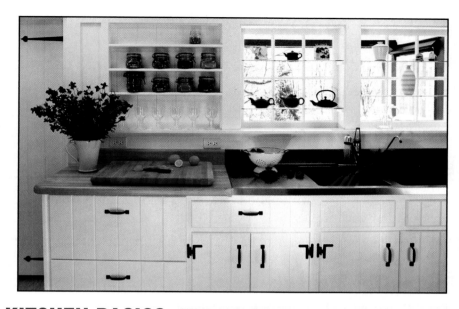

Unit 5: KITCHEN BASICS

Chapter 20: Food Safety & Storage.................... 278

• Foodborne Illness • Cleanliness in the Kitchen • Don't Cross-Contaminate
• Cook Food Thoroughly • Refrigerate Food Promptly • Storing Food
• Safeguarding the Food Supply

Career Pathways *Home Economist—Charla Draper*.................... 293

Chapter 21: Preventing Kitchen Accidents 296

• Kitchen Safety Basics • Preventing Falls • Handling Sharp Edges
• Preventing Fires and Burns • Using Electricity Safely • Hazardous
Household Chemicals • Cooking Outdoors Safely • Protecting Family
Members • In Case of Accident

Career Prep *Choosing Entrepreneurship* 302

Chapter 22: Equipping the Kitchen.................... 306

• Kitchen Design Basics • Kitchen Components • Buying for the Kitchen
• Major Appliances • Small Appliances • Cookware and Bakeware • Food
Preparation Tools • The Outdoor Kitchen

Career Pathways *CEO—Helen Chen*.................... 327

Chapter 23: Conserving Resources 330

• Why Conserve? • Using Energy Efficiently • Using Water Wisely • Taking
Out the Trash • A World Perspective

Career Prep *Preparing a Resumé* 336

Unit 6: THE ART OF COOKING

Chapter 24: Using Recipes 342

• The Well-Written Recipe • Weights and Measures • Changing a Recipe
• Collecting Recipes

Career Prep *Applying for a Job*.................. 350

Chapter 25: Preparation Techniques.................. 354

• Measuring Ingredients • Cutting Foods • Mixing Ingredients • Coating
Techniques • Other Techniques

Career Prep *Job Interviews* 362

Chapter 26: Cooking Methods.................. 366

• How Food Cooks • Cooking Rates • Moist-Heat Cooking • Cooking in Fat
• Dry-Heat Cooking • Microwave Cooking

Career Pathways *Radio Show Host—Lynne Rossetto Kasper*.................. 379

Chapter 27: Developing a Work Plan 382

• The Work Plan • Teamwork in the School Foods Lab • Teamwork at Home

Career Prep *Dressing for Work*.................. 386

Chapter 28: Creative Additions 390

• Seasonings • Garnishes • Freshening Up Favorites • Food as Gifts

Career Pathways *Graphic Designer—Leigh-Anne Tompkins*.................. 397

Chapter 29: Preserving Food at Home.................. 400

• Praise of Preserving • Preparing to Preserve • Freezing Fruits and Vegetables
• Canning Fruits and Vegetables • Drying Food
• Using Home-Preserved Food

Career Prep *Wages and Benefits*.................. 406

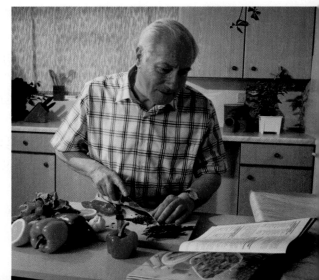

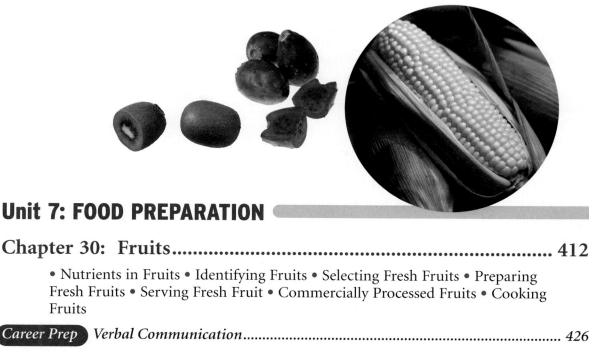

Unit 7: FOOD PREPARATION

Chapter 30: Fruits.. 412

• Nutrients in Fruits • Identifying Fruits • Selecting Fresh Fruits • Preparing Fresh Fruits • Serving Fresh Fruit • Commercially Processed Fruits • Cooking Fruits

Career Prep *Verbal Communication*.. 426

Chapter 31: Vegetables 430

• Nutrients in Vegetables • Types of Vegetables • Fresh Vegetables • Convenience Forms of Vegetables • Using Leftover Vegetables

Career Pathways *Television Chef—Curtis Aikens*............................ 445

Chapter 32: Grain Products............................... 448

• What Are Grains? • Nutrients in Grains • Grains and Grain Products • Convenience Forms of Grains • Buying and Storing Grains • Preparing Grains

Career Prep *Nonverbal Communication* 458

Chapter 33: Legumes, Nuts & Seeds 462

• Legumes • Nuts • Seeds

Career Prep *Electronic Communication* 472

Chapter 34: Dairy Foods 476

• Nutrients in Dairy Foods • Milk and Milk Products • Cheese • Dairy Substitutes • Buying Dairy Foods • Storing Dairy Foods • Using Dairy Foods

Career Prep *Technology in the Workplace* 486

Chapter 35: Eggs 490

• The Structure of Eggs • Nutrients in Eggs • Buying Eggs • Storing Eggs
• Egg Substitutes • Egg Science • Preparing Eggs for Cooking • Cooking
with Eggs

Career Prep *A Work Ethic* 502

Chapter 36: Meat 506

• Nutrients in Meat • Makeup of Meat • Identifying Meat Cuts • Inspection
and Grading • Judging Meat Tenderness • Ground Meat • Variety Meats
• Processed Meats • Convenience Forms • Buying Meat • Storing Meat
• Cooking Meat

Career Pathways *Executive Director—Dina Chacón-Reitzel* 517

Chapter 37: Poultry 520

• Nutrients • Types of Poultry • Forms of Poultry • Inspection and Grading
• Buying Poultry • Storing Poultry • Cooking Poultry

Career Prep *Responsible Leadership* 528

Chapter 38: Fish & Shellfish 532

• Fish and Shellfish Nutrition • Types of Fish and Shellfish • Inspection and
Grading • Buying Fish and Shellfish • Storing Fish and Shellfish • Cooking
Fish • Cooking Shellfish • Microwaving Methods

Career Prep *Setting Priorities* 540

Chapter 39: Beverages 544

• Water • Juices • Coffee • Tea • Dairy-Based Beverages • Punch • Soft
Drinks • Microwaving Beverages

Career Prep *A Positive Attitude* 552

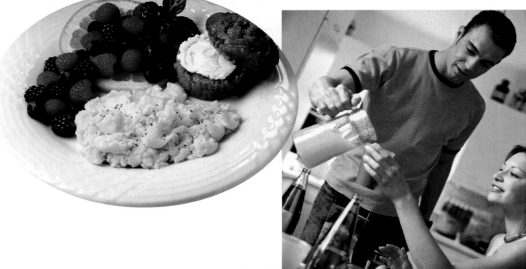

Unit 8: FOOD COMBINATIONS

Chapter 40: Sandwiches & Pizza 558
• What Is a Sandwich? • Pizza

Career Pathways *Marketer—Santiago Ogradón Cortés* 567

Chapter 41: Salads & Dressings 570
• Types of Salads • Choosing Salad Greens • Choosing Salad Dressings
• Making and Serving Salads

Career Prep *Business Etiquette* 578

Chapter 42: Stir-Fries & Casseroles 582
• Stir-Fries • Casseroles

Career Prep *Positive Work Relationships* 588

Chapter 43: Soups, Stews & Sauces 592
• Liquids • Thickening Methods • Soups • Stews • Sauces • Storage

Career Pathways *Television Co-Host—Aaron Sanchez* 603

Unit 9: THE ART OF BAKING

Chapter 44: Baking Basics 608
• Ingredients for Baking • The Baking Process • Storing Baked Products

Career Prep *Anger Management* 618

Chapter 45: Quick & Yeast Breads 622
• Making Quick Breads • The Marvel of Yeast Bread • Making Yeast Bread

Career Prep *Problem Solving* 630

Chapter 46: Cakes, Cookies & Candies 634
• Making Cakes • Making Cookies • Making Candies

Career Pathways *Food Photographer—Lois Ellen Frank* 645

Chapter 47: Pies & Tarts 648
• Pies • Tarts • Baking Pies and Tarts • Convenience Pies and Tarts

Career Prep *Ethics on the Job* 654

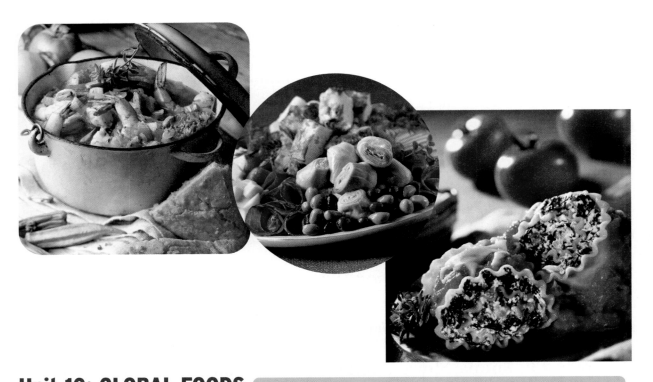

Unit 10: GLOBAL FOODS

Chapter 48: Foods of the United States & Canada 660

• The United States • Canada

Career Pathways *Restaurant Owner—Derrick Robinson*...................................... 669

Chapter 49: Foods of Latin America & the Caribbean 672

• Latin America • The Caribbean

Career Pathways *Entrepreneur—Park Kerr* 679

Chapter 50: Foods of Western & Northern Europe.................... 682

• Western Europe • Northern Europe

Career Prep *Working with the Public* 690

Chapter 51: Foods of Southern Europe 694

• Mediterranean Cuisines • Spain • Portugal • Italy • Greece

Career Pathways *On-Line Editor—Kate Heyhoe*.. 703

Chapter 52: Foods of Eastern Europe & Russia......................... 706

• Eastern Europe • Russia • The Independent Republics

Career Prep *Managing Life's Demands*.. 712

Chapter 53: Foods of Southwest Asia & Africa............ 716

• Southwest Asia • North Africa • Sub-Saharan Africa

Career Prep *Managing Stress* 722

Chapter 54: Foods of South & Eastern Asia.................. 726

• South Asia • East Asia • Southeast Asia

Career Prep *Workplace Laws*.. 734

Chapter 55: Foods of Australia & Oceania.................... 738

• Australia • Oceania

Career Prep *Career Advancement* 742

Glossary............................ 746

Credits 757

Index................................ 759

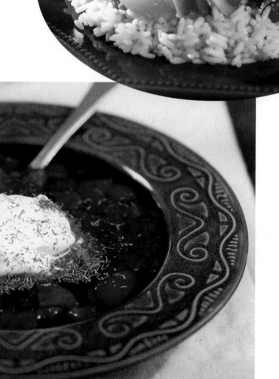

HIGHLIGHTED TOPICS

Celebrations Around the World 42
Dietary Reference Intakes for Teens 80
Daily Values 81
Calories in Nutrients 85
Approximate Daily Calories for Teens 86
Nutrient Sources for Calories 86
Sugar Ingredients in Foods 96
Dietary Fiber in Selected Foods 98
Approximate Protein in Selected
    Foods 106
Approximate Cholesterol in Selected
    Foods 109
Approximate Fat in Selected Foods 111
Food Sources of Water-Soluble
    Vitamins 118
Food Sources of Fat-Soluble Vitamins 121
Food Sources of Major Minerals 123
Food Sources of Trace Minerals 125
Approximate Water Content of Food 133
Summary of Dietary Guidelines for
    Americans 144
Selected Calorie Levels from USDA
    Food Guide 145
Sample Serving Sizes 146
Nutrition Facts Panel 148
Sample Nutrient Ranges for Teens 149
Checking Up on Nutrients 150
Calories Used in Activities 165
Food Terms to Know 204
Sample Meal Plan 228
Decoding the Food Label 240
Servings per Pound of Meat, Poultry,
    and Fish 244
How Much to Tip 271
Some Bacteria That Cause Foodborne
    Illness 280
Cold Temperature Storage of Meats,
    Poultry, and Fish 287
Cold Temperature Storage of Dairy
    Products and Miscellaneous Foods 287
Cookware and Bakeware Materials 318
Units of Measurement 346

Volume and Weight Equivalents.................. 347
Conversion Chart 348
Ingredient Substitutions 349
Microwave Power Levels 376
Sunday Brunch Timetable 384
Work Plan for Sunday Brunch 385
Commonly Used Herbs 392
Commonly Used Spices 394
Have You Tried These Fruits? 414
Fruit Descriptions and Uses 415
Vegetable Descriptions and Uses 432
Common Sea Vegetables 438
Grain Forms 450
Common Pasta Shapes 455
Dried Pasta Yields 457
Grain Cooking Times and Yields................. 459
A Guide to Legumes 465
A Guide to Nuts 470
Ripened Cheeses 482
Types of Meat.. 508
Wholesale Cuts of Meat 509
Bone Shapes: The Clue to Tenderness 511
Internal Doneness Temperatures for
    Meat 515
How to Cut Up a Whole Chicken 523
Low-Fat Fish.. 534
Fatty Fish 535
How Much Caffeine? 545
A Guide to Salad Greens 576
Starch Amount for Thickening Liquids 595
Baking Pan Equivalents 637
Stages in Cold Water Test 643
How to Make a Lattice Piecrust................... 653

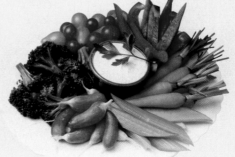

Fruit Punch 262

Granola 344

Griddled Potato Scones 345

Kiwifruit Leather 402

Peach-Blueberry Crisp 424

Sautéed Greens 442

Apple and Spice Oatmeal 451

Molded Pasta Salad 457

Boston Baked Beans 468

Easy Macaroni and Cheese 487

Italian Frittata 500

Chili 512

Chicken with Pasta and Horseradish

    Cream Sauce 524

Fish and Vegetables en Papillote 539

Strawberry Yogurt Splendor 551

Italian Sandwiches 561

Pizza Snacks 565

Homestyle Coleslaw 572

Fresh 'n' Fast Fried Rice 585

French Oven Beef Stew 595

White Sauce 601

Cranberry Almond Muffins 625

Buttermilk Biscuits 626

Sunny Carrot Cake 636

Lemony Sugar Cookies 639

Chocolate Peanut Clusters 642

Chocolate Pie 650

Pie Shell 651

Soft Pretzels 663

Maple Ice Cream Sandwiches 668

Chayotes Rellenos con Queso 677

Cuban Black Bean Soup 678

Lemon Curd 684

Ratatouille 686

Blaukraut 688

Gazpacho 697

Gnocchi 700

Fresh Tomato Sauce 701

Avgolemono (Egg-Lemon Soup) 702

Goulash 708

Kasha 710

Hummus 719

Moroccan Fruited Couscous 720

Dal 728

Asian Fried Rice with Peas 731

Edamame Salad 732

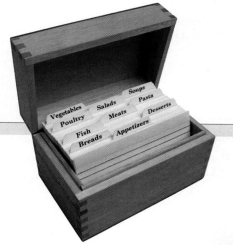

Nutrition Connection

Make a nutrition connection by learning how much you need of different foods in order to eat healthfully.

Career Pathways

Author: Madhur Jaffrey......................... 45

Food Scientist: Craig "Skip" Julius 71

Nutrition Consultant: Sylvia
    Meléndez-Klinger 87

Chef: John Rivera Sedlar 99

Food Editor: Andria Scott Hurst 155

Fitness Consultant: Peter Nielsen 169

Publicist: Dick Dace 207

Professor: Bill Quain 263

Home Economist: Charla Draper 293

CEO: Helen Chen 327

Radio Show Host: Lynne Rossetto Kasper..... 379

Graphic Designer: Leigh-Anne Tompkins 397

Television Chef: Curtis Aikens 445

Executive Director: Dina Chacón-Reitzel 517

Marketer: Santiago Ogradón Cortés............. 567

Television Co-Host: Aaron Sanchez 603

Food Photographer: Lois Ellen Frank 645

Restaurant Owner: Derrick Robinson 669

Entrepreneur: Park Kerr 679

On-Line Editor: Kate Heyhoe 703

Career Prep

About the Career Features.......................... 30

Career Opportunities................................ 58

Aspects of Industry 112

Using Knowledge and Skills 126

Preparing for the Work World 136

FCCLA Opportunities 178

Interests and Aptitudes............................. 190

Goal Setting 216

Education and Training.............................. 230

Managing Resources 246

Locating Job Opportunities 272

Choosing Entrepreneurship 302

Preparing a Resumé 336

Applying for a Job 350

Job Interviews... 362

Dressing for Work 386

Wages and Benefits 406

Verbal Communication 426

Unspoken Communication 458

Electronic Communication 472

Technology in the Workplace........................ 486

A Work Ethic 502

Responsible Leadership 528

Setting Priorities... 540

A Positive Attitude 552

Business Etiquette 578

Positive Work Relationships.......................... 588

Anger Management..................................... 618

Problem Solving.. 630

Ethics on the Job 654

Working with the Public............................... 690

Managing Life's Demands 712

Managing Stress 722

Workplace Laws... 734

Career Advancement................................... 742

TRENDS in TECHNOLOGY

New Ways with Waste 52
Ready—or Not? 70
Nutrition Analysis Software 152
Big Steps in Baby Foods 186
"Milking Soybeans" 215
Groceries in Your Computer 237
Nonstick Finishes 322
"Green" Plastics 335

Recipe Files 351
Talented 'Taters 441
New Dairy Technologies 485
Egg Laying Technology 493
Salads in Space 573
Cryogenics in the Kitchen 615
Bush Tucker 740

Consumer FYI

Snacking for Health 202
Dining Out 216
Hectic Lives Versus Healthful Meals 225
Farmers Markets 236
Policing the Food Supply 290
Childproofing the Kitchen 301
Clay-Pot Cooking 321
Recipe Trends 343
Cooking Classes 370
Cookie Cutter Art 396
Square Watermelons? 420
Baby Vegetables 439
Adding Oats 453
Soy for Dessert? 469
Eggshells 493
Tea and Health 549
Creative Condiments 560
"Casseroles" to Go 587
Fats for Baking 613
Bread Machines 628

food science

Look for this logo beside text passages that provide food science information.

SAFETY ALERT

This important feature will alert you to safety issues involving food consumption and preparation.

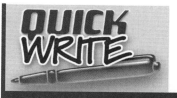

QUICK WRITE

Practice your writing skills by starting each chapter with the writing idea provided. Each exercise is linked to a writing technique.

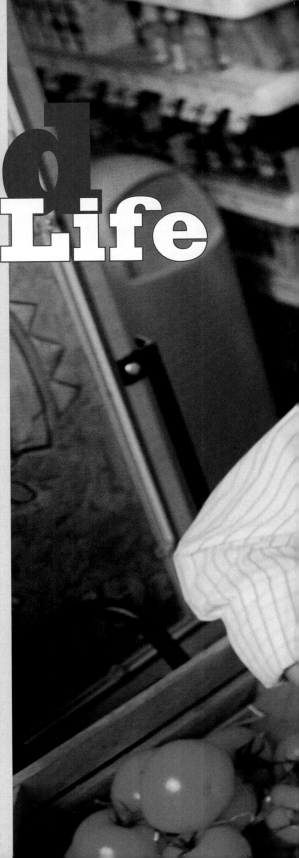

UNIT 1

Food in Your Life

CHAPTER 1 The Amazing World of Food

CHAPTER 2 Diversity at the Table

CHAPTER 3 The Food Supply

CHAPTER 4 Food Science & Technology

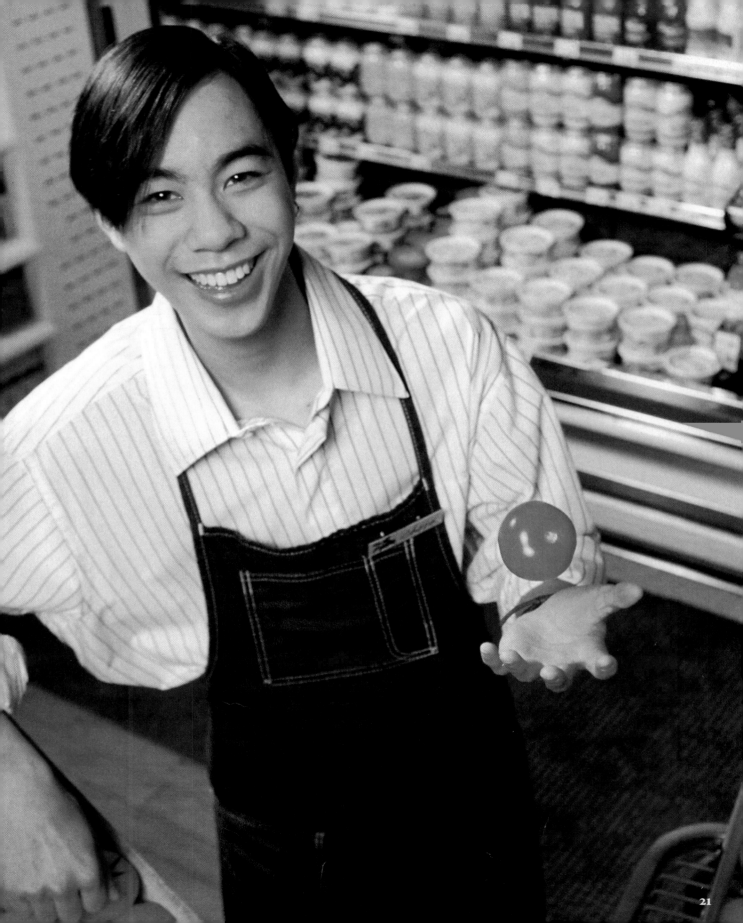

The Amazing World of Food

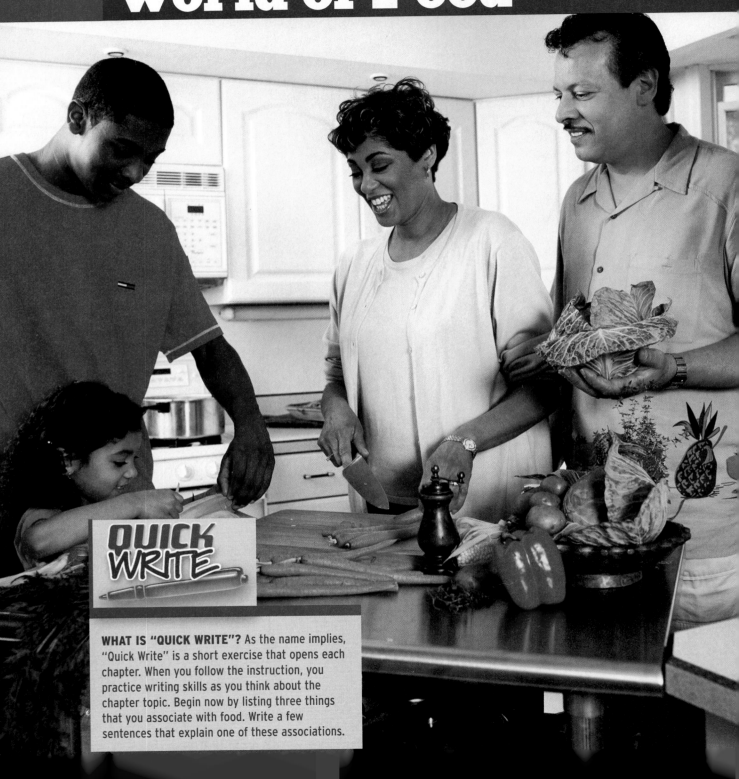

QUICK WRITE

WHAT IS "QUICK WRITE"? As the name implies, "Quick Write" is a short exercise that opens each chapter. When you follow the instruction, you practice writing skills as you think about the chapter topic. Begin now by listing three things that you associate with food. Write a few sentences that explain one of these associations.

Objectives

▶ Explain what makes food powerful.

▶ Describe ways that foods bring pleasure.

▶ Explain the connection between careers and the world of food.

▶ Summarize the food challenge humanity faces globally.

▶ Describe skills and qualities you can build during your foods course.

Terms

comfort foods
critical thinking
leadership
management
nonverbal communication
nutrients
nutrition
self-esteem
verbal communication
wellness

A T THE BREAKFAST TABLE, A TEEN IS thinking about a history test at school. She barely notices the cereal she's eating. During lunch, she munches a sandwich, but she's so involved in talking to a friend that thoughts of the sandwich hardly enter her mind. Sometimes food is taken for granted, but if you stop and think about it, you'll see that food has a huge impact on your life. Food is truly amazing, and the incredible story of food begins with its power to help keep you alive and healthy.

THE POWER OF FOOD

Food is essential for life, for without it people perish. That pang of hunger that sends you to the refrigerator is there for a reason. It tells you that it's time to eat. Food not only helps you live, but it also affects the quality of your life. If you make poor food choices, you pay a price—physically, mentally, and emotionally.

Nutrition

Picture in your mind a few of your favorite foods. Do you see pizza, yogurt, an apple, or maybe a bagel? What you can't see is that food is made of many different chemicals that your body can use. Now imagine each food breaking apart into thousands of particles. This actually happens when you eat. Food is made of many different chemicals that are released when food breaks down. These chemicals are life-sustaining compounds known as **nutrients**. The body must have them to function, grow, repair itself, and create energy. See **Fig. 1-1**.

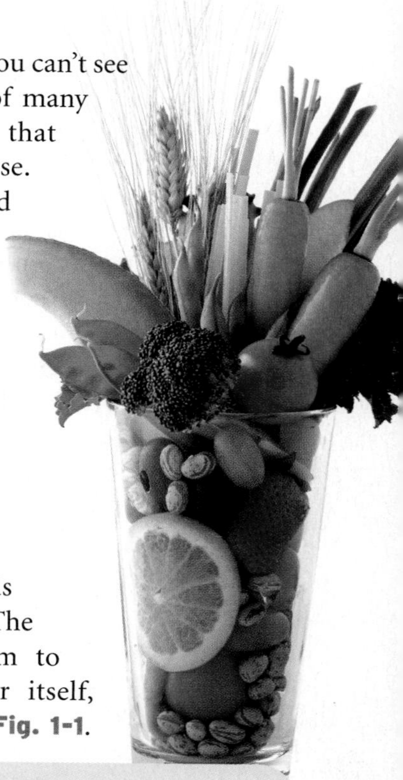

Fig. 1-1 Foods contain substances that people need. What are they?

These chemicals are so important that they have given rise to a branch of science called nutrition. **Nutrition** is the study of nutrients and how the body uses them.

People often think of nutrition in a slightly different sense. They relate nutrition to how food choices affect health. You are said to practice good nutrition if you eat foods that provide all the nutrients needed and in the right amounts.

Although many people consciously try to make healthy food choices, some don't. Those who know little about nutrition or aren't interested in improving their eating habits make poor food choices. This can lead to problems with nutrition and health. The way food affects health demonstrates the power of food like nothing else. You can harness this power by making healthful food choices, which can help you experience wellness.

Wellness

When should you think about your health? Some people wait until they develop health problems to ask what they should have done differently. Today many people prefer to do their best to stay healthy. The word "wellness" is commonly used to explain this approach.

Wellness is a person's total health, including physical, mental, and emotional well-being. With wellness, you're not just free from illness; you're practicing preventive care that helps you stay at your peak of good health. Wellness is a philosophy that encourages people to take responsibility for their own health before they become ill. It is reflected in both attitudes and behavior. See **Fig. 1-2.**

Your health is influenced by heredity, lifestyle, and the food you eat. You may be an average, healthy person or you may have been born with a physical weakness. Within this framework, however, you have the potential for good health.

Practicing wellness is not a guarantee against sickness. It is, however, a way to help you achieve the highest level of health possible for you. Moreover, it may reduce your risk of developing such chronic diseases as diabetes and heart disease. While practicing wellness, many decisions influence your health. They include decisions in all these areas:

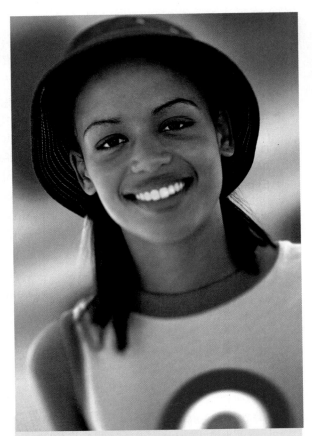

Fig. 1-2 Practicing wellness can help you stay at your peak of good health. What can you do to influence your wellness in positive ways?

- The food choices you make.
- The amount of physical activity you get.
- How you manage your feelings and emotions.
- Decisions to stay free of alcohol and other drugs.

By developing habits that promote wellness, you have a better chance to remain healthy and happy throughout your life. The food choices you make are a powerful part of this effort.

The Role of Science

What difference does it make whether you choose to eat french fries once in a while or you eat them every day? It makes a big difference, and science can tell you why.

Through research, scientists continue to discover much about the nutrients in food and their importance to good health. What chemicals are in food? How are they processed in your body? What do they do for you, and how do they work together? As you learn more about the science of nutrition, your eating decisions can be made more wisely.

Science can also help you in the kitchen. Why does yeast dough have to be kneaded? How can you keep an apple from turning brown? Science has answers to questions like these. Your cooking skills and confidence improve when you understand kitchen science. See **Fig. 1-3**.

These are not the only ways that science links to food. Think about the foods available in supermarkets. That wide assortment is there partly due to science.

- **Agriculture.** Farmers are supplied with the latest information to help them increase the food supply and grow top-quality food.
- **Food processing.** Improvements in processing methods help insure a bountiful supply of nutritious food throughout the year.
- **Food safety.** Scientists provide the latest information on safe food handling methods and also monitor the quality of the nation's food supply.

Without science, food would be less available and less understood. With science, you have many healthful foods to eat and the knowledge to choose them.

THE PLEASURES OF FOOD

In today's world, food offers much more than nutrition. It is an amazing source of pleasure. Creative minds have found countless ways to make good food one of the delights of living.

Enjoyment

To most people, food is more than a necessity—it's a source of enjoyment. Food satisfies the senses and makes you feel good.

A few studies suggest that people who enjoy their food absorb more nutrients from it. Some scientists reason that the digestive process is involved. Before eating and even when you see or smell food, your brain reacts. It instructs your

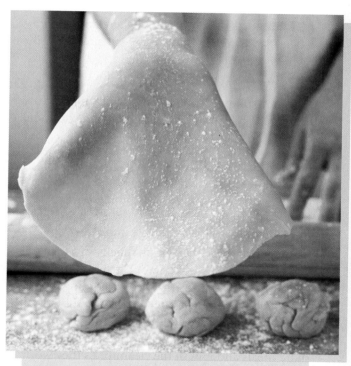

Fig. 1-3 In many ways, the kitchen is like a science lab. Learning how yeast reacts in dough, for example, can help you bake successfully.

mouth and stomach to get ready to digest the food by making chemicals to help break the food down. If you don't like the food or it looks unappetizing, however, the brain may be reluctant to tell the body to start the digestive process. As a result, fewer nutrients become available.

Many countries recognize the importance of enjoying food and making mealtimes pleasant. Some have issued dietary guidelines that not only recommend what to eat but also encourage people to enjoy food. Here are some examples:

- **Japan.** Make all activities pertaining to food pleasurable ones. Sit down and eat together and talk. Enjoy cooking at home.
- **Great Britain.** Enjoy good food.
- **Norway.** Food + joy = health.
- **Korea.** Enjoy meals. Keep harmony between the diet and daily life.

- **Thailand.** A happy family is when family members eat together and enjoy treasured family tastes and good home cooking.
- **South Africa.** Enjoy a variety of foods.

When you take time to enjoy your meals, you help your body to good health. This is a common message around the world.

Family and Social Ties

"I don't know exactly why, but every time my family has people over for dinner or a party, everyone gathers in the kitchen." Do you share this teen's observation? Guests seem to be drawn to kitchens, where they enjoy snacks and conversation while food is prepared. Kitchens are warm and busy, with aromas that are welcoming.

For many families, the kitchen is the social center of the home. That's where family members fix meals and talk about the day's events. They share meals and join in the cleanup. As they work and eat together, family bonds strengthen.

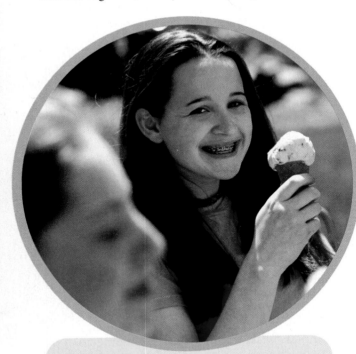

Fig. 1-4 People often enjoy sharing food with friends at special events. Why do you think food is part of so many social gatherings?

The social significance of food stretches far beyond the kitchen. See **Fig. 1-4**. If you think about the pleasant times you've had, chances are many of them involved food. Food is part of such social events as weddings, birthday parties, and holiday celebrations. Certain foods, like hot dogs at a baseball game, are linked to sporting events. Food adds a bright spot and a break during a busy committee meeting. A Super Bowl party just wouldn't seem right without food. Sharing a pizza with friends is fun. Even when a friend comes to your house, you may offer something to eat or drink.

Why is it that most social occasions include food? Food makes people feel welcome and at ease. Food can be a focus of conversation and activity. It can create a warm feeling of hospitality, making it easier for people to socialize.

Comfort

When stressed, troubled, bored, or unhappy, people often turn to food for comfort. **Comfort foods**, which are usually creamy, soft, and rich, are familiar foods that make people feel good.

Common comfort foods are ice cream, chocolate, macaroni and cheese, mashed or fried potatoes, fresh bread with butter, pizza, fried chicken, spaghetti, potato chips, and rice pudding. Comfort foods are often high in fat and calories. See **Fig. 1-5**.

Frequently, comfort foods remind people of times during childhood, when life was simple and carefree. Recent scientific research suggests that comfort foods may slow the release of stress-related hormones, making people feel better. Do any foods comfort you when you're unhappy or stressed?

Entertainment

Your ancestors probably didn't think of food as entertainment, but today food entertains in many ways. Eating out is one form of entertainment. Restaurants are all around, serving everything from fast food to elegant culinary specialties. Some people eat out regularly, perhaps once a week. Some enjoy spending a whole evening at their favorite restaurant. One mother and daughter decided to try every ethnic restaurant in their

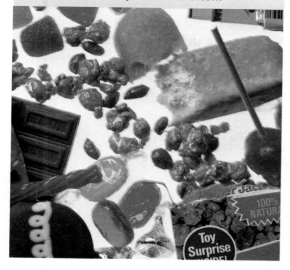

Fig. 1-5 Some foods give people feelings of comfort. What might happen if these foods "comfort" a person too often?

tion and ones that specialize in such foods as bread or poultry. Many cookbooks cover regional and ethnic cooking. Some books are devoted to the science behind foods and cooking. Reading about foods is one more way that food entertains people today.

Adventure

Do you long for adventure? Food can help by bringing you new and different experiences. You might try a new food you've never tasted before. To start, look for unusual fruits and vegetables in the produce department of a supermarket. You can also experiment with recipes and cooking techniques. If you're ambitious, prepare a chocolate mousse or learn to debone a chicken.

city as a way to spend time together. (The term ethnic refers to different nationalities.)

Who would think that food could be the topic for a whole cable channel? It is, and you can watch everything from a professional chef at work, to the way restaurants around the world prepare foods, to how candies are made. You can even visit farms in many countries to see how foods are grown and harvested, all from the comfort of your living room.

In many areas of the country, food festivals are annual events that draw crowds. People celebrate the pumpkin, strawberry, blueberry, watermelon, peach, corn, lobster, and crawfish, to name a few. See **Fig. 1-6**. You might never know all the inventive ways to prepare pumpkin until you go to a pumpkin festival. Ethnic festivals offer an opportunity to taste new foods or to put your own family's culture in the spotlight.

Many people enjoy reading magazines on food preparation—even though they might never prepare the recipes. Avid cookbook collectors find hours of pleasure in browsing through their favorites. The demand for cookbooks is so great that bookstores offer a wide selection. You can buy cookbooks that cover general food prepara-

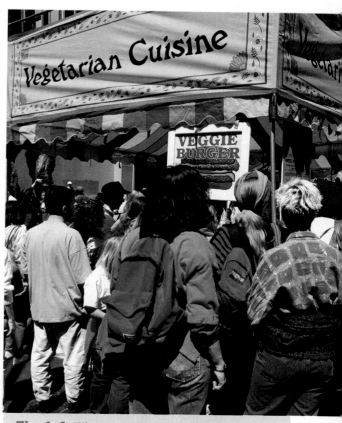

Fig. 1-6 When you think about it, food is surprisingly entertaining these days. People gather at all sorts of festivals to enjoy featured foods. How else do food and entertainment go together?

Many adventurous people like to explore ethnic foods and global food customs. Browsing an ethnic market may introduce you to different foods and seasonings to try. In ethnic restaurants, you could sample something unfamiliar on the menu. Friends with different ethnic backgrounds might explain their food customs to you. All of these ideas can bring the adventure of food into your life.

THE CREATIVE SIDE OF FOOD

If you're not yet convinced that food is amazing, watch professional chefs create desserts in competition. The elaborate structures of spun sugar and chocolate are truly artistic. People who appreciate food as an art form can turn ordinary recipes into dishes that are as appealing to the eye as they are flavorful. Presenting and serving food attractively becomes as important as proper preparation. See **Fig. 1-7**.

Many people express their creativity as they prepare and serve food. Turning an assortment of ingredients into a delicious dish can be quite sat-

isfying. Sharing the dish with others makes the enjoyment even greater.

The food preparation methods you'll learn in this course are based on scientific principles. They form the foundation for all cooking. Once you learn and understand them, you can experiment with your own food combinations. You can show your own creativity. You might even head for a cooking contest or a county fair to show your skills.

THE CAREER POSSIBILITIES OF FOOD

If you're starting to appreciate how interesting the world of food is, a food career could be in your future. How would you like to be the person who creates ideas for new ice cream flavors? Maybe you'd like to decorate beautiful wedding cakes in your own bakery. Does making delicious dishes as a chef sound appealing? If none of these seems right for you, maybe another of the many food-related careers is.

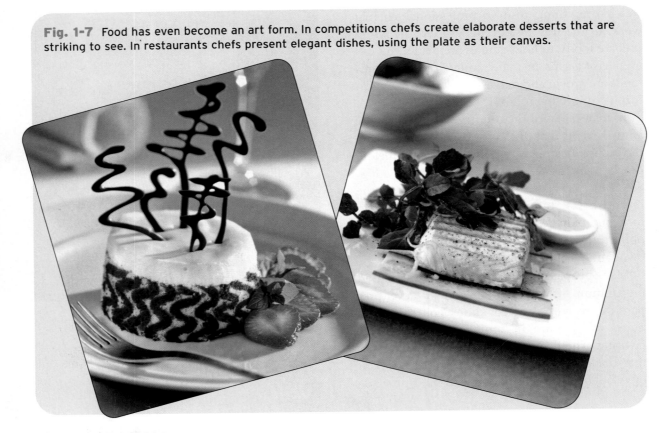

Fig. 1-7 Food has even become an art form. In competitions chefs create elaborate desserts that are striking to see. In restaurants chefs present elegant dishes, using the plate as their canvas.

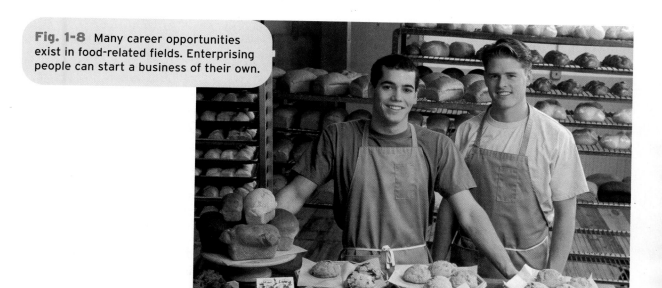

Fig. 1-8 Many career opportunities exist in food-related fields. Enterprising people can start a business of their own.

Too often, people choose a line of work without really knowing much about it. This important decision may be left to chance, when it should be carefully thought out. To find a satisfying career, let this course be an opportunity for exploration.

Many careers today are food-related. If you like science, food science is fascinating. If you're interested in nutrition, you might find out about dietetics. If you like the outdoors, you might like agriculture. You can teach, cook, write, or take pictures. That's just the beginning. As you learn about food, learn about related careers too. You just might find the right match for your life's work. See **Fig. 1-8**.

THE GLOBAL VIEW OF FOOD

No discussion about food would be complete without looking at the global view. As technology brings people closer around the world, perspectives on food are changing. Through television and international travel, Americans are learning more and more about faraway foods and customs. As immigrants move from one country into another, they bring along their food customs, which are shared and sometimes blended with customs in the new environment. One result is increased interest in global foods, making ethnic restaurants more popular than ever. See **Fig. 1-9**.

Modern transportation makes it possible to import foods from even the most remote areas of the globe. Therefore ethnic foods are now sold in supermarkets side by side with traditional American favorites. Ethnic foods are changing the way many Americans cook.

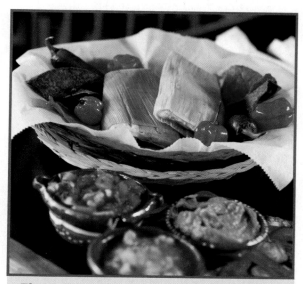

Fig. 1-9 Greater availability of ethnic foods has opened the door to trying many dishes that were unfamiliar to previous generations. You can sample foods from different cultures in restaurants or make them yourself.

At the same time people have also become aware of the inequality in the global food supply. Some nations have more food than they need, while people in other nations are starving. The challenge facing humanity is to ensure an adequate food supply for every person on the planet so that no one goes hungry.

FOOD IN YOUR FUTURE

Your adventure in food is about to begin. There is so much more to learn about the many ways that food impacts your life. As you work with food during this course, you have an extra bonus. You'll build skills and qualities that are useful in all areas of your life. See **Fig. 1-10**.

- **Self-esteem. Self-esteem** is the feeling that you are a worthwhile, capable person. Building food preparation skills and sharing your efforts with others can help raise your self-esteem.
- **Critical thinking.** Through **critical thinking**, you analyze and evaluate what you hear and

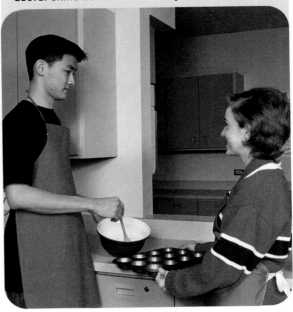

Fig. 1-10 In the foods lab, you won't just learn to prepare foods. You'll learn other useful skills as well. What might those be?

Career Prep

About the Career Features

AS YOU'VE SEEN IN THIS CHAPTER, topics in foods and nutrition are everywhere today. Books tell you how to lose weight and improve fitness. Television cooking shows bring you a world of cuisines. Internet chat rooms buzz with health information—and misinformation. If all this interest in foods and health has you interested in a career in the foods industry, the two career features in this book will be a valuable guide. One of the two career features is located at the end of each chapter.

In the feature you're reading now, called "Career Prep," you'll find insights into what it takes to succeed in a career today. What qualities do employers look for? What skills will you need? How can you start preparing for a career

while still in school? You'll also learn the "nuts and bolts" of tracking down jobs, writing a resumé, and using e-mail at work. Other articles deal with issues that affect life, both on the job and off, such as reaching goals and resolving conflict. Each article includes a "Career Connection" activity that encourages you to explore the topic further or apply the discussion in a realistic situation.

"Career Pathways" is the other career feature in your text. It contains profiles about successful people in the foods world and gives you a real-life look at the food industry, as described by people who work in it. How does a home economist come to own her own consulting firm? Where does a cookbook author find all

read. You become better able to understand and interpret information. For example, you recognize when a health claim for a food product sounds too good to be true. You notice and resist negative influences on your food choices.

- **Communication.** Working in the foods lab can increase your ability to communicate well. **Verbal communication** includes speaking, listening, writing, and reading. You send and receive messages about thoughts, feelings, and information. A good communicator in the foods lab listens to what the teacher says, relays instructions to others, and follows directions. **Nonverbal communication** sends messages without words. Facial expressions offer quick clues to what you're thinking and feeling. For example, if you taste something you don't like when you're with others, you might say nothing even though your feelings show in your expression.

- **Leadership.** **Leadership** is a person's ability to guide or direct people. As you learn more about nutrition, you could show leadership by helping others choose healthful foods.

- **Management.** Using specific techniques to handle resources wisely as you reach for goals is called **management**. In your foods class, you will learn to manage time so that several dishes are ready to eat at a meal. You will learn about managing a food budget and sticking to it. You will also learn to keep a food record for evaluating your eating habits. In addition, you will learn to plan meals. Good organization is part of management. It shows when you arrange food and equipment in an orderly and logical way for quick and efficient meal preparation.

People enjoy foods classes so much these days. What better place to learn skills for life while sampling delicious foods? So get ready for exploration. The amazing world of food awaits you.

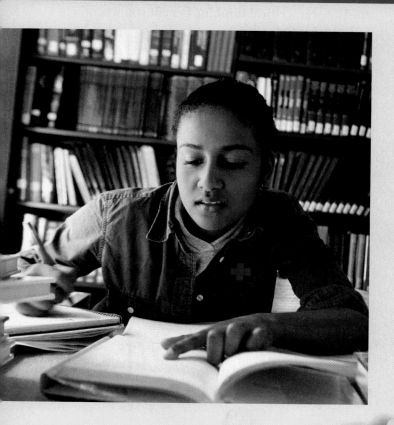

those recipes? What's it like to be a food photographer? As you meet the people in this feature, you'll encounter both information and inspiration.

Together, "Career Prep" and "Career Pathways" may help you decide whether a job in foods and nutrition is waiting for you. If so, who knows? Your own experience and insight might someday be included in a textbook for future foods professionals.

Career Connection

Questions and answers. Write at least five questions you have about foods and nutrition careers. Compare questions in class and create a master list of questions that your class will answer throughout this course. Keep the list in a visible place for regular reference. You may find many answers in the career features. If not, search other references for answers.

Summarize Your Reading

▶ Food contains life-sustaining compounds that contribute to wellness. Through research, scientists have learned how foods affect health, what happens when foods are cooked, and ways to increase and improve the food supply. All of this shows the power of food.

▶ Food brings pleasure to people by offering enjoyment at mealtimes, creating a focal point for family and social gatherings, providing a sense of comfort during difficult times, contributing entertainment via food festivals, and adding adventure through new food experiences.

▶ Food offers different ways to show creativity.

▶ A wide variety of career possibilities are available in the foods field.

▶ For many reasons, people today are taking a global view of food.

▶ A foods course provides many opportunities to build useful life skills.

Check Your Knowledge

1. If you could break food down into its components, what would you find?

2. Why are **nutrients** essential?

3. How can you practice good **nutrition**?

4. When should people become interested in **wellness**? Why?

5. What decisions are involved in practicing wellness?

6. Describe three ways that science impacts foods.

7. What might happen if you don't like the appearance or taste of the food you're eating?

8. In what ways is food socially significant?

9. Why do some foods actually make people feel more comfortable?

10. Compare the past and present significance of restaurants in people's lives.

11. How are cookbooks used today?

12. In what ways can food add adventure to life?

13. What shows the creativity of a chef?

14. What mistake do many people make when getting ready to enter a career?

15. **CRITICAL THINKING** Why is the challenge that humanity faces regarding the global food supply so difficult?

16. How can **critical thinking** benefit you when it comes to foods?

17. Compare **verbal communication** and **nonverbal communication**.

18. How can you learn **management** skills in a foods class?

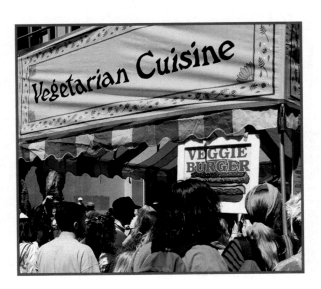

Apply Your Learning

1. **LANGUAGE ARTS** **Memories.** Food is often part of memorable holidays and celebrations. Write about a special event in your life in which food played a role. You might think of something humorous (a dish that didn't turn out right), something sentimental (the beautiful cake at a family wedding), or another idea you have.

2. **Comfort Foods.** What food or foods make you feel better when you're stressed or feeling down? Compare your response to others in class. Discuss why such foods offer comfort and the pitfalls of relying on these foods too often.

3. **Food Festivals.** On the Internet learn about the many different kinds of food festivals that take place around the country. Choose one to describe to the class.

4. **Creative Food Presentations.** Look through food magazines to see the creative ways that chefs plate foods. With a partner, come up with creative alternatives to the presentations you see.

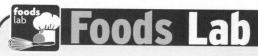 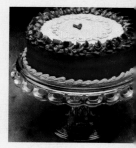

Foods Lab

Foods and Emotions

Procedure: Bring in a food that people often consider to be "comfort food" or "party food." With the class, set out a buffet of these foods for sampling.

Analyzing Results

❶ What qualities, such as those related to taste and texture, do the foods have in common?

❷ How would you rate the overall healthfulness of this food selection? What might this suggest about food and emotions?

❸ Suppose this activity were done by students of a different culture. Would you expect the foods to be more similar to or different from the ones your class brought in? Explain.

Food Science Experiment

Food Preferences

Objective: To learn how expectations affect food preferences.

Procedure:

1. Pour equal amounts of four different types of orange juice—from concentrate or bottled, for example—into four separate, clear glasses. Tint three glasses with one drop of food dye to create four different colored samples. Write down the dye used in each sample.

2. Ask a classmate to inspect the samples and rank them in order of preference, based on appearance. Record the responses.

3. Have your classmate taste each sample while blindfolded and rank them again. Record the responses and compare them to those from Step 2.

Analyzing Results

❶ Which colors were most visually appealing to the tester? Least appealing? What might explain this preference?

❷ Did the samples ranked highest on appearance also rate highly on taste? Explain.

❸ Suppose you had used grape juice instead of orange. Do you think the results would have been different? In what way?

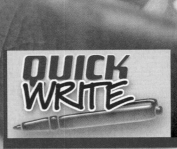

QUICK WRITE

USING NARRATIVE. A narrative is a sequence of related events—in other words, a story. Write a short narrative about your first encounter with a new food. What were the circumstances? What do you recall about your reaction? How did the experience affect your feelings about the food today?

To Guide Your Reading:

Objectives

▶ Explain how a culture is defined.

▶ Give examples of food customs.

▶ Describe how various influences shape a culture's food customs.

▶ Explain similarities among foods in different cultures.

▶ Explain why some food customs carry on over time, yet some change.

▶ Explain why American cuisine is a "melting pot."

Terms

cuisine
culture
custom
ethnic
fasting
fusion cuisine
staple foods

Have you ever been to an international Food Fair? Strolling from booth to booth, you can sample dishes from around the world. Some have exotic flavors and names you might not recognize, from the artistic Chinese morsels called dim sum, to the hearty chicken-and-seafood paella (pie-AY-yuh) from Spain. Food festivals are more than a pleasure for the senses. They're also a delicious way for people to share their own culture and learn about others. See **Fig. 2-1**.

WHAT IS CULTURE?

Culture is a set of customs, traditions, and beliefs shared by a large group of people. Through culture, a group's identity is defined. Language, style of dress, form of government, and other aspects of a society's way of life make up culture.

Cultures are often linked to countries of the world. People who live in Japan and Scotland, for example, have cultural traits that are unique to each country. While nations create culture, religions and races do too as people come together to share what they have in common.

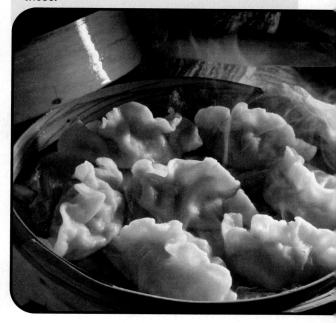

Fig. 2-1 In China, people enjoy gathering to eat a variety of snack foods called dim sum. The delicacies include stuffed dumplings like these.

When people move around the world, they carry culture with them and pass it on to new generations. In this way, those with a common history or heritage preserve their culture in new settings. The Inuit people have lived in the Arctic region for thousands of years. Some now live in Canada and some in the United States, but the cultural bond of their heritage remains strong.

In one society, it's not unusual to find multiple cultures. People who move to a different country may adopt customs in the new culture while still preserving the culture of their former home. In a strong society, people respect the cultural differences around them.

You'll often hear the term **ethnic** used to describe cultures. Ethnic clothing, for example, refers to the garments associated with a culture. Ethnic food describes food that is typical of a culture.

Food and Culture

Interest in ethnic foods is high today. In fact, the entire last unit of this text will take you around the globe to learn about foods of the world and to sample some. This chapter just sets the stage for more exploration.

As you learn about the foods of different cultures, you'll hear the word **cuisine** (kwih-ZEEN). Cuisine refers to a culture's representative foods and the specific styles for preparing them. A cuisine may be particular to a country or a region within a country, or it may be a blend from different areas. Tex-Mex cuisine combines foods from Texas and Mexico to create such specialties as tacos, burritos, and nachos. See **Fig. 2-2**.

Along with cuisines, food customs develop in a culture. A **custom** is an established practice that is repeated over time. Food customs include how and when foods are eaten. Depending on the culture, food might be eaten with chopsticks, a fork, or the fingers. In some cultures, the main meal is taken at midday; in others, it's served in the evening. Table manners are also among food customs. You may have learned that smacking your lips while you eat is rude; in some countries it's taken as a compliment.

How have food cuisines and customs evolved? Just as many different recipes start with the same basic ingredients, different customs originate from the same basic influences.

INFLUENCES ON CUISINES AND CUSTOMS

Cuisines and food customs are shaped by influences both inside and outside of a society. Many have developed over centuries. Some influences that have had great historical impact on food cuisines and customs are described here.

Geography

Compared to the tens of thousands of items in supermarkets today, the grocery list for earlier generations was short indeed. For much of history, geographic location determined diet. Geography—climate, soil, and amount of sunlight—influenced growing conditions, and people

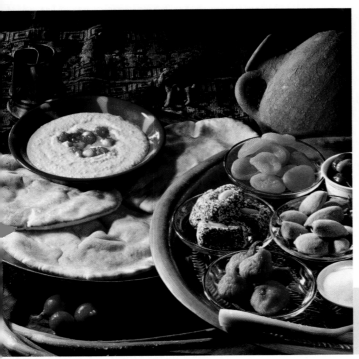

Fig. 2-2 When you see certain foods, you may think of a particular cuisine. Does one come to mind here?

ate only what could grow locally. These plants and animals became **staple foods**, the most widely produced and eaten foods in an area.

Grains have long been a common staple food worldwide, but the kind of grain varied, depending on the climate. The primary grain in southeastern Asia was rice, which is ideally suited to the hot, humid conditions found in much of that area. See **Fig. 2-3**. In the same way, drought-resistant sorghum grew well in the hot, dry regions of Africa, India, and China.

Crops that require a more temperate climate, including wheat, rye, barley, and oats, became the main grains in the cooler zones of Europe and parts of Asia and Africa. Corn, also called maize, thrived in North and South America. Millet was found in almost every country on the globe.

Geography also played the deciding role in hunting and raising animals for meat or milk. In regions with long coastlines and inland lakes and rivers, people came to depend largely on fishing for their food. Salmon, cod, and other cold-water fish were staples in Finland and Norway. In the islands of the Pacific Ocean, such as Japan, daily meals might include squid, octopus, sea urchins, shark fin, and seaweed.

On land, the woods and meadows of North America offered large and small game, from squirrel to bison. Inhabitants of the African plain hunted zebra and antelope. Where grazing land was good, people raised cattle. Where pasture was scarce or the land was hilly, as in eastern Mediterranean countries, sheep and goats were better adapted. In harsher climates, camels, yaks, or llamas might be found.

Finally, geography affected how foods were prepared. Since its earliest days, cooking involved an open fire. If fuel for a fire was easy to come by, foods could cook slowly. Meals might feature long-simmering stews, from a Hungarian goulash to a Louisiana gumbo. In contrast, cooking fuel was scarce in many Asian countries. Food was cut into small pieces that cooked quickly. Frying in small amounts of fat and steaming were faster methods than roasting and baking. Parts of a meal might be cooked at the same time, stacked in containers, to conserve fuel.

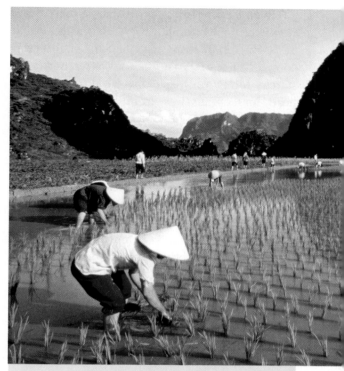

Fig. 2-3 Throughout history, the foods typically eaten have been linked to the geography of an area. What geographic characteristic would be needed to grow rice?

Economics

Until relatively recent times, most societies had two distinct classes: a small group of wealthy, powerful aristocrats and large numbers of "working poor," who just made ends meet. Two kinds of cuisines emerged from this economic difference.

The wealthy dined on fattened meat and fowl and a choice of fresh fruits and vegetables. They could afford the cost to refine grain into white flour. Meals for common people were meager and usually monotonous. They consisted of porridges and dark breads made from whole or coarsely ground grains. Soups and stews were based on whatever a family could hunt, catch, or raise. Wild berries and dried fruit satisfied the sweet tooth. Some people grew food for local markets, but they sold the best crops and meatiest parts of the animals.

Given economic hardship, cooks grew resourceful in adding variety to meals. Edible odds and ends, from pig's feet to oxtails, were cooked into zesty stews and stretched with starchy, filling root vegetables. Meat from the feet, head, and organs was ground and stuffed into casings made from hog intestines—the recipe for a sausage. Different seasonings, combinations of ingredients, and processing methods produced an assortment of these meats. Have you heard of headcheese? That's not a cheese at all, but a sausage made with the meat and gelatin from a calf or pig's head.

Cooks were equally inventive with grains. Oats, corn, and barley could be baked into breads, steamed into puddings, cooked with milk, and sweetened with raisins.

Recipes created out of economic necessity are still popular today. Some of today's favorite comfort foods started as "peasant" foods, including meatloaf, chicken noodle soup, rice pudding, and mashed potatoes.

As a prosperous middle class developed in societies, characteristics from both types of cooking merged. In southern France, fish merchants would offer their unsold fish at a cheap price to housewives, who made a simple stew. Eventually, those cooks who had the means transformed the fish stew into bouillabaisse (BOOL-yuh-bayz), adding costly shellfish to a tomato-based broth seasoned with select herbs. See **Fig. 2-4**.

Foreign Contacts

You may not think of bagels and cheesecake as "foreign foods." Before the turn of the twentieth century, however, they were little known in the United States until several million Jewish people immigrated from Eastern Europe and Russia. The new citizens shared a rich cooking tradition of rye breads, noodle puddings, corned beef—and bagels and cheesecake. See **Fig. 2-5**.

Immigration is one event that promotes food borrowing. Exploration is another. European explorers who reached the Americas found unfamiliar foods in abundance. They brought back samples and seeds of these "strange" plants: dry beans, corn, peanuts, vanilla, tomatoes, potatoes, sweet potatoes, sweet and hot peppers, chocolate,

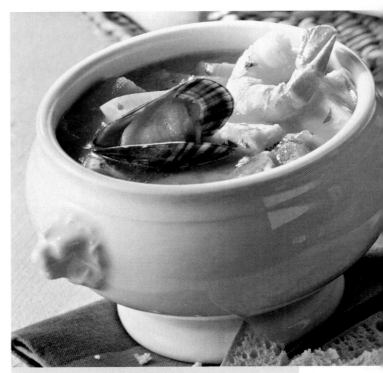

Fig. 2-4 Bouillabaisse is a highly seasoned stew made with at least two kinds of seafood. This celebrated and festive dish from France was preceded by a more economical version than the one often made today.

and cassava, a type of root. Over the centuries, many of these items became popular in Europe.

Meanwhile, colonists learned to grow many of their favorite foods in the "New World." In time, they introduced Native Americans to wheat, barley, chickpeas, cattle, and assorted vegetables.

As explorers discovered new routes to Asia, trade with that area increased. Tea, which had been popular in China since ancient times, arrived in Europe early in the seventeenth century. Before long, it had become the national beverage in both England and Russia.

War and conquest have a similar impact on a culture's cuisine, with sometimes unexpected results. From the twelfth to the seventeenth century, the Ottoman Turks swept through the Mediterranean and southeastern Europe. They advanced government, architecture—and pastry. From the Persians they learned the art of making

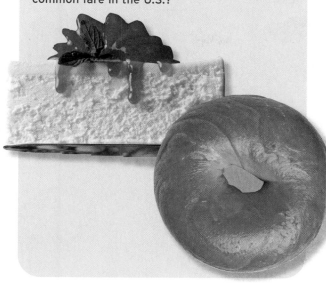

Fig. 2-5 As people around the world come together, they share foods of their cultures. How did cheesecake and bagels become common fare in the U.S.?

delicate, tissue-thin leaves of dough. The Turks layered this dough with spiced, ground nuts and steeped it in honey to make baklava (bah-kluh-VAH). As the Ottoman Empire spread into Hungary around 1535, the Hungarians adapted the technique to make a fruit-filled pastry roll called strudel.

Religious Beliefs

Many religions, directly or indirectly, teach about the use of food. Hindus do not eat beef because they consider cattle to be sacred animals. "Keeping kosher" in the Jewish faith requires that some foods be prepared in certain ways and that some foods be avoided altogether. Buddhism urges "mindfulness" about one's diet, which leads some followers to vegetarianism. Seventh Day Adventists often choose vegetarianism to express the value of simplicity and respect for the body.

Fasting, or abstaining from all or certain foods for a period of time, is a practice in some religions. Catholics fast or refrain from eating meat on some holy days. During Ramadan, a month-long religious observance, Muslims neither eat nor drink during daylight hours. Jewish people observe Yom Kippur, the Day of Atonement, by fasting from sunset the day before.

Technology

What technology has had the biggest impact on food cuisines and customs? Some young people might say microwave cooking. Their grandparents might mention electricity. A historian might suggest crafting the first pots and pans, or even learning to build a fire.

In every age, advances in technology have drastically changed the way people eat and cook. See **Fig. 2-6.** The stove, for example, allowed cooks to control the amount of heat applied to food, which was a challenge over an open fire. They could leave food in an oven, knowing it would maintain a steady temperature without constant supervision, or simmer meat for hours on a cooktop without fear of burning. Milk, eggs, cheese, and other delicate foods could be used to create rich sauces and tender desserts. The broiler gave food open-flame qualities without the inconvenience of an open flame.

Before refrigerators and freezers were widely available, "stocking up" on food meant canning it yourself. Most leftovers couldn't be saved for long. Ice cream was an infrequent treat that required a lot of work, as well as fresh eggs and cream.

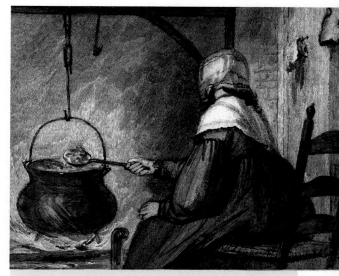

Fig. 2-6 Technology has changed the way people cook. A colonial mother started baking beans on Saturday and cooked them over the fire all night for Sunday's meal.

These appliances and many other innovations not only increased food choices, but they also helped move cooking methods beyond the bare basics. Improved technology, and the leisure time it gave, allowed people to develop new techniques and recipes. Previously, preparing food had been seen mostly as a necessity. Technology opened the way to cooking as creative expression.

SIMILARITIES IN GLOBAL CUISINES

Although cuisines and food customs developed independently in different cultures, similarities are noticeable. Are Chinese rice noodles really much different from Italian spaghetti? Do Greek feta cheese and Mexican queso fresca seem alike? Despite the variations, many foods from around the world have commonalities. That's not so surprising. The same principles of preparing food apply in every culture, and people the world over have the same basic needs that foods meet.

Preparation Methods

In many cuisines similar preparation methods arose in different locations. For example, all cultures learned to grind grains into flour. Cooks mixed the flour with water to make dough, which they shaped into breads, rolls, and noodles. Raised, or leavened, breads grew popular throughout Europe and parts of Asia. Flatbreads, which are rolled or patted into a circle and cooked on a griddle, were found from Southwest Asia, to North Africa, to South America. See **Fig. 2-7**.

Filled dumplings also appeared in cuisines worldwide. Thin sheets of noodle dough were made into pockets stuffed with cooked chopped meat, seafood, or vegetables. They were sealed and then steamed, boiled, or baked. Italians called them ravioli (ra-vee-OH-lee), the Chinese called them wontons (WAHN-tahns), and Jewish people named them kreplach (KREHP-luk).

Many cuisines preserved meats by drying and smoking. This is how the Italians made pepperoni and the Chinese produced lop chong (lahp chung). A Spanish version is chorizo (chuh-REE-zoh), while a Polish variety is called kielbasa (keel-BAH-suh).

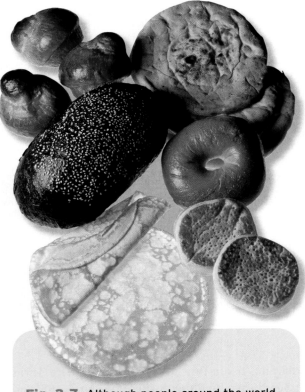

Fig. 2-7 Although people around the world discovered how to make flour from grains, they prepared their breads in different ways. Some made flatbreads, while others made their bread dough rise.

Unless forbidden by religion, thrifty cooks in many cultures saved the blood of butchered animals as a food ingredient. In parts of Europe, highly seasoned blood sausages combined animal blood with barley, oats, or rice. The English called their version blood pudding. In Poland, a nutritious soup, czernina (chehr-NEE-nah), was made with duck blood and dried fruits. All of these foods are still eaten today.

Social Meanings

Food plays a symbolic role in social activities the world over. It's a universal sign of hospitality. In some cultures, the "care and feeding" of guests is a duty, with precise customs related to entertaining. Hosts who fail to offer food to visitors—and visitors who refuse the offer—commit a social offense. Rules are less rigid in the United States,

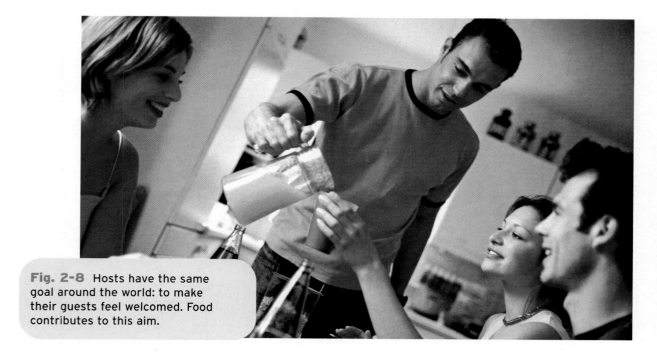

Fig. 2-8 Hosts have the same goal around the world: to make their guests feel welcomed. Food contributes to this aim.

but the message is the same: sharing food is a way to show friendship and acceptance. See **Fig. 2-8**.

Every culture has festivals for special occasions, and traditional foods are often part of the festivities, as shown in **Fig. 2-9** on pages 42 to 43. In some countries, the religious feast of Easter is celebrated with spring lamb and new spring vegetables. People in Poland and Ukraine color eggs in intricate designs. Italian Easter bread is a ring-shaped, braided coffeecake with colored eggs tucked into the top.

Fittingly, foods highlight harvest festivals in any culture. The Scottish festival of Lammas features breads made with flour from the first cutting of wheat. In the Czech Republic, people celebrate Obzinsky with sauerkraut and a cheese-filled pastry called kolacke (koh-LAH-chee). A spring harvest celebration in Nigeria includes a fishing derby.

FOOD CUSTOMS TODAY

It may seem that the food customs you follow now are the same ones you've always followed. That's probably true, to a degree. Maybe you've always eaten with a knife and fork—but the food at the other end of those utensils may have changed considerably, just over the course of your lifetime.

Maintaining Food Customs

Some food customs are handed down as a matter of cultural pride. Even if the original reason no longer exists, the custom is part of the people's tradition and identity.

In the Mexican tradition, for example, tamales are made by spreading the tamale dough on cornhusks and then folding the husks over the filling. Aluminum foil and coffee filters, which are more available and easier to work with, make practical substitutes. Taking the time to learn and teach the original skill, however, shows pride and respect for Mexican heritage. It says that the old ways are valuable and worth saving.

Keeping food customs can also provide a sense of cultural security, just as family food customs give a sense of personal security. When they carry on food traditions, many people feel a sense of connectedness, a belonging to something larger than themselves.

Of course, some traditions continue because people have grown to enjoy them. Chocolate remains a staple in Mexican cuisine, as it has been since the time of the Aztecs. It's essential to the hot pepper paste used to make mole (MOH-lay), a sauce served with chicken. Chocolate syrup is a favorite topping for fried bananas.

Fig. 2-9
Celebrations
Around the World

All around the world, foods are part of many different celebrations. Holidays, special occasions, and various customs give reason for such celebrations.

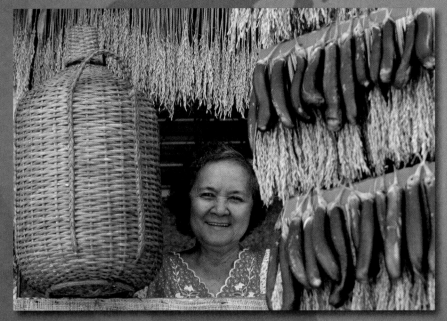

In the Philippines, people celebrate the Agawan festival to give thanks for a good harvest. This Filipino woman smiles as she peers through a window adorned with vegetables during the festivities.

Songkran is the New Year celebration in Thailand. Festivities include such varied events as religious ceremonies, beauty pageants, water fights to wash away bad luck, and traditional foods sold by vendors.

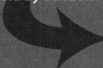

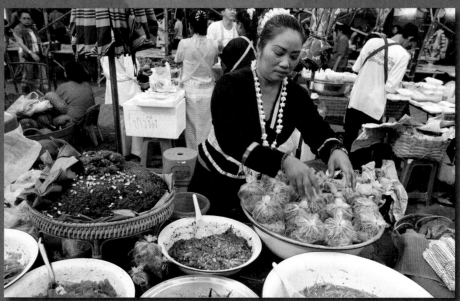

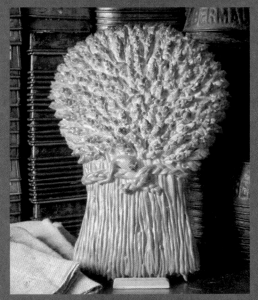

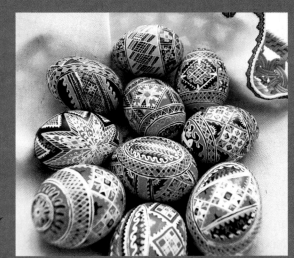

These beautiful and intricately designed eggs, called pysanky (PEH-san-keh), are an ancient art form in Ukraine. The eggs are part of the Easter celebration.

In many European countries an abundant harvest is celebrated by baking festival bread shaped in the form of a wheat sheaf, or bundle. This one is made in the United Kingdom.

Dressed in the traditional attire of Denmark, this young girl eats a breakfast of aebleskivers (eh-bleh-SKEE-vors) during Danish Days. Aebleskivers are tasty pancake-like spheres dipped in fresh jams or sprinkled with powdered sugar.

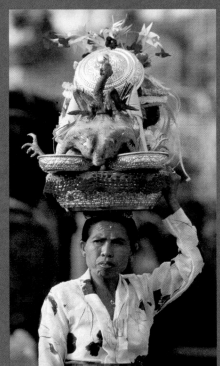

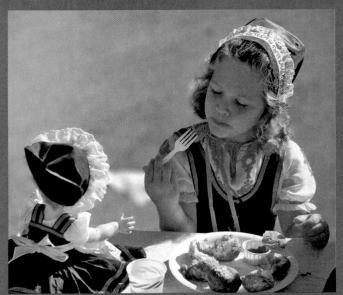

On the island of Bali in Indonesia, this woman carries food and decorations on her head during a harvest festival. In her village people celebrate the Ngusaba festival to give thanks for their rice crop.

Think About It:
Why do you think harvest is a common theme for celebrations in so many countries?

Changing Food Customs

The forces that help create customs can help change them, and even eliminate them. With the rapid advances of the last century, technology especially is changing what and how people eat.

With so many modern methods to process, transport, and store foods, the supermarket is increasingly a global market. Foods can be flown thousands of miles in a few hours, so Florida oranges can be sold fresh in Norwegian groceries. Norwegian cod can be frozen while still on the fishing vessel and arrive frozen at a restaurant in New York City.

Improved communications may be having an even greater impact. As exploration did hundreds of years ago, communication technology allows people to share and experience the foods of many cultures. Satellite links and the Internet allow instant access, even to remote corners of the globe. A cook in rural Georgia can watch a chef in England make an Indian yogurt sauce on a television show or "Webcast."

The trend of experimenting with foreign cuisines has given rise to a new school of cooking called **fusion cuisine**. See **Fig. 2-10**. With it, new recipes are created by mixing the influences of different food traditions. For example, you might find French crepes filled with Caribbean-style shrimp in a coconut-lime sauce.

FOOD CUSTOMS IN THE U.S.

The United States has become home to people of countless ethnic backgrounds. This cultural blend is often called a "melting pot." Each food custom adds to the overall flavor of American cooking, yet none disappears entirely. Some recipes retain their cultural identity. Hummus is still considered a Middle Eastern dish, for example. Others have melded into the American food "landscape." Pretzels and doughnuts, two popular snacks, and coleslaw, a favorite at Fourth of July picnics, were all contributed by the Dutch.

At the same time, groups blended their foods, techniques, and flavors with others. The practice continues today. Pizza was originally an Italian dish. Now you can order a Tex-Mex pizza filled with refried beans and salsa, or a Creole pizza covered with shrimp, eggplant, and hot pepper sauce to taste.

Likewise, restaurants featuring ethnic cuisines are gaining in popularity. Menus often include standard American dishes as well as international choices. Such foods as beef kebabs (kuh-BAHBS) and pita (PEE-tuh) bread may become as familiar as steak and dinner rolls. You might even enjoy foods from different cuisines at the same meal. If you start with curried chicken and rice and finish with a slice of Black Forest cake, you've sampled cuisines of India, China, and Germany, respectively.

Cultures also share their holiday celebrations. Many Asian Americans celebrate the Lunar New Year, which falls on the second new moon after the winter solstice, with elaborate banquets featuring traditional foods: watermelon seeds; spring rolls filled with minced vegetables; and rice dumplings filled with minced meat, beans, and peanuts. American friends are invited as special guests. When celebrating the Irish holiday of St. Patrick's Day, many people, whether Irish or not, enjoy the traditional corned beef and cabbage meal.

With this "recipe swapping," many people see American cuisine as a work in progress, a continually updated cookbook that blends the best of all cultures.

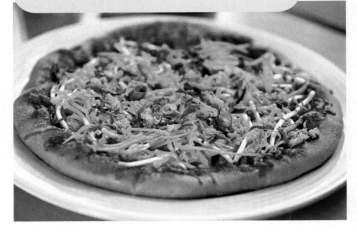

Fig. 2-10 Creativity shows when chefs, professional and amateur, experiment with fusion cooking. A Thai chicken pizza, for example, blends cuisines.

Author

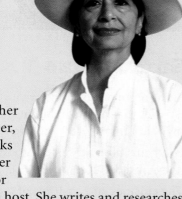

MADHUR JAFFREY: Madhur Jaffrey's careers give new meaning to the term "transferable skills." A flair for artistry and drama has brought her success in both the world of acting and the world of cooking.

Born in Delhi, India, Madhur earned several scholarships to study at the Royal Academy of Dramatic Art in London, England. Building on her success, she came to the United States in the late 1950s, appearing in short films and off-Broadway plays. Finding few roles for Indian actors, Madhur turned to her degree in English literature and love for writing to help pay the bills. She began writing magazine articles on two subjects she knew well: the arts and food. Her reputation as a master of Indian cuisine led to her first cookbook, *An Invitation to Indian Cooking*. Published in 1973, it was reissued in 1999 and is still in print today, a rare feat.

Since then, acting and writing have occupied much of Madhur's time, energy, and talents. She has starred in motion pictures, onstage in New York City and London, and in numerous drama series for British television. Her writing credits include magazines as diverse as the scholarly *Smithsonian* and the trendy *Vogue*, as well as the food publications *Saveur* and *Bon Appetit*. Her equally wide-ranging subjects include Indian cave paintings and Soviet restaurants. She has also authored several children's books.

Cuisine and Culture. It is for her lively exploration of Eastern cuisine, however, that food fans know Madhur Jaffrey best. Two of her cookbooks (she has written over a dozen) have won the prestigious James Beard Foundation Award for Best International Cookbook. Her many series of cooking shows are immensely popular in England and have aired around the world, from the United States to New Zealand.

As with her acting career, Madhur sinks herself into her roles as author and television host. She writes and researches, she travels and tests recipes, to bring her audience authentic East Asian culture, as well as authentic foods. For Madhur, cooking has always been about more than food. It's a gateway to a nation's history, traditions, values, and geography. She gives her audience more than information on cooking. She gives them a better understanding of the world.

"You can do anything." Achievements like these do not come by accident. Madhur prepared by developing a range of skills through a solid education. She pursued interests and new experiences. She read widely. As an immigrant, she was not always welcomed by others, yet she worked and persevered, never letting limited attitudes limit her goals or her pride in her Indian heritage. "Concentrate," she says, "and you can do anything. Do something that excites and fulfills you. If you're lucky enough to find it, your cup will be filled for the rest of your life."

On-line Connections

1. To learn more about topics in this article, search the Internet for these key words: James Beard Foundation; Indian cuisine; East Asian cuisine; writing cookbooks.

2. To learn about related careers, search the Internet for these key words: recipe developer; food anthropologist.

Summarize Your Reading

▶ A nation may have unique cultural characteristics that define it, but at the same time it may contain multiple cultures.

▶ Food cuisines and customs offer ways to describe a culture.

▶ The cuisines and customs of a culture are influenced by geography, economics, foreign contacts, religious beliefs, and technology.

▶ All over the world, people use similar principles in preparing foods and use food to meet the same basic needs.

▶ Today food customs continue to be handed down to new generations. At the same time, circumstances cause some customs to change.

▶ Ethnic restaurants and celebrations are evidence of the different food customs and cuisines in the United States.

Check Your Knowledge

1. What is **culture**?

2. What makes **cuisines** different?

3. What are some examples of food customs in a culture? Compare these to customs in your community.

4. Historically, what determined the **staple foods** in regions of the world?

5. **CRITICAL THINKING** Why do you think early people in history may have cooked their foods quickly?

6. How did class distinctions determine what people ate in historical times?

7. What effect did world exploration have on the foods people ate?

8. How have wars throughout history had impact on the foods people eat?

9. What is **fasting**?

10. What allowed food preparation to become more creative? Why?

11. **CRITICAL THINKING** Why are the breads of different cultures around the world both similar and different?

12. Compare ravioli and wontons.

13. Why is food part of social activities around the world?

14. For what reasons are food customs handed down to new generations?

15. How does communication around the world affect food customs?

16. What is **fusion cuisine**?

17. Why is the United States considered a "melting pot"?

18. **CRITICAL THINKING** Why do you think ethnic restaurants have gained popularity in the U.S.?

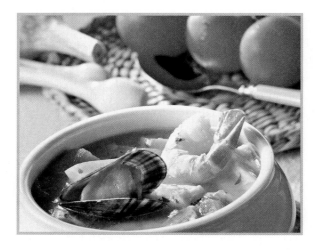

Apply Your Learning

1. **SOCIAL STUDIES** **Custom Awareness.** When business people travel around the world, they often learn about food customs so that they don't make mistakes that might offend their hosts. Choose a country and investigate what food customs you would need to know if you were going there.

2. **Dinner Invitation.** Matt has been invited to a friend's home for dinner. The friend's cultural background is different from Matt's, which means the food may be quite different from what's familiar to Matt. He is concerned about going and can't decide what to do. How would you advise him?

3. **Food Origins.** Identify a food or dish commonly eaten in America but with origins elsewhere in the world, such as yogurt, oranges, hot chocolate, meatballs, or stews. Find information that traces the origin of the food or dish and describes how it arrived in America.

4. **SOCIAL STUDIES** **Cultural Celebrations.** Search the Internet to learn about a holiday celebrated in another country. What foods are associated with the holiday? How are they prepared and served?

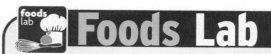

Foods Lab

Using Regional Foods
Procedure: Choose and prepare a recipe that features one or more foods for which your region is known. Rate the recipe on meal appeal and ease or difficulty of preparation. Serve samples to the class.

Analyzing Results
❶ What regional foods did lab teams choose? How were they used in different recipes?

❷ What cultural influences are shown in the recipes prepared?

❸ Suppose you are moving to a different part of the country. Select an area and describe how you could change your recipe to take advantage of that area's local foods.

5. **Prediction.** What do you think cultures will be like in 100 years? Will they be more distinct or less so? Why?

Food Science Experiment

Comparing Cuisines
Objective: To compare traditional foods in different cultures.

Procedure:
1. With your lab group, find five recipes typical of the cuisine assigned by your teacher. Include both main and side dishes.
2. List those ingredients that appear most often. Categorize these as protein foods, fruits, vegetables, and seasonings.
3. Compile this information with the findings of other teams to create a class chart.

Analyzing Results
❶ What foods appear most often in each category? What might explain the cross-cultural appeal of these foods?

❷ Which foods are common to only one or two cuisines? How do you explain their limited use?

❸ What foods in the chart are commonly served in meals in your region? Based on the chart, compare the ways these foods are prepared in your region to their use in other cultures.

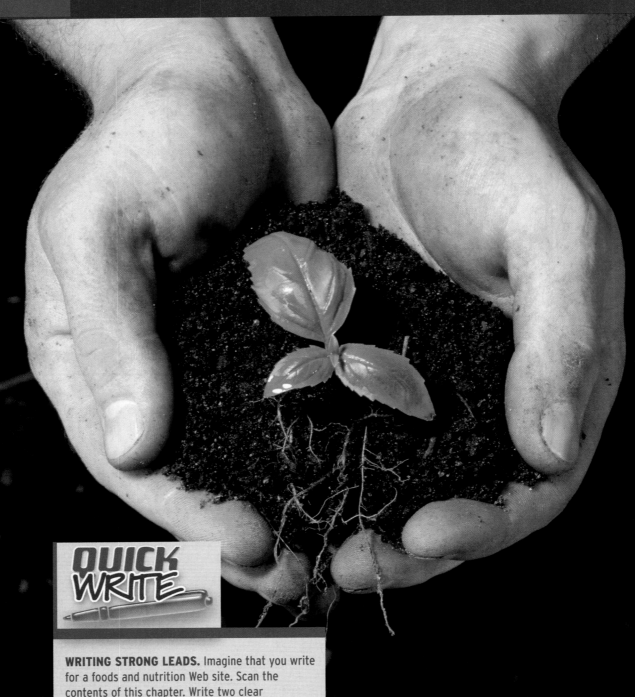

QUICK WRITE

WRITING STRONG LEADS. Imagine that you write for a foods and nutrition Web site. Scan the contents of this chapter. Write two clear sentences that summarize what the chapter is about while capturing your readers' interest.

H AVE YOU EVER THOUGHT TO APPRECIATE the vast food selection the typical American enjoys? Foods from near and far, common and exotic, fill the shelves of farmers markets, supermarkets, and ethnic groceries. All of these foods are part of a food supply made available through the efforts of many people, but the story begins with biology.

THE FOOD CHAIN

In the biological world, organisms live as communities in particular environments. An environment can be as small as a pond or as large as a forest or ocean. Scientists call an environment that contains a community of organisms that interact and depend upon each other an **ecosystem**.

In an ecosystem, organisms get food from other organisms and the environment. This process is called the **food chain**. The food chain is actually a cycle, one part of a more complex web. The cycle has four main components.

• **Sun.** The sun supplies the original energy for the planet in the form of light. This energy is needed to make food. See **Fig. 3-1**.

• **Producers.** Certain members of a community make, or produce, food. In some communities, producers include all green plants. Using the sun's energy, plants produce their own food in their leaves. Some of this food sustains the plant, but some is stored as energy for future needs—or for anything that eats the plant. Thus

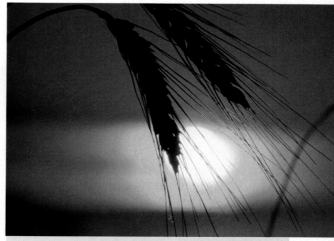

Fig. 3-1 Energy from the sun is needed to make food.

plants not only produce their own food but also make food available for consumers.

- **Consumers.** Oganisms that eat food and convert it into usable energy are consumers. In the ecosystem that includes humans, consumers are of three types. Most consumers are **herbivores** (HUR-buh-vors), which eat only plants. They include all farm animals, such as cattle, sheep, and poultry. A second group of consumers, the **carnivores** (CAHR-nuh-vors), feed almost entirely on animals. Most humans fall into the smallest group, **omnivores** (AHM-nih-vors). They eat both plants and animals.
- **Decomposers.** Decomposers are such organisms as bacteria and fungi, which break down dead matter and return the components to the environment as nutrients. They might well be called "recyclers," for they provide producers with the raw materials needed to start the cycle again.

Biodiversity

As you can see, in a healthy ecosystem nothing is wasted. All elements work together to sustain life. Relationships within and between ecosystems are not only efficient, but also interdependent. If any part fails, food chains may be disrupted and food supplies threatened. That's why an ecosystem needs **biodiversity**, a wide variety of plant and animal species.

Biodiversity lessens the risk of a break in the chain, because a role is filled by more than one organism. For example, butterflies carry pollen from plant to plant so they can produce fruit. Recently, an unusually harsh winter killed many monarch butterflies in North America. With biodiversity, other butterfly species, as well as bees, could carry on the role of pollinating plants. See **Fig. 3-2**.

Natural Resources

Every ecosystem is supported by natural resources. Without these, the ecosystem could not survive. Essential resources include the following:

- **Land.** Nutrient-rich soil is needed for plant life, even underwater. In land that's cultivated to raise crops or graze animals, fertilizers are added to supply needed nutrients.

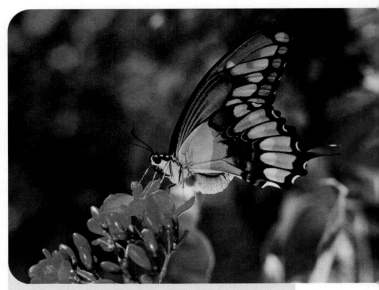

Fig. 3-2 Butterflies enable plants to produce fruit. What might happen if the butterflies in an ecosystem die?

- **Water.** Water is the "life's blood" of any ecosystem. Marine life, of course, needs ample amounts of clean fresh or salt water. Rainfall and snowmelt provide moisture to land. If needed on farms and ranches, land may be irrigated, artificially watered by using pipes or diverting a stream. For instance, dates grow naturally in California's hot, dry regions. Growing hay and providing water for cows in those areas requires irrigation.
- **Climate.** Most foods grow in a range of moderate air temperatures. Mushrooms thrive in cool surroundings. Grapes prefer hotter conditions. In some areas, seasonal changes limit the growing season to warmer months. In milder climates, different crops may grow year-round. Animals too are naturally suited to certain temperatures. Brahman cattle are well adapted for the heat and humidity of their native India, a climate where sheep would suffer.

The earth provides resources in abundance, but they are not evenly distributed. As a result, the size and quality of food supplies are affected around the world.

THE FOOD SUPPLY IN THE UNITED STATES

The United States is fortunate to have abundant resources for raising food. Along with a temperate climate and a plentiful water supply, the U.S. has a wide expanse of good farmland and pastureland.

Food Producers

Food usually begins its journey on the farms, ranches, and fisheries that produce much of the food you eat. Some foods may have traveled great distances, even from other countries, to get to your table.

Farmers in the United States have long produced enough food not only for domestic use but also for export. A century ago, rural America was dotted with many small family farms. As agriculture has become more industrialized, these farms have dwindled, many absorbed into large operations. See **Fig. 3-3**.

Large farms have certain advantages, one being efficiency. Such farms can specialize in a single crop, while small farmers raise several different crops and often livestock as well. Large operations may be better able to absorb the costs of farming and produce greater quantities of food for increasing needs around the world.

On the other hand, some people worry about the loss of small farms and the impact large operations may have on the environment if proper stewardship of the land doesn't occur. High-producing crops may need more fertilizer and pesticides, making them more expensive to grow. Food shipped from great distances may have reduced quality and flavor.

In many areas of the country, interest in local food supplies is growing. Many people are turning to farmers markets, community supported agriculture projects, urban gardens, and many other programs that link consumers directly with the farmers who produce their food.

Food Processors

Once harvested, food is shipped to processors. Processing ranges from simple to intense, depending on the food and the selling form. To

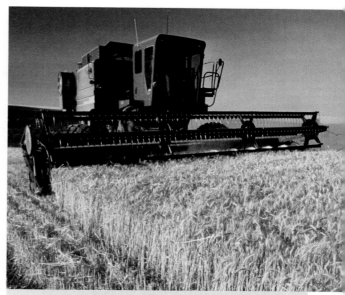

Fig. 3-3 Farms have long been part of the rural American scene. What difficulties do they face today?

sell as fresh produce, an ear of corn is merely cleaned and packaged. To make cornmeal, the kernels are dried and ground. Kernels can also be soaked, pulverized, and treated with acids to release corn oil. Further processing creates a sweetener, corn syrup.

Some processing helps keep perishable foods from spoilage. These foods become **shelf-stable**—they can be stored at room temperature in their original, unopened containers. Such foods also have a longer **shelf life**, the length of time food holds its original flavor and quality. Some common preservation processes are described here:

- **Canning.** Canning seals food in airtight metal or glass containers, which are then heated to destroy microorganisms that could cause spoilage or illness.
- **Freezing.** Through freezing, foods are frozen quickly to slow the growth of any harmful organisms.
- **Curing.** Such ingredients as salt, spices, sugar, and sodium nitrite are added when foods are cured. This method is most commonly used

NEW WAYS WITH WASTE

Just as you must throw out banana peels and egg shells, food makers also deal with inedible food parts. Some food "scraps," such as grain and animal by-products, end up in pet foods. Many waste products, however, are just that—wasted—at an economic cost to food makers and an environmental cost to the planet.

To help solve both problems, researchers in Australia are refining a complex technology that includes nanofiltration and crystallization. The process purifies some waste products to recover higher quality components. For example, to make cheese, the liquid part of milk is normally drained off. Some is powdered and sold for gravy and hot cocoa mixes, but it's often cheaper to throw it out. The new technology allows scientists to extract a finer-grade powder that's valuable for use in medicines. Minerals and salts can also be saved.

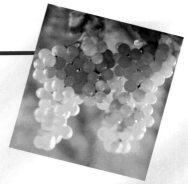

The technology holds exciting possibilities. It's already used to recover waste water left from food manufacturing. It may also save costly natural colors, flavors, and nutrients usually lost in processing sugars, fruits, and vegetables. Equally important for manufacturers, the system is cost effective: the profits from selling the food products recovered are greater than the expense of the technology.

__Think Beyond>> Now, natural grape flavoring is expensive and hard to come by. If this technology becomes widespread, what might the impact on grape growers be? On consumers?

with meats, but also with fish, pickles, and some vegetables. Pork, for instance, may be cured to make sausage or salami.

- **Drying.** This process removes moisture from food, inhibiting the growth of harmful organisms. Grains, beans, milk, and fruit are often dried.
- **Freeze-drying.** Freeze-drying first freezes and then dries food. The process retains more flavor, texture, and nutrients than does drying alone. Freeze-drying is used to make instant coffee and dried soup mixes.
- **Controlled atmosphere storage.** This technique extends shelf life by holding foods in a cold area with specific amounts of nitrogen, oxygen, and carbon dioxide. It is especially useful for fruits.

Food Additives

Have you ever wondered how jellybeans get their brilliant colors? Food additives are the answer. A **food additive** is a substance added to food for a specific reason during processing. Some additives occur naturally. Others are chemical combinations created in laboratories. Altogether, food processors now use over 3,000 such ingredients. The U.S. Food and Drug Administration monitors their safe use. Besides coloring, additives are used for the following:

- **Flavoring.** Growing and processing conditions can affect a food's flavor. For example, added flavorings ensure that cans of cherry pie filling taste alike.
- **Improving nutrition.** Nutrients are added to some foods. Many of the vitamins and minerals listed on cereal boxes come from additives.
- **Increasing shelf life.** Working alone or with other processing methods, certain additives delay spoilage. Raisins are preserved by both drying and sulfur dioxide.
- **Maintaining texture.** Processing often changes a food's texture. With additives, pickles keep crisp even after canning.

- **Helping foods age.** Foods ranging from cheese to flour may be aged before they are sold. Additives can speed this process.

Food additives are not new to the food supply. Salts and spices, you'll recall, have been used to cure meats for thousands of years. Additive use, however, has increased. Some people believe that many added chemicals are unnecessary, and some may even be harmful to health. As a result, a few food processors make products that are free of chemical additives.

Packaging

Packaging is an essential part of processing. Containers help preserve the quality, shape, and appearance of food. Familiar packaging materials include paper, plastic, aluminum, and lightweight steel. Packaging methods are continually updated, allowing food manufacturers and processors to offer an expanded line of products.

Food Distributors

From the processor, food is shipped by a vast network of trucks, trains, and planes to distribution centers throughout the country and world. Distribution facilities are essentially huge warehouses with controlled-atmosphere zones. There, food awaits the last leg of its journey, to the store where you buy it. See **Fig. 3-4**.

Types of distributors vary. Some distribute regionally; others deal internationally. Some distributors handle a certain cuisine. Others specialize in baked goods, frozen foods, or gourmet items. Some facilities are owned by the store's company. Others are separate businesses that contract out space to different food sellers.

Food Retailers

The distributor ships food to the many different food retailers. Supermarkets, with their wide selection of products, are the most popular retail food outlet in the United States.

Fig. 3-4 Foods pass through several stages before reaching a location where you can buy products and take them home for your table.

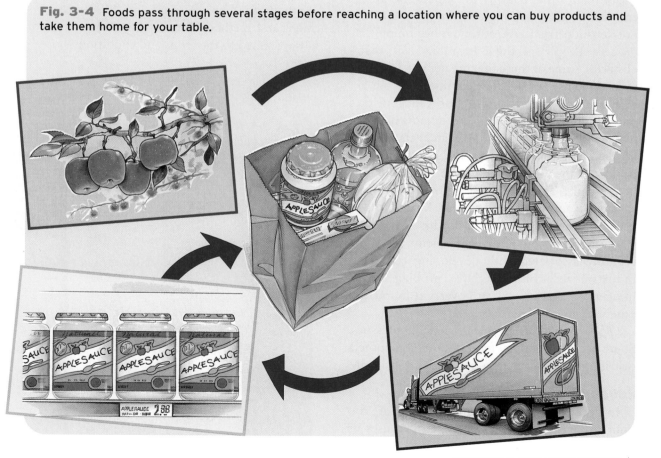

A retailer's primary job is to offer customers a wide range of foods. Retailers certainly don't lack for items because food processors and manufacturers constantly develop new products in an effort to win consumers. Some stores review as many as 100 new products a week. Because shelf space is limited, however, only the most promising items are accepted. New foods that don't sell well are pulled from the shelves.

GLOBAL FOOD PROBLEMS

While some countries enjoy an abundant food supply, many other nations do not. In **industrialized nations**, or developed countries, a sophisticated, organized food industry provides people with a varied and nutritious diet. A fishing vessel captain may locate a school of flounder using sonar and then locate buyers for the catch using the Internet. Meanwhile, the crew starts to process the fish onboard. Industrialized nations that cannot produce enough food, such as Japan, Kuwait, and Switzerland, can afford to import it.

For many other nations, the situation is different. **Developing nations** are countries that are not yet industrialized or are just beginning that process. People in these locations face many obstacles, some of them life threatening, in trying to feed themselves and their families.

To see world hunger more clearly, imagine that one out of every seven people you know has only one meager meal on a good day and eats nothing for days at a time. That's the reality for about 15 percent of the world's population, some 800 million people. The most severe form of a food shortage is **famine**, which can last for months or years and cause thousands of deaths.

Although serious hunger problems are more typically associated with developing countries, industrialized countries have problems with hunger too. Anywhere that poverty is found, the potential for hunger exists.

Global hunger involves a tangled web of issues. Some factors concern food production, others distribution. Some are related to certain social ills.

Economics

In developing countries, many people are too poor to buy food. Instead, each family raises its own food on a small plot of land, a practice known as **subsistence farming**. Families live on whatever they can produce, usually a limited supply, with little variety and inadequate nutrition.

Some farmers accumulate enough land to grow cash crops—crops they can sell. Local shortages often occur, however, because large food exporters pay farmers the best price for their crop. Since world food prices change frequently, cash-crop farmers can't depend on a steady income.

In many countries, governments and utility companies can't afford to provide the services needed for a reliable food supply. Imagine trying to run a grocery store where aging, overloaded electricity plants are shut down for a few hours every day.

Inefficient Methods

Subsistence farming makes use of ancient methods. Animals supply the power. Farm tools are simple, their designs dating back hundreds of years. See **Fig. 3-5**. With such outdated tools and methods, food production is low. Modern equipment and methods are costly, however, and not always suited to the crops and conditions.

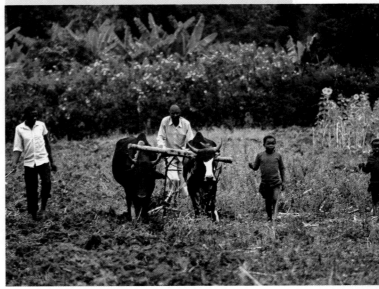

Fig. 3-5 Farming is difficult in countries where people must use outdated techniques.

Developing countries also lack modern food storage facilities. Food is stored unprotected, where it can be damaged by animals, insects, and mildew. Refrigeration is unavailable, so such basic items as dairy foods, fresh produce, and meat spoil quickly.

Good roads are rare in developing nations, especially in the countryside. Bicycles and donkey carts are more common than trucks. You can imagine the impact on food distribution. City dwellers may have enough to eat, while villagers a few miles away are struggling. In times of famine, poor distribution keeps food aid from reaching starving people.

Natural Disasters

A natural disaster can cripple a region's food supply for years. A drought, an unusually long period without rain, damages crops and kills animals. Floods and hurricanes wash away soil and roads. People in developing countries are most vulnerable. In areas where food production and distribution are already shaky, this destruction brings about famine and starvation.

Rapid Population Growth

Experts predict that the world population, which has been growing steadily, will increase to 9 billion by 2025. The most rapid increase has been, and will continue to be, in developing countries. As populations grow, so does the demand for food. At the same time, more land is taken for housing, leaving less land for farming. The population in most developing nations is outgrowing the food supply. See **Fig. 3-6**.

Fuel Shortages

Because most food must be cooked to be eaten, cooking fuel is essential. In developing countries, wood is the main fuel source. In many areas, the wood supply is dwindling as forests are cut for farming or development to support the growing population. Gathering enough wood for a day's meal can mean walking for half a day. Without trees and shrubs for fuel, people use dung, dried animal manure. While it's free and plentiful, dung produces a lot of smoke and little heat.

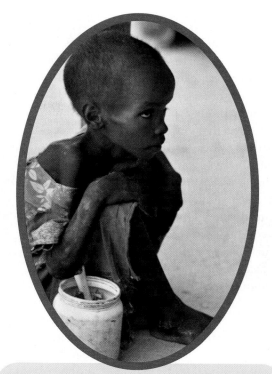

Fig. 3-6 Hunger is a serious problem in some parts of the world.

Conflict and Politics

Armed conflict can devastate food supplies. Animals are killed and crops destroyed. Farmers are driven from their land, and fighting disrupts food distribution.

To escape the danger, many people flee to nearby regions. Thousands of refugees stream into an area, where the local food supply cannot support the surge in population. Everyone suffers.

Food is also used as a political weapon, to punish opponents or reward supporters. A ruling party may limit food distribution only to urban areas, forcing people to leave rural properties, which are then given to political party members. Food aid may be stolen and sold on the black market, never reaching those in need. In recent decades, such tactics have left millions starving in Uganda, Congo, and other African countries, and in Bosnia in southeastern Europe.

GLOBAL WATER PROBLEMS

Looking at a globe, you see that water covers about three-fourths of the earth's surface; however, 98 percent of it is salt water, and undrinkable for humans, crops, and farm animals alike. The remaining 2 percent is fresh water, but 75 percent of that is frozen in the polar regions. Of the total water on this planet, then, less than 1 percent is available for human needs.

Fresh water flows in lakes, rivers, and streams. It's also found beneath the earth's surface as **groundwater**. Groundwater fills the cracks and spaces between rocks and sediment, much as water fills holes in a sponge. It's brought to the surface by digging wells.

Some areas have ample water, such as those along the Amazon River in South America and the Great Lakes in North America. Supplies in desert countries are far less dependable.

As with the food supply, the earth's growing population will strain its water supply. About 70 percent of the world's fresh water is now used for agriculture. See **Fig. 3-7**. As populations grow, however, urban demands for water are expected to exceed rural ones.

In 2003, the United Nations issued a report on the global water supply. It predicted that by 2050, up to 7 billion people in 60 countries will face a water scarcity. The poor will suffer most.

Water Contamination

Water can, and must, be used over and over. In industrialized countries, with advanced sanitation systems and water treatment plants, people often take clean water for granted. These very systems, however, can endanger the water supply.

Waste from a variety of sources is pumped into sewage systems and directly into waterways. In cities, rainwater runs off lawns and streets, carrying oil, gasoline, and garden chemicals into storm sewers. Chemicals and animal waste from farms and fish farms may also wash into streams. People pour toxic chemicals down sink drains, unaware that sewage treatment plants may not be able to handle those pollutants.

In developing countries the story is different. More than 2 billion people have no sanitary sys-

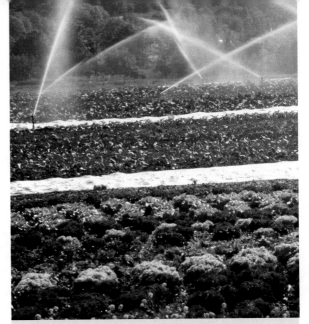

Fig. 3-7 Much of the world's water supply helps grow crops to feed an ever-increasing population.

tem at all. Despite this fact, many of these nations dispose of toxic chemicals in their waterways as they attempt to industrialize. In fact, 90 percent of the wastewater in developing countries is dumped untreated into rivers and lakes, which feed the village wells and streams where people draw water. Every year, contaminated water causes the deaths of 1.4 million children under age five.

WHAT CAN BE DONE?

Some threats to the food and water supply can't be controlled. Those that result from human activity are being countered by human effort. Such groups as the Peace Corps, Food and Agriculture Organization (FAO) of the UN, and Oxfam International contribute their expertise, from nutrition education to livestock vaccination. Their common goal is improving food security, the state of having a steady food supply, both now and in the future. To achieve this, people must learn the skills to improve their lives permanently through careful resource management and development. See **Fig. 3-8**.

Over time, food producers in developing countries will not only support themselves but

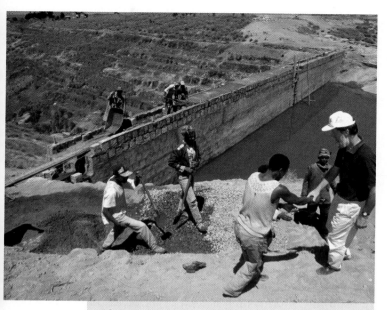

Fig. 3-8 Volunteers bring their expertise to help people in a developing country build a dam.

also contribute to their nation's economy. Already, people who once depended on food aid are starting bakeries, fishing cooperatives, and other small businesses.

Technology is a great asset in this work, combined with knowledge of the ecosystem. Solutions must suit the land and the culture and be affordable to small food producers. For instance, farmers in developing countries are encouraged to create village seed banks of native crops to preserve the area's biodiversity. This approach promotes not only a healthy ecosystem, but also a heritage and a way of family life, whether in Kenya or Kansas.

Increase Food Supplies

Different strategies help people grow more food from limited resources. Researchers are developing tougher grain varieties and other plant foods that can resist disease and pests plus tolerate drought and poor soil. Engineers have designed an irrigation system that uses a foot-powered pump to water a family garden—vastly more efficient than hauling water in buckets.

Organic Food Production

Raising foods organically has been valuable in improving food quality in wealthy and impoverished countries alike. **Organic farming** methods do not use pesticides, hormones, or artificial fertilizers; they stress resource conservation. Soil is fertilized with compost and animal manure. Weeds may be cut and fed to cattle. Farmers curb pests with biological controls called integrated pest management (IPM), such as letting harmless weeds grow to keep more threatening varieties in check.

Organic production has opened opportunities for smaller producers, processors, and retailers. While methods are often cheaper, they aren't cost-effective for large-scale use. Organic foods command a higher price.

Alternative Farming Methods

Alternative farming methods may help increase food supplies. **Agroforestry** is an ancient practice of raising shade-loving crops, such as mushrooms and cocoa, under the shelter of trees. Besides giving protection, the trees also control erosion, improve the soil, and preserve forest habitats. In addition, some trees provide lumber, oils, and extracts for medicine.

Agroforestry offers two benefits. First, it improves the food supply and the income of small farmers. It also encourages farmers to protect the environment, especially rainforests, as vital to their own welfare.

Other, less traditional types of farming show promise as well. In **hydroponic farming** (heye-druh-PAH-nik), plants are grown without soil. Instead, they're held in water, gravel, or sand and fed with nutrient-enriched water. See **Fig. 3-9** on page 58. Using hydroponics, foods can even be grown on rooftops.

Aquaculture is a method of raising seafood in enclosed areas of water. Fish farms may be specially designed ponds or stretches of coastal waters. Aquaculture is one of the world's fastest growing industries, due in part to restrictions that protect some fish populations from overfishing. The U.S. Department of Commerce predicts that

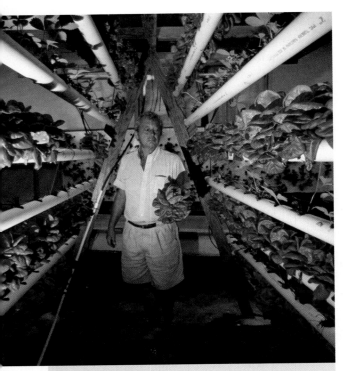

Fig. 3-9 Food that is grown through hydroponics doesn't use soil.

by 2010, aquaculture will provide over one-third of all the fish eaten in the United States. Fish farming may help combat overfishing if care is taken to avoid upsetting native species and habitats.

Develop Alternative Fuel Sources

Agroforestry is one way to increase fuel supplies. Harnessing existing supplies more effectively can also ease the shortage. For example, simple wood-burning stoves are more efficient than open fires. They might burn briquettes made of compressed sawdust, which is often dumped into streams, clogging and polluting the water supply.

Solar Energy

Estimates say the earth gets more energy from the sun in a month than is held in all of its oil, coal, and gas reserves. Solar power is renewable, easy to access, nonpolluting, and it's practical. It takes no wood for utility poles or land for power lines.

Solar energy is functional for both food production and cooking. Screened, enclosed solar dryers dry grains and other crops away from

Career Prep

Career Opportunities

THE FIELD OF FOODS AND NUTRITION is wide-ranging and rapidly growing. Advances in technology are constantly creating new jobs. Each job you see is linked to many, less obvious occupations. You know a rice farmer is part of the food industry. Do you also think of the research scientist who develops the rice seed, the seed dealer who sells it, or the test kitchen worker who helps develop new rice recipes?

In this book, you'll read about specific jobs. You'll see how jobs can link in a career path with a series of related jobs in a field of work. To explore career opportunities, remember these sources of information:

- Your school counselor is a good starting point. Counselors provide information about all kinds of jobs. They also give tests and checklists to help you discover your skills and interests, which often suggest jobs you might enjoy.

- The United States Department of Labor offers several impressive resources, found in print or at the Department's Web site. The *Occupational Outlook Handbook* and the *Career Guide to Industries* list the typical duties, required training, and average earnings of thousands of jobs. The *Occupational Outlook Quarterly* has articles on specific occupations and the job market.

birds and pests. Skylights in henhouses reduce the need for electrical lighting, which increases egg laying.

Simple solar cookers are used successfully in India, China, Africa, and Central America. Inexpensively made from cardboard and aluminum, these cookers perform basic tasks, from baking potatoes to simmering rice and stews. They can even pasteurize water and milk.

Wind Power

Wind power, another renewable resource, might be a solution for farms set on open stretches of land. Giant windmills, shown on page 60, and turbines turn wind power into electricity that can run irrigation pumps and water cattle. Crops can be planted up to the very base of these structures.

U.S. farmers who install turbines are paid by their utility company for any excess electricity they produce. Farmers who can't afford this machinery may lease parcels of land to "wind developers." As the technology is refined, it may be more available to developing countries.

Practice Sustainable Living

Many people believe that solving global food and water supply problems takes a global change in looking at the situation—and in living. They advocate **sustainable living**, achieving economic growth while protecting the environment and promoting human well-being. People see themselves as managers of the world's resources, not only consumers. Sustainable living de-emphasizes material goods as the basis for "the good life," while acting with concern for the needs and quality of life of all people.

Because the word green is associated with environmentally friendly practices, sustainable living is sometimes called green living. You might think of it as low-impact living. For instance, buying locally grown foods—"green shopping"—promotes biodiversity in the ecosystem. Transporting the foods uses less fuel, and preservatives aren't needed, thus limiting the damage to the environment. Everyday choices and habits such as these help ensure that future generations can count on the same resources you use today.

- Trade groups promote their professions through pamphlets, videotapes, and Web sites. They describe jobs in the field and education required.

- Food manufacturers' Web sites often feature employees describing their jobs. While these may feature the positive aspects, they do give you an idea of the types of jobs available.

- Likewise, schools and training institutes like to show how and where their graduates are employed and the career success they enjoy.

- The time-tested, personal approach is still valuable, especially for insights into a certain area of foods and nutrition, from catering to plant science. Talking to people who have a particular job can give you "inside information" about a typical day at work. Job shadowing, or following them through part of the day, can be even more revealing.

Learning about foods and nutrition can be interesting, useful, and fun. Finding a job that excites you can make your studies even more rewarding.

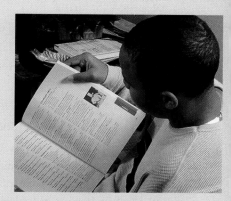

Career Connection

Identifying jobs. Using Internet and other sources, explain the skills and duties required for one of the following jobs: baker, food service manager, dietetic technician, or food scientist. Compare information in class. From your discussion, what can you conclude about opportunities in foods and nutrition?

Summarize Your Reading

▶ The food chain is a cycle that is part of a very complex web that depends on biodiversity and natural resources.

▶ The food supply in the United States reaches you by going through a journey from production to processing, distribution, and retailing.

▶ Food scarcity is a large problem in developing nations.

▶ Some countries have water problems because they have no sewage system at all; others have sewage systems that cannot handle all the substances that drain into them.

▶ Alternative farming methods, fuel sources, and ways of living can help increase food supplies.

Check Your Knowledge

1. What is an **ecosystem**?

2. How do the components of a food chain function?

3. Why is **biodiversity** necessary?

4. How do natural resources impact food supplies around the world?

5. What are the advantages and disadvantages of large U.S. farms?

6. How does food processing impact food spoilage?

7. Describe six common preservation processes.

8. Why are additives used in foods?

9. What is the purpose of a food distributor?

10. **CRITICAL THINKING** Why do you think retail food operations have become so much larger in recent years?

11. Compare **industrialized** and **developing nations**.

12. What problems do people who practice **subsistence farming** face?

13. How do natural disasters affect developing countries?

14. **CRITICAL THINKING** What food impacts might result if a war in a developing nation sends refugees to a nearby developing country?

15. Why is water a global concern?

16. What is the basic goal of such organizations as the Peace Corps, FAO, and Oxfam International?

17. How are organic foods different from other foods?

18. Describe alternative farming methods.

19. How can wind impact the world's energy needs?

20. What is the basic thinking of people who practice **sustainable living**?

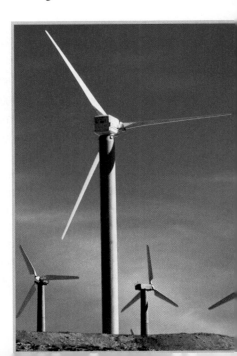

Apply Your Learning

1. **SCIENCE** **Food Chain.** Use biology books to learn what different food chains look like.

2. **Farm Research.** Learn more about how farming has changed in recent years. Report on the difficulties faced by farmers who own small operations, or family farms. Why have such changes occurred?

3. **SOCIAL STUDIES** **Developing Nations.** Investigate conditions in a developing nation. Report on food availability and the specific events and situations that are having impact. What actions are in place to help?

4. **Solar Power.** Find directions for making a simple solar cooker. Make one and try it out. Share the results in class, explaining how the cooker works.

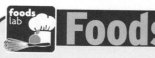

Foods Lab

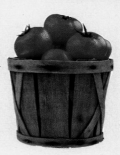

Comparing Food Forms

Procedure: Compare a fresh fruit or vegetable with one of its processed forms. Prepare each food as needed for serving. Evaluate on appearance, taste, texture, and amount of preparation required.

Analyzing Results

❶ Which form of the food did you find more appealing? Why?

❷ How did the foods compare in amount and difficulty of preparation?

❸ In what types of recipes would you use each form you tried? Why?

Food Science Experiment

Home-Processed Foods

Objective: To compare home processing and commercial processing methods.

Procedure:

1. Pare, core, and slice one large apple. Cook with a small amount of water until tender, using medium-low heat on a cooktop or 100 percent power in a microwave oven.

2. Mash the apple. Continue cooking, stirring frequently, until most of the water has evaporated. Don't burn the apple.

3. Scrape the mashed apple into a blender and process into a sauce.

4. Measure ½ cup homemade applesauce and ½ cup commercially prepared applesauce from a newly opened container. Weigh each sample and record.

5. Evaluate each sample for appearance, taste, and texture. Write down your observations.

6. Cover and refrigerate both samples. Observe and evaluate again after two days.

Analyzing Results

❶ How did the samples compare in weight? What might account for any differences?

❷ How did the samples compare on appearance, taste, and texture on the first day? After two days? What might explain any changes?

❸ What kind of processing did both types of applesauce undergo? What additional processing was the commercial applesauce subjected to? What effect did this have?

Food Science & Technology

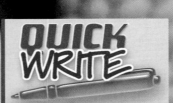

PERSUASIVE WRITING. What do you think is the most useful technological development in foods? Canning food? The microwave oven? Fat-free products? Write a paragraph stating and explaining your choice.

To Guide Your Reading:

Objectives
▶ Relate technological advances to their impact on food production and availability.
▶ Compare the potential positive and negative impacts of genetically modified foods.
▶ Explain how science and technology have led to improved nutrition.
▶ Assess the usefulness of technology in meal preparation.

Terms
analogs
aseptic packages
clone
enrichment
ergonomics
food science
formed products
fortification
functional foods
genetic engineering
manufactured food
MAP packaging
retort pouches
science
technology

Take a minute to jot down ten foods you would serve at a party for friends. Would you have microwave popcorn? Cheese-filled pretzels? Ready-to-bake cookies? Fruit-flavored bottled water? To add nutrition, would you offer low-fat sour cream and a package of ready-to-eat, fresh vegetables for dipping? If making your list is easy, thank a food scientist and food technologist. Their many contributions to the food supply make parties—and mealtimes—both interesting and nutritious. See **Fig. 4-1**.

THE SCIENTIFIC SIDE OF FOOD

Science is a very broad term. One general definition of **science** is the study of the physical world at all levels, including the findings and knowledge that result from such studies. A related concept is **technology**, which is the practical application of scientific knowledge. Technology is science in action.

The relationship between food, science, and technology goes back about half a million years, when people discovered that certain foods were more edible when held over a fire for a while—in

other words, when they were cooked. In a sense, early people practiced a very simple form of **food science**, the scientific study of food and its preparation. Ever since those days, applying science to food has produced marvelous, even life-saving, results.

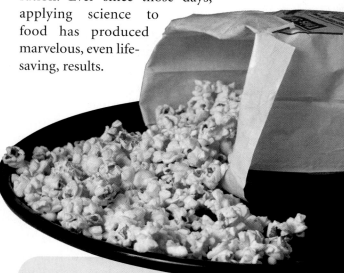

Fig. 4-1 Many foods are available and easy to prepare and serve due to the work of food scientists.

EXPANDING THE FOOD SUPPLY

You've seen how the food supply moves from production to the stores near you. Another look reveals the role that technology plays in this chain of events.

Food Production

Suppose a time machine whisked you 125 years into the past. As you watch people producing food, what would you see? At that time, methods were simple, a combination of animal power, human labor, and handmade tools. Natural mishaps could spell hardship, whether a hurricane, chicken flu, or an infestation of potato beetles.

With today's engineering, farming is more efficient. A single piece of machinery does the work of a dozen farmhands. On a wheat farm in the spring, a planter drops hundreds of pounds of seed in rows at the precise depth and spacing. At harvest time, a huge combine (KAHM-byn) rolls up and down the field, simultaneously picking, threshing, and cleaning the grain. A grain elevator system measures the yield from each acre. The farmer can pinpoint less productive areas, using global positioning satellites, and then treat them as needed with fertilizers or pesticides.

Advances in other sciences have reduced some of the risk in food production. Climatologists are better able to predict weather patterns so that farmers can plan and manage better. For example, when anticipating a drought, a farmer might conserve water at planting. Veterinarians inspect and immunize livestock. Diseases that once wiped out entire herds are prevented with a dose of vaccine.

Food Processing and Distribution

Did you know that a typical supermarket carries around 20,000 different items? Technology has been a leader in creating and meeting the demand for variety. Scientists work with ingredients and processes to develop new foods and improve existing ones. They look for ways to deliver foods more safely and efficiently to a wider market.

New Food Choices

If you're like most people, chances are good that you ate something today that didn't exist when your grandparents were your age. Fat-free, low-calorie, and flavored foods are relatively new products of technology. Perhaps you ate a **manufactured food**, a product developed as a substitute for another food. Manufactured foods increase choices for people on restricted diets or restricted incomes, as the following examples illustrate:

- **Analogs.** Analogs (A-nuhl-awgs) are foods made to imitate actual foods. Some meat and dairy analogs are made from a vegetable protein, processed to replace animal-derived products. They may contain textured soy protein (TSP), tofu, vegetables, or grains. They can be made into meatless patties, bacon-flavored breakfast links, and imitation cheese. TSP granules can be purchased for homemade dishes. See **Fig. 4-2**.

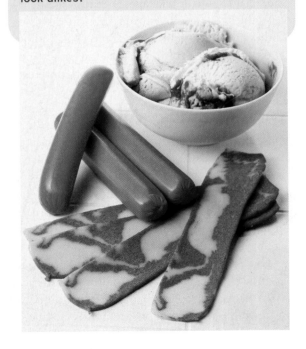

Fig. 4-2 When is a food not what it appears to be? When it's an analog. Analogs look like specific foods, but they're made with different ingredients. Why might people choose these look-alikes?

- **Formed products.** Foods made from an inexpensive source and processed to imitate a more expensive food are **formed products.** Surimi (soo-REE-mee), for example, is white fish flavored and shaped to resemble lobster or crab.
- **Egg substitutes.** These are made from egg white and other ingredients. Because they have no yolks, they have little or no fat or cholesterol. See **Fig. 4-3**.

Egg substitutes and other manufactured foods sometimes replace more expensive or fragile ingredients in prepared items. Frozen blueberry waffles cost less and keep better when they contain blueberry "buds"—a mixture of sugar, oil, salt, dyes, and artificial flavor—rather than real berries.

Packaging

Almost every food you eat, from the time it leaves the producer until it's sold in the store, relies on packaging—or packaging "systems," to use the industry term—to preserve quality and safety, and to add convenience. Some of these methods and their uses are described here. See **Fig. 4-4**.

- **Modified atmosphere packaging (MAP).** With **MAP packaging**, a mixture of carbon dioxide, oxygen, and nitrogen is inserted into

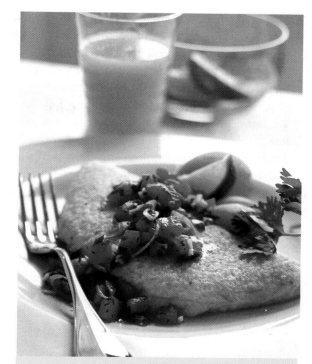

Fig. 4-3 People who can't eat whole eggs for health reasons may buy egg substitutes. How are egg substitutes different from real eggs?

the package before sealing to slow bacterial growth. The ratio of gases depends on the product. Food retains more quality since it isn't sub-

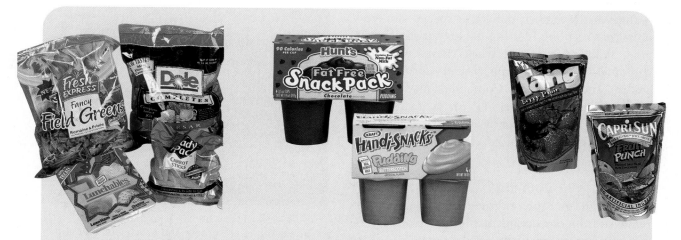

Fig. 4-4 Today's food packaging systems offer improved storage options while keeping the quality and safety of the foods. Here are examples of MAP packaging (left), aseptic packaging (center), and retort pouches (right).

jected to long periods of damaging heat, as with canning. With MAP, cooked meats and fresh pasta keep in a refrigerator for weeks.

- **Aseptic packages.** Also called "juice boxes," **aseptic packages** (ay-SEP-tik) consist of layers of plastic, paperboard, and aluminum foil. The food and package are sterilized separately and rapidly. The food is then packaged under sterile conditions. This technology meets a growing demand for shelf-stable foods. It's a popular packaging for liquids and may be used for cereals, grains, and other dry goods.
- **Retort pouches. Retort pouches** are flexible packages also made of aluminum foil and plastic film. As with canning, food is placed in the pouch and both are heat-processed. Unlike cans, however, retort pouches can store foods after opening. Some are adapted for use in the microwave.

Packaging technechnologists continually refine and develop variations of these basic processes. Slider zippers improve the seal on plastic bags. Fresh, pre-washed spinach comes ready to cook in microwavable plastic. Peanut butter and jelly are sold in side-by-side squeeze tubes.

Transportation

Transportation and packaging technology combine to bring you foods from around the world. See **Fig. 4-5**. Foods commonly travel over 1,000 miles. People in Minnesota can enjoy fresh oranges in December, thanks to special storage units that keep foods at top quality during shipping. Railroad cars and trucks have separate, computer-controlled compartments for frozen, chilled, and dry foods. Containers made with vacuum insulation panels (VIP), an extremely thin plastic or Styrofoam™ layer coated with a metallic film, can keep ice cream frozen for a week.

Genetic Engineering

Through **genetic engineering**, genes are removed from one organism, such as a plant, animal, or microorganism, and transferred to another one. Foods that are genetically engineered are known as genetically modified organisms (GMOs), genetically modified foods (GMFs), or bioengineered foods. So far, genetic engineering has been limited to plants and fish.

Genetic engineering can give a food a characteristic it doesn't normally have. For example, genes from a pesticide or weed killer can be inserted into corn and soybeans to make them resistant to pests and weed killers. Plants can also be changed to grow better under poor growing conditions. Another use is to change the texture of a food so that it is not easily damaged during handling and shipping. Experiments are under

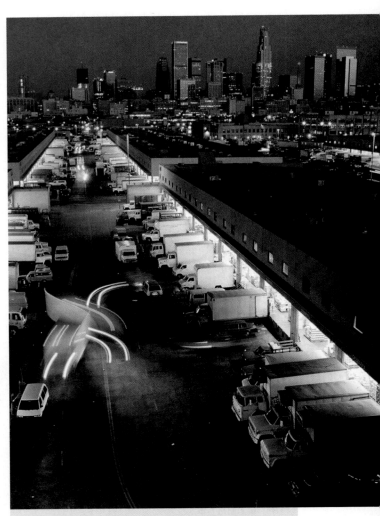

Fig. 4-5 Today people who live far from where foods are grown and processed can still enjoy them. Modern transportation systems make that possible.

way to produce fruit that ripens without becoming mushy. Other experiments are attempting to create naturally decaffeinated coffee.

Genetic engineering has both advantages and disadvantages. Advantages include:

- A larger food supply because more crops survive pest and weed damage and because poor soil can be used as farmland. World hunger could be lessened.
- Improved nutrition and taste of some foods. Substances that cause allergies might be removed.
- Greater resistance to spoilage.
- Reduced use of pesticides as a benefit to the environment. Plants can ward off pests that attack them.
- New and better varieties of food. See **Fig. 4-6**.

Disadvantages of genetic engineering include:

- Possible health problems, such as allergic reactions. For example, if genes from Brazil nuts are used in other foods, people with allergies to nuts might become seriously ill. In addition, some experts worry that introducing foreign genes into a food might create new toxins.
- Potential threat to the environment and food supply. Pollen might drift on the wind and spread to standard crops, destroying the biodiversity of the ecosystem.
- Creation of super weeds that resist herbicides. Such weeds may result when herbicide-resistant plants pollinate weeds. Insects feeding on pesticide-resistant plants could become immune to the pesticide.
- Inability of developing countries to buy the very expensive seeds.

To date, GMOs have not proven harmful to human health. Many people are concerned, however, that they have not been tested adequately. For instance, no long-term studies have been conducted to determine any effects on human health. Many consumer groups would like to see GMOs identified on food labels so people know what they're buying. They also want better testing to determine safety. They urge tighter controls on

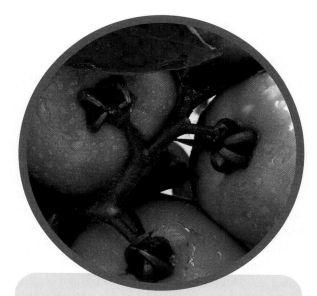

Fig. 4-6 An early plant biotechnology technique slowed down the softening process in tomatoes. Since tomatoes can stay on the vine longer, without being picked at the green stage, they develop fuller flavor.

farming and processing GMOs so the rest of the food supply is not contaminated.

Some food processors refuse to use GMOs in their products because of consumer resistance. Because of public pressure, the European Union has banned them.

Cloning

A **clone** is a genetic copy of an organism. Natural cloning produces identical twins. Scientists can also create clones through special procedures with genetic materials. Cloning took a major step in 1996 when Dolly the sheep was born, the first mammal cloned from an adult cell. Since then, the technology has been extended to cattle and pigs, as well as other animals.

Advocates believe cloning will expand and improve the food supply and prevent hunger as populations increase. Critics point out that it could destroy the biodiversity of a species. Many people oppose the process on ethical and religious grounds.

IMPROVING HEALTH

At one time, a book on foods and nutrition would have been very short. Little was known about the relationship between diet and health. Now nutrition science frequently reveals new facts, and technology devises new ways to apply the growing body of information.

Better Nutrition in Foods

Improving the nutrition of foods is a common use of technology. One standard practice is **enrichment**, which restores nutrients that were lost in processing to near original levels. For example, the iron and B vitamins found in whole grains are returned to breakfast cereals, white bread, and other foods made with refined grains. Another process, **fortification**, adds a nutrient that is not normally found in a food. Milk, for instance, is fortified with vitamin D. See **Fig. 4-7**.

Functional Foods

Calcium-fortified orange juice is just one of the many functional foods available today. **Functional foods** are those that provide health benefits beyond basic nutrition. Many aim at disease prevention. Soy protein is thought to reduce the risk of heart disease, so it is added to many foods.

Functional foods fit into four categories.

- **Natural whole foods.** Grapes, broccoli, salmon, garlic, and oats are among the foods that appear to have certain health advantages because of chemical compounds they naturally contain. Studies indicate that oats, for example, can help lower cholesterol levels, thereby reducing the risk of coronary heart disease.
- **Enhanced foods.** Some foods have nutrients and other substances added. A cereal with added fiber is an example.
- **New food products.** Food scientists continue to develop new foods with particular health benefits. For instance, people can buy a specially made margarine that lowers cholesterol.
- **Foods created by science.** Through biotechnology, scientists create some foods with special functions. A tomato, for example, may be genetically engineered to contain more of a substance (lycopene) that is linked to cancer reduction.

Functional foods are one of the fastest growing markets in U.S. food sales. Currently, there are no special regulations governing them. They must only meet the existing FDA rules for food and supplements.

Functional foods that are natural fit well into a healthful diet. The use of functional foods that have been modified or created is less clear. Known as designer foods or nutraceuticals (noo-truh-SOO-tih-kuhls), these functional foods need long-term study to determine safe use. Some health experts are concerned that these foods may pose health problems. Eating several foods that have been enhanced with the same nutrient, for example, could create a harmful excess of that nutrient in the body. Experts also warn against relying too heavily on modified foods at the expense of other nutritious foods. Functional foods aren't likely to offer a quick fix to health problems.

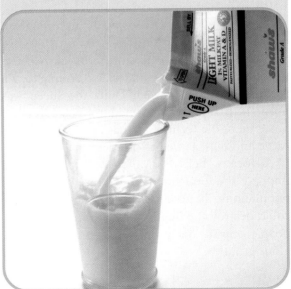

Fig. 4-7 When you drink milk, you are consuming a fortified food. Vitamin D has been added to help your body make use of the calcium in milk.

Nutrition Research

So far, nutrition research has uncovered about 40 nutrients and hundreds of chemical compounds, all essential to good health. No one knows how many others await discovery.

Discovering a nutrient is only the beginning of the research process. Scientists spend years determining the role each nutrient plays in human health. See **Fig. 4-8**. Exactly how does the body use the nutrient? How much is needed, and which foods are the best sources? What are the effects on the nutrient of processing and storage, of heat and light? Researchers also analyze the nutrient's chemical formula so that it can be manufactured.

Nutrition research extends into the food chain. For example, scientists try to improve soil and animal feed so that cattle produce leaner beef.

Ergonomics

Have you ever had a backache after working at a computer for a long time? If so, you understand the value of ergonomics. **Ergonomics** (ur-guh-NAH-miks) is the study of ways to make space and equipment easier and more comfortable to use.

Ergonomics is essential in designing kitchens, appliances, and cookware that minimize strain on muscles, bones, and joints. Ergonomically designed countertops can be adjusted to different heights. Handles on tools are shaped to fit comfortably in the hand. Some are covered in soft plastic to cushion the grip.

Work simplification, an important part of ergonomics, means using the most efficient ways to get a job done. Work simplification in the kitchen or foods lab can save time and energy.

IMPROVING MEAL PREPARATION

All cooks, whether on television or in your school cafeteria, owe their culinary creations largely to food science and technology. Consider the following contributions:

- **Cooking techniques.** A delicious, tempting meal is not the result of kitchen secrets, but of natural laws and hard science. Foods are chemicals, and a recipe is a chemical formula. Even a

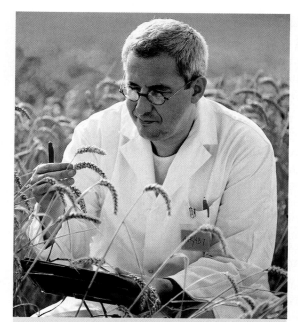

Fig. 4-8 Scientists study foods to learn more about how they impact health. Their work extends from farm to laboratory.

slight change in one ingredient or condition is apt to create a different product. Scientific study reveals how different foods react chemically and physically when they're heated, chilled, chopped, or mixed. Cooks who understand the science can choose the ingredients and preparation methods that yield the best results.

- **Appliances.** From the wood-burning cook stove of the 1800s to today's twin-chambered oven with eight cooking functions, technology continually offers kitchen appliances that make meal preparation easier and more successful. See **Fig. 4-9** on page 70. Tasks that were once done by hand are now done by food processors and dishwashers. Appliances are also more reliable, easier to use, and energy efficient. "Smart" appliances contain a computer chip "brain" that monitors their own workings and lets you program their features. Some even alert you when repairs are needed.

- **Personal computers.** Personal computers and the Internet are changing the way professional

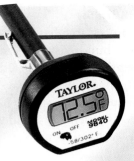

TRENDS in TECHNOLOGY

READY—OR NOT?

A good idea isn't always enough to get technology out of the laboratory and into the kitchen. Timing and value are deciding factors. For example, problem-solving, "smart" appliances have been available since the 1980s. Refrigerators flash a warning when the door is left open. Microwave ovens can be programmed for multi-stage cooking. Other, more impressive features, however, might not catch on. You may never see a refrigerator that tells you when you're running low on an item inside. Since features come at a price, consumers may decide that the current, simpler technology that makes foods visible through clear plastic shelves and bins is just fine.

Another mostly unrealized innovation is the "Web-enhanced" kitchen. Here, appliances are linked electronically and accessible by the Internet. You program or command them by going on-line. Coordinating appliances in this way takes extensive and expensive computerization—embedding microprocessors in countertops, for instance—which must be included during home construction. Thus, it's an option only to upper-income families who are buying new homes.

Will such kitchens be common someday? Possibly, especially if a simpler technology to build them can be found.

__Think Beyond>> If you were designing a kitchen item, how would you decide which features are worthwhile?

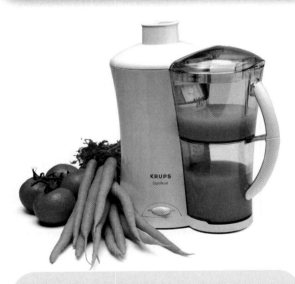

Fig. 4-9 How would you decide whether to buy a new appliance on the market?

and home cooks shop, plan, and prepare meals. Computers conveniently store recipes, create menus, and organize shopping lists. They can help keep track of what's in your kitchen and what you spent on it. You can evaluate one food or an entire meal for its nutrition content. The Internet gives people information about food choices. You can find up-to-date information on diets and nutrition research, as well as recipes and cooking hints. You may be able to order milk and cereal through the Web site of your local supermarket, or Peruvian potatoes from a food importer.

FOOD TECHNOLOGY TRADE-OFFS

Food technology offers exciting possibilities, but not without drawbacks. The modern processing and transportation system that brings you many nutritious foods also creates by-products to manage. On-line shopping benefits those who are physically challenged but hurts smaller grocers who can't offer the service.

New technology brings new decisions. With more products of technology available every day, you need to educate yourself on the latest innovations. Learning to identify pros and cons and being able to evaluate what's worthwhile will be useful skills in the years ahead.

Food Scientist

CRAIG "SKIP" JULIUS: Food scientist Craig Julius has an alphabet soup of letters after his name: CFE, CRC, CCS, and more. They stand for various certifications that recognize experience, knowledge, and professional development. They also represent a fascination with food that began, literally, in grandma's kitchen. As a child, Craig watched his grandmother work her homemade wonders. The interest carried into his teens, when he worked in a bakery while in high school.

The Chief Chef. With a bachelor's degree in food science and nutrition, Craig set out to see what opportunities awaited. He soon found them, working his way up to chef de cuisine at the Pontiac Silverdome, an 80,000-seat arena near Detroit, Michigan. At the same time, he completed coursework in buffet preparation and presentation at the internationally recognized Culinary Institute of America. Over the next twelve years, Craig worked as executive chef in several Detroit-area restaurants.

It was a course in nutrition that turned his career. Until then, he recalls, "I never wondered what happened to the food after people ate it. I was only concerned that they enjoy it. This opened up a whole new world for me. I got interested in the food science aspect. It was natural to progress from the culinary plus the food science into product development."

Build a Better Salsa. A few years later, Craig's fascination with creating recipes took him from kitchen to lab. He became director of research and development for a large food service corporation that owned a chain of restaurants worldwide and fed fans at major U.S. sporting events. Craig oversaw the formulation of recipes and techniques to produce quality foods in each setting. His division also tested new products from manufacturers—over 2,000 items each year. His work in food science earned him another credential, Certified Food Service Executive (CFE).

The career climb didn't end there. In 1997, Craig took on an even greater challenge, as corporate executive chef for Nestlé USA. Now manager of product innovation, he plays a leading role in the risky venture of launching new food products. Being involved in every aspect adds variety to his work. One day he might tinker with a salsa recipe in the test kitchen. The next day, he confers with marketing analysts on how to sell the new product. Rounding out his professional growth, Craig earned titles as Certified Research Chef (CRC) and Certified Culinary Scientist (CCS).

As you might guess, Craig is enthusiastic about the value of experience as education. "Every food company I know either has or is looking for someone with culinary or food science experience. Work at different restaurants. Go to a good culinary school, the best you can afford. With a few more years of experience, the sky's the limit!"

On-line Connections

1. To learn more about topics in this article, search the Internet for these key words: culinologist; food scientist; certified research chef.

2. To learn about related careers, search the Internet for these key words: culinary consultant; packaging technologist.

Summarize Your Reading

▶ Through science and technology, the food supply today has become more plentiful, varied, interesting, and even more healthful.

▶ Genetic engineering has both advantages and disadvantages, leading to differences of opinion on the subject.

▶ Technology aims to improve health by improving food nutrition, doing nutrition research, and creating equipment that makes working with foods more comfortable.

▶ Many improvements in meal preparation have been made through technology.

Check Your Knowledge

1. How does the term **technology** relate to **science**?

2. What is **food science**?

3. How has technology impacted food production?

4. Describe three types of **manufactured foods**.

5. Why does **MAP** retain more quality in foods?

6. What type of packaging has helped meet the increasing demand for shelf-stable foods?

7. What advantage do **retort pouches** have over cans?

8. How has transportation changed in its ability to ship foods over greater distances?

9. How are organisms **genetically engineered**?

10. What are some qualities that have been given to foods through genetic engineering?

11. What are the arguments for and against **cloning** foods?

12. Yummy Crunch cereal contains vitamins that were put back after their loss during processing. What is this procedure called?

13. If a nutrient is added to a food that didn't have the nutrient before, what is this procedure called?

14. Why are some foods called functional?

15. Should you make all **functional foods** part of your diet? Explain.

16. How is technology involved in nutrition?

17. What are the advantages of applying **ergonomics** to kitchen design?

18. Technology has improved meal preparation in what ways?

19. **CRITICAL THINKING** "It always seems that right after I buy a new appliance, they come out with a newer version that does more." Do you agree with this person's statement? How do you suggest individuals and society manage this situation?

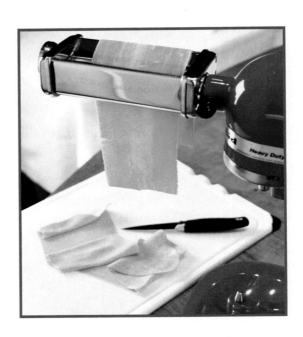

Apply Your Learning

1. **LANGUAGE ARTS** **Sentence Completion.** Complete this sentence in writing: "To me, technology means …" Share responses in class.

2. **Interview.** Talk with an older adult, possibly a grandparent, to learn how technology has changed foods and kitchens over the years. How were meals prepared when the interviewee was young? What foods were available? What do you think about the changes?

3. **Ergonomic Exploration.** Look at kitchen tools in a store. Compare different styles of such tools as can openers and hand utensils. What differences do you see? Which items have better ergonomic design? How do they compare to similar items you have at home?

4. **Technology Trade-Offs.** Make a list of kitchen appliances that have multiple features. Read advertisements, or look at those you have at home. Which features do you think are least useful? Why do you think appliances have these features? How do they relate to cost? What can you learn from this?

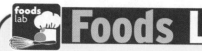 **Foods Lab**

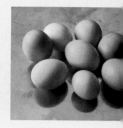

Evaluating Manufactured Food

Procedure: Prepare a food and its manufactured food replacement. Evaluate the foods on appeal and nutritional value.

Analyzing Results

❶ How does the manufactured food compare to the original in taste, texture, and appearance? How do costs compare?

❷ What nutritional advantages does each food offer?

❸ Read the ingredient list of the manufactured food. What do you think each ingredient adds in sensory qualities and nutrition?

❹ When might each food be a good choice for meals or recipes?

 Food Science Experiment

Comparing Packaging

Objective: To evaluate the effectiveness of different types of packaging.

Procedure:

1. Use a newly opened container of potato chips. Place five chips in a plastic storage bag. Seal the bag tightly, squeezing out as much air as possible without crushing the chips.

2. Wrap five chips in a piece of aluminum foil. Fold the ends of the foil to seal tightly, gently forcing out as much air as possible without crushing the chips.

3. Leave both samples in the same location for three days. Then observe and evaluate the samples, comparing them on taste and texture.

Analyzing Results

❶ Which potato chips were crisper? Less crisp?

❷ Which chips had the more agreeable taste? Less agreeable?

❸ What do you think caused the results you noted in questions 1 and 2?

❹ Based on your findings, explain why potato chips are packaged as they are.

UNIT 2
Nutrition Basics

CHAPTER 5   **Nutrients at Work**

CHAPTER 6   **Carbohydrates**

CHAPTER 7   **Proteins & Fats**

CHAPTER 8   **Vitamins & Minerals**

CHAPTER 9   **Water & Phytochemicals**

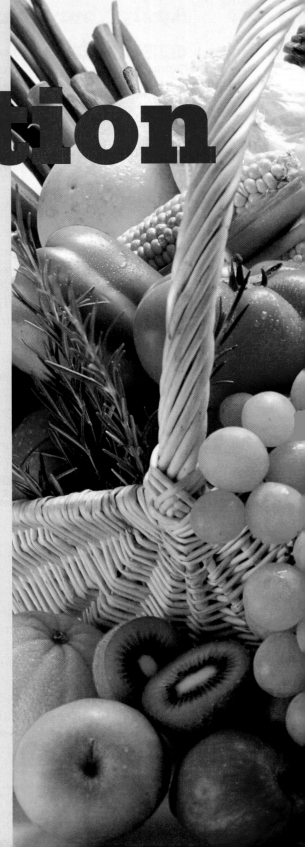

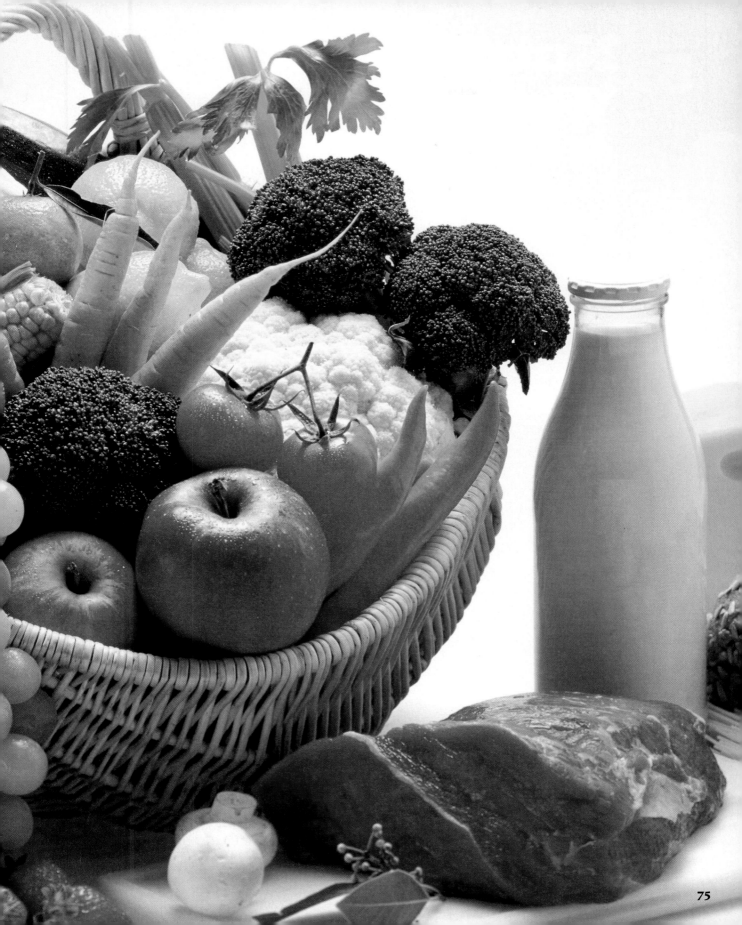

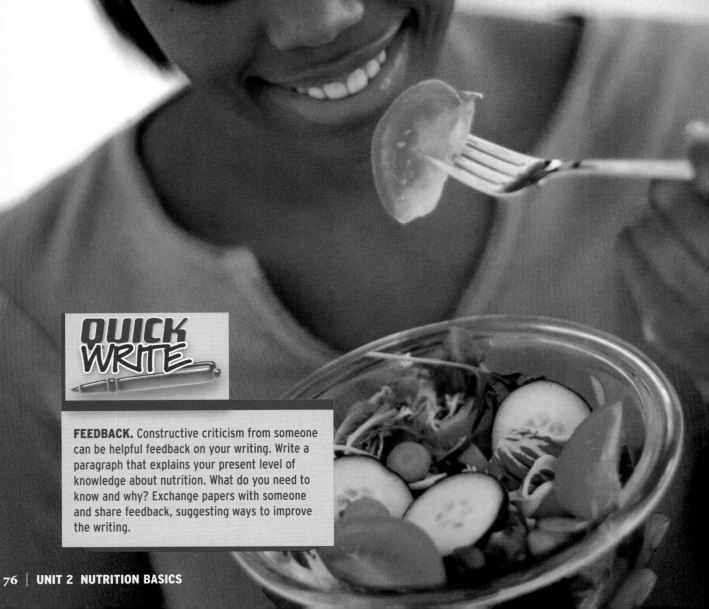

Nutrients at Work

QUICK WRITE

FEEDBACK. Constructive criticism from someone can be helpful feedback on your writing. Write a paragraph that explains your present level of knowledge about nutrition. What do you need to know and why? Exchange papers with someone and share feedback, suggesting ways to improve the writing.

To Guide Your Reading:

Objectives

- ▶ Explain the impact of nutrients on your body and health.
- ▶ Describe standards and guidelines that provide information about nutrient requirements.
- ▶ Summarize the steps in the digestive process.
- ▶ Explain how nutrients are absorbed, transported, and stored in the body.
- ▶ Discuss the role of metabolism in the body.

Terms

absorption	esophagus
Adequate Intakes (AI)	glucose
anemia	glycogen
basal metabolism	malnutrition
calorie	metabolism
chyme	oxidation
Dietary Reference Intakes (DRI)	pancreas
digestion	peristalsis
enzyme	Recommended Dietary Allowances (RDA)
	villi

T HE HUMAN BODY IS AN INCREDIBLE organism. Although your outward appearance changes little from day to day, the atoms, molecules, and cells inside your body are constantly moving and changing.

Without any instructions from you, thousands of vital processes are carried out automatically at every moment. Your brain sends and receives signals so you can think, remember, and reason. Your lungs inhale oxygen from the air and exhale waste products. Cells are constantly repaired and replaced in order to keep you active and healthy. In fact, during the time it takes to read this paragraph, about 100 million of your body cells will die, and new ones will be built to take their place. See **Fig. 5-1**. How is all this possible? Foods and the nutrients they contain help your body carry out these processes continuously.

THE NUTRIENTS IN FOODS

If you take a chemical look at food, what will you find? First, food contains water in amounts that vary from 5 to 90 percent depending on the

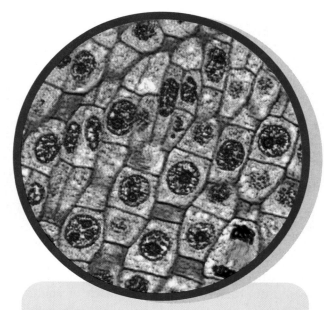

Fig. 5-1 Cells are the basic units that make up your body. Nutrients from foods help repair cells and replace those that die.

food. The remaining solid materials are mostly carbohydrates (kahr-boh-HY-drayts), fats, and proteins. A very small amount of vitamins, minerals, and other compounds make up the rest of food. Together, these food components are known as nutrients. Your body uses nutrients in many ways, including these basic functions:

- **Carbohydrates.** Provide the body's main source of energy.
- **Fats.** Provide a concentrated source of stored energy as well as insulation for the body.
- **Proteins.** Help build, repair, and maintain body tissues.
- **Vitamins.** Help regulate many vital processes.
- **Minerals.** Help the body work properly.
- **Water.** Participates in chemical reactions in the body and helps transport materials to and from cells.

Besides nutrients, foods also contain small amounts of substances called phytochemicals (fy-toh-KE-mih-kuhls), a topic for a later chapter. These compounds may help reduce the risk of developing certain chronic health problems. Ongoing research continues to reveal more about them.

Nutrients and Health

Trillions of cells make up the tissues in your body, and healthy cells make healthy tissues. To function properly, cells need nutrients.

When it comes to nutrients, not all foods are alike. One food may supply vitamin C, yet another doesn't. As long as you choose a healthful variety of foods in the recommended amounts, the nutrients that your body needs will be available for the important work to be done.

Faulty or inadequate nutrition can lead to **malnutrition**. A deficiency or severe shortage of a nutrient is one form of malnutrition. For example, not getting the recommended amount of iron can cause **anemia** (uh-NEE-mee-uh), a blood disorder characterized by lack of energy, weakness, shortness of breath, and cold hands and feet. In some developing countries, chronic malnutrition is a serious problem. Anywhere that poverty exists, however, malnutrition is possible, even in the United States.

Another form of malnutrition is caused by overeating and gaining many extra pounds that lead to overweight. Eating extra-large portions of food and excess amounts of sugars and fats instead of fruits, vegetables, and lean meat can cause this problem.

Can you stay healthy by eating varied foods with the nutrients you need? That depends. To begin with, your health is influenced by your heredity, lifestyle, and food choices. You can't change heredity, but you can do something about lifestyle and food choices. See **Fig. 5-2**.

Anyone who has destructive habits can't expect good nutrition to perform miracles. If you abuse your body with alcohol or other drugs, good nutrition can't keep you healthy. If you don't get enough sleep, good nutrition can't give you more energy. When your lifestyle includes healthy habits as well as good nutrition, however, you can enjoy these benefits within the framework of your wellness potential:

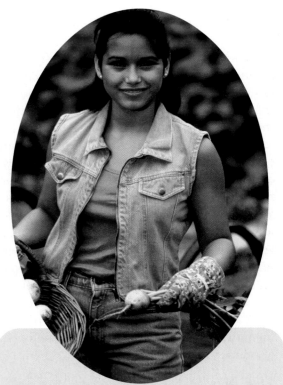

Fig. 5-2 You have many more foods to choose from than people have ever had. How can you tell which foods contribute to good health?

- **Appearance.** Shiny hair, bright eyes, healthy nails and teeth, and smooth, clear skin all link to good nutrition.
- **Fitness.** Good nutrition helps you stay active and alert. You have the energy to perform your best, whether in school or at work. You maintain energy throughout the day, without feeling dragged out.
- **Weight.** Within your body limitations, you can have a healthy weight.
- **Illness.** Research shows that many illnesses are related to poor nutrition. Keeping the body well usually takes less time and effort than curing a minor sickness. Good nutrition can help you lower the likelihood of developing some problems.
- **Healing.** With good nutrition, the body heals more easily. Medicine and surgery alone cannot heal the body. Rather, they provide conditions that help healing take place. For example, surgery might remove a diseased area, allowing the body to repair or replace remaining damaged cells. If you break an arm, the physician lines up the broken ends and puts the arm in a cast to keep the bones from moving. In time, the body manufactures all the new cells needed to mend the break.
- **Emotions.** Dealing with pressures can be a challenge. Sometimes people can't concentrate or study. Stress can lead to feelings of weariness or even depression. Good nutrition can lessen feelings like these and help people cope more effectively.
- **Future health.** Many serious health problems, such as heart disease and some cancers, can result from years of poor eating habits. Good nutrition today may help you avoid these problems in the future. See **Fig. 5-3**.

Nutrient Teamwork

Scientists have discovered that even though nutrients perform distinct functions in the body, these functions interact. Therefore a single nutrient is not totally responsible for any one process.

Instead, nutrients work together as teams. For example, proteins are an important part of bone structure, but certain minerals strengthen the

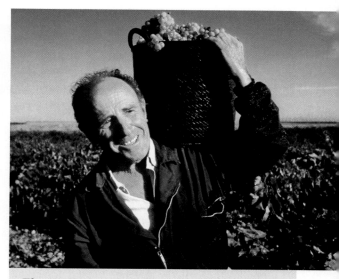

Fig. 5-3 Over time, poor eating habits can lead to health problems. On the other hand, good nutrition helps people live a healthier life now and in the future.

bones. Nutrient teamwork means your body must have an adequate supply of all nutrients. Do you see why limiting your food choices could lead to problems?

Nutrient Requirements

A question people often ask about nutrients is: "How much do I need?" You, your family, and friends all need the same nutrients, but not necessarily in the same amounts. Females, for instance, require more iron than males. Athletes and others who are physically active need more carbohydrates for energy than inactive people do. Because teens are growing, they require larger amounts of certain nutrients than adults need.

Most nutrients are needed in relatively small amounts. The metric system is the easiest way to measure nutrients. This system includes small units of measure, such as the milligram (mg). For example, female teens need 15 mg of the mineral iron each day.

Scientists have developed a series of standards for assessing nutrient needs among people of different age and gender groups. These standards have different names but are known under the general label, **Dietary Reference Intakes (DRIs)**.

Fig. 5-4

Dietary Reference Intakes for Teens (RDA OR AI)

Nutrient	Males 9-13	Males 14-18	Females 9-13	Females 14-18
Protein	34 g	52 g	34 g	46 g
Carbohydrate (total)	130 g	130 g	130 g	130 g
Dietary fiber	31 g	38 g	26 g	26 g
Fat (total)	*	*	*	*
Saturated fat	*	*	*	*
Cholesterol	*	*	*	*
Vitamin A	600 µg RAE	900 µg RAE	600 µg RAE	700 µg RAE
Thiamin	0.9 mg	1.2 mg	0.9 mg	1.0 mg
Riboflavin	0.9 mg	1.3 mg	0.9 mg	1.0 mg
Niacin	12 mg NE	16 mg NE	12 mg NE	14 mg NE
Vitamin B_6	1.0 mg	1.3 mg	1.0 mg	1.2 mg
Vitamin B_{12}	1.8 µg	2.4 µg	1.8 µg	2.4 µg
Folate	300 µg DFE	400 µg DFE	300 µg DFE	400 µg DFE
Biotin	20 µg	25 µg	20 µg	25 µg
Pantothenic acid	4 mg	5 mg	4 mg	5 mg
Vitamin C	45 mg	75 mg	45 mg	65 mg
Vitamin D	5 µg	5 µg	5 µg	5 µg
Vitamin E	11 mg α-TE	15 mg α-TE	11 mg α-TE	15 mg α-TE
Vitamin K	60 µg	75 µg	60 µg	75 µg
Calcium	1,300 mg	1,300 mg	1,300 mg	1,300 mg
Copper	700 µg	890 µg	700 µg	890 µg
Iodine	120 µg	150 µg	120 µg	150 µg
Iron	8 mg	11 mg	8 mg	15 mg
Magnesium	240 mg	410 mg	240 mg	360 mg
Phosphorus	1,250 mg	1,250 mg	1,250 mg	1,250 mg
Potassium	*	*	*	*
Selenium	40 µg	55 µg	40 µg	55 µg
Sodium	*	*	*	*
Zinc	8 mg	11 mg	8 mg	9 mg

*No value estalished

Key to nutrient measures

g   gram
mg   milligram (1,000 mg = 1 g)
µg   microgram (1,000 µg = 1 mg; 1,000,000 µg = 1 g)
RAE   retinol activity equivalents (a measure of Vitamin A activity)
NE   niacin equivalents (a measure of niacin activity)
DFE   dietary folate equivalents (a measure of folate activity)
α-TE   alpha-tocopherol equivalents (a measure of Vitamin E activity)

Two examples of DRIs are **Recommended Dietary Allowances (RDAs)** and **Adequate Intakes (AIs)**. An RDA is the amount of a nutrient needed by 98 percent of the people in a given age and gender group. An AI is used when a lack of scientific information makes it impossible to establish the RDA for a particular nutrient. The DRIs, which include RDAs and AIs, are updated periodically as new information becomes available. **Fig. 5-4** shows the DRIs for teens.

Dietitians, nutritionists, and other health professionals use DRIs to help shape U.S. nutrition policy and develop educational programs. The food industry also uses this information for product development.

The U.S. Food and Drug Administration (FDA) uses the DRIs as the basis for another set of guidelines. Known as Daily Values (DVs), they are used on nutrition labels. See **Fig. 5-5.**

THE DIGESTIVE PROCESS

When you eat food, your body needs to use the nutrients. The cells in body tissues, however, are so small that only very tiny substances can enter them. Therefore food must be broken down to make nutrients available. One meal can provide

Fig. 5-5

Daily Values

Nutrient	Daily Value	Nutrient	Daily Value
Protein	50 g*	Vitamin C	60 mg
Carbohydrate (total)	300 g*	Vitamin D	400 IU (6.5 µg)
Dietary fiber	25 g	Vitamin E	30 IU (9 mg α-TE)
Fat (total)	65 g*	Vitamin K	80 µg
Saturated fat	20 g*	Calcium	1,000 mg
Cholesterol	300 mg	Copper	2 mg
Vitamin A	5,000 IU (875 µg RAE)	Iodine	150 µg
Thiamin	1.5 mg	Iron	18 mg
Riboflavin	1.7 mg	Magnesium	400 mg
Niacin	20 mg NE	Phosphorus	1,000 mg
Vitamin B_6	2 mg	Potassium	3,500 mg
Vitamin B_{12}	6 µg	Selenium	70 µg
Folate	400 µg	Sodium	2,400 mg
Biotin	300 µg	Zinc	15 mg
Pantothenic acid	10 mg		

*Based on a diet of 2,000 calories per day

Key to nutrient measures

g	gram
mg	milligram (1,000 mg = 1 g)
µg	microgram (1,000 µg = 1 mg; 1,000,000 µg = 1 g)
IU	International Unit (an old measure of vitamin activity)
RAE	retinol activity equivalents (a measure of Vitamin A activity)
NE	niacin equivalents (a measure of niacin activity)
α-TE	alpha-tocopherol equivalents (a measure of Vitamin E activity)

millions of nutrient molecules, but how does that happen and where do they go? Your digestive system has the answer.

Digestion is the mechanical and chemical process that breaks food down to release nutrients in forms your body can absorb for use.

Digestion takes place in the digestive tract, a hollow tube about 26 feet long. This flexible tube extends from the mouth to the rectum (REK-tum), winding around mostly within the abdomen. See **Fig. 5-6**.

The Digestive System

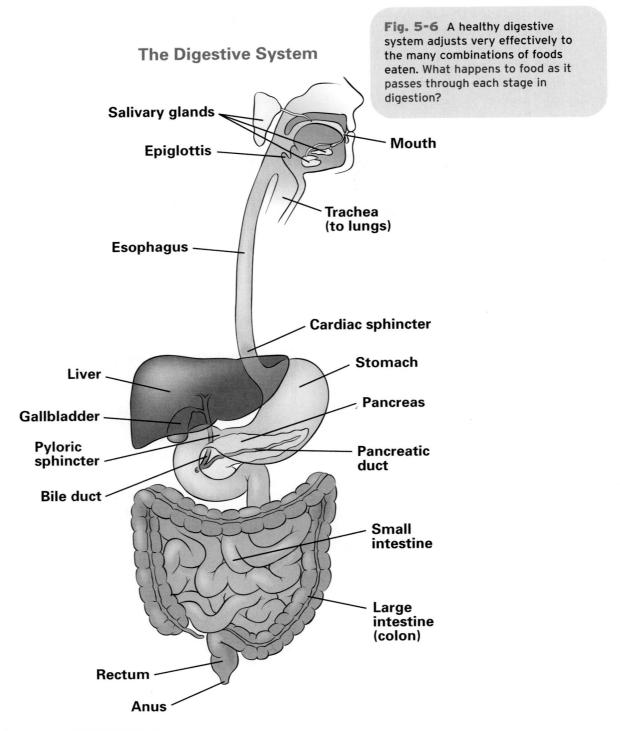

Fig. 5-6 A healthy digestive system adjusts very effectively to the many combinations of foods eaten. What happens to food as it passes through each stage in digestion?

Salivary glands

Epiglottis

Mouth

Trachea (to lungs)

Esophagus

Cardiac sphincter

Stomach

Liver

Pancreas

Gallbladder

Pyloric sphincter

Pancreatic duct

Bile duct

Small intestine

Large intestine (colon)

Rectum

Anus

The Mouth

Digestion begins in the mouth. As you chew, your teeth grind food down into smaller pieces that are easier to swallow and digest. This mechanical part of digestion increases the surface area of food, yielding more space for chemical reactions to occur.

Chewing solid food to the consistency of applesauce is recommended. If you swallow larger pieces, your stomach won't be able to digest them completely, and you will lose the benefits of some nutrients.

The chemical part of digestion begins as saliva is released in the mouth. Saliva contains the enzyme ptyalin (TY-uh-lun), which mixes with food and continues to break it down. **Enzymes** are special proteins that help chemical reactions take place. Carbohydrates are the first nutrients to break down chemically. The ptyalin in saliva helps change carbohydrates into sugars.

Even before you take a bite of food, what happens? The sight, aroma, or the thought of food can start saliva flowing in your mouth—your mouth "waters." The taste of food continues to produce saliva. Taste buds on the tongue can identify four general flavors: salty, bitter, sour, and sweet. Some researchers also list a savory fifth flavor, called umami (yoo-MAH-mee).

People prefer foods that taste good, but enjoying the flavors also depends on your nose. Only your sense of smell enables you to identify the specific food you're eating. If this sounds far-fetched, think about the last time you had a cold. You might not have felt like eating because the food didn't taste good.

Try this experiment. The next time you eat, pinch your nostrils together firmly with your fingers and breathe through your mouth. Then take a bite of flavorful food. What do you taste? You probably taste one of the flavors the tongue senses but not the characteristic flavor of the food you're eating. Release your nostrils and breathe through your nose. What do you taste now?

The Esophagus

Once swallowed, food passes into the **esophagus** (ih-SAH-fuh-gus), the part of the tube that

Peristalsis

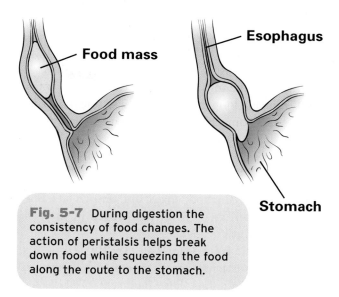

Food mass

Esophagus

Stomach

Fig. 5-7 During digestion the consistency of food changes. The action of peristalsis helps break down food while squeezing the food along the route to the stomach.

connects the mouth and stomach. Food moves through the esophagus by **peristalsis** (pehr-uh-STAHL-sus). Through peristalsis, the muscles of the esophagus contract and relax, creating a series of wavelike movements that force the food into the stomach. See **Fig. 5-7**. This action continues the physical breakdown of the food. A valve at the end of the esophagus closes to prevent food from moving back up the tube.

The Stomach

The stomach is the widest part of the digestive system. This hollow, muscular pouch is just below the rib cage. On average, the stomach can hold about 6 cups of food.

The stomach produces gastric juices—acids and enzymes that help food break down chemically. A film of sticky mucus lines the stomach walls, protecting them from damage by acids. Although carbohydrates began to break down in the mouth, proteins and fats start this process in the stomach.

The stomach also breaks food down mechanically through peristalsis. The churned food turns into a thick liquid called **chyme** (KIME).

Different foods take different amounts of time to break down and leave the stomach. Carbohydrates take the shortest time, usually 1 to 2 hours. Proteins take longer, about 3 to 5 hours. Fats take the longest time to digest, up to 12 hours.

The Small Intestine

After processing in the stomach, food moves a little at a time into the small intestine. The small intestine is a long, narrow, winding tube that connects the stomach and large intestine. Here, three types of digestive juices act on the chyme as the breakdown of carbohydrates, proteins, and fats continues.

- **Bile.** Helps the body digest and absorb fats. Bile is produced in the liver and stored in the gall bladder until needed.
- **Pancreatic juice** (pan-kree-AH-tik). Contains enzymes that help break down carbohydrates, proteins, and fats. The **pancreas** (PAN-kree-us), a gland connected to the small intestine, produces this substance.
- **Intestinal juice.** Works with other juices to break down food. It is produced in the small intestine.

ABSORPTION OF NUTRIENTS

Once food has been broken down, it must be absorbed. Through **absorption**, nutrients move into the blood stream. Most absorption takes place through the surface of the small intestine. The inner wall of the small intestine is arranged in folds, which are lined with billions of tiny, fingerlike projections called **villi** (VIH-leye). The villi increase the surface area of the intestine so that more nutrients can be absorbed. Although the small intestine is only about ten feet long, the surface area is equal to about one quarter of a football field. See **Fig. 5-8.**

After absorption, waste material, including dietary fiber, is left in the small intestine. Fiber is the indigestible portion of food that helps with digestion and absorption. This waste moves into the large intestine, also called the colon. The colon removes water, potassium, and sodium from the waste. The remainder is stored as a semisolid in the rectum, or lower part of the large intestine, until elimination.

Enlargement of Intestinal Wall

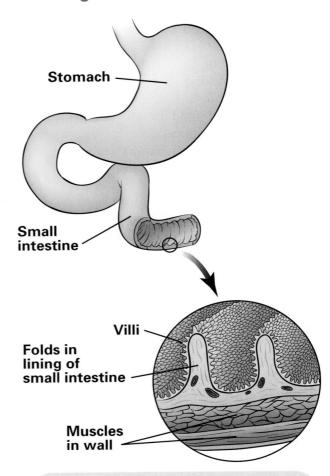

Fig. 5-8 The lining of the small intestine has a wrinkled surface with millions of finger-shaped projections called villi. What is their purpose?

NUTRIENT TRANSPORTATION

After nutrients are absorbed by the villi of the small intestine, they are carried to the liver through a blood vessel, called the portal vein. One of the liver's many jobs is to turn nutrients into forms the body can use.

When fully broken down chemically, carbohydrates become a simple sugar called **glucose** (GLOO-kohs), or blood sugar. Glucose is the body's basic fuel. Fats are changed into fatty acids. Proteins are broken down into amino acids.

You may have noticed that the breakdown of only three nutrients has been mentioned so far. That's because vitamins, minerals, water, and phytochemicals do not break down. They are used by the body in the same form they have in food.

After any necessary breakdown, nutrients are ready for travel. As part of the circulatory system, the bloodstream carries nutrients and oxygen to individual cells, where they are put to work.

NUTRIENT STORAGE

If not needed immediately, some nutrients can be stored for future use. For example, the liver converts extra glucose into **glycogen** (GLY-kuh-juhn), a storage form of glucose.

If the glucose supply is more than can be stored as glycogen, the rest is converted to body fat. Excess fatty acids and amino acids are also converted into body fat. Fats are deposited throughout the body as an energy reserve.

Minerals and vitamins are stored in various ways. For instance, iron is stored in the liver and in bone marrow. Vitamins that dissolve in fat are stored mainly in the liver and in body fat. Some nutrients, including vitamins that dissolve in water, are not stored for long periods. If not needed soon, they are removed from the body with the wastes.

METABOLISM

After nutrients arrive at their destinations, they are put to work by way of another process—metabolism (muh-TA-buh-lih-zum). Through **metabolism** living cells use nutrients in many chemical reactions that provide energy for vital processes and activities. You may wonder how this happens.

Remember the glucose made from carbohydrates? The body uses glucose as a fuel to produce energy. Glucose in the cells combines chemically with oxygen to produce energy and heat. This process is called **oxidation** (ahk-suh-DAY-shun), a term for chemical reactions that combine elements with oxygen. A fireplace illustrates oxidation, with wood as the fuel. To burn, the wood uses oxygen from the air and produces light and heat. See **Fig. 5-9**.

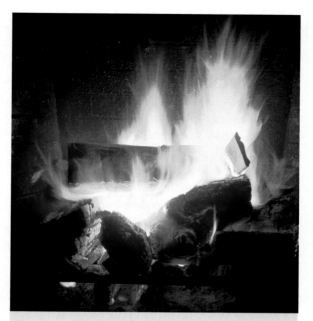

Fig. 5-9 A fireplace creates heat energy by chemically combining oxygen with the fuel wood. Your body cells create energy for all your activities by combining oxygen with the fuel glucose, which carbohydrates provide.

Energy is measured in units called kilocalories (kih-loh-KA-luh-reez), better known as calories. A **calorie** is the amount of energy needed to raise the temperature of 1 kilogram of water (a little more than 4 cups) 1 degree Celsius. In the metric system, energy is measured in kilojoules (KJ). A calorie can measure the amount of energy available in food or the amount of energy used by the body for activities.

Scientists have determined that pure forms of nutrients have the calories shown in **Fig. 5-10**. As you can see, fat has a little more than twice the number of calories as carbohydrate and protein.

Fig. 5-10

Calories in Nutrients

Nutrient	Calories
1 gram pure carbohydrate	4 calories
1 gram pure protein	4 calories
1 gram pure fat	9 calories

Your body needs energy for every activity. All foods provide energy, but carbohydrates are the main source.

Basal Metabolism

Your body uses energy for automatic processes as well as for physical activities. Automatic processes that sustain life include breathing, digesting food, and building and repairing tissue. Because these processes go on 24 hours a day, your body uses small amounts of energy even when you are resting and sleeping. The minimum amount of energy you need to maintain these basic processes in the body is called **basal metabolism** (BAY-zuhl muh-TA-buh-lih-zum).

The amount of energy used for basal metabolism is called basal metabolic rate, or BMR. Everyone's body works at its own speed, so all individuals have their own personal basal metabolic rate. That's why energy needs vary greatly from person to person. Generally, about two-thirds of calories consumed are used for basal metabolism, but this varies with the individual. Remaining calories are used for physical activities, such as work and exercise.

Energy Requirements

The number of calories people need for energy in a given day varies. Age, weight, and gender all have impact. If you're still growing, for example, you need more calories for the extra energy it takes to build muscles and bones. In general, the U.S. Department of Agriculture recommends the daily calorie amounts in **Fig. 5-11** for teens.

Activity level also affects calorie guidelines. The more active you are, the more energy you use. For instance, you would use more energy walking up a flight of stairs than riding in an elevator. A teen who spends leisure time at the computer needs fewer calories than one who spends the same amount of time swimming or playing soccer.

Recommended Sources of Calories

Health experts recommend what percentage of calories should come from carbohydrates, proteins, and fats. This ratio provides the healthiest balance of the three nutrients. **Fig. 5-12** shows the amounts recommended for teens and adults.

Fig. 5-11

Approximate Daily Calories for Teens		
Activity Level*	Males Ages 14 to 18	Females Ages 14 to 18
Sedentary	2,000 to 2,400	1,800
Moderately Active	2,400 to 2,800	2,000
Active	2,800 to 3,200	2,400

*Sedentary: less than 30 minutes of physical activity daily. Moderately active: 30 to 60 minutes. Active: over 60 minutes.

As an example, suppose one teen needs about 2,200 calories a day. If she limits fat to 30 percent of her day's calories, that allows her 660 calories from fat (2,200 3 .30 = 660). How many grams of fat will supply 660 calories? Since there are 9 calories in 1 gram of fat, divide 660 by 9. The answer is 73 grams. If the teen eats a bagel with cream cheese and a glass of orange juice for breakfast and a fish sandwich with medium fries for lunch, the total amount of fat is about 58 grams. To stay within her fat limit, she will have to make careful food choices for the rest of the day.

AN INCREDIBLE JOURNEY

If you didn't realize before, you now see what an incredible journey your most recent meal is taking at this very moment. The events that convert food from a meal to the chemical substances that help keep you healthy are remarkable. Making use of the nutrients in food is your body's responsibility, but choosing foods that have the needed nutrients is yours. Learning more about nutrients will make it easier for you to understand and manage this responsibility.

Fig. 5-12

Nutrient Sources for Calories		
Nutrient	Teens	Adults
Carbohydrates	45-65%	45-65%
Proteins	10-30%	10-35%
Fats	25-35%	20-35%

Career Pathways

Nutrition Consultant

SYLVIA MELÉNDEZ-KLINGER: Suppose you're a bakery sales executive who wants to tap the growing Hispanic market. How do you increase bread sales to Hispanic consumers? First, you call Sylvia Meléndez-Klinger. Sylvia is founder of Hispanic Food Communications, a company that helps segments of the food industry understand the needs of this rapidly emerging ethnic group.

Career Paths Converge. Owning a nutrition consulting firm specializing in the Hispanic market wasn't part of Sylvia's career plan when she started in dietetics. Given her personal and professional background, however, it seems a natural destination. Born in Mayaguez, Puerto Rico, and raised in Mexico City, she "fell in love with food and nutrition" while in high school in Monterrey, Mexico. She earned her bachelor's degree in dietetics and nutrition and later a master's degree in public administration. Her work as a research dietitian included nutrition surveys of different populations. At the University of California, she counseled and monitored patients in a study to determine the effects of a heart medication. She did nutrition assessment research in children with high blood cholesterol at Northwestern University in Chicago.

As Sylvia says, "Every day I learned, and am still learning, something that prepared me for my business career—from managers who taught me responsibility and perseverance, to jobs that require you to meet deadlines."

Sylvia's last position before entrepreneurship was with Quaker Oats in Chicago. As culinary development specialist and supervisor of consumer test kitchens, her duties were as impressive as the job title. From conducting consumer research, to coordinating sales training, to creating "signature" recipes, Sylvia probably had something to do with any Quaker Oats products you may have eaten in the 1990s. Finally, with encouragement from colleagues, she started Hispanic Food Communications in 2000.

Closing Culture Gaps. So how could Sylvia's company help the would-be bread seller? Her recipe analysts might suggest changes to make the bread a better fit for Hispanic cooking. Sales staff might lay out an appealing, culturally aware advertising campaign, with a translator fine-tuning the message to convey the right tone and meaning. If a bilingual spokesperson is needed for media events, Sylvia supplies one.

The nutrition component has not been forgotten either. "Providing the correct nutrition and health information so consumers can start a healthier lifestyle" is not just good marketing sense. It is also one of her job's most rewarding aspects. "I really love my career and will never get tired of talking about food and nutrition." That, she believes, is a key to success: stay close to what first excites you about a career, whatever field you choose. Of foods and nutrition she says, "The opportunities and avenues are there. All you need is energy and a love for the game!"

On-line Connections

1. To learn more about topics in this article, search the Internet for these key words: Hispanic cuisine; nutrition research; master's degree in public administration.

2. To learn about related careers, search the Internet for these key words: research dietitian; brand manager.

Summarize Your Reading

▶ Food is made of nutrients that have varied functions that are essential to keep the body working properly. Nutrients, along with healthy habits, lead to many benefits.

▶ When nutrition is inadequate or faulty, malnutrition can result.

▶ The Dietary Reference Intakes (DRIs) were developed to help people assess their nutri-ent needs. Daily Values also provide infor-mation for consumers.

▶ Through the processes of digestion, absorp-tion, transportation, and metabolism, the body is able to use the nutrients in foods in many different ways.

Check Your Knowledge

1. What basic functions do the six nutrients provide?

2. Are there different types of **malnutrition**? Explain.

3. How can people benefit from healthy habits and good nutrition?

4. If you limit your food choices, how is nutri-ent teamwork affected?

5. Name and describe the two components of the **Dietary Reference Intakes (DRIs)**.

6. What is the relationship between DRIs and nutrition labels?

7. What is the purpose of **digestion**?

8. What role do **enzymes** play in digestion?

9. Does gravity force foods through the diges-tive system? Explain.

10. Compare the rates that carbohydrates, pro-teins, and fats take to break down before leaving the stomach.

11. **CRITICAL THINKING** Predict what might happen if food passes through the digestive system more quickly than normal.

12. During digestion, what happens in the small intestine?

13. How do **villi** aid **absorption**?

14. What is **glucose** and how is it used?

15. What happens to glucose if it isn't needed right away?

16. What is **metabolism**?

17. What do **calories** measure?

18. If two people have different basal metabolic rates, what does that mean?

19. How do calories relate to activity level?

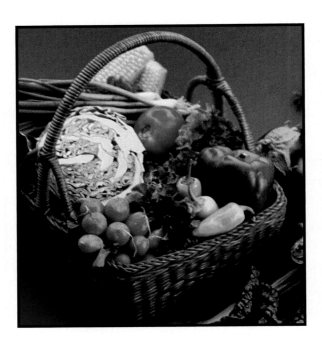

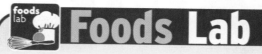
Apply Your Learning

1. **Nutrient Chart Comparison.** Using the charts in the chapter, compare the DRIs for you with the Daily Values. What differences do you find? Why do you think there are differences?

2. **Digestive System Model.** Construct a 3-D model of the digestive system, using readily available materials. Label the parts and outline the steps in the digestive process.

3. **MATH Calorie Calculation.** Calculate the number of calories from protein, carbohydrates, and fat in one serving each of three to five foods that you regularly eat. Make a chart to show your results. Where do most of the calories come from in these foods?

4. **MATH Fat Grams.** If a teen needs 2,600 calories each day and limits fat to 30 percent of a day's calories, how many grams of fat can he consume?

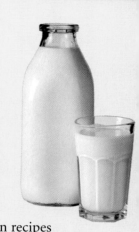

Foods Lab

Meeting Nutrient Needs

Procedure: With your lab team, choose a nutrient or use one that's assigned. Locate several foods in the lab (or bring in examples) that provide at least 15 percent of the daily requirement per serving for the nutrient. Display the items and give a presentation that explains how the foods might be used in recipes and meals to meet or help meet the daily requirement for this nutrient.

Analyzing Results

❶ How varied were the types of foods you chose? Give examples.

❷ How appealing, practical, and economical were your meal and recipe ideas?

❸ Based on the presentations of all lab teams, do you think it's easy or difficult to meet nutrient needs from readily available foods?

Food Science Experiment

Acids in Digestion

Objective: To explore the effect of acids and food surface area on digestion.

Procedure:

1. Cut a single piece of uncooked meat, about 1½ inches cubed. Place in a plastic container.

2. Add 1 Tbsp. vinegar to the meat. Seal and refrigerate the container.

3. Repeat Steps 1 and 2, but cut the meat into four, ¾-inch cubes.

4. After two days, slice all the pieces of meat in half. Evaluate and compare the two samples on appearance and texture.

Analyzing Results

❶ Describe the outer surface of the samples. What changes, if any, occurred?

❷ Describe the interior of the samples. Again note any changes.

❸ How would you explain the results you recorded in questions 1 and 2?

❹ How does this experiment relate to digesting food? What does it suggest about promoting thorough digestion?

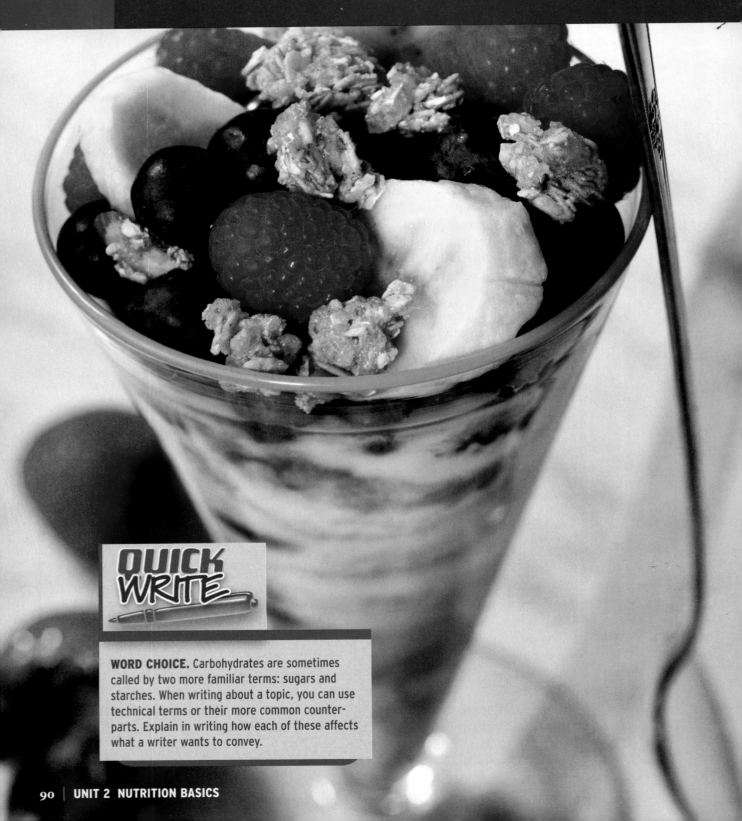

QUICK WRITE

WORD CHOICE. Carbohydrates are sometimes called by two more familiar terms: sugars and starches. When writing about a topic, you can use technical terms or their more common counterparts. Explain in writing how each of these affects what a writer wants to convey.

To Guide Your Reading:

Objectives

- ▶ Explain how carbohydrates are made.
- ▶ Compare simple and complex carbohydrates and relate them to sugars and starches.
- ▶ Describe how carbohydrates are digested in the body.
- ▶ Identify what type of carbohydrate is provided by different plant foods.
- ▶ Explain the roles of each type of carbohydrate in the diet.

Terms

added sugars
carbohydrates
chlorophyll
complex carbohydrates
dietary fiber
disaccharides
monosaccharides
photosynthesis
polysaccharides
simple carbohydrates
starches
sugars
sugar substitutes

D O YOU THINK ALL CARBOHYDRATES ARE THE same? Is fiber useful? Are starchy foods fattening? If you're not sure how to answer these questions, this chapter will help you. Adding to your understanding of carbohydrates (kahr-boh-HY-drayts) may clear up some confusion. Even better, you'll be able to make smarter health decisions.

WHAT ARE CARBOHYDRATES?

Whether you're climbing the stairs or pondering a tough test question, you're using energy. **Carbohydrates** are your main source of energy. Although some carbohydrates are in milk, they are mostly in plant foods. Fruits, vegetables, grain products, dry beans, nuts, and seeds all have this nutrient. Generally, foods like these are the least expensive food energy you can buy. See **Fig. 6-1**.

Three carbohydrates play a role in your health: sugars, starches, and fiber. Plants make all of these.

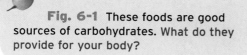

Fig. 6-1 These foods are good sources of carbohydrates. What do they provide for your body?

MAKING CARBOHYDRATES

The chemical process that makes carbohydrates is called **photosynthesis** (foh-toh-SIN-thuh-sus). Using the sun's energy, plants convert carbon dioxide and water into oxygen and the sugar glucose. The green pigment **chlorophyll** (KLOR-uh-fil) must be in the plant for photosynthesis to occur. See **Fig. 6-2**.

Plants produce glucose at great speed—millions of new sugar units every second. Glucose is the building block for all carbohydrates. Plants use glucose to build leaves, flowers, fruits, and seeds. They also use it to help form the fiber that strengthens and supports cell walls. Plants store extra glucose as starch in roots, stems, and leaves.

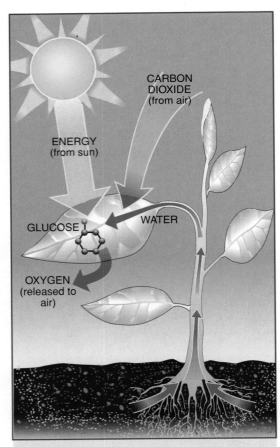

Fig. 6-2 Through photosynthesis plants make carbohydrates. What do plants need for this process?

Sugars: Simple Carbohydrates

To make glucose, plants absorb water (H_2O) through their roots and take in carbon dioxide (CO_2) from the air. These sources provide carbon (C), hydrogen (H), and oxygen (O), the chemical elements needed to build **sugars**. Plants make different kinds of sugars. See **Fig. 6-3**. Some are single units called **monosaccharides** (mah-nuh-SA-kuh-ryds). Mono means "one" and saccharide means "sugar." The following sugars have a single-unit chemical structure:

- **Glucose.** This mildly sweet sugar exists naturally in fruits and vegetables. It's also in honey, corn syrup, and the sugars used to sweeten food products. Glucose is also known as dextrose.
- **Fructose.** Fruits, many vegetables, and honey contain fructose, a highly sweet sugar.
- **Galactose.** This sugar is seldom found naturally in foods. It is in milk and helps create milk sugar (lactose). Galactose is not very sweet.

When two monosaccharides combine chemically, a **disaccharide** (dy-SA-kuh-ryd) forms. *Di* means "two." Sugars with two-unit structures always include glucose, as shown in these common disaccharides:

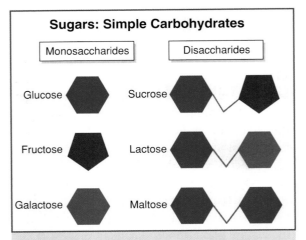

Fig. 6-3 Sugars, or simple carbohydrates, have simple chemical structures. The six shown here are important in nutrition. What do you notice about glucose and disaccharides?

- **Sucrose.** Sucrose (glucose + fructose) is found in fruits, sugar cane, and sugar beets.
- **Lactose.** Lactose (glucose + galactose) is found only in milk and milk products.
- **Maltose.** Maltose (glucose + glucose) forms when starch is digested.

In nutrition, the most important sugars are the six just described. Because their one- and two-unit structures are chemically simple, sugars are called **simple carbohydrates**.

Note the ending of each sugar name, *ose*. When you read food labels, this word ending will help you identify ingredients that are sugars.

Starches: Complex Carbohydrates

To build **starches**, plants combine single glucose units into more complicated chemical arrangements called **polysaccharides** (pah-lee-SA-kuh-ryds). *Poly* means "many." Some structures link as many as several thousand chemical units. Because of the more complicated structures, starches are classified as **complex carbohydrates**. See **Fig. 6-4**.

Dietary Fiber

Dietary fiber consists of plant materials that can't be digested by human enzymes. Although sugars and starches are nutrients, fiber is not, but it is essential for good health.

DIGESTING CARBOHYDRATES

While plants are excellent glucose producers, humans and animals can't make it. They need glucose, however, to create energy for many vital processes. There is a simple way for people to get glucose—by eating foods that come from plants.

After you eat foods that have carbohydrates, your body converts them mostly back to glucose during digestion. In the mouth the enzymes in saliva begin to break down starches. Digestive enzymes in the intestines continue the process. The starch is eventually broken down into glucose, the single-unit sugar that can then be absorbed into the blood stream.

Digestive enzymes also help break disaccharides down into single units. For example, the enzyme lactase breaks down the disaccharide

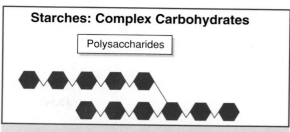

Fig. 6-4 Starches, or complex carbohydrates, have complex chemical structures. What simple sugar makes up starches?

lactose. People who don't have enough lactase may become lactose intolerant. Their body can't break down the lactose in dairy products, which causes digestive discomfort.

Since digestive enzymes can't break down dietary fiber, it passes through the system undigested. Bacteria in the digestive tract, however, can alter the material somewhat.

CARBOHYDRATES IN FOOD

When you eat foods from plants, you get carbohydrates in all forms. Since fiber gives shape to plants, it's present to some degree in all plant foods. For example, fiber keeps celery stalks and broccoli stems rigid and strong. The amount of sugars and starches in plant foods varies.

Sugars in Food

An apple tastes sweet because of the sugar produced by the tree. The sugars made by apple trees and other plants occur naturally. Throughout history, people have satisfied their "sweet tooth" with naturally occurring sugars. Strawberries, oranges, and other fruits have an appealing sweet taste that comes from the sugar put there by nature. Natural sugar also occurs in milk.

Early people probably chewed on sugarcane for the sweet taste. Sugarcane is a tall grass grown in warm climates. See **Fig. 6-5** on page 94. Eventually, people discovered ways to refine sugar, which means extracting naturally occurring sucrose from sugarcane and sugar beets.

Sugars that are extracted from plants and used to sweeten foods are called **added sugars**. After

Starches in Food

In a plant, glucose is stored as starch. Grains are a rich source of starch, making them a valuable supplier of energy around the world. Such vegetables as peas, corn, lima beans, winter squash, and potatoes also contain starch. In addition, starch is in dry beans, peas, and lentils.

You may have heard someone say, "I like corn best early in the season when it's nice and sweet." Why did the corn's taste change? In a young plant, glucose usually forms other sugars first. As the plant matures, these become starches. That's why the earliest ear of corn usually tastes sweeter than the ears harvested later. See **Fig. 6-6**.

Since starches are made of sugars, wouldn't you expect starchy foods to taste sweet? They don't because starch molecules are too large to fit your taste buds' receptors. As starches break down in your mouth, however, you may notice a sweeter taste. Try chewing a cracker slowly to observe this change.

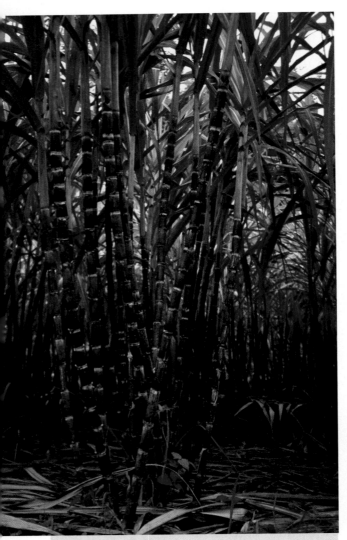

Fig. 6-5 About 30 percent of the world's sugar supply comes from sugar beets. The other 70 percent comes from sugar cane, shown here. The large stems, or canes, look like bamboo. Sucrose is inside these canes.

extraction, the sugar sucrose is made into the brown, white, and powdered sugars sold in supermarkets. The table sugar people put in tea has been refined for use as a sweetener. Other added sugars include high-fructose corn syrup, corn syrup, honey, maple syrup, and molasses. Cookies, cakes, pastries, candies, fruit drinks, and soft drinks taste sweet due to added sugars.

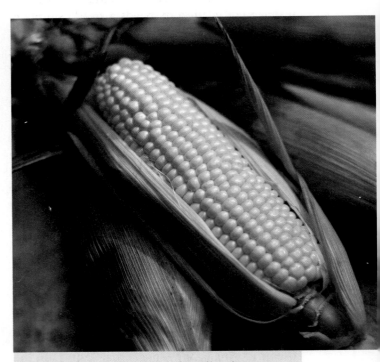

Fig. 6-6 Sweet corn is a favorite at many dinner tables. When standard sweet corn is mature and ready for sale, it contains about 5 to 6 percent sugar and 10 to 11 percent starch.

THE NEED FOR CARBOHYDRATES

When one teen gained extra weight, he decided to cut most carbohydrates from his diet. He blamed those particular foods for the gain. With a better understanding of what carbohydrates do for him, he might have thought differently.

If you don't eat enough foods with carbohydrates, your body won't have a good supply of glucose. Glucose circulates in your bloodstream, destined for all the cells in your body. Within the cells, glucose participates in billions of chemical reactions that release energy, or calories, to keep body systems like digestion going. Glucose powers your breathing, walking, running, and thinking skills. You can learn a new math principle because your brain splits millions of glucose units every second to provide energy. Limiting glucose limits how well your body can function. For example, brain cells depend on glucose to function properly. Therefore carbohydrates are essential for these cells to do their work. See **Fig. 6-7**.

Some glucose is stored in the muscles and liver as glycogen. Your body needs a steady supply of glucose, so it retrieves stored amounts as needed. When your body needs energy, it converts the glycogen back into glucose and returns it to the bloodstream. To get through the last quarter in the basketball game, a player's body can call upon glycogen for a fresh supply of energy.

In the absence of carbohydrates, the body uses fat and protein for energy, but that takes protein away from building and repairing tissues. There is concern that a very low carbohydrate diet may result in bone mineral loss, an increase in blood cholesterol levels, and an increased risk of kidney stones. It may also affect the functioning of the central nervous system.

CARBOHYDRATES IN THE DIET

According to health experts, teens and adults should get 45 to 65 percent of their daily calories from carbohydrates. If your body turns carbohydrates into glucose for energy, does it matter which carbohydrate foods you eat? It definitely does. Although most carbohydrate foods are rich in vitamins, minerals, and fiber, some are not.

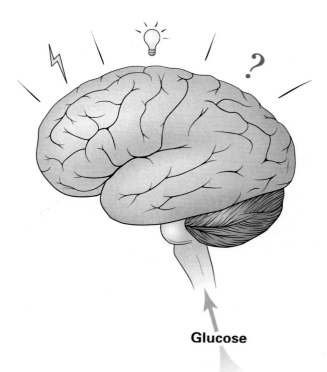

Glucose

Fig. 6-7 Your brain runs on glucose. Although the brain is only a small part of the human body, some researchers believe it consumes over 20 percent of the body's energy. What could happen if your supply of glucose is low?

Health experts suggest that your daily carbohydrate allowance be mostly from complex carbohydrates and naturally occurring sugars rather than added sugars.

Bacteria in the mouth produce acid from carbohydrate foods, especially sticky ones that remain on the teeth. This acid can cause tooth decay. Therefore regular brushing is essential for healthy teeth and gums.

Added Sugar in the Diet

For most people, foods with added sugar can be part of a healthy eating plan. Used in moderation, sugar adds flavor to food without causing health issues. Most people, however, eat far too much added sugar, which can lead to overweight and other health problems.

Foods with added sugar include soft drinks, cakes, cookies, and candy. Foods that supply calories and have little or no nutrients are called empty-calorie foods. Often their calorie count is high. A 12-ounce soft drink, for example, can contain as much as 10 teaspoons of sugar. Since 1 teaspoon of table sugar equals about 15 calories, the drink has about 150 calories and no other nutrients. See **Fig. 6-8**.

Nutrition experts recommend that healthy people use only moderate amounts of added sugars, but what does that mean? The U.S. Department of Agriculture suggests an average limit of 10 teaspoons of added sugars per day on a 2,000-calorie diet and 18 teaspoons on a 2,800-calorie diet. This includes sugar in processed foods. Very active people with high-energy needs may be able to consume more sugar than those with low-energy needs.

Even if you don't eat candy and cookies, you may still get more calories from sugar than you realize. Sugar is often used to flavor processed foods, such as ketchup, salad dressings, and convenience foods. You can estimate the sugar in food by converting the grams of sugar on a food label to teaspoons. Since 4 grams of sugar equal 1 teaspoon, 8 grams equal 2 teaspoons. A tablespoon of ketchup and a tablespoon of some jams each contain about 2 teaspoons of sugar.

Read the ingredient list on the food label. If any of the terms in **Fig. 6-9** appear in an ingredient list, you know that the product contains added sugar. When these names are listed as the first or second ingredient or when several names appear, the food is probably high in added sugar.

Limiting foods with added sugars helps control calories. Calories can be spent on more healthful foods instead. Fruits are a good alternative to empty-calorie foods. Their natural sweetness is often lower in calories. An orange has 60 calories plus vitamins, minerals, phytochemicals, and fiber. A candy bar might have over 200 calories and be high in fat but have few other nutrients. For people who like a sweet treat, satisfying that taste with fruit is a healthful option.

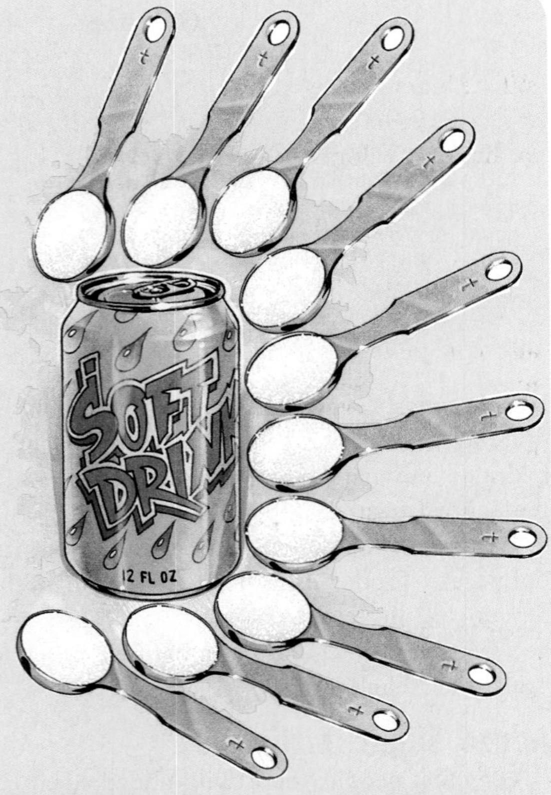

Fig. 6-8 When your parents were growing up, teens drank more milk than soft drinks. Today the reverse is true. Some teens drink as many as three to five soft drinks every day. How does that translate to sugar intake? What are the risks?

Fig. 6-9

Sugar Ingredients in Foods	
Brown sugar	Lactose
Corn sweetener	Malt syrup
Corn syrup	Maltose
Dextrose	Maple sugar
Fructose	Molasses
Fruit juice concentrate	Raw sugar
Glucose	Sucrose
High-fructose corn syrup	Syrup
Honey	Table sugar
Invert sugar	Turbinado

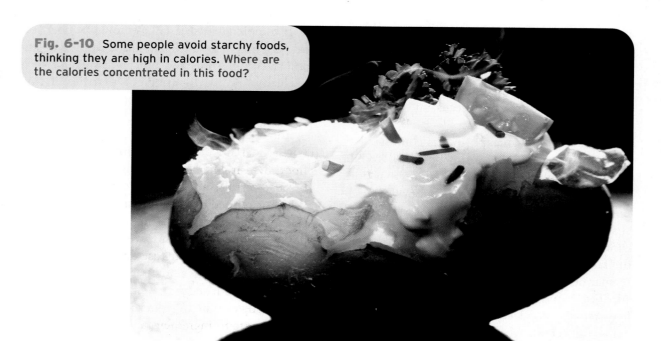

Fig. 6-10 Some people avoid starchy foods, thinking they are high in calories. Where are the calories concentrated in this food?

Sugar Substitutes

Can foods taste sweet without providing calories? Yes, because food producers use **sugar substitutes** to sweeten many foods, while adding few or no calories. Artificial sweeteners and sugar alcohols are commonly used substitutes.

- **Artificial sweeteners.** These non-nutritive sweeteners are calorie-free. Currently, four artificial sweeteners are approved for consumer use. They are aspartame (AS-puhr-taym), acesulfame-K (a-suh-SUHL-faym-kay), saccharin (SA-kuh-ruhn), and sucralose (SOO-kruhlohs). Over the years, critics have raised questions about the safety of artificial sweeteners. To date, these concerns have not been proven.
- **Sugar alcohols.** These occur naturally in fruits and vegetables, but they are also manufactured from carbohydrates for use in sugar-free foods. Sugar alcohols do not contain sugar or alcohol. They provide about one-half to one-third fewer calories than regular sugar. Some common sugar alcohols include sorbitol (SOR-buhtawl), mannitol (MA-nuh-tawl), and isomalt (EYE-soh-mawlt). They are used in sugar-free candies, cookies, ice cream, and chewing gum. Excessive use of sugar alcohols may cause diarrhea.

Foods sweetened with sugar substitutes may still be high in calories. For instance, many sugar-free cookies are high in fat, and you'll recall that fat has nine calories per gram.

Starch in the Diet

Most of the carbohydrates you consume should be complex. Starchy foods not only provide glucose to keep your body running, but they also contribute protein, vitamins, minerals, phytochemicals, and fiber.

Some people believe that starchy foods are high in calories. Often bread, potatoes, and pasta are blamed for a weight increase. By themselves, these foods are not high calorie. Topping them with high-fat spreads, sauces, and gravies, however, greatly increases the overall calorie count. See **Fig. 6-10**.

As an example, one teen always buttered her bread liberally. She ate pasta with rich cream sauces and hearty meat sauces, sprinkled heavily with grated cheese. She always drenched a baked potato with butter and sour cream. When she gained weight, she blamed the carbohydrates, but they were not the problem. The toppings were.

Complex carbohydrates can actually help people manage weight. These foods are generally very filling and low in fat and added sugars.

Fiber in the Diet

Dietary fiber is sometimes called bulk, cellulose, or roughage. Fiber is only found in foods from plant sources, including fruits; vegetables; whole-grain products; nuts; seeds; and dry beans, peas, and lentils.

You've read that dietary fiber is eliminated as waste. In that case, how can it be useful? While fiber is the only form of carbohydrate that does not provide energy, it does serve important functions. Fiber is vital to human digestion. Fiber absorbs water, much like a sponge. As a result, it contributes bulk, which helps food move through the large intestine at a normal rate. It promotes regular bowel movements and helps prevent constipation. Studies show that dietary fiber may help reduce blood cholesterol levels. Fiber also helps you feel full, which helps prevent overeating and weight gain.

Teens need anywhere from 26 to 38 grams of dietary fiber a day, depending on their age and gender. Adults need 19 to 38 grams. **Fig. 6-11** shows the amount of fiber in some common foods.

If you plan to increase the amount of fiber you eat, do so gradually. This allows your body to adjust. Adding fiber too quickly can cause such problems as gas, bloating, or diarrhea. Drink more water as you increase the amount of fiber you eat.

To get enough fiber in your diet, look for certain foods. Since whole-grain foods have more fiber than refined grains, choose whole-grain breads, cereals, and crackers instead of white bread or refined cereals and crackers. Try brown rice instead of white. You might add wheat germ, barley, or bulgur to soups, stews, and casseroles. Another suggestion is to eat more dry beans, peas, and lentils. You could choose bean burritos and chili with beans. Finally, include more cooked vegetables in your diet by eating such foods as stir-fries and vegetable pizza. By choosing foods like these, you get the benefits of fiber along with the nutrients that complex carbohydrates provide.

Fig. 6-11

Dietary Fiber in Selected Foods

Food	Approximate Measure	Grams of Dietary Fiber	Food	Approximate Measure	Grams of Dietary Fiber
Apple or pear	1	4	Refried beans	½ cup	6
Orange	1	3	Split pea soup	10 oz.	4
Strawberries	1 cup	4	Raisin bran	1 cup	8
Orange juice	¾ cup	0-1	Cooked oatmeal	1 cup	4
Baked potato with skin	1 medium	4	Bran muffin	1	4
Corn, cooked	½ cup	3	Whole wheat bread	2 slices	4
Broccoli or spinach, cooked	½ cup	2	White bread or bagel	2 slices 1 bagel	1
Peanut butter	2 Tbsp.	2	Brown rice, cooked	1 cup	3
Mixed nuts	¼ cup	2	White rice, cooked	1 cup	1
Black-eyed peas, cooked	½ cup	8	Spaghetti, cooked	1 cup	2
Baked beans	½ cup	7	Air-popped popcorn	3 cups	4

Chef

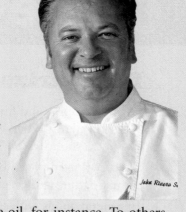

JOHN RIVERA SEDLAR: John Rivera Sedlar's title as "Tamale King" is one he takes to heart. He has built a career on stretching the popular Latin American dish to its culinary limits.

Food has played a special role in John's heritage, going back three generations. His great-grandparents farmed the rich soil near the New Mexico village of Abiquiu (Ah-bih-CUE), raising apricots, chiles, pinto beans, and corn. Growing up, John saw how his grandmother and great-aunt used these ingredients in traditional dishes of the American Southwest.

John's own career began humbly but advanced swiftly. At age fifteen, he started bussing tables at restaurants in his hometown of Santa Fe, New Mexico. At eighteen, he moved to take a restaurant job in Los Angeles. By his twenties, he was apprentice chef at the renowned L'Ermitage, where he immersed himself in classic French cuisine.

Shaking Up the Southwest. Beginning in the early 1980s, John owned and cooked for a string of successful Los Angeles restaurants. He earned a reputation as an innovator of fusion cooking, transforming the Southwestern foods he loved through the artistry of French techniques. Tamales became the focus of his imagination. He filled them with striking combinations like asparagus and lobster. He integrated salad greens and herbs right into the masa.

In 1994, following a powerful earthquake in Southern California, John sold the restaurants he owned and set his sights on other dreams. In 1999 he started a specialty food company. Marketed under the name Sedlar's Southwest Kitchen, the line shows his flair for reinventing Latin American staples. Adventurous eaters can sample taco shells in assorted flavors and chocolate-filled dessert tamales. They can decorate plates with hot sauce "paints." Some recipes John updated to meet modern health concerns—replacing the traditional lard with olive oil, for instance. To others he added distinctive ingredients from other cuisines. Travel, reading, and collaborating with colleagues provide a steady stream of inspiration.

The Treasure of Tamales. Today, developing recipes for the Southwest Kitchen line and for his cookbooks and catering business fills John's professional plate, yet the tamale remains a passion. The food, he says, is literally "wrapped in tradition." The basic recipe is common to all of Latin America, yet each region is proud of its own variation.

To preserve that link between food history and heritage, John plans to open a "Tamale Museum" that will actually celebrate all aspects of Southwestern cuisine. Exhibits will range from the Native American diet of a thousand years ago to the food vendor's brilliantly painted "taco wagon" in today's working-class Los Angeles neighborhoods. For the "Tamale King," the museum will be a fitting tribute to a food treasure in his life.

On-line Connections

1. To learn more about topics in this article, search the Internet for these key words: tamales; Native American foods; Sedlar's Southwest Kitchen.

2. To learn about related careers, search the Internet for these key words: food stylist; food marketing.

Summarize Your Reading

▶ Sugars, starches, and fiber are carbohydrates made by plants. When you eat plant foods, you get carbohydrates.

▶ Glucose is a simple carbohydrate that occurs in many fruits and vegetables.

▶ In general, foods with simple carbohydrates, such as oranges and melons, taste sweet, and foods with complex carbohydrates, such as potatoes and pasta, don't taste sweet.

▶ For many reasons, carbohydrates are an essential part of the diet.

▶ Sugars provide energy whether they're in a fruit or a candy bar. The fruit, however, usually has other nutrients and fewer calories.

Check Your Knowledge

1. What kinds of foods provide **carbohydrates**?

2. Describe **photosynthesis**.

3. What makes glucose and sucrose different?

4. If you saw the word dextrose on a food label, what would you know about that particular ingredient?

5. What is the difference between **sugars** and **starches**?

6. Why isn't **dietary fiber** a nutrient?

7. **CRITICAL THINKING** A teen had a long bike ride coming up the next day, so he decided to get ready by eating a big steak the night before. Explain your opinion of his decision.

8. During digestion, what happens to the carbohydrates you have eaten?

9. How is the sugar in an apple different from the sugar in a cookie?

10. Since sugars are used to make starch in a plant, why don't such starchy foods as potatoes taste sweet?

11. Predict what might happen if a person eliminated all carbohydrates from his or her diet.

12. Why might a lack of glycogen be a problem?

13. **CRITICAL THINKING** A friend says to you: "I'm supposed to cut down on carbohydrates, so I don't eat many starchy foods now." Thinking of health, how might you respond?

14. If someone on a 2,000-calorie diet drinks a 12-ounce soft drink, how much more sugar could the person eat during the day if following USDA suggestions?

15. Suppose a cereal bar has 16 g of sugar. How many teaspoons of sugar is that?

16. How can a food that replaces sugar with a sugar substitute be high in calories?

17. Why do some people think that starchy foods make people gain weight?

18. If fiber is just eliminated as waste, why is it needed?

19. What kinds of foods contribute fiber to the diet?

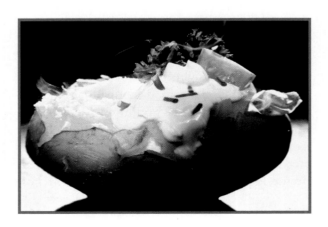

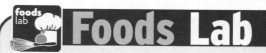
Apply Your Learning

1. **SOCIAL STUDIES** **Survey.** Take a survey of students' favorite snack foods and categorize them into simple and complex carbohydrates. What do the results show about students' eating habits and health?

2. **Natural or Added.** Read food labels to find out whether sugars in food you eat are natural or added. What surprises did you find?

3. **MATH** **Calculating Carbohydrates.** Recall that 1 gram of carbohydrates has 4 calories. If a person on a 2400-calorie diet gets 55 percent of those calories from carbohydrates, how many grams of carbohydrates are consumed each day?

4. **Fiber Diary.** Keep a food diary for three days. Circle the foods you ate that are high in fiber. Calculate how much fiber you eat in a typical day. Is that enough? How could you get more in your diet if needed?

Foods Lab

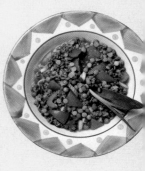

Carbohydrate Recipes

Procedure: Create a simple, easy-to-prepare recipe that uses at least two good sources of complex carbohydrates. It may be a sandwich, salad, main dish, or dessert. Prepare and evaluate your recipe.

Analyzing Results

1. What types of foods did you choose as carbohydrate sources? How did they add to the recipe's appeal?

2. What combinations of foods did other teams use? Which do you think were most appealing?

3. Based on the recipes you saw, what do you think are other advantages of choosing carbohydrate-rich foods?

Food Science Experiment

Artificial Sweeteners

Objective: To compare the sweetness and taste of artificial sweeteners.

Procedure:

1. Label four identical cups for identification, using random letters or numbers. Into each cup pour ½ cup of lemon juice.

2. To each cup, add one of the following sweeteners: one packet of aspartame; one packet of saccharin; one packet of sucralose; or 2 tsp. sugar. Stir to dissolve. Write down each cup's identification code and the sweetener it contains.

3. Ask a classmate to taste the juice samples and to rank them in order of sweetness.

Then have the tester taste the samples again and rank them from most pleasing to least pleasing taste. Have the tester eat a cracker after each tasting.

4. Compile your findings with those of other students in a chart on the board.

Analyzing Results

1. Overall, which sweeteners were judged the sweetest? Least sweet?

2. Which sweeteners were judged most pleasing? Least pleasing?

3. Compare the answers to questions 1 and 2. Do those results surprise you? Explain.

4. What might account for different perceptions of sweetness in different people?

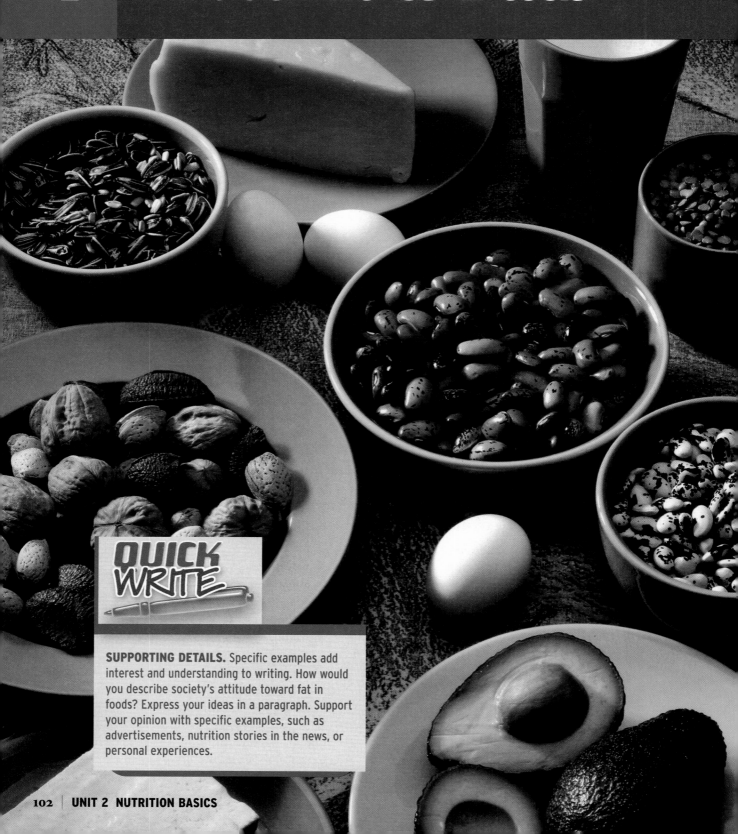

QUICK WRITE

SUPPORTING DETAILS. Specific examples add interest and understanding to writing. How would you describe society's attitude toward fat in foods? Express your ideas in a paragraph. Support your opinion with specific examples, such as advertisements, nutrition stories in the news, or personal experiences.

I<small>N THIS CHAPTER YOU'LL GET TO KNOW TWO</small> more nutrients—proteins and fats. Much has been written about them. If you learn the basics about these nutrients, you'll be better able to evaluate what you read and hear.

PROTEIN

Without proteins, life could not exist. Proteins contribute to your growth and development. They also help your body repair itself.

Proteins are found in many foods. Some are from animal sources, including meat, poultry, fish, eggs, and dairy products. Proteins are also found in food from plant sources, especially dry beans and peas, nuts, vegetables, and grain products.

The Structure of Proteins

You might be surprised to learn that proteins make up about one-fifth of your body's total weight. As part of every cell, proteins are in all tissues and organs. In fact, a single cell may contain thousands of different proteins.

Although proteins are very small, scientists consider them to be complex. That's because proteins are made from chemical building blocks that are called **amino** (uh-MEE-noh) **acids**, which link together in many different arrangements. Genetic information in cells—DNA—provides instructions for making each protein. See **Fig. 7-1**.

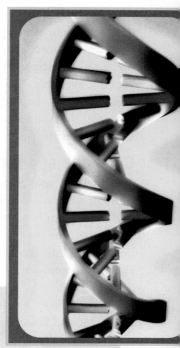

Fig. 7-1 Your cells contain DNA, which has the genetic information for making all the proteins in your body.

To date, 22 amino acids have been identified in protein foods. Imagine how many different arrangements they can make. For comparison, think how many words are created from the 26 letters in the alphabet. It's easy to see why hundreds of thousands of proteins exist.

When amino acids chain together to make proteins, they take different shapes. Shape determines function. Some amino acids wind together in long, rope-like spirals. These proteins form structures in your body, including tendons and ligaments. Some amino acids combine and fold into globular shapes, producing proteins that can carry chemical compounds. **Hemoglobin** (HEE-muh-gloh-buhn), a protein with a globular shape, transports oxygen in the blood to all the cells in your body. Each protein has a specialized job in the body.

Protein Digestion

How does the protein in food become the protein in your body? Once you've eaten a protein food, your body breaks the protein down into amino acids. Then the amino acids can be reassembled as human body protein. Here's how that works.

Protein digestion starts in the stomach. First, strong stomach acid changes the shape of the proteins. Then stomach enzymes break the proteins down more. Protein digestion continues in the small intestine until individual amino acids become available. The amino acids can then be absorbed into the bloodstream. Upon reaching the cells, the amino acids are used to make proteins for specific purposes.

Complete and Incomplete Proteins

Your body makes many amino acids for itself. Even in healthy people, however, the body can't make some amino acids or can't make them in sufficient amounts. The amino acids that your body needs but cannot provide are called **essential amino acids**. You must get these from foods. See **Fig. 7-2**.

Some protein foods contain all the essential amino acids. Since foods from animal sources have them all, they are known as **complete proteins**.

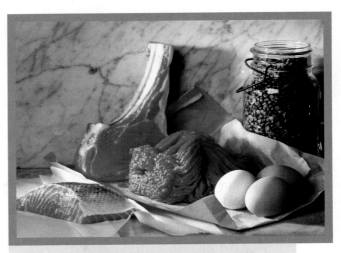

Fig. 7-2 Good sources of protein include animal foods, which have complete proteins, and plant foods, which have incomplete proteins. Soy beans are the only plant food with complete protein.

By contrast, foods from plant sources lack at least one essential amino acid. Therefore plant proteins are called **incomplete proteins**. Soy beans, which are a complete protein, are the only exception. Dry beans, peas, lentils, nuts, and seeds have nearly all the amino acids. Grains and also many vegetables are missing more of them. As you can see, plant proteins are incomplete in different ways.

When your body doesn't have the right quantity and proportion of amino acids, it can't build the proteins you need. The work of some proteins may not get done, which can lead to health problems. Making protein foods part of your diet helps protect your health. People who don't eat foods from animal sources need to get all the essential amino acids from incomplete proteins. By choosing a variety of plant foods, especially grain products, dry beans and peas, and nuts and seeds, they can easily get what they need. What's missing in one plant food, they get by eating another. See **Fig. 7-3**.

The Need for Protein

Proteins have so many roles to play in the body that only a few can be highlighted here. These, however, are enough to underscore the value of proteins:

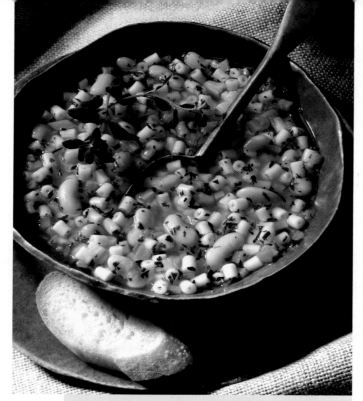

Fig. 7-3 Plant foods don't have all the amino acids you need. By eating a variety of plant foods, however, you can get them all. They don't need to be eaten in the same meal.

- **Growth and maintenance.** Your body is a major construction zone of building and rebuilding. In children and young adults, new cells are needed for growth. Your hair, eyes, teeth, skin, muscles, and bones are all made of proteins. The proteins you eat help keep these structures in good condition. Most proteins in a healthy body are constantly broken down and replaced. New skin cells from beneath the surface continually replace old cells. The cells in your intestinal tract live for only a few days, calling for regular replacement. People who are ill need new cells to replace damaged ones. For all these functions, the body needs a continuous supply of proteins to grow and repair worn-out and damaged parts.
- **Enzymes.** Chemical reactions are constantly going on in the cells of your body. Without the special proteins called enzymes, these reactions couldn't take place at the necessary rate.

- **Hormones.** Hormones are chemical messengers that help regulate conditions in the body. Some hormones in the body are made from amino acids. One of these is the thyroid hormone that regulates body metabolism. Another is insulin, which helps maintain the level of glucose (sugar) in your blood.
- **Antibodies.** Antibodies are proteins that fight invaders. The body creates them when a need arises. For example, if you get the flu, the body makes antibodies to fight it. If you get the same strain of flu again, your body "remembers" what to make and fights off the illness more quickly. In this way, proteins are part of the immune system. They play a major role in fighting disease.
- **Fluid balance.** A cell's life depends on having fluid in the right amount. Too much fluid causes cells to rupture, and too little stops their activity. Cells can't move fluids directly themselves, so they build proteins inside cells to attract water, and they send proteins into the blood stream to maintain fluid levels there.

Normally, proteins provide very little energy. If you don't eat enough carbohydrates and fats to meet your energy needs, however, the body can use proteins for energy. As a result, that means the vital work of proteins doesn't get done.

How Much Do You Need?

Health experts recommend that teens get 10 to 30 percent of their calories from proteins and that adults get 10 to 35 percent. A larger person needs more proteins than someone smaller. Suppose a teen's daily calorie requirement is 2,800 calories. The appropriate daily protein range for him would be between 70 and 210 grams.

$$2,800 \times .10 = 280 \text{ calories} \div 4 \text{ calories per gram} = 70$$

$$2,800 \times .30 = 840 \text{ calories} \div 4 \text{ calories per gram} = 210$$

Use **Fig. 7-4** on page 106 to see how some foods might fit this range.

During certain periods in life, a person's need for proteins is higher. For instance, pregnant women and nursing mothers need extra proteins to build new cells. Infants, children, and teens

Fig. 7-4

Approximate Protein in Selected Foods		
Food	Approximate Measure	Protein (Grams)
Beans, baked	½ cup	7
Beans, white, dried, cooked	1 cup	17
Beef, ground	3 oz.	22
Beef, roast	4 oz.	31
Bread	1 slice	2-5
Cheese, cheddar	1 oz.	7
Chicken, roasted	3 oz.	27
Egg	1	6
Green beans	½ cup	1
Halibut	3 oz	23
Milk	1 cup	8
Nuts, mixed	1 oz.	5-6
Peanut butter	2 Tbsp.	7-9
Peas	½ cup	2-4
Pasta	1 cup	7
Tofu	3 oz.	4-7
Yogurt, plain	8 oz.	8

need proteins to help them grow. When people are ill or injured, proteins help rebuild damaged cells.

Excess Protein

Although protein is essential, nutrition experts agree that too much can be harmful. Excess amounts are broken down and stored by the body as fat. Also, if you eat huge amounts, your body must work overtime to break down the extra protein and remove the byproducts.

Healthy people don't need protein or amino acid supplements. Most people get plenty of protein by choosing a variety of foods.

Inadequate Protein

Although getting enough protein is not typically a problem for people in developed countries, it's a serious problem in other parts of the world. Where food supplies are inadequate, people may not get enough protein and calories.

Protein-energy malnutrition (PEM) is a leading form of malnutrition in the world. Children are especially affected. With PEM they lose weight and don't grow properly. Some die of starvation. Even in developed countries, PEM can affect people who have eating disorders or drug addictions.

Protein Food Choices

Most Americans get the largest amount of their protein from animal sources. Health experts recommend, however, that people get more of their protein from plant sources. Generally, plant sources have less fat and usually cost less too.

Popular dishes based on plant foods include rice and beans, a peanut butter sandwich, and baked beans with brown bread. Soybean products are a high-protein option. You could use tofu, tempeh (TEM-pay), and soy milk in preparing main dishes.

Plant foods can also be mixed with a little animal protein to create dishes. Macaroni and cheese, tuna-noodle casserole, and vegetable and chicken stir-fry provide complete protein in reasonable amounts.

THE LIPID FAMILY

Lipids are a family of chemical compounds in every living cell, both in foods and in the human body. Two types of lipids are especially important in nutrition because of how they affect health. One is **triglycerides** (try-GLIH-suh-ryds), commonly called fats. Sterols, another type of lipid, include the well-known, fat-like substance cholesterol (kuh-LES-tuh-rawl). Levels of triglycerides and cholesterol in the body can be checked through medical blood tests.

Fats

Fats are greasy substances, either solid or liquid, that will not dissolve in water. Liquid fats are called oils. Foods high in fat include butter, margarine, oils, cream, salad dressings, gravies, fried foods, some baked goods, ice cream, nuts and seeds, egg yolks, whole milk, some cheeses, and meat products, including bacon, sausage, and hotdogs.

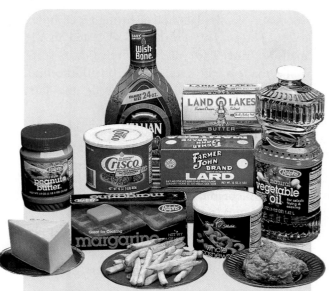

Fig. 7-5 In these foods, fat is apparent. What other foods have visible fat? What are some foods that contain invisible fats?

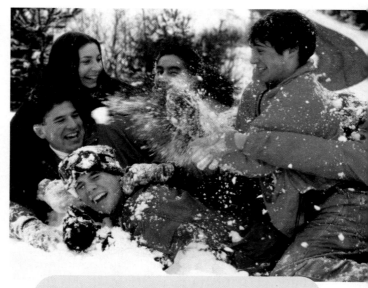

Fig. 7-6 Fat gives you energy for activities. Body fat not only supplies reserve energy but also insulates against cold and protects the bones and internal organs from injury.

Some fats are easy to see. The white portions around and through meats are fat. Fats in butter, margarine, and oil are also apparent. When fats can be seen, they're called visible fats. See **Fig. 7-5**.

Many foods contain fats that cannot be seen because they are part of the food's chemical composition. These are invisible fats. Such foods as egg yolks, nuts, whole milk, baked goods, and avocados do not look greasy or oily, yet they are all high in fat. This means that you cannot judge the amount of fat in a food by appearance alone.

Much of the fat eaten in foods is converted and stored throughout the body. **Adipose cells** are the warehouses for this fat. The cells in adipose tissue grow larger as they store additional fat.

Why Fats Are Needed

With all that is written about the negative side of fats in the diet, it's easy to conclude that fats are "bad." That's not actually true. Fats have several important functions in the body. See **Fig. 7-6**.

- Fat helps the body absorb vitamins A, D, E, and K.
- Body fat serves as a reserve supply of energy.

- Body fat cushions and protects the heart and other vital organs. It protects bones from injury.
- A layer of body fat under the skin provides insulation for warmth.
- Fat is a component of cell membranes.
- Because fats move slowly through the digestive system, they help you feel full longer after eating.

The fats in foods have value too. Food flavor and texture is often enhanced by a little fat. Fats add moisture and tenderness to some foods and crispiness to others.

Structure of Fats

Fats are made from chemical structures known as **fatty acids**. It takes three fatty acids plus glycerol to make a triglyceride. *Tri* means three. Fatty acids are not all the same. For one thing, some form longer chemical chains than others.

Another difference among fatty acids is their degree of saturation. The chemical structure of a fatty acid includes hydrogen. When a fatty acid contains all the hydrogen it can chemically hold, it is a **saturated fatty acid** (SA-chuh-ray-tud).

Sometimes hydrogen is missing from a fatty acid structure, creating an unsaturated fatty acid. If only one hydrogen unit is missing, the result is a **monounsaturated fatty acid** (mah-no-un-SA-chuh-ray-tud). *Mono* means one. If two or more hydrogen units are missing, a **polyunsaturated fatty acid** (pah-lee-un-SA-chuh-ray-tud) forms. *Poly* means many.

The fats found in foods generally have all three basic fatty acids, but in varying amounts. For example, a saturated fat has mostly saturated fatty acids. Fats that are solid at room temperature, such as butter and the fat on meat, are made up mainly of saturated fatty acids. Fats that are liquid at room temperature, such as corn oil and olive oil, are primarily composed of unsaturated fatty acids. See **Fig. 7-7**. Melting does not change saturation. For instance, butter solidifies again at room temperature.

Essential Fatty Acids

Your body can't make all the fatty acids it needs, so some are considered essential. These

Fig. 7-7 Some fats are solid and some are liquid. Which are more likely to be saturated?

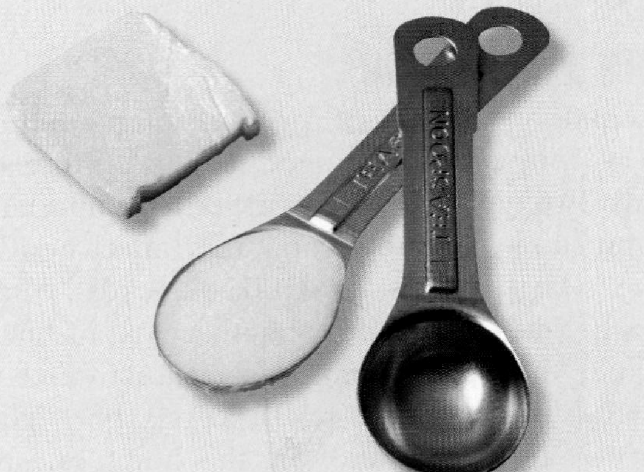

must be obtained through foods. One important fatty acid is linolenic acid (li-nuh-LEE-nik), also identified as **omega-3 fatty acid** (oh-MAY-guh). This fatty acid may lower the risk of heart disease. It is found in fish oils, especially in fatty fish, such as salmon, sardines, mackerel, trout, and herring. Plant sources include flax seeds and walnuts.

Fat Digestion

When you eat foods with fats, the digestive process breaks the fats down through a complex series of steps. Fats are mainly digested in the small intestine. The gallbladder releases its store of bile, made by the liver, into the small intestine. Components in bile help dismantle the fats, which break down into fatty acids.

Fatty acids are absorbed into the bloodstream, where they travel to the liver and to tissues that need them. Not all fatty acids can travel alone, so some re-form into triglycerides and join with protein in chemical "packages" that transport them through the bloodstream. These travel packages are called **lipoproteins** (leye-poh-PROH-teens). Many triglycerides travel to fat cells throughout the body for storage.

Cholesterol

Cholesterol, a fat-like substance present in all body cells, is needed for many essential body processes. Cholesterol is used for digesting fat and making vitamin D, as well as making some hormones and building cells. Too much cholesterol, however, is linked to heart disease.

Your body manufactures cholesterol. In fact, it makes all the cholesterol you need. You also get cholesterol, however, from foods. All foods from animal sources contain cholesterol. Some have higher amounts than others, such as fatty meat and poultry, egg yolks, liver and other organ meats, shrimp, and squid. See Fig. 7-8. Foods from plant sources have no cholesterol.

LDL and HDL

A certain amount of cholesterol circulates in the blood. Cholesterol does not float through the bloodstream on its own, however. Like some fats, it is transported in two types of lipoprotein packages—LDL and HDL.

- **LDL.** Low-density lipoprotein, or **LDL**, takes cholesterol from the liver to wherever it is needed in the body. If too much LDL cholesterol is circulating, excess amounts can build up in the artery walls. This buildup increases the risk of heart disease and stroke, which earns LDL cholesterol the "bad" cholesterol reputation.
- **HDL.** High-density lipoprotein, or **HDL**, is more helpful. It picks up excess cholesterol and takes it back to the liver for excretion, keeping the cholesterol from harming the body. For this reason, HDL cholesterol is known as "good" cholesterol. (To remember that HDL is the "good" one, you might associate the letter "H" with a positive word like "healthy" or "happy.") On a blood test, you would want your level of HDL to be high but your level of LDL to be low.

Fat Affects Cholesterol

The relationship between fats and cholesterol can be confusing. By eating foods that contain

Fig. 7-8

Approximate Cholesterol in Selected Foods

Food	Approximate Measure	Cholesterol (Milligrams)
Beef, ground, extra lean, broiled well done	3 oz.	84
Butter	1 Tbsp.	30
Candy bar	1	5
Chicken, roasted breast, with skin	3.4 oz.	83
Doughnut	1	25
Egg yolk	1	213
Liver, pan-fried beef	3 oz.	410
Mayonnaise	1 Tbsp.	5
Milk, whole	1 cup	35
Milk, nonfat	1 cup	5
Shrimp, fresh cooked	3 oz.	166

cholesterol, you obviously take cholesterol into your body. This dietary cholesterol contributes to the cholesterol that builds up in the blood.

On the other hand, dietary fat is believed to have an even greater effect on the level of blood cholesterol. The liver uses fats as fuel to make cholesterol. The types of fat affect cholesterol levels in different ways.

- **Saturated fat.** Foods with saturated fat appear to raise the level of LDL (bad) cholesterol in the bloodstream. Foods relatively high in saturated fat include fatty meat, poultry skin, whole-milk dairy products, and the tropical oils—coconut oil, palm oil, and palm kernel oil.
- **Polyunsaturated fat.** Foods with polyunsaturated fat may help lower cholesterol levels if they are used instead of saturated fats. Many vegetable oils, such as corn oil, soybean oil, and safflower oil, are high in polyunsaturated fat. Fats in seafood are mostly of this type.
- **Monounsaturated fat.** Foods with monounsaturated fat appear to lower LDL (bad) cholesterol levels and may help raise levels of HDL

(good) cholesterol. Foods relatively high in monounsaturated fat include olives, olive oil, avocados, nuts, peanut oil, and canola oil. See **Fig. 7-9**.

As you can see, the type of fat you eat affects your cholesterol level. Cooking with olive oil, for example, has health advantages over using a tropical oil. Even though both oils are fats, the olive oil has a positive impact on cholesterol. Check food labels to see how much total fat and saturated fat a product contains.

Trans Fats

Here's a riddle for you: when is a vegetable oil not an oil? The answer is: when it's hydrogenated. The chemical process of **hydrogenation** (hydrah-juh-NAY-shun) turns vegetable oils into solids. The missing hydrogen is added to the unsaturated fat, which increases saturation. Shortening and most margarines are hydrogenated vegetable oils.

Food producers often use hydrogenated fats to give products a longer shelf life and extra flavor. Many restaurants also use them when frying foods. For consumers, there's a health price to pay. Hydrogenation forms trans fatty acids, also called trans fats. **Trans fats** function like saturated fats in the body. They increase LDL cholesterol levels in the blood and may lower HDL.

Trans fats are common in margarine, salad dressings, crackers, snack foods, baked goods, fast foods, and convenience foods. You can often figure out where they are by reading ingredient lists on food labels. Such terms as "vegetable shortening," "hydrogenated," and "partially hydrogenated" alert you to the presence of trans fats in the food.

As of January 1, 2006, food producers are required to put trans fat amounts on nutrition labels. Some food producers are changing their foods to reduce the amount of trans fats. In the future they may use new processes that turn liquids to solids without creating trans fats.

How Much Do You Need?

Studies show that most Americans eat too much fat and the wrong kinds. As a result, their risk of heart disease and cancer increases. Since

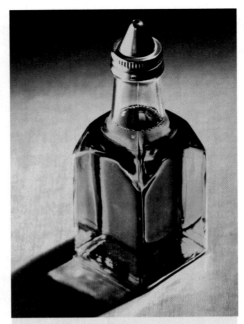

Fig. 7-9 The oils you cook with can have very different impacts on cholesterol. Why is olive oil more healthful than tropical oils?

foods with fat tend to be high in calories, too much fat can contribute to overweight and obesity, along with more health risks.

With all the concerns about fat in food, some people have gone to an extreme. A fat-free diet isn't the answer. You need fats to be healthy, but eating them in moderation and using your knowledge to make good choices is the best approach.

You can lower health risks by choosing foods that are moderate in total fat. See **Fig. 7-10** for selected examples of fat in foods. As you've read, health experts recommend that teens get 25 to 35 percent of their calories from fats and adults get 20 to 35 percent. For a teen who consumes about 2,400 calories each day, total fat should be in the range of 67 to 93 grams.

2,400 × .25 = 600 calories ÷ 9 calories per
gram = 67 grams

2,400 × .35 = 840 calories ÷ 9 calories per
gram = 93 grams

For saturated fat, trans fats, and cholesterol, health experts recommend keeping these intakes low. Of the fats eaten, trans fats and saturated fats together should be less than 10 percent of total calories. For a 2,000-calorie diet, that's a total of about 22 grams.

$$2,000 \times .10 = 200 \text{ calories} \div 9 \text{ calories per gram} = 22 \text{ grams}$$

Fig. 7-10

Approximate Fat in Selected Foods

Food	Approximate Measure	Fat (Grams)	Saturated Fat (Grams)	Food	Approximate Measure	Fat (Grams)	Saturated Fat (Grams)
Almonds, dry roasted	1 oz.	15	1	Cookies, chocolate chip with butter	1	5	2
Apple, fresh	1 cup	Trace	Trace	Cookies, oatmeal	1	3	1
Bagel, plain	1 (3½ in.)	1	Trace	Doughnut, cake	1	11	2
Banana, fresh	1	1	0	Egg	1	5	2
Beef, ground, extra lean	3 oz.	14	5	French fried potatoes	Medium	27	7
Bread	1 slice	1	Trace	Green beans, fresh	½ cup	Trace	Trace
Brownie, plain	1 (0.8 oz.)	7	2	Ice cream, chocolate	½ cup	7	4
Butter	1 Tbsp.	11	7	Margarine, stick	1 Tbsp.	11	2
Cake, angel food	1 piece	Trace	Trace	Margarine, tub	1 Tbsp.	7	1
Cheesecake	1 piece	18	9	Mayonnaise	1 Tbsp.	11	1.5
Chocolate, plain, milk	1 oz.	9	5.2	Milk, 1%	1 cup	3	2
Chocolate cake, no frosting	1 piece	14	5	Milk, whole	1 cup	8	5
Cheese, cheddar	1 oz.	9	6	Olive oil	1 Tbsp.	14	2
Cheese, mozzarella	1 oz.	6	4	Potato chips	Small bag	11	2
Chicken breast, roasted with skin	½ breast	8	2	Salad dressing, french, homemade	1 Tbsp.	10	2
Chicken breast, with skin, batter dipped, fried	½ breast	18	5	Shortening	1 Tbsp.	13	3.6

Cholesterol in the diet should be limited to less than 300 milligrams per day. Since your body makes what it needs, you don't really need any from food.

Controlling Fat

To many people, foods with fat taste good. Excluding all fats in an eating plan would take some of the enjoyment away and could make foods with fat more tantalizing. Eating fat in moderation allows you to enjoy the taste and protect your health at the same time.

When you control fat, you can actually eat more food without adding calories to your diet. Try substituting carbohydrates and proteins for some fat. Per gram, these foods have about half the calories of fat. Cutting fat without substituting other foods can help with weight loss.

Some people have actually gained weight when trying to cut fat. They thought they could eat larger quantities of fat-free and low-fat foods, not realizing that such foods often have the same or more calories.

These suggestions can help you control the amount of fat you eat:

- Eat plenty of fruits, vegetables, and whole-grain products.
- Choose fat-free or low-fat milk, yogurt, and cheese.

Aspects of Industry

AS EVERY GOOD COOK KNOWS, EACH ingredient in a dish affects the other ingredients, and so, the final product. Sweetening a cake with honey instead of sugar changes its texture, moistness, and flavor.

The same holds true for workers in an industry, whether it's foods or home furnishings. Each aspect of an industry affects other aspects, and thus has an impact on the business itself. Understanding these elements helps you see how they affect your job.

What are these elements that are of concern in all industries? Experts have identified eight main areas, according to the type of related tasks in each one.

- **Planning.** Identifying product or service to provide; setting goals; developing general policies and procedures.
- **Management.** Establishing a "chain of command" for employees and general methods of operation.

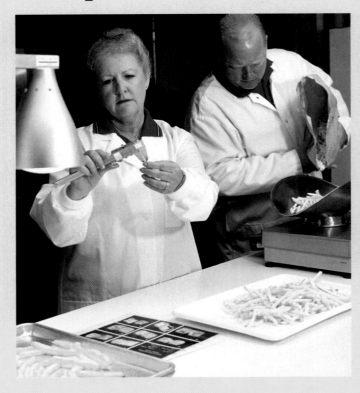

- Remove the skin from chicken and turkey before eating. Most of the fat is located just under the skin.
- Choose lean cuts of meat. Trim off and drain off fat.
- Choose lean ground beef or ground turkey.
- Watch portion sizes. A giant steak or hamburger includes much more fat than one with just a few ounces of meat.
- Choose fish instead of meat for some meals.
- Limit fried foods.
- Add fewer fats at the table. Using smaller amounts of butter, margarine, oily salad dressings, sour cream, gravy, and rich sauces makes a big difference. For example, 1 tablespoon of sour cream has 2 grams of saturated fat. How would 4 tablespoons affect your daily limit of saturated fat?
- Look for margarine and other processed foods that are free of trans fats.
- Eat high-fat desserts only occasionally. Make servings small.

Sorting out the facts about fats may seem like a challenge. When you read food labels, however, and learn what the numbers mean, it's easier than you might think.

- **Finance.** Making budgeting decisions; choosing accounting methods.
- **Technical and production skills.** Developing job skills needed by employees, such as teamwork, communication, and using machines and computers.
- **Underlying principles of technology.** Identifying useful technology; determining the impacts of technology; staying current on technology.
- **Labor and personnel issues.** Identifying employee rights and responsibilities; developing policies concerning labor organizations, cultural sensitivity, and other employee needs.
- **Community issues.** Identifying the industry's impact on the community; establishing good relations with different community groups; contributing to the community's well-being.
- **Health, safety, and environmental issues.** Avoiding or eliminating potentially harmful working conditions; establishing employer and employee responsibilities for workplace safety; identifying the industry's impact on the environment; implementing environmentally safe practices.

You can probably imagine how all these areas of industry and jobs relate. Suppose new machinery allows an industry to produce more with fewer workers. Employers in this industry may raise their production goals. They might increase spending to buy the machines. They may eliminate some jobs while adding others. The change in technology had a "domino effect" on planning, finance, production, and labor.

Whatever field you choose, it's wise to stay informed about developments in the industry. Appreciating the forces that shape the industry's direction can make you a more knowledgeable and effective worker.

Career Connection

Planning for outcomes. Increasingly, restaurants are offering customers more healthful meal choices. Create a flow chart showing three ways that this trend might affect the aspects of industry described above. If you were a restaurant worker, what actions might you take to use this trend to help your employer and make yourself a more valued employee?

Summarize Your Reading

▶ Proteins are essential for life. Your body can't build the proteins it needs without the right quantity and proportion of amino acids.

▶ The lipid family of chemical compounds in every living cell contains two that are important to health: triglycerides (or fats) and sterols (mainly cholesterol).

▶ Excess fat is stored in adipose cells that enlarge and produce weight gain.

▶ You need fat in your diet, but only in moderation.

▶ The type of fat you eat affects levels of good and bad cholesterol in the blood.

▶ Trans fats, which are made by food producers, appear to have a negative impact on cholesterol levels.

Check Your Knowledge

1. Chemically speaking, what is protein?

2. What is **hemoglobin**?

3. How does protein in food become protein in the body?

4. Compare **complete** and **incomplete proteins**.

5. Summarize the work of proteins in your body.

6. For teens, what percentage of calories should come from proteins?

7. What can happen if you eat too much protein?

8. What is a health expert likely to recommend as good food sources for protein? Why?

9. After a blood test, if someone says his **triglyceride** level is high, what does he mean?

10. Can you see fat in foods? Explain.

11. Why is it important to include some fat in the diet?

12. **CRITICAL THINKING** Use chemistry to theorize why foods heavy in **saturated fatty acids** are solid at room temperature.

13. If butter melts, does it become **polyunsaturated**? Explain.

14. What happens to fats during digestion?

15. What is **cholesterol** and how do you get it?

16. Compare **LDL** and **HDL**.

17. What effect does fat have on cholesterol?

18. How is a **trans fat** made?

19. If a teen needs 2,500 calories each day, how many grams of fat does that allow?

20. Why do some people gain weight when cutting down on fat?

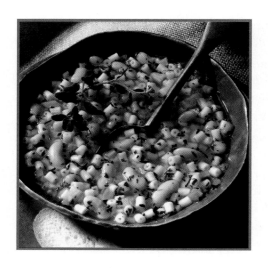

Apply Your Learning

1. **Protein Requirements.** Plan a day's meals to meet, but not go over, your protein requirement, using foods from animal sources. Do the same again, but use foods from plant sources. Compare the two approaches. What adaptations could you make to include both food sources?

2. **MATH** **Fat Calculations.** On a 2,300-calorie diet, one teen limits fat to 30 percent of her calories. How many grams of fat is this? How many of these grams can be from trans fats and saturated fats combined?

3. **Menu Analysis.** Using a sample restaurant menu, look for low-fat menu selections. Which menu choices are best when limiting fat? Compare results in class.

4. **Omega-3 Research.** Research the amount of omega-3 fatty acids in a variety of foods and chart results.

5. **Fat Comparison.** Compare total fat and saturated fat in at least ten of your favorite foods, charting the information. What generalizations can you draw?

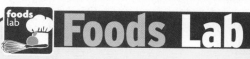

Foods Lab

Reduced-Fat Recipes

Procedure: Evaluate a regular dairy product and its reduced-fat variety, comparing the foods on taste, texture, and appear ance. Then prepare two versions of a simple recipe, such pas a cream cheese dip or a bread pudding, using one of the foods in each version. Compare the finished products.

Analyzing Results

❶ What differences, if any, did you detect between the food's regular and reduced-fat varieties?

❷ Were any differences more noticeable, or less so, in the recipe? What might explain this result?

❸ What advice would you give for using the lower-fat product in this and similar recipes?

Food Science Experiment

Properties of Gelatin

Objective: To compare how temperature and beating affect the protein gelatin.

Procedure:

1. Completely dissolve a 3-oz. box of powdered gelatin dessert in 1 cup of boiling water.

2. Add 1 cup of ice cubes and stir until melted.

3. Chill for *one* of these assigned variation times: 5 minutes; 10 minutes; 20 minutes.

4. Remove from the refrigerator and record the mixture's consistency.

5. Beat with an electric mixer at high speed for one minute. Refrigerate for 15 minutes.

6. Remove the mixture. Compare class results, putting observations in a board chart.

Analyzing Results

❶ Why was it necessary to dissolve the gelatin before adding ice?

❷ How did cooling affect the gelatin's consistency before and after beating?

❸ Research "denaturation" as it applies to proteins in food. How does this help explain what happened in the experiment?

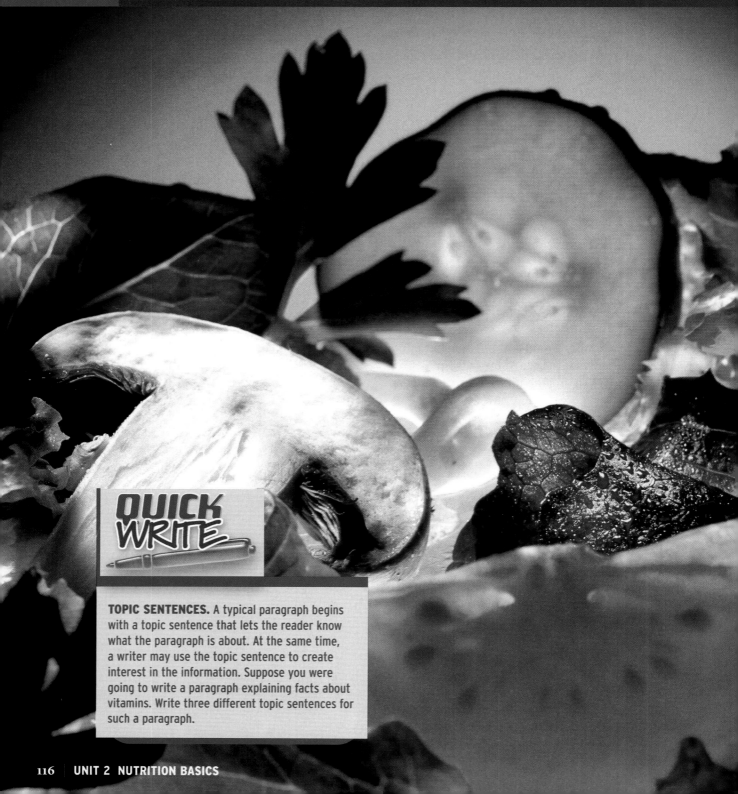

CHAPTER
8 Vitamins & Minerals

QUICK WRITE

TOPIC SENTENCES. A typical paragraph begins with a topic sentence that lets the reader know what the paragraph is about. At the same time, a writer may use the topic sentence to create interest in the information. Suppose you were going to write a paragraph explaining facts about vitamins. Write three different topic sentences for such a paragraph.

Objectives

▶ Identify vitamins and minerals needed by the body.

▶ Explain the functions of various vitamins and minerals.

▶ Suggest good sources for specific vitamins and minerals.

▶ Describe conditions that can result from certain vitamin and mineral deficiencies.

Terms

antioxidants

electrolyte minerals

fat-soluble vitamins

free radicals

hypertension

iron-deficiency anemia

major minerals

osteomalacia

osteoporosis

pica

toxicity

trace minerals

water-soluble vitamins

COMPARED TO OTHER NUTRIENTS, VITAMINS and minerals are needed in much smaller amounts. That's why they are called micronutrients. Nevertheless, vitamins and minerals are essential for good health. Without these assistants, carbohydrates, proteins, and fats could not do their work. Moreover, many processes in the body can't take place if micronutrients are missing.

WHAT ARE VITAMINS?

Vitamins are complex substances in food. Some vitamins are found in a wide range of foods. See **Fig. 8-1**. Others are limited to just a few food sources. By themselves, vitamins don't supply energy, nor do they become any part of the body's structure. They are important because they support many chemical reactions that go on constantly in your body.

You've read about enzymes, the special proteins that help chemical reactions take place in body cells. Enzymes can't work alone. Vitamins team with them to keep cellular activity going. If vitamins are consistently absent, imagine what can happen. Cellular slowdowns and malfunctions will eventually affect the way your body operates.

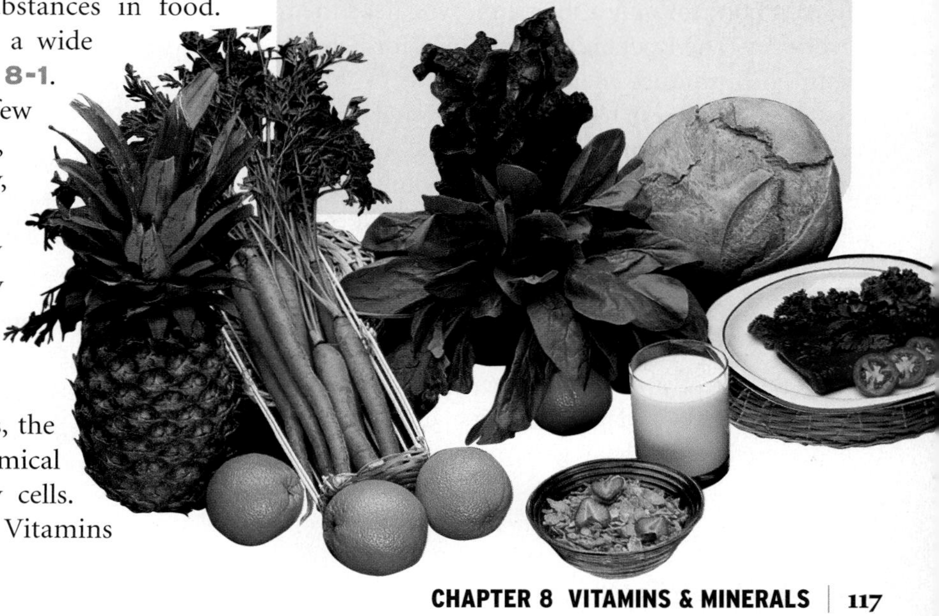

Fig. 8-1 Foods that are high in vitamins and minerals usually contain other nutrients as well. Why does your body need vitamins and minerals?

Some nutrients, including vitamins C and E, act as antioxidants (an-tee-AHK-suh-dunts). **Antioxidants** are substances that protect body cells and the immune system from damage that can be done by harmful chemicals in the air and in foods. Research suggests that antioxidants may help prevent certain diseases, including heart diseases and cancer.

Like paint protecting your car from rust, antioxidants protect your body's cells. When cells burn oxygen to produce energy, substances called **free radicals** are a by-product. Free radicals can damage body cells. Antioxidants are thought to transform the free radicals into less damaging compounds or even repair the damaged cell itself.

When vitamins were first discovered, letters of the alphabet identified them, as in vitamins A and B. Research eventually proved that vitamins are chemicals, so chemical names were assigned to replace the letters. Today some vitamins are still known by letter. Ascorbic acid, for example, is commonly called vitamin C.

Vitamins are classified into two groups: water-soluble and fat-soluble. These categories indicate how vitamins are absorbed and transported in the bloodstream.

Water-Soluble Vitamins

Water-soluble vitamins dissolve in water and pass easily into the bloodstream during digestion. **Fig. 8-2** lists the water-soluble vitamins and their food sources. Because these vitamins remain in your body for only a short time, you need them every day. The B vitamins are known for helping your body produce energy.

The body doesn't usually store water-soluble vitamins. Excess amounts are removed with waste products. Consuming excessive amounts isn't a good idea, however, since research shows some evidence of possible health problems. Health professionals can give advice on supplement use.

Vitamin C (Ascorbic Acid)

Well over two hundred years ago, a disease named "scurvy" plagued sailors at sea. As an experiment, a physician gave many of them citrus

Fig. 8-2

Food Sources of Water-Soluble Vitamins

Vitamin C (Ascorbic Acid)

Citrus fruits, including oranges, grapefruit, and tangerines; other fruits, including cantaloupe, guava, kiwi, mango, papaya, and strawberries; vegetables, including bell peppers, broccoli, cabbage, kale, plantains, potatoes, and tomatoes.

Thiamin (Vitamin B_1)

Enriched and whole-grain breads and cereals; dry beans and peas; lean pork and liver.

Riboflavin (Vitamin B_2)

Enriched breads and cereals; milk and other dairy products; green leafy vegetables; eggs; meat; poultry; fish.

Niacin (Vitamin B_3)

Meat; poultry; fish; enriched and whole-grain breads and cereals; dry beans and peas; peanuts and peanut butter.

Vitamin B_6 (Pyridoxine)

Poultry; fish; pork; dry beans and peas; nuts; whole grains; some fruits and vegetables; liver and kidneys.

Folate (Folacin, Folic acid, Vitamin B_9)

Green leafy vegetables; dry beans and peas; fruits; enriched and whole-grain breads.

Vitamin B_{12} (Cobalamin)

Meat; poultry; fish; shellfish; eggs; dairy products; some fortified foods; some nutritional yeasts.

Pantothenic acid (Vitamin B_5)

Meat; poultry; fish; eggs; dry beans and peas; whole-grain breads and cereals; milk; some fruits and vegetables.

Biotin (Vitamin H)

Green leafy vegetables; whole-grain breads and cereals; liver; egg yolks.

fruits to eat, which cured the illness. Since lime juice became a regular preventative, sailors became known as "limeys." When vitamin C was eventually identified, it was named ascorbic acid.

What does vitamin C do for you? This vitamin helps maintain healthy capillaries, bones, skin, and teeth. The enzyme that forms and takes care of collagen, a tissue protein, depends on vitamin C. Collagen gives structure to bones, cartilage, muscle, and blood vessels. Vitamin C helps your body heal wounds and resist infections. In addition, it aids in the absorption of iron and works as an antioxidant.

A lack of vitamin C can cause problems. Among these are poor appetite, weakness, bruising, and soreness in the joints. Although some people believe taking large amounts of vitamin C can help cure colds, no scientific evidence supports this belief. Large doses may cause nausea, cramps, and diarrhea.

Thiamin (Vitamin B₁)

Thiamin helps turn carbohydrates into energy. It is needed for muscle coordination and a healthy nervous system.

Thiamin deficiency was first noticed in the disease beriberi. In East Asia before 1900, prisoners were stiff and weak from beriberi. A physician noticed that chickens at the prison displayed similar symptoms. When the chickens ate the discarded bran removed from the prisoners' rice, the chickens' symptoms disappeared. When the prisoners were convinced to eat the discarded bran, they also improved. This early observation led to the identification of something valuable in the bran of whole grains—thiamin.

Nausea, apathy, and loss of appetite are early symptoms of a thiamin deficiency. Today most people get the thiamin they need by eating a variety of nutritious foods, including enriched and whole-grain breads and cereals.

Riboflavin (Vitamin B₂)

Riboflavin helps the body release energy from carbohydrates, fats, and proteins. It contributes to

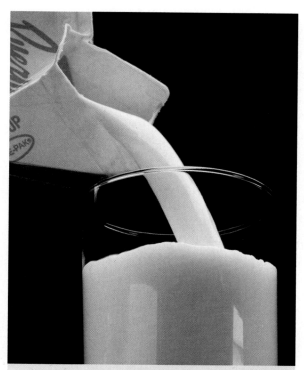

Fig. 8-3 Milk is sold in containers that don't let the light enter. What is the purpose?

body growth and red cell production. Although deficiency is rare, signs include light sensitivity, gritty eyes, sore tongue, mouth and lip sores, and dry, flaky skin.

Most people get riboflavin from milk and milk products. Since riboflavin is easily destroyed by light, milk containers that prevent light from entering offer protection. See **Fig. 8-3.**

Niacin (Vitamin B₃)

Niacin helps your body release energy from carbohydrates, fats, and proteins. You need it for a healthy nervous system and mucous membranes.

Pellagra (puh-LA-gruh), a disease that results in skin lesions and mental and digestive problems, is caused by a lack of niacin. This disease was rampant in parts of the U.S. during the early 1900s. At the time, diets were based mainly on cornmeal, which is low in protein and lacks the essential amino acid tryptophan (TRIP-tuh-fan). Tryptophan is present, however, in most other protein foods. The human body uses tryptophan to make niacin. Without this amino acid, people developed pellagra because their bodies couldn't produce niacin. Although pellagra occurs today in some developing countries, it is rare where people eat enough protein foods.

Vitamin B$_6$ (Pyridoxine)

Vitamin B$_6$ helps the body release energy from carbohydrates, proteins, and fats. It promotes a healthy nervous system. B$_6$ also helps make nonessential amino acids, which are used to build body cells. The conversion of tryptophan to niacin is aided by B$_6$.

Although deficiency is rare, symptoms include skin disorders, confusion, irritability, and insomnia. Serious deficiencies can produce convulsions. Taking excess amounts in supplements may cause nerve problems, such as difficulty in walking.

Folate (B$_9$)

Folate, also called folic acid and folacin, teams with vitamin B$_{12}$ to help build red blood cells and form genetic material (DNA). It also helps the body use proteins and may help protect against heart disease.

Folate has gained particular attention for its helpful role in preventing birth defects that damage the brain and spinal cord. Since defects can occur even before a woman realizes she's pregnant, folate is now added to grain products. A health professional may prescribe additional folate before and during pregnancy and lactation (milk production). See **Fig. 8-4**.

The name *folate* comes from the word *foliage*, meaning leafy green vegetables. As you might expect, these are good food sources of folate.

Without adequate folate, a person can develop anemia, which alters red blood cells so they carry less oxygen. Symptoms include feeling tired and weak. People may also develop diarrhea and lose weight.

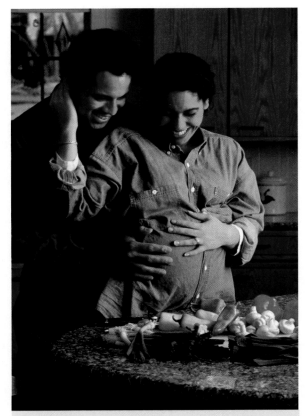

Fig. 8-4 Folate is particularly important for women who may become pregnant. Why do they need it?

Vitamin B$_{12}$

Vitamin B$_{12}$ is needed to process carbohydrates, proteins, and fats. It helps maintain healthy nerve cells and red blood cells and is used in making genetic material. Vitamin B$_{12}$ and folate rely on each other to do their work.

Other than in fortified cereals, vitamin B$_{12}$ is not found in plant foods. For this reason, a strict vegetarian needs to choose foods that provide the nutrient. Some older adults take B$_{12}$ supplements because they have trouble absorbing the vitamin. Most diets provide adequate amounts of this vitamin.

A B_{12} deficiency is characterized by fatigue, weakness, nausea, sore mouth or tongue, loss of appetite, weight loss, and numbness or tingling in the hands and feet. Pernicious anemia is a chronic condition in people who cannot absorb B_{12}. This has serious effects if not treated.

Pantothenic Acid (Vitamin B₅)

Pantothenic acid helps the body release energy from carbohydrates, fats, and proteins. It helps the body produce cholesterol and promotes normal growth and development. It is needed for a healthy nervous system. Deficiencies are rare because the vitamin is abundant in food. It can also be manufactured by intestinal bacteria.

Biotin

Biotin deficiency is also rare because it's widely available. This vitamin helps your body use carbohydrates, fats, and proteins.

Fat-Soluble Vitamins

As the term implies, **fat-soluble vitamins** are absorbed and transported by fat. These vitamins

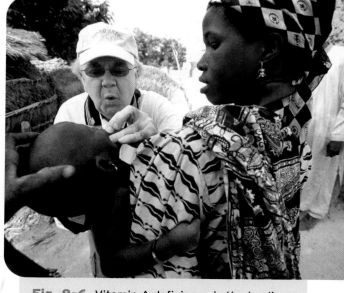

Fig. 8-6 Vitamin A deficiency is the leading cause of preventable blindness in children. This is a public health problem in many developing countries of the world. The World Health Organization (WHO) and its major partners are working to supply supplements to children who need this nutrient.

Fig. 8-5

Food Sources of Fat-Soluble Vitamins

Vitamin A

Dairy products; liver; egg yolks; foods high in beta-carotene, such as carrots, sweet potatoes, broccoli, and dark green, leafy vegetables.

Vitamin D

Fortified dairy products; egg yolks; fatty fish, such as herring, salmon, and mackerel; fortified breakfast cereals.

Vitamin E

Nuts; seeds; green leafy vegetables; wheat germ; vegetable oils and products made from them; soybean oil.

Vitamin K

Green leafy vegetables; other vegetables; some fruits.

include A, D, E, and K. **Fig. 8-5** lists food sources for each of these vitamins.

If you take in more fat-soluble vitamins than you need, they are stored in the liver. Your body can draw on these vitamins when needed, so daily replacement isn't essential. If large amounts of fat-soluble vitamins accumulate in the body, the effects can be damaging. Use caution with vitamin supplements.

Vitamin A

Three forms of vitamin A are active in the body: retinol, retinal, and retinoic acid. Together, they promote good vision and help maintain tissues and skin. Vitamin A also supports reproduction and growth.

Vitamin A deficiency can cause rough, scaly skin and infections in the respiratory tract and other areas of the body. Deficiency is a serious problem in developing countries. In these areas, lack of vitamin A causes night blindness and even total blindness in many children. See **Fig. 8-6**.

A balanced diet is unlikely to produce vitamin A **toxicity**, an excessive amount that is poisonous in the body. Too many supplements, however, can create excessive amounts that cause headaches, vomiting, double vision, abnormal bones, and liver damage.

Many vegetables and some fruits contain the phytochemical beta-carotene (bay-tuh-CARE-uh-teen), which can produce vitamin A in the body. A deep orange or dark green color, as in carrots and broccoli, indicates the presence of beta-carotene. Too much beta-carotene may turn the skin yellow, but it's harmless.

Vitamin D

You've probably heard that the mineral calcium builds strong bones, but calcium has a partner in vitamin D. Vitamin D maintains levels of calcium and phosphorus in the blood. It makes calcium available for proper bone growth.

You can get vitamin D in two ways. The body makes some vitamin D through the action of sunlight on the skin, which is why it's called the "sunshine vitamin." In general, 10 to 15 minutes of sun on the hands, face, and arms three times a week is enough. The time of year, sunscreen, and skin color affect the amount of vitamin D produced.

Fortified milk is one of the best sources of vitamin D. Since the 1930s, this nutrient has been added to milk to help ensure that people get what they need. If you don't drink milk, be sure to get enough vitamin D from other sources, such as egg yolks and fatty fish.

Before the 1930s, rickets, a disease caused by vitamin D deficiency, was a serious problem among children in the United States. In adults, a vitamin D deficiency causes **osteomalacia** (ahs-tee-oh-muh-LAY-shuh). With both diseases, bones are weak and sometimes deformed. Children with rickets may have bowed legs.

Too much vitamin D can have serious health effects, including nausea, vomiting, and hardening of soft body tissues. Supplements, rather than food, are linked to excesses. Extra sun exposure doesn't produce excess vitamin D; however, too much sun can cause skin damage, even skin cancer. See **Fig. 8-7**.

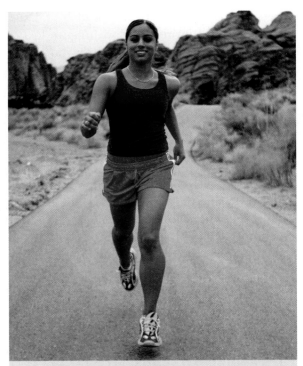

Fig. 8-7 Your body can make vitamin D from sunlight on your skin. Outdoor activities can help you fill this need. Can you get too much vitamin D if you stay outside for a long time?

Vitamin E

Vitamin E is valued as an antioxidant. It protects cells from oxidation damage, particularly in the lungs. Research suggests that vitamin E may reduce the risk of heart disease and possibly some cancers. Through ongoing studies, researchers hope to learn more about the health roles of this nutrient.

Vitamin E deficiency is rare because the vitamin is found in many foods; however, processing, storage, and cooking may affect vitamin E content. Toxicity from excess amounts is also rare.

Vitamin K

Without vitamin K, even a tiny cut on your skin would bleed endlessly. Vitamin K helps blood clot so that wounds stop bleeding. Bone health may also be influenced by this vitamin, which assists certain proteins.

Like vitamin E, vitamin K deficiency and toxicity are rare with a healthy diet. A number of food sources provide the vitamin, but vegetables are standouts. Vitamin K is another vitamin that the body can produce.

WHAT ARE MINERALS?

Although minerals make up only about four to five percent of your body weight, they are vital for good health. Most minerals become part of your body structure, such as your teeth and bones. Others make substances that your body needs. Often minerals team with vitamins in chemical reactions. For example, vitamin C boosts iron absorption.

Minerals are classified as either major or trace. You need smaller amounts of trace minerals than of major minerals.

Major Minerals

Each **major mineral**, sometimes called macromineral, has special duties to perform in your body. **Fig. 8-8** lists major minerals and their food sources.

Calcium

Calcium helps regulate blood clotting, nerve activity, and other body processes. It is needed for muscle contraction, including the heart. It helps keep teeth and gums healthy.

Above all, however, calcium is essential for keeping your bones strong. If you don't get enough calcium throughout your life, you risk developing **osteoporosis** (ahs-tee-oh-puh-ROH-sus). This condition causes bones to become porous, making them weak and fragile. As a result, people may develop a stooped posture and their bones can break easily. About 10 million Americans, both men and women, have osteoporosis. Another 34 million are at risk for developing it. See **Fig. 8-9**.

To lower your risk of osteoporosis, you need to start now. Bone mass builds up during childhood, the teen years, and young adulthood. The more you do to build strong, healthy bones now, the less likely you will develop osteoporosis when you are older. These tips will help you build strong bones:

Fig. 8-8

Food Sources of Major Minerals

Calcium
Dairy products; canned fish with edible bones; dry beans, peas, and lentils; dark green, leafy vegetables, such as broccoli, spinach, and turnip greens; tofu made with calcium sulfate; calcium-fortified orange juice and soy milk.

Phosphorus
Meat; poultry; fish; eggs; nuts; dry beans and peas; dairy products; grain products.

Magnesium
Whole-grain products; green vegetables; dry beans and peas; nuts and seeds.

Sodium (Electrolyte)
Table salt; processed foods.

Chloride (Electrolyte)
Table salt.

Potassium (Electrolyte)
Fruits, including bananas and oranges; vegetables; meat; poultry; fish; dry beans and peas; dairy products.

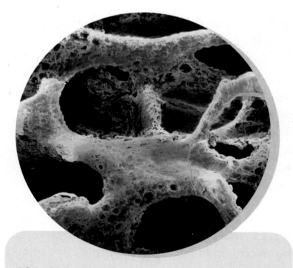

Fig. 8-9 This photo shows unhealthy bone, which may break easily. How can you build strong bones for the years ahead?

- Eat plenty of calcium-rich foods, including dairy products, dry beans and peas, and dark green, leafy vegetables.
- Follow other basic guidelines for healthy eating. Since nutrients work in teams, you need vitamin D and other nutrients to build healthy bones.
- Take part in vigorous activities, such as a sport or exercise routine. Weight-bearing exercises help build and maintain strong bones. Walking or jogging and weight training are examples.
- Avoid excess caffeine, which is found in coffee, tea, and some soft drinks. Don't use tobacco products and alcohol. All may contribute to osteoporosis.

Phosphorus

Phosphorus works with calcium to build strong bones and teeth. It helps release energy from carbohydrates, fats, and proteins. In addition, it helps build body cells and tissues. Because protein foods are rich in phosphorus, deficiencies are unknown.

Magnesium

Magnesium helps build bones and make proteins. It helps nerves and muscles work normally. Magnesium also contributes to proper heart function. Deficiency isn't common.

Sodium, Chloride, and Potassium

In your body, fluids flow in and out of cells through cell walls. The fluids on the inside and outside must be in balance, or cells will burst or collapse. Since cells can't control fluid flow directly, sodium, chloride, and potassium offer help. These major minerals are among those known as **electrolyte minerals** (ih-LEK-truh-lyt) because they form chemical particles called electrolytes. Electrolytes are in all body fluids, and cells can move them through cell walls as needed. Since electrolytes attract fluid, they pull fluid with them to new locations. As a result, electrolytes and fluids remain in balance, preventing cell damage.

These three minerals also have other functions. Sodium helps with muscle and nerve action and helps regulate blood pressure. Chloride helps transmit nerve signals. In the stomach, chloride helps maintain the acidity level needed to digest food. Potassium helps maintain a steady heartbeat and helps with muscle and nerve action. In addition, it helps maintain normal blood pressure.

Since table salt is a chemical combination of sodium and chloride, you get both of these minerals when you eat salt. Some foods naturally contain sodium, but it is also added to many foods during processing.

Generally, getting too much potassium is not a problem, but experts agree that too much sodium is. **Hypertension**, or high blood pressure, has been linked to high salt intake. This condition can lead to cardiovascular disease and strokes. Too much sodium can cause loss of calcium and increase the risk of kidney stones.

For these reasons, health experts recommend eating no more than 2,300 milligrams of sodium each day. Most people take in much more. One rounded teaspoon of table salt contains about 2,300 milligrams of sodium. To limit your sodium intake, try these suggestions:

- Choose foods that are naturally low in sodium, including fresh fruits and vegetables, fresh meats and poultry, and such grains as brown rice and bulgur.
- Limit the amount of processed foods you eat: frozen meals, packaged mixes, cured meats, canned foods, cereals, breads, salad dressings, and sauces. Choose processed foods with the lowest sodium.
- Limit such condiments as soy sauce, ketchup, mustard, pickles, and olives, which are high in sodium.
- Limit salty snacks, such as chips, crackers, pretzels, and nuts, or choose unsalted ones.
- Instead of salt, use herbs and spices to flavor food. See **Fig. 8-10**. Many spice and herb mixes are available to use as substitutes.

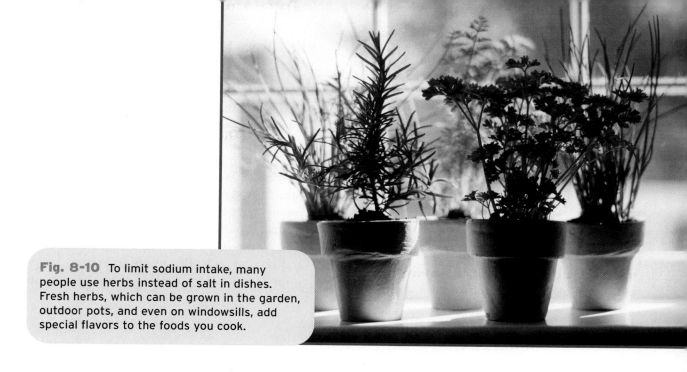

Fig. 8-10 To limit sodium intake, many people use herbs instead of salt in dishes. Fresh herbs, which can be grown in the garden, outdoor pots, and even on windowsills, add special flavors to the foods you cook.

- Add little or no salt to food when cooking and at the table.

Sodium, chloride, and potassium deficiencies are uncommon. If an illness, such as vomiting or diarrhea, causes excessive fluid loss, electrolytes will be lost and must be replaced.

Trace Minerals

Trace minerals are sometimes called microminerals. Even though you need only small amounts of these minerals, they serve vital functions. You can get all the trace minerals you need from food. Excess amounts can be harmful, so be careful in using mineral supplements unless under the direction of a health professional. **Fig. 8-11** shows trace minerals and their food sources.

Iron

Iron is essential for making hemoglobin, the substance in red blood cells that carries oxygen to all body cells. If you don't get enough iron, your blood may not be able to carry enough oxygen to your cells. The resulting condition is called **iron-deficiency anemia**. People with anemia are often tired, weak, short of breath, and pale. They may feel cold.

Fig. 8-11

Food Sources of Trace Minerals

Iron
Meat; fish; shellfish; egg yolks; dark green, leafy vegetables; dry beans and peas; enriched and whole-grain products; dried fruits.

Iodine
Saltwater fish; iodized salt.

Zinc
Meat; liver; poultry; fish; shellfish; dairy products; dry beans and peas; peanuts; whole-grain breads and cereals; eggs; miso (fermented soybean paste).

Selenium
Whole-grain breads and cereals; vegetables (amount varies with content in soil); meat; variety meats; fish; shellfish.

Copper
Whole-grain products; seafood; variety meats; dry beans and peas; nuts; seeds.

Fluoride
Water supplies in many communities (added to help improve dental health); also in some bottled waters.

Anemia is common around the world. Since females who are menstruating need more iron than males, they are particularly prone to this problem.

Some people who are iron deficient have an unusual appetite for ice, clay, or other nonfood items. This condition is called **pica**, and it usually diminishes after the need for iron is identified and addressed.

If you eat foods rich in vitamin C at the same time as plant foods rich in iron, your body can absorb more of the iron from these foods. Food cooked in an iron skillet absorbs some of the iron. Researchers disagree, however, on how much iron food can absorb from this source.

Other Trace Minerals

Besides iron, you need a number of other trace minerals.

- **Iodine.** Iodine is stored in the thyroid gland. This gland, located in the neck, produces substances needed for growth and development. Too much or too little iodine can cause thyroid problems. Without enough iodine, a lump called a goiter can form at the front of the neck. Infants can be born with mental retardation if a woman is iodine deficient during pregnancy.
- **Zinc.** Zinc helps enzymes do their work. In addition, it aids the immune system, helps wounds heal, and promotes normal growth in

Career Prep

Using Knowledge and Skills

HAVE YOU EVER HEARD A FELLOW student say: "Why do I have to study algebra? I'll never use the quadratic formula in the real world." That may be true about particular facts, but look a little deeper for the whole truth.

With so much information available today, how much do you need to know? That's up to you. Some people stop learning before they get through high school and then operate at that level for life. Others soak up learning and become more interesting people who leap ahead in life.

Although you can't learn everything there is to know, your brain does have an amazing capacity to store information—even facts that don't seem relevant at the moment. Since lives and careers take so many twists and turns, you never know when you might need something that was once stored away. A journalist recalled chemistry basics when working on a food science feature for the newspaper. The new owner of a deli restaurant relied on math skills to help understand accounting and tax

paperwork for the business. As a high school student, neither person would have foreseen these particular needs.

Those who are scornful of learning risk later regrets. For instance, an employee who was assigned to escort foreign visitors on a tour regretted paying so little attention in history class. Someone else regretted never learning to read and write well when trying to create a résumé and fill out job applications. Since no one knows exactly what the future holds, wasting opportunities to learn is definitely risky.

If you think learning is only about absorbing facts, think again. Just as it takes effort and practice to become a good volleyball player, your brain needs a workout to move to higher levels of understanding and ability. Learning a math concept prepares your brain to tackle a more difficult one. As you "practice" learning in school, your brain builds new skills. Through math formulas and scientific principles, you learn logic, problem solving, and creativity, skills you can use far beyond the classroom. Language arts classes

children. Zinc deficiency has wide-ranging effects on the body, including growth retardation, poor appetite, loss of taste, dry skin, and depression.

- **Selenium.** Selenium (suh-LEE-nee-um) is an antioxidant. It maintains the structure of muscles, red blood cells, hair, and nails. Scientific evidence shows that it may protect against certain cancers.
- **Copper.** Certain enzymes rely on copper to do their work. Copper helps form hemoglobin and collagen. Deficiencies are rare.
- **Fluoride.** The main function of fluoride is to prevent tooth decay and strengthen bones.

Since foods contain little fluoride, many communities add the mineral to drinking water when it doesn't occur naturally. Some toothpastes have added fluoride. See **Fig. 8-12**.

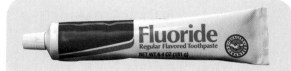

Fig. 8-12 Fluoride helps prevent tooth decay. Does your drinking water contain fluoride?

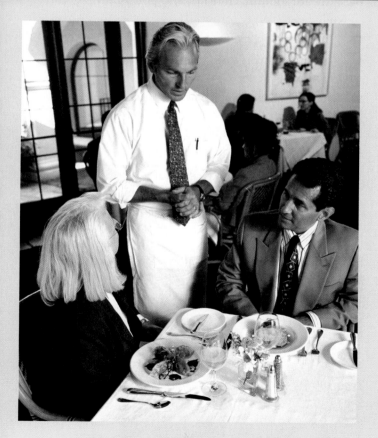

prepare you to communicate effectively. Social studies classes teach you to put events of the day into perspective and to understand people from many backgrounds. Through research and study, you increase your ability to find and interpret information—both valuable skills. When harnessed, brain power can give you an edge in countless ways throughout life.

PRACTICAL SKILLS

Much of what you learn actually has direct links to the real world. Take a foods and nutrition class, for example. The practical skills you learn can be directly applied to personal and professional life. For one thing, nutrition knowledge arms you to make wise eating choices. Learning to choose and prepare foods is a skill you need for independence and good health. Consumer skills can help you reduce waste—in the budget, in the kitchen, and even on the planet. If a career in foods or nutrition is your choice, the information and skills in related courses can provide useful education, experiences, and other resources to help you realize your career dreams.

Career Connection

Skills at work. Observe a nutrition or food service professional at work. Record instances when the person uses math, thinking, and communication skills. Share observations in class.

Summarize Your Reading

▶ Many processes in the body could not take place without the assistance of vitamins and minerals.

▶ Vitamins are named by letter, but they also have chemical names that describe them.

▶ Eating a wide variety of foods is the best way to get most of the vitamins and minerals you need.

▶ Some vitamin and mineral deficiencies can result in serious threats to health.

▶ With knowledge about vitamins and minerals, you can make food choices that help you get what you need in the right amounts, without deficiencies or excesses.

Check Your Knowledge

1. Why are vitamins and minerals called micronutrients?

2. Why are some vitamins considered to be **antioxidants**?

3. Compare **water-soluble** and **fat-soluble vitamins**.

4. What does vitamin C do for you?

5. **CRITICAL THINKING** One family stored milk in small, clear containers. What do you think of this practice?

6. What function in the body do riboflavin, niacin, vitamin B_6, vitamin B_{12}, vitamin B_5, and biotin have in common?

7. Why is folate a very important vitamin?

8. What can occur with vitamin A deficiency?

9. What is **toxicity**?

10. What are two ways to get vitamin D?

11. **CRITICAL THINKING** Why do cooks need to pay particular attention to the ways that foods are prepared?

12. Compare **major** and **trace minerals**.

13. Why do teens need to think about **osteoporosis**?

14. Why are sodium, chloride, and potassium called **electrolyte minerals**?

15. What can help reduce **hypertension**?

16. What are some signs of **iron-deficiency anemia**?

17. One teen chewed on ice to the point that her friends noticed and commented on the frequency. What might be wrong?

18. Why is fluoride needed in the diet?

19. **CRITICAL THINKING** What do you think about the trend to fortify many food products with vitamins and minerals?

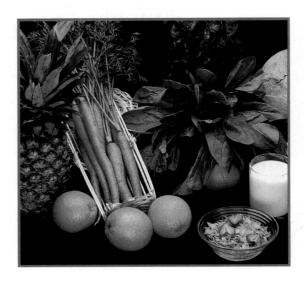

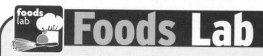

Apply Your Learning

1. **Label Comparison.** Compare the label of a multiple vitamin and mineral supplement with the recommended amounts of vitamins and minerals needed daily. What conclusions can you draw? What might be the consequences of overusing supplements?

2. **LANGUAGE ARTS** **Read and Report.** Read a news article about vitamins and minerals and summarize the article for class.

3. **MATH** **Sodium Comparison.** Compare the amount of sodium in selected fresh vegetables and their canned versions. Chart your results. What conclusions can you draw?

4. **Taste Test.** Find recipes for herb mixes and seasoning mixes that can be used in place of salt in certain foods. Prepare one and taste test it with your classmates.

5. **Menu Planning.** Plan a day's menus, including a variety of foods that supply your vitamin requirements for the day and at least some mineral requirements.

6. **SOCIAL STUDIES** **Developing Countries.** Find information on vitamin and mineral deficiencies in developing countries. Research the health problems

Foods Lab

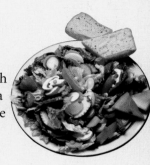

Vitamin Salad

Procedure: With your lab team, create a recipe for a vitamin- or mineral-rich salad. It may be a main dish or a side dish. Try to plan a dish that is appealing to the eye as well as nutritious. Prepare and evaluate your salad.

Analyzing Results

❶ What foods did you choose for your salad? What vitamins or minerals did each provide?

❷ How did you prepare these foods to promote appearance, taste, and texture?

❸ What other nutrients does the salad supply?

associated with one specific deficiency and report on any actions intended to solve the problem.

Food Science Experiment

Functions of Salt

Objective: To identify one action of salt in food and in the body.

Procedure:

1. Cut two, ¼-inch slices from an eggplant. Set each slice on a plate.

2. Sprinkle one slice with ¼ tsp. of salt. Let both slices sit for 30 minutes. Then observe.

Analyzing Results

❶ What changes do you notice in each slice of eggplant? What do you think caused this change?

❷ Based on this experiment, explain why salt is used to dry foods, such as ham, for preserving.

❸ How do you think salt affects fluids in the body?

Water & Phytochemicals

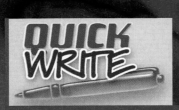

DESCRIPTIVE WRITING. Vivid descriptions help a reader "see" or "feel" what the writer is describing. Think of a time when you were extremely thirsty for some reason. During a sports event? On a hot camping trip? When the heat reached 100 degrees? Write a paragraph that uses descriptive words to make your experience very real to readers.

Objectives

▶ Explain how the body uses water.

▶ Compare your own water requirement to what you actually consume.

▶ Suggest ways to increase water intake.

▶ Define phytochemicals and, in general, explain their possible benefits.

▶ Relate specific phytochemicals to their possible benefits and food sources.

▶ Summarize how phytochemicals can be included in the diet.

Terms

| beta-carotene
| cruciferous vegetables
| dehydrated
| hydration
| phytochemicals

SCIENTIFIC RESEARCH REGULARLY REVEALS new theories and facts about nutrients. As a result, basic nutrition concepts change from time to time. For example, years ago no one thought of water as a nutrient. Today, health experts classify water as one of the six nutrients needed to sustain life.

Phytochemicals, on the other hand, are not called nutrients. Although these substances appear to help prevent certain diseases, scientists don't classify them as nutrients—at least not yet. As research uncovers more about their role in the human body, these substances may eventually be called nutrients too.

THE NUTRIENT WATER

Think about the many ways that water is part of your life. In this text, you'll explore some of those impacts: how water affects weight, water conservation, and water as a beverage. The topic for now is water as a nutrient.

You might be surprised to hear that water makes up about 55 to 75 percent of a mature body. The amount varies, depending on age, gender, and body composition. It's easy to see that water is critical for survival. People can live for about six weeks without food but only a few days without water. See **Fig. 9-1.**

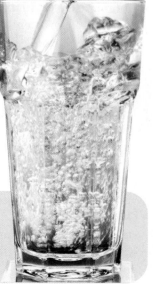

Fig. 9-1 Water is vital. Without this nutrient, life wouldn't last for more than a few days.

The Need for Water

Water is part of every cell, tissue, and organ in your body. Not only do cells contain water, but they are also bathed in it. Without water in the right balance, body cells would die. As the main component of all body fluids, water is in blood, saliva, digestive juices, and urine. Wherever water is in the body, it has work to do.

- **Chemical reactions.** Within the cells, water participates in chemical reactions that sustain the body. For example, water helps break food down into nutrients before passing them through the intestinal wall and into the bloodstream.
- **Transportation.** Minerals, vitamins, glucose, and other substances dissolve in water. Blood carries oxygen and nutrients to the cells that need them.
- **Cushioning and moisturizing.** Moisture from water cushions joints, tissues, and organs to protect them from shock. For example, your spinal cord needs this protection. Water also moisturizes your eyes, mouth, and nose and keeps your skin soft.
- **Waste removal.** Water helps filter out pollutants and toxins and get rid of waste products. Some substances are excreted through the water in urine. Water keeps solid wastes in the intestines moist for ease in elimination, thereby preventing constipation.
- **Temperature regulation.** You perspire to cool your body and keep a normal temperature of about 98.6°F. Exercise warms the body and produces perspiration. As perspiration evaporates from the skin, the process cools the body. See **Fig. 9-2**.
- **Breathing.** When you inhale, your body adds moisture to the air so the lungs can process it. As you exhale, water is removed from the lungs. On a cold day, this water is visible. The low temperature condenses the warm water vapor in your breath, so you see a small cloud.
- **Overall well-being.** You feel better and stronger and have more energy when enough water is available for all the tasks it performs in your body.

How Much Do You Need?

Water enters the body in liquids and food. Through metabolism, the body also makes some water. Water exits the body in four ways: through sweat, breathing, urine, and feces. On average you lose about 2 to 3 quarts of water each day. You need to input enough water to balance what the body needs for output. **Hydration** (hy-DRAY-shun) means getting enough water to meet all the body's needs. When you consume enough water, you are hydrated.

To get the water needed, health experts recommend that teens and adults drink 8 to 12 cups of water every day. You can determine the daily minimum you need by dividing your weight (as pounds) in half. The result is the number of ounces of water you need. For example, someone who weighs 130 pounds needs at least 65 ounces of water (130 divided by 2 = 65), or approximately 8 cups (65 ounces divided by 8 ounces per cup = 8.1). This formula applies only to people who weigh more than 100 pounds.

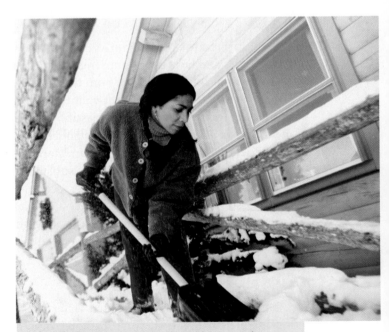

Fig. 9-2 When physically active, people perspire in cold as well as warm weather. When is it more noticeable? You need to stay hydrated no matter what the season.

To be sure you drink enough water, measure the amount in the glass you normally use. Then determine the number of glasses you need to get your daily quota of water.

You can also estimate the amount by counting gulps, which are hearty swallows. One gulp usually equals about one ounce of water.

Under certain conditions, people may need more than the recommended amount. Strenuous work and exercise increase perspiration. An illness with fever or diarrhea can cause water loss. So can some medications. Exposure to extremely hot or cold weather, pregnancy, breast-feeding a baby, and eating high-fiber foods can all increase water needs.

A healthy body does not store water as a reserve supply. If you drink more than you need, your body will get rid of it.

Dehydration

People who don't drink enough water every day become **dehydrated**. Signs of dehydration include dark-colored urine, dry lips and skin, and constipation. Dehydration can also cause headaches, dizziness, nausea, and light-headedness. Muscle fatigue is also possible, leaving you tired much of the time. You need to drink enough water to balance what the body uses each day. Extreme dehydration can produce seizures, brain damage, and even death.

Thirst is one of the warning signs of dehydration. By the time you feel thirsty, however, you have already lost a significant amount of water. To prevent dehydration, drink water regularly throughout the day and not just when you're thirsty.

Other Fluids

At least half of the fluids you drink should be plain water. The remainder can come from milk, juice, and other beverages. Beverages that contain caffeine don't count toward your water requirement. Coffee, tea, and most cola soft drinks have caffeine, which promotes water loss by increasing the flow of urine. See **Fig. 9-3**.

Most solid foods contain water in varying amounts. In general, fruits and vegetables have a higher percentage of water than other foods. See

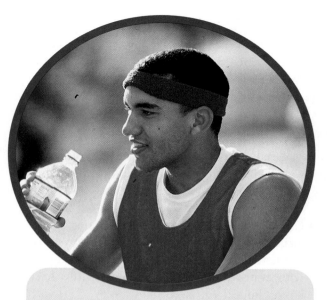

Fig. 9-3 Health experts suggest drinking water rather than soft drinks. Beverages with caffeine tend to remove water from the body and may keep water from entering body cells.

Fig. 9-4. Consider the water in foods as a bonus rather than part of your daily requirement. Then you'll be sure to get the amount of water your body needs to function well.

Fig. 9-4

Approximate Water Content of Food	
Food	**Percentage of Water**
Fruits and vegetables	80–90%
Milk	90%
Cooked cereals	85%
Eggs	75%
Pasta	65%
Seafood	60–85%
Meats	45–65%
Cheeses	35%
Breads	35–40%
Nuts	2–5%
Oils	0%

Drinking More Water

Like many other people, you may need to increase the amount of water you drink. Adopting a few new habits can help you increase your water intake. Try these suggestions:

- If you haven't been drinking enough water, increase the amount gradually.
- Make a habit of drinking at least eight ounces of water when you get up in the morning, when you go to bed, and before each meal. That alone supplies five cups of water.
- Carry a sports bottle filled with water. If you feel like having a beverage, reach for the sports bottle instead of a soft drink. Refill the bottle with water as needed and add a little fresh lemon juice if you like.
- Take a water break instead of a soft drink or coffee break.
- Drink water before, during, and after you mow the grass, shovel snow, roller blade, or participate in any other physical activity.

PHYTOCHEMICALS

When you drink water and eat healthfully, you benefit from all the nutrients that you've studied—but there's more. In plant-based foods, scientists have discovered additional substances that appear to have many positive impacts on health. These naturally occurring chemical compounds are called **phytochemicals**. *Phyto* comes from the Greek word *phyton*, meaning plant.

Plants produce phytochemicals for protection from insects, viruses, fungi, and the sun. Some phytochemicals give plants color, flavor, and aroma. Scientists have identified thousands of phytochemicals in plant foods, and the list continues to grow. Recent estimates suggest that every plant contains at least 200 different phytochemicals.

Since phytochemicals are not considered essential for life, they are not classified as nutrients. As research reveals more about what these substances can do, however, they could earn nutrient status. Even now, some people call them phytonutrients because of their possible influences on health.

Benefits of Phytochemicals

Phytochemical research has been going on for years. Most investigation has focused on identifying and classifying these compounds. Only recently have scientists begun to discover the critical roles phytochemicals are believed to play in the human body. These are some of the possible benefits:

- Act as antioxidants.
- Enhance immunity.
- Keep cancer cells from forming and also from multiplying.
- Influence the body's production of cholesterol.
- Protect the body against such diseases as cancer, diabetes, heart disease, high blood pressure, and blindness caused by aging.

How do specific phytochemicals act in the body? How much of each one do you need? Do these compounds work alone or together? To answer these questions, scientists are conducting extensive research on phytochemicals. For example, some scientists now believe that the unique mix of compounds in each food makes them effective because they act as a team. Scientists must study one compound at a time, however, to discover the answers.

Examples of Phytochemicals

As phytochemicals are identified and studied, scientists categorize them according to characteristics and functions. Unless you're a scientist, the scientific names, categories, and subdivisions can be confusing. Several phytochemical categories are described here.

Carotenoids

Hundreds of compounds make up the carotenoids (kuh-RAH-tuhn-oids). Scientists probably know more about this phytochemical cateogory than any other. You may recognize these well-known carotenoids:

- **Beta-carotene.** One of the earliest phytochemicals discovered was **beta-carotene** (bay-tuh-CARE-uh-teen). The body uses beta-carotene to make vitamin A whenever it's needed. Beta-carotene also acts as an antioxidant and may

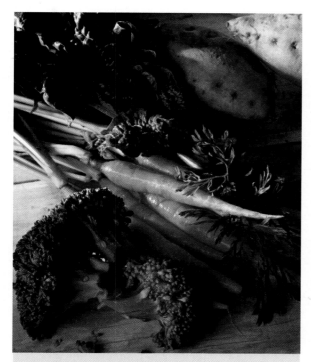

Fig. 9-5 Color is a clue to beta-carotene. These carrots have the orange color typically associated with beta-carotene. How can broccoli have beta-carotene since it's not orange?

help prevent cancer. Beta-carotene and other carotenes in the carotenoid category are found in colorful fruits and vegetables. These include yellow and orange fruits and vegetables, such as apricots, cantaloupes, papayas, peaches, carrots, pumpkins, sweet potatoes, and winter squash. Although beta-carotene is basically orange, chlorophyll in green plants can mask this color. Therefore green vegetables are also good sources, including spinach, mustard greens, green peppers, broccoli, green peas, and kale. See **Fig. 9-5**.

- **Lycopene.** Red fruits and vegetables contain lycopene (LY-kuh-peen). Tomatoes and tomato products are good sources. Others are pink grapefruit, guava, and watermelon. Lycopene may reduce the risk of cancer and heart disease.
- **Lutein.** Another well-known carotenoid is lutein (LOO-tee-uhn), which is found in kale, spinach, collard greens, romaine lettuce, broccoli, and brussels sprouts. Kiwifruit and egg yolks are other sources. Lutein may help protect against blindness.

Flavonoids

The flavonoids (FLAY-vuh-noids) make up another phytochemical category. See **Fig. 9-6**. Flavonoids include the following:

- **Anthocyanins.** Anthocyanins (an-thuh-SY-uh-nuns) are found in blackberries, blueberries, cherries, cranberries, kiwifruit, strawberries, eggplant skin, plums, red cabbage, and red or purple grapes. They are antioxidants and may lower cancer risk.
- **Isoflavones.** Soybeans and soy-based foods contain isoflavones (eye-soh-FLAY-vohns). They may prevent cancer, lower cholesterol, and help reduce symptoms of menopause, the point in life when a woman's menstrual cycle slows and stops.
- **Quercetin.** Quercetin (KWUR-suh-tun) is found in onions, tea, and many vegetables. Besides acting as an antioxidant, it may reduce growth of cancer cells.
- **Resveratrol.** Red grapes and juice have resveratrol (rez-VAIR-uh-trawl). It's an antioxidant and may contribute to heart health and reduce cancer risk.

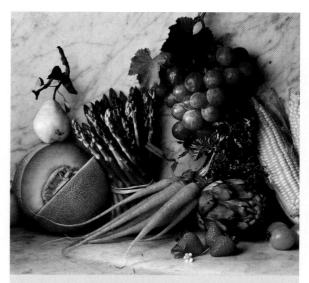

Fig. 9-6 Flavonoids have several potential benefits. Which of these foods contain flavonoids? Which contain other phytochemicals?

Other Phytochemical Categories

Besides carotenoids and flavonoids, a few other notable phytochemical categories are:

- **Allyl sulfides.** Allyl sulfides (A-lul sul-fyds) are found in garlic, onions, chives, leeks, and shallots. They may prevent cancer and lower blood pressure and cholesterol.
- **Indoles.** Indoles (IN-dohls) are found in **cruciferous vegetables** (kroo-SIH-fuh-rus). These include all vegetables from the cabbage family: cabbage, broccoli, brussels sprouts, cauliflower, kale, Swiss chard, and bok choy. See **Fig. 9-7**. Indoles are antioxidants. In addition, they may reduce some cancer risks.
- **Phytosterols.** Phytosterols (FEYE-tahs-tuh-rawls) are found in vegetable oils. They may have a positive effect on cholesterol levels.
- **Saponins.** Whole-grain products, soy products, and dry beans, peas, and lentils contain saponins (SA-puh-nuns). They may lower cholesterol and prevent cancer.

How Much Do You Need?

As public interest in phytochemicals grows, manufacturers are creating supplements that supply them. These are often called nutraceuticals. Since phytochemicals in each plant may work as a team, you can get all the phytochemicals in the right combinations just by eating plant foods. You'll also get phytochemicals that haven't been identified yet.

Health experts don't recommend taking supplements because research hasn't determined how much of each phytochemical is needed and what quantity is safe to take. Only a few studies have been done on the effectiveness and safety of taking just one phytochemical. For example, as one of the earliest phytochemical supplements produced, beta-carotene became very popular.

Career Prep

Preparing for the Work World

YOU MAY HAVE HEARD THAT HAVING many interests makes a good impression on a job application or at an interview. This is true, to a point. Employers aren't impressed by numbers alone. They look for involvement in organizations and events, which shows that a person has the skills to be a good worker.

In this sense, your interests and activities can complement your studies and personal qualities in preparing for a job. The ideas below can help you enhance work skills and promote yourself as a potential employee:

- **Leadership.** Look for leadership opportunities, not merely membership, in clubs and organizations. You might take on the duties of a specific office, such as president or treasurer, or a task, such as chairing a committee to put

on an awards banquet. If you belong to a book club, mention if you started the club or have led any discussions.

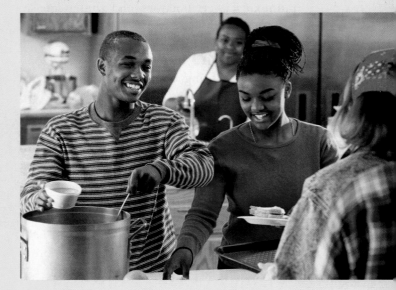

Eventually, studies showed that these supplements are actually harmful to people who smoke or work with asbestos.

Getting Phytochemicals

Some foods are stars on the phytochemical stage. Color counts when choosing fruits and vegetables: the brighter the color, the greater the supply of phytochemicals tends to be. Aim for at least five to nine servings of fruits and vegetables each day—in different colors. Include cruciferous vegetables regularly.

Whole-grain products offer many phytochemicals. Besides whole-grain breads, cereals, pasta, and crackers, you could try brown rice, kasha, bulgur, and millet. Dry beans, peas, and lentils are good phytochemical sources, as are herbs, spices, and tea. You can eat soy in tofu, soy nuts, and soy milk. By including plenty of foods like these for meals and snacks, you will get the benefits of

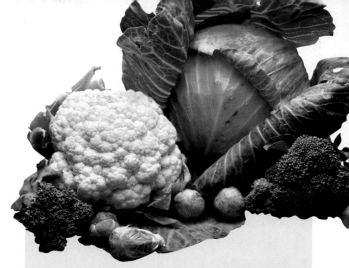

Fig. 9-7 Cruciferous vegetables belong to the cabbage family. What phytochemicals do they contain?

many different phytochemicals. These foods offer a delicious way to help protect your health.

- **Commitment.** In volunteer work, strive for deeper commitment to fewer groups, instead of occasionally helping many groups. Show your willingness to get involved at several levels of an organization. You not only demonstrate an ability to understand group relationships and management but also make yourself more useful to the organization. Of course, this doesn't mean that you shouldn't help other causes when a need arises.

- **Career match.** Give priority to activities that most resemble the career you want to follow. If your professional goal is to run a restaurant, consider volunteering in a nursing home kitchen.

- **Teamwork.** If competitive sports are your game, remember that employers are less concerned with your team's win-loss record than with your contribution to the effort, regardless of success. Point out ways that you showed teamwork and helped teammates play their best.

- **Health.** If you enjoy recreational sports or other physical activities, such as jogging or gardening, stress that you appreciate the benefits to physical and mental health. This shows an understanding of, and commitment to, good health. This quality helps address employers' concerns about employee productivity and insurance costs.

Of course, you shouldn't choose interests and activities only on their value as work preparation. The point of these pursuits is to do something that makes you happy and calls forth your best effort. If they also give a sense of success and confidence that helps prepare you for a career, that's a bonus.

Career Connection

Making pastimes pay. List three interests you have or activities you take part in. For each one, describe one thing you can do to improve or develop a skill or quality that may be useful in the workplace.

Summarize Your Reading

▶ Water, which makes up a large part of the human body, is at work in many ways throughout the body.

▶ If water isn't in the right balance within the body, cells will die.

▶ The amount of water people need varies according to activity level, illness, medications, weather, pregnancy, breast-feeding, and the high-fiber foods eaten.

▶ Phytochemicals are produced by plants for their own protection and may offer certain protections to humans who eat the plants.

▶ Many phytochemicals have been identified in foods, and scientists are continually discovering more.

Check Your Knowledge

1. What does water have in common with carbohydrates, proteins, fats, vitamins, and minerals?

2. How much of a mature body is water?

3. Describe the ways that the body makes use of water.

4. How does water exit the body?

5. How much water do you lose every day?

6. What is the condition of a properly **hydrated** body?

7. How can you estimate the daily amount of water you need to consume?

8. What are some signs of **dehydration**?

9. Should you wait until you're thirsty to drink? Explain.

10. How much of the fluids you drink should be plain water?

11. What effect do coffee, tea, and cola drinks have on water in your body?

12. Give tips to increase water intake.

13. What are **phytochemicals**?

14. Why are phytochemicals not currently classified as nutrients?

15. What are some possible benefits of phytochemicals?

16. How do you explain why many green vegetables have **beta-carotene** even though this phytochemical's color is basically orange?

17. What color do you associate with lycopene and why?

18. What phytochemicals might you get by eating blueberries, soybeans, onions, and red grapes?

19. What foods are good sources of indoles?

20. **CRITICAL THINKING** Relate this statement to phytochemicals: "Eat a variety of foods to stay healthy."

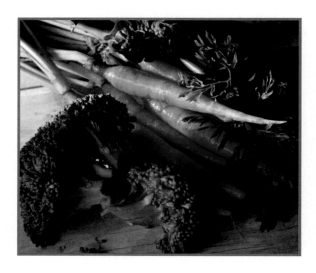

Apply Your Learning

1. **MATH** **Water Calculation.** For three days, keep track of the plain water you drink. Compute the average number of cups you drink in a day. Calculate how many cups of water you need every day, using the formula in the text. Compare the figures. Are you getting enough water? Was your record realistic, or did you drink more just because you were keeping track? What adjustments, if any, do you need to make in your water intake?

2. **Water Estimate.** Put one cup (8 ounces) of water in a drinking glass. Then take gulps until the water is gone, counting gulps as you go. How many gulps make a cup for you? Repeat to check your consistency. You can use this information throughout the day, even at drinking fountains.

3. **LANGUAGE ARTS** **Phytochemical Handout.** Write a one-page grocery store handout or make a poster to inform shoppers about the benefits of including foods with phytochemicals in the diet.

Foods Lab

Water Taste Test

Procedure: With members of your lab team, conduct a blind taste test of bottled, softened, and regular tap water. Include tap water from different parts of your community, if possible. Serve all samples at the same temperature. Evaluate and rank the samples in order of preference. Try to distinguish each type.

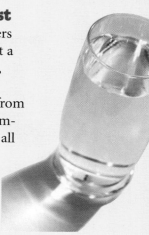

Analyzing Results

❶ What qualities of the water did you notice?

❷ Could any team members tell one type of water from another? If so, how?

❸ Overall, did your team prefer varieties of bottled water more than, less than, or equally to tap water?

❹ Did this test change your opinion of bottled and tap water, or confirm it? In what way?

Food Science Experiment

Water in Foods

Objective: To identify and compare the water content of different types of food.

Procedure:

1. Weigh one carrot, one hamburger bun, and one hot dog (or other foods supplied by your teacher). Record the weight of each.

2. Cut each food into chunks and process individually in a blender until smooth or pulpy.

3. Scrape each food into a strainer. Force out as much liquid as possible. Retain the liquid; measure and weigh it.

4. Find the percentage of water in each food by dividing the weight of the food's water by its total weight.

Analyzing Results

❶ Which food was highest in liquid content? Lowest?

❷ How do you think each food "held" its liquid?

❸ Suppose you ate all three foods in one day. How useful would they be in contributing to your daily need for water?

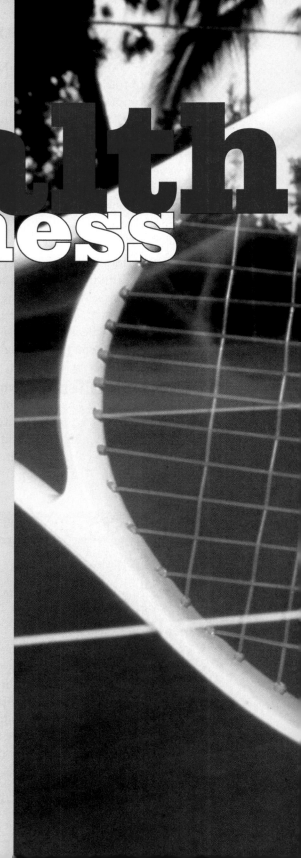

UNIT 3

Health

& Wellness

CHAPTER 10 **Nutrition Guidelines**

CHAPTER 11 **Keeping a Healthy Weight**

CHAPTER 12 **Health Challenges**

CHAPTER 13 **Life-Span Nutrition**

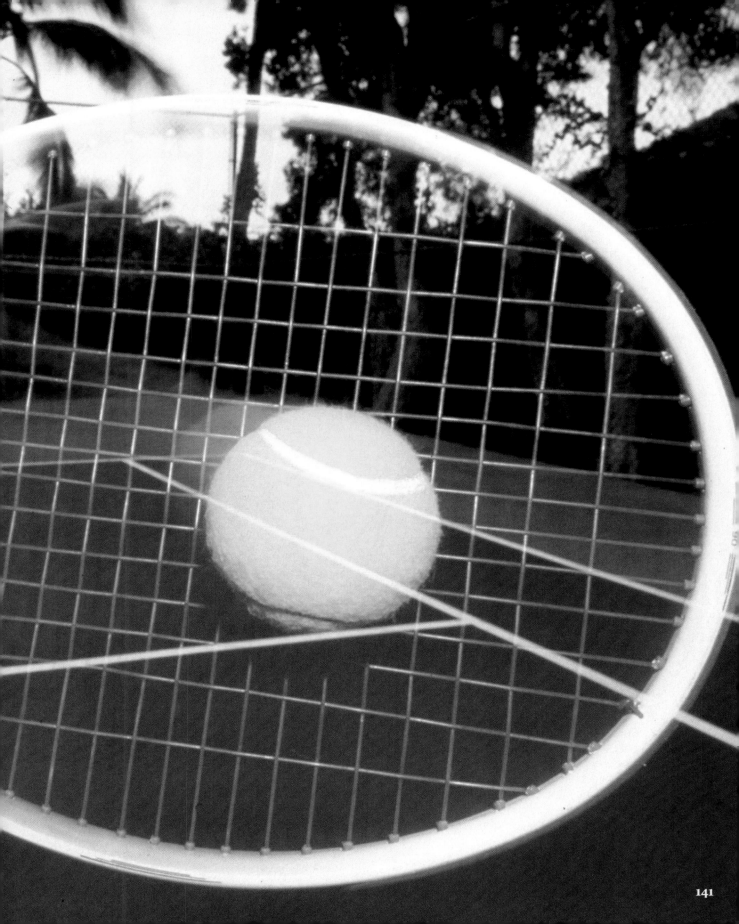

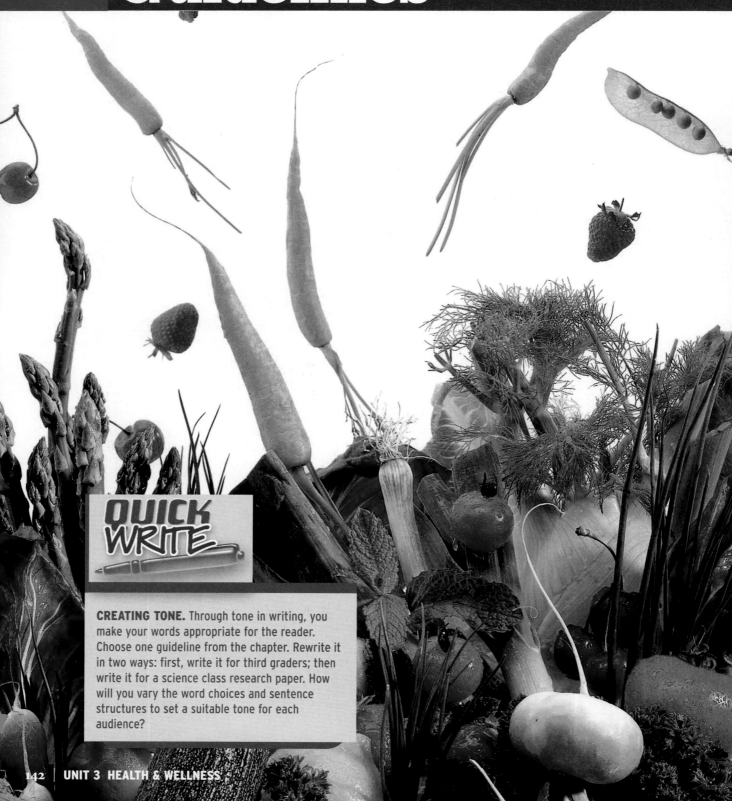

Nutrition Guidelines

QUICK WRITE

CREATING TONE. Through tone in writing, you make your words appropriate for the reader. Choose one guideline from the chapter. Rewrite it in two ways: first, write it for third graders; then write it for a science class research paper. How will you vary the word choices and sentence structures to set a suitable tone for each audience?

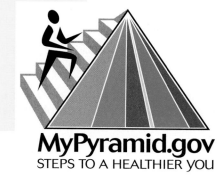

MyPyramid.gov
STEPS TO A HEALTHIER you

"THE MORE I READ AND HEAR IN THE NEWS about nutrition, the more I wonder what's true and what isn't. Even when I think I'm making the best food choices for my health, a new study or book comes out to say something different."

Many people share this person's frustration. Books and news stories regularly contradict each other. Instead of giving up on health advice, people need to use common sense and reliable resources.

RELIABLE RESOURCES

The U.S. Department of Agriculture (USDA) provides diet and health guidelines for consumers. These include the Dietary Guidelines for Americans, MyPyramid, and the Nutrition Facts panel.

Dietary Guidelines for Americans

The **Dietary Guidelines for Americans** offer sound advice on nutrition and fitness. They provide the most current, science-based information to help people live healthy lives and reduce their risk of chronic disease. The guidelines, updated in 2005, are the basis for federal nutrition policies and programs. **Fig. 10-1** on page 144 summarizes main topics in the guidelines.

The Dietary Guidelines are supported by information throughout this text. For example, you've already studied nutrients, and you'll learn about healthy weights and physical activity in the next chapter. Food safety is another topic in the guidelines. Chapter 20 teaches this information.

MyPyramid

In 2005, the USDA replaced the old Food Guide Pyramid with **MyPyramid**, shown at the top of this page. MyPyramid is divided into vertical bands of different colors. The bands represent five food groups (plus oils). The varying widths of the bands show that you need to eat different relative amounts of food from the groups. Since food needs are not the same for everyone, MyPyramid can be accessed on the Internet so that you can tailor the tool to reflect your own food needs. To stress the importance of exercise, MyPyramid also shows a figure walking upstairs.

Fig. 10-1

Summary of Dietary Guidelines for Americans

Main Topics	Key Recommendations
Adequate nutrients within calorie needs	• Eat a variety of nutritious foods and beverages. • Choose foods that limit saturated and trans fats, cholesterol, added sugars, and salt.
Weight management	• Balance calories consumed with calories used for energy needs to maintain a healthy weight. • Adjust calories and activity to prevent weight gain.
Physical activity	• Engage in regular physical activity and limit sedentary activities. Teens should get at least 60 minutes of physical activity on most, but preferably all, days of the week. For adults the recommendation is 30 minutes. • Increase exercise for weight reduction and added health benefits.
Food groups to encourage	• Consume a variety of foods from the different food groups. Eat the recommended amounts each day but in balance with energy needs.
Fats	• Choose lean, low-fat, and fat-free when selecting and preparing foods. • Limit intake of fats and oils high in saturated and trans fat. • Consume less than 10 percent of calories from saturated and *trans* fat. • Teens should keep total fat intake between 25 and 35 percent of calories.
Carbohydrates	• Choose fiber-rich fruits, vegetables, and whole grains often. • Limit foods and beverages with added sugars.
Sodium and potassium	• Consume less than 2,300 mg (about 1 teaspoon) of sodium per day by preparing foods with little salt. • Consume potassium-rich foods, such as fruits and vegetables.

Food Groups

To use MyPyramid effectively, you need to be familiar with the food groups. As you read the descriptions that follow, find each group in **Fig. 10-2.** Different calorie levels are shown at the top of this chart. For each level, you'll see suggested amounts of food to eat from the food groups, subgroups, and oils in order to meet recommended nutrient intakes.

The following descriptions include color names in parentheses. These colors correspond to the color bands in MyPyramid.

• **Fruit Group (red).** Choose a variety of fruits, whether fresh, frozen, canned, or dried. Most of the time, these are a better choice than fruit juice.

• **Vegetable Group (green).** Eat a variety of vegetables too. This group has several subgroups, with weekly amounts to eat for these. You should focus on eating more dark green vegetables, such as broccoli and dark leafy greens. Orange vegetables include carrots, sweet potatoes, and pumpkin. Examples of starchy vegetables are white potatoes, corn, and green peas. Vegetables in the "other" category include tomatoes, tomato juice, lettuce, green beans, and onions. Notice that dry beans are listed under vegetables and also with meats. They are considered to be part of both groups but should be counted in only one group when figuring your daily intake.

Fig. 10-2

Selected Calorie Levels from USDA Food Guide

Food Groups*	Calorie Levels						
	1,600	1,800	2,000	2,200	2,400	2,600	2,800
Fruits	1.5 c (3 srv)	1.5 c (3 srv)	2 c (4 srv)	2 c (4 srv)	2 c (4 srv)	2 c (4 srv)	2.5 c (5 srv)
Vegetables	2 c (4 srv)	2.5 c (5 srv)	2.5 c (5 srv)	3 c (6 srv)	3 c (6 srv)	3.5 c (7 srv)	3.5 c (7 srv)
Dark Green	2 c/wk	3 c/wk	3 c/wk	3 c/wk	3 c/wk	3 c/wk	3 c/wk
Orange	1.5 c/wk	2 c/wk	2 c/wk	2 c/wk	2 c/wk	2.5 c/wk	2.5 c/wk
Dry beans/peas	2.5 c/wk	3 c/wk	3 c/wk	3 c/wk	3 c/wk	3.5 c/wk	3.5 c/wk
Starchy	2.5 c/wk	3 c/wk	3 c/wk	6 c/wk	6 c/wk	7 c/wk	7 c/wk
Other	5.5 c/wk	6.5 c/wk	6.5 c/wk	7 c/wk	7 c/wk	8.5 c/wk	8.5 c/wk
Grains	5 oz-eq	6 oz-eq	6 oz-eq	7 oz-eq	8 oz-eq	9 oz-eq	10 oz-eq
Whole	3	3	3	3.5	4	4.5	5
Other	2	3	3	3.5	4	4.5	5
Meat, poultry, fish, dry beans, eggs, nuts, and seeds	5 oz-eq	5 oz-eq	5.5 oz-eq	6 oz-eq	6.5 oz-eq	6.5 oz-eq	7 oz-eq
Milk, yogurt, and cheese	3 c	3 c	3 c	3 c	3 c	3 c	3 c
Oils	22 g	24 g	27 g	29 g	31 g	34 g	36 g
Discretionary calorie allowance**	132	195	267	290	362	410	426

* Food group amounts are shown in cups per day (c), cups per week (c/wk), and ounce-equivalents per day (oz-eq). Where it applies, the number of servings (srv) is in parentheses. Oils are shown in grams (g).

** This number shows calories that can be eaten in addition to the amounts of nutrient-dense foods in each group. Any solid fats and added sugars in foods are counted here.

- **Grain Group (orange).** Half of the grains you eat in a day should be whole grains. Read the label to find grains that are whole.
- **Meat and Beans Group (purple).** Choose lean protein foods and vary your choices. Include more fish, beans, nuts, and seeds than meats and poultry.
- **Milk Group (blue).** As you know, foods in this group are calcium-rich. As a teen, you need 3 cups of low-fat or fat-free milk or an equivalent amount of low-fat yogurt or cheese. Choose lactose-free products or foods that are calcium-fortified if you can't digest milk.
- **Oils (yellow).** Use limited amounts and choose liquid rather than solid.

Nutrient Density

The USDA Food Guide is based on choosing foods that are nutrient dense. **Nutrient density** is the relationship between nutrients and calories in a food. Foods with low nutrient density are relatively low in nutrients and high in calories. They are high in fat and added sugars. For example, candies and sweet desserts are high in calories from fat and sugar and supply little or no vitamins, minerals, and phytochemicals. Soft drinks are high in sugar but provide no nutrients.

Foods with high nutrient density offer more nutrients and fewer calories. They are low in fat and refined sugars. Some food preparations can quickly turn a food from high to low nutrient density. What happens when you bake apples into a pie? The apples, which are nutrient dense, join with fat in the crust and added sugar in the filling to make a food with much lower nutrient density.

How Many Calories for You?

How much food should you eat in a day? To figure this out, you need to know what number of calories per day is right for you. People have different needs for calories and nutrients, depending on their age, gender, body size, and activity level. Extremely active people, including athletes, may need more calories for their energy needs. Someone who wants to gain or lose weight has to adjust calories. A health expert can help you determine your requirements.

To estimate your calorie needs, check MyPyramid on the Internet. In general, females age 14 to 18 need 1,800 daily calories if sedentary; 2,000 if moderately active; and 2,400 if active. Males age 14 to 18 need 2,000 to 2,400 daily calories if sedentary; 2,400 to 2,800 if moderately active; and 2,800 to 3,200 if active.

Sedentary people get less than 30 minutes of physical activity each day. Moderately active people get 30 to 60 minutes of physical activity daily, and active people get more than 60 minutes.

Food Amounts

With daily calories in mind, you can fit food amounts into your eating plan. Look again at **Fig. 10-2**. Under the calorie levels supplied, you'll see how much food in each group is recommended per day. For example at 2,200 calories, 2 cups of fruit (four ½-cup servings) and 7 ounces of grains are listed. As you can see, MyPyramid uses cups to measure fruits, vegetables, and milk. Ounces are used for grains, meat, and beans.

Fig. 10-3

Sample Serving Sizes

Food Groups	Servings and Equivalents
Fruits	• 1 small orange (½ cup) • ½ cup fresh, frozen, or canned fruit • ¼ cup dried fruit (½ cup) • ½ cup fruit juice
Vegetables	• 1 cup raw, leafy vegetable (½ cup) • ½ cup cooked or chopped raw vegetable • ½ cup vegetable juice
Grains	• 1 slice bread (1 oz.) • 1 cup dry cereal (1 oz.) • ½ cup cooked rice, pasta, or cereal (1 oz.) • 1 oz. dry pasta or rice
Meat, poultry, fish, dry beans, eggs, nuts, and seeds	• 3 oz. cooked lean meat, poultry, or fish • ½ cup cooked, dry beans or peas (2 oz.) • 1 egg (1 oz.) • 2 Tbsp. peanut butter (2 oz.) • ⅓ cup nuts (1½ oz.) • 2 Tbsp. seeds (½ oz.)
Milk, yogurt, and cheese (low fat or fat free)	• 1 cup milk or yogurt • 1½ oz. natural cheese (1 cup) • 2 oz. processed cheese (1 cup)
Oils	• 1 tsp. soft margarine (4½ g) • 1 Tbsp. low-fat mayonnaise (4½ g) • 1 tsp. vegetable oil (4½ g)

Fig. 10-3 shows how to compare servings you might eat to MyPyramid amounts. For the servings given, cup- and ounce-equivalents are shown in parentheses when needed. For example, ¼ cup of dried fruit equals ½ cup of the daily fruit requirement.

To see how this works, suppose someone on a 2,200-calorie diet eats a small orange and a slice of toast for breakfast. Since a small orange equals ½ cup of fruit in MyPyramid, 1½ additional cups of fruit (or the equivalent) are needed during the day. Since the toast counts as 1 ounce, the person needs 6 more ounces of grains.

When estimating food amounts, sometimes you have to take the food apart in your mind. Stir-fries, stews, pizza, and other foods include ingredients from more than one food group. For example, a bowl of cereal with milk covers what two food groups? Other mixtures may take a bit more thought, but classifying them gets easier with practice. How would you break down tacos, for example?

Portion Sizes

While eating out with his family, one teen looked with amazement at the pasta dish he had been served. The pasta came in a bowl that was as large as some serving bowls his family used at home. As this teen noticed, the size of food portions in restaurants can be huge. In fact, portion sizes have increased dramatically in recent years.

As people have become accustomed to large portions, the trend has increased. For instance, many foods sold in supermarkets are bigger than ever. Some bananas and apples are much larger than what you could count as ½ cup. A small bagel might be only 2 or 3 ounces, yet the large size might be 4 or 5. Snacks are sold in larger packages today.

Even for meals at home, people often eat large portions. Although ½ cup of cooked spaghetti (equal to 1 ounce) is a reasonable serving, at least 2 cups often cover a dinner plate.

Many people eat all the food on their plate. As a result, they eat too much and gain weight. An extra 100 calories a day without added exercise can increase your weight by 10 pounds in a year.

Whether it's a restaurant or home portion, amounts are often much larger than the serving sizes in **Fig. 10-3**. A quantity that's too large can put you well over what you need in a day. What impact would a half-pound hamburger have on a 2,200-calorie diet?

You can use several methods to judge food amounts. At home, measure a reasonable serving size of food and put it on a plate. Make a mental note of how much of the plate is covered. Another method compares the food to something familiar, like your whole hand, fist, palm, or fingertip.

Still another method compares amounts to familiar objects. Some examples are shown in **Fig. 10-4**. Once you know what a serving should look like, you won't have to measure the food.

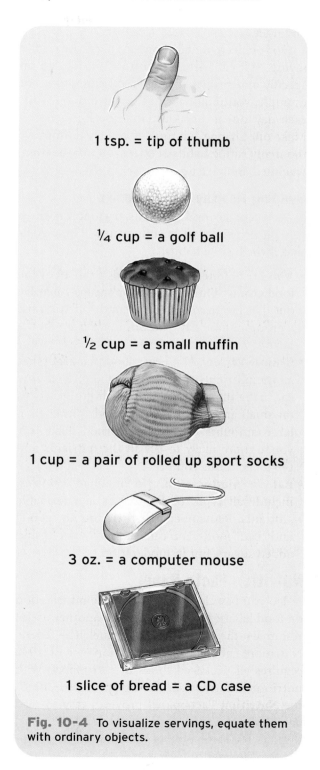

1 tsp. = tip of thumb

¼ cup = a golf ball

½ cup = a small muffin

1 cup = a pair of rolled up sport socks

3 oz. = a computer mouse

1 slice of bread = a CD case

Fig. 10-4 To visualize servings, equate them with ordinary objects.

Checking What You Eat

Using what you've learned, you can evaluate your eating habits. Keep track of what you eat for several days. Then compare total amounts to those in **Fig. 10-2** to see whether you're staying on target.

Do you need to make some changes? Instead of saying, "I'll eat better from now on," decide on specific and realistic changes you can make. For example, you might say, "I'll eat two more fruits each day, one at breakfast and one for a snack." Make one change at a time. If you try to improve too many eating habits at once, you may be overwhelmed and give up.

Building Healthy Eating Habits

As you make food decisions, try to follow three general principles of healthy eating. These goals make worthwhile habits:

- **Aim for balance.** Choose foods from all of the food groups. Omitting a group means you leave out that group's nutrient strengths. If you miss a group on one day, you can make it up on the next.
- **Choose variety.** Not every food in a group has all the nutrients the group provides. Therefore eat many different foods in each group. Focus on small amounts of varied foods rather than large amounts of a few favorites. That way you're more likely to get all the nutrients and phytochemicals you need.
- **Eat in moderation.** To manage calories, include all types of foods, but in reasonable amounts. Remember that there are no "good" and "bad" foods. You can eat foods with fat and added sugars, but in moderation.

Nutrition Facts Panel

Do you pay close attention to the information on food labels? If so, you've found another useful resource—the Nutrition Facts panel. The federal Nutrition Labeling and Education Act of 1990 requires all packaged foods to carry labels with nutrition information. As shown in **Fig. 10-5**, the **Nutrition Facts panel** provides easy-to-read data about the food in the container. Each panel displays the same type of information in a standardized format.

Nutrition Facts

Serving Size   1 cup (228g)
Servings Per Container   2

Amount Per Serving

Calories 260   Calories from Fat 120

	% Daily Value*
Total Fat 13g	**20%**
Saturated Fat 5g	**25%**
Trans Fat 2g	
Cholesterol 30mg	**10%**
Sodium 660mg	**28%**
Total Carbohydrate 31g	**10%**
Dietary Fiber 0g	**0%**
Sugars 5g	
Protein 5g	

Vitamin A 4%	Vitamin C 2%
Calcium 15%	Iron 4%

*Percent Daily Values are based on a 2000 calorie diet. Your daily values may be higher or lower depending on your calorie needs:

		Calories:	2,000	2,500
Total Fat	Less than		65g	80g
Sat Fat	Less than		20g	25g
Cholesterol	Less than		300mg	300mg
Sodium	Less than		2,400mg	2,400mg
Total Carbohydrate			300g	375g
Dietary Fiber			25g	30g

Calories per gram:
Fat 9   •   Carbohydrate 4   •   Protein 4

Fig. 10-5 Nutrition Facts panels can help you identify what nutrients are in a food and how much of each nutrient the food contains.

What's on the Panel?

Near the top of the Nutrition Facts panel, you'll see "Serving Size" and "Servings Per Container." A container with 3 servings of ½ cup each has about 1½ cups in all.

The rest of the label information is based on the single-serving amount shown. You'll see total calories per serving as well as the number of calories from fat per serving. You can use this information to keep track of the number of total calories you eat throughout the day.

The nutrition label also gives per-serving information about some of the nutrients that are significant in a healthy eating plan. Amounts shown (in grams or milligrams) include total fat, saturated fat, trans fat, cholesterol, sodium, total carbohydrates, dietary fiber, sugars, and protein.

For most nutrients and for certain vitamins and minerals, the label also lists "% Daily Value." Expressed as a percentage, **Daily Value** (DV) is set by the federal government and reflects current nutrition recommendations based on a 2,000-calorie diet. DV can be used to compare food products.

Using the Panel

Do you always eat precise serving amounts? Like most people, you probably don't, so you need to adjust label numbers accordingly. Suppose the label on a 46-ounce jar of vegetable juice lists 6 servings of about 8 fluid ounces each. If you drink more or less than the stated serving size, the label data doesn't match what you drank. The vegetable juice label lists 50 calories and 1 gram of protein per serving. If you drink 2 servings (16 fluid ounces), you're actually consuming 100 calories and 2 grams of protein.

The Nutrition Facts panel and other resources can help you evaluate your nutrient intake. See **Fig. 10-6** on pages 150–151. Use **Fig. 10-7** as a guide for estimating some of your nutrient needs.

DIETARY SUPPLEMENTS

"I don't think you should be skipping meals the way you do," one teen said to another. "It's okay," the other teen replied. "I take vitamins." What the second teen didn't realize is that a vitamin tablet isn't a good replacement for real food.

Dietary supplements are substances taken in addition to the foods people eat. Supplements include vitamins, minerals, amino acids, and herbals. They are available as tablets, capsules, liquids, and powders.

For some people, dietary supplements may be useful. People taking certain types of medication, pregnant and nursing women, those recovering from illness, infants, the elderly, and people with special nutrition needs might not be able to get enough nutrients from foods.

Fig. 10-7

Sample Calories for Teens	Carbohydrates (45-65% of Total Calories)	Protein (10-30% of Total Calories)	Total Fat (Limit of 25-35% of Total Calories)
2,800	315-455 g	70-210 g	78-109 g
2,600	293-423 g	65-195 g	72-101 g
2,400	270-390 g	60-180 g	67-93 g
2,200	248-358 g	55-165 g	61-86 g
2,000	225-325 g	50-150 g	56-78 g
1,800	203-293 g	45-135 g	50-70 g

Sample Nutrient Ranges for Teens*

*Ranges computed by multiplying calories times percentage and dividing by the number of calories per gram. Carbohydrates and proteins have 4 calories per gram. Fat has 9 calories per gram.

Most people, however, don't need supplements. They can get all the nutrients they need through balanced and varied eating. Supplements lack the great variety of compounds in foods. People need phytochemicals, fiber, and the whole range of nutrients that foods contain. If they rely on supplements as a substitute for poor food choices, they may be short-changing themselves.

Nutrient Megadoses

Some people take megadoses (MEH-guh-doh-sehs) of dietary supplements. A **megadose** is a very large amount of a supplement that people believe will prevent or cure a disease. Such supplements are sometimes called high-potency.

Excess amounts of some nutrients can accumulate in the body and cause harm. Those that are not stored simply pass out of the body unused, wasting your money. If you need to take supplements for some reason, avoid megadoses. They could be harmful to your health.

Herbals

Herbals are plants used for medicinal purposes. Many have been used for generations and are linked to folklore about their effectiveness.

Fig. 10-6

Checking Up on Nutrients

Don't you wish you had a quarter for every time a parent has said, "Eat your vegetables; they're good for you"? Learning to connect foods with nutrients is a lesson that starts early. You can use nutrition tools and data to build on that lesson.

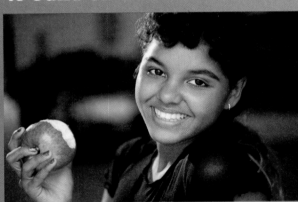

Understanding Nutrient Charts

Nutrition Facts panels are an excellent resource for checking the nutrients in foods. If you eat an orange, however, there's no label. What if a food label has been thrown away? You can learn what nutrients are in foods from charts in references and on the Internet. Fig. A is a sample of a Nutritive Values of Foods chart. Use it to answer these questions:

1. If you eat 1½ cups of vanilla soft serve ice cream, how many grams of total fat and saturated fat did you consume?

2. Which foods have the highest amount of: potassium, vitamin A, niacin?

3. How many calories are in a sandwich made with 2 slices of whole wheat bread and 3 Tbsp. of peanut butter?

4. Of the foods listed, which one has the most sodium?

5. From the chart, what food groups contain the most vitamin C?

Fig. A Sample Chart Showing Nutrient Values of Foods

Food Description	Approx. Measure	Weight	Food Energy	Protein	Carbo-hydrates	Dietary Fiber	Fat	Saturated Fat	Cholesterol
		g	cal	g	g	g	g	g	mg
Banana	1	118	109	1	28	3	1	.2	0
Bread, whole wheat	1 slice	28	69	3	13	2	1	.3	0
Carrots, cooked from raw	½ cup	78	35	1	8	3	<1	t	0
Chicken breast, roasted, no skin	1	172	284	53	0	0	6	1.7	146
Ice cream, vanilla soft serve	1 cup	172	370	7	38	0	22	12.9	157
Peanut butter	2 Tbsp.	32	190	8	6	2	16	3.3	0

< = less than; t = trace; g = grams; mg = milligrams; mcg = micrograms; cal = calories

Examine Your Nutrient Intake

Analyzing what you eat can be informative even though detailed tracking isn't needed all the time. To get a general idea about your nutrient intake, list the amounts of each food and beverage you consume for three to five typical days, including a weekend. Use nutrition analysis software to compare your intake to recommended nutrient amounts, or try this:

1. Create a chart like the one in Fig. A, and list the foods and amounts along the left.

2. Enter nutrient data for each food. Use food labels and nutritive values charts.

3. Total each nutrient and divide by the number of days recorded to get average daily amounts.

4. Compare results to the appropriate DRI recommendations on page 80. Estimate your calorie needs based on Chapter 5. Estimate carbohydrate, protein, and fat amounts, guided by Fig. 10-8 on page 149. Of total fat, no more than 10 percent of calories should be from saturated and trans fats.

5. Analyze the results. Why might these results vary from an analysis done for you by a health professional?

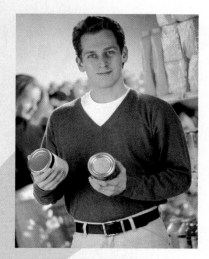

Using Nutritive Values

A Nutritive Values of Foods chart can be used to check the nutrients in meals.

1. Create menus and snacks for one day or use existing meal plans.

2. Make a chart like Fig. A, listing foods along the left.

3. Use a nutritive values chart to fill in nutrient data for the foods listed.

4. Total each nutrient for the whole day, and compare the results to the DRIs on page 80 for an older teen female and male. Remember that individual nutrient needs vary and are balanced over several days.

Calcium	Iron	Magnesium	Potassium	Sodium	Vitamin A	Thiamin	Vitamin E	Riboflavin	Niacin	Folate	Vitamin C
mg	mg	mg	mg	mg	mcg	mg	mg	mg	mg	mcg	mg
7	.37	34	467	1	5	.05	.32	.12	.64	22	11
20	.92	24	71	148	0	.1	.24	.06	1.07	14	0
24	.48	10	177	51	957	.03	.33	.04	.39	11	2
26	1.79	50	440	127	10	.12	.45	.2	23.6	7	0
225	.36	21	304	105	265	.08	.64	.31	.16	15	1
12	.59	51	214	149	0	.03	3.2	.03	4.29	24	0

NUTRITION ANALYSIS SOFTWARE

To make nutrition analysis easier, computer software developers put nutrient data into programs that do the math for you. You enter information about your physical condition, including age, height, weight, gender, and activity level. From this data, the program creates your nutrition needs profile. When you enter a type of food and serving size, the program computes the major nutrients and calories provided, both as a figure and a percentage of your daily needs. This feature helps you analyze menus and plan meals that meet nutrition goals.

Analysis software also has other conveniences. It might create and analyze recipes and generate shopping lists. It may include recipes for specific diets, such as vegan or low-sodium. You can learn your healthful weight range, a recommended caloric intake, and how many calories are burned during various activities.

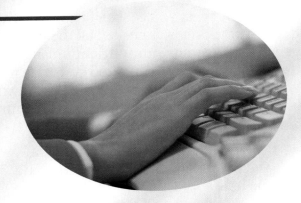

Software must be based on accurate data and is most effective if it has an extensive data bank. Figures from the USDA's nutrient databases are reliable. Programs may list from 5,000 to 20,000 individual food items.

Remember that nutrition analysis software can't replace personal advice from a physician or dietitian. It's simply one more tool for managing your health.

__Think Beyond>> Use nutrition analysis software to create menus for three days. Follow the guidelines in the Dietary Guidelines for Americans.

Many modern medicines are made from plants. One is digitalis (dih-juh-TA-lus), which is used to treat heart failure.

While some herbal products are safe and may be effective, many others can endanger health. Many do not contain the active herbs or are contaminated, which makes them unsafe. They can also interfere with medications. Not enough long-term studies have been done to determine the safety of herbals.

Buying Dietary Supplements

Before taking any supplement, check with a reliable health professional. If you need to buy supplements, read the "Supplement Facts" label, which must appear on the container. It shows the serving size and number of servings in the container. It also lists the amount of each nutrient and other ingredients in each serving and the percentage of the DV. An expiration date is included.

Health experts recommend that people avoid any supplements with more than 100 percent of the DV. Also avoid supplements that contain unfamiliar ingredients.

SEPARATING FACT FROM FICTION

Whether you're watching television, reading a magazine, or surfing the Internet, chances are you'll find information about nutrition. An advertisement promotes a new snack treat. A Web site sells a long list of dietary supplements. A report claims new conclusions in a recent nutrition study. How do you know what to believe? To separate fact from fiction, learn about different types of food information and how to evaluate them.

Food Myths

Do apple cider vinegar and honey have curative powers? For centuries some people believed so. Such food myths persist as they're passed from one generation to another. See **Fig. 10-8**.

Many myths misinterpret information. Are brown eggs more nutritious than white? Actually, egg color depends on the breed of hen. Brown

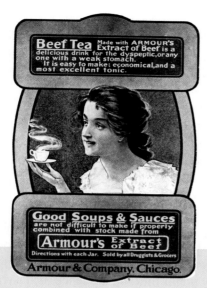

Fig. 10-8 As far back as the 1800s, sellers traveling in wagons from town to town promoted products that could "cure" almost anything. Would they be successful today?

and white eggs are produced by different breeds, but the eggs have the same nutrients.

Another common myth claims sea salt is more nutritious than regular salt. In truth, both have the same amount of sodium chloride, but table salt comes from salt mines and sea salt comes from evaporated seawater. Sea salt may have a few minerals found in the ocean, but not enough to make a difference.

Advertising

Advertising informs and entertains, but its main purpose is to sell a product. Food ads usually emphasize flavor and the pleasure of eating. Nutrition information is secondary—often missing completely. Advertisers want to convince you that their product is good for you and better than the competition, so they may use tactics like these:

- **Limited information.** Advertisements often give only facts that encourage you to buy. A snack food, for instance, may be praised for its flavor and crispiness, but nothing is said about the amount of fat inside.
- **Positive images.** Some advertisers use positive images, including friendship and a pleasing appearance, to convince you that their product will make you feel or look better. The advertiser

hopes you'll associate these images and feelings with the product.

- **Celebrity endorsement.** Some ads show popular performers or athletes promoting a product. Does the person actually use the product? The ad might not tell you.
- **Scare tactics.** Advertisers may play on people's fears of aging or disease by claiming their product can prevent or relieve symptoms.
- **Studies.** Advertisers sometimes use findings from nutrition studies to support product claims. A study quoted may be the only one to disagree with all other studies, but the advertisement doesn't tell you that.
- **Infomercials.** These ads look like regular consumer programs on television or ordinary stories in a magazine or newspaper. Unless you look carefully, you may believe you're watching a television program or reading an article.
- **False claims.** Be alert for statements that are not true. "Fast results guaranteed!" "Eat all the desserts you want and still lose weight!" Remember, if a claim sounds too good to be true, it probably isn't true. See **Fig. 10-9**.

Companies also use other techniques to promote products. A soft drink company may lend its name to a sports event or arrange to have its product shown in a movie. Coupons and eye-catching store displays encourage consumers to buy. Even product packages are a form of advertising.

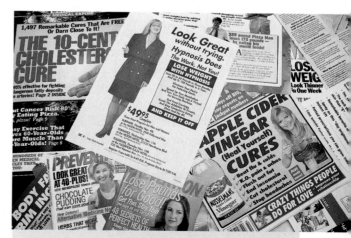

Fig. 10-9 Advertisements and media messages can be hard to resist. What makes them that way?

The Internet

Although the Internet is packed with information, not everything is reliable. Anyone can create a site to inform and sell products. Since Web sites are not screened for accuracy, some have incorrect, even deceptive, information.

Nutrition Fraud

As consumers look for more ways to deal with health problems, nutrition and health fraud becomes a growing concern in society. **Fraud** occurs when people gain something of value, often money, by deceiving others.

Fraudulent schemes appear on the Internet and in advertising claims in newspapers, magazines, and mailings. They may be as basic as selling a useless supplement or as serious as promoting an ineffective cancer cure that causes people to skip the medical care they need.

When someone complains to the Food and Drug Administration (FDA) or the Federal Trade Commission (FTC) about fraud, deceptive information, or unfair business practices, the agencies step in. Until someone complains, however, the offense continues.

Evaluating Information

In today's world you face an endless supply of information. Your challenge is to identify what is accurate and useful. Learning this skill can save you time and money and also help you avoid harm. See **Fig. 10-10**. To evaluate information, put these ideas into practice:

- **Look for the source.** If you hear or read something that seems questionable, be inquisitive. Find the original source of the information. Then investigate. Most food producers have a toll-free number for their consumer service department, or you can contact them on their Web site.
- **Identify Web sites.** Beware of nutrition information on Web sites operated by commercial interests. Look for sites operated by federal, state, and local governments; hospitals; universities; and professional health organizations.
- **Read carefully.** Check dates to find current information. As you read, ask yourself whether

this is a personal opinion or factual information backed up by credible science and research. For studies, read the whole report, not just the headline, which is designed to get your attention but may be misleading. If the report is based on preliminary findings, wait for further evidence. Look for follow-up reports, and compare several studies.

- **Identify funding.** Most studies are done by universities, colleges, and independent research groups, but funding is usually provided by industry and special interest groups. For example, a university study claiming that salt doesn't raise blood pressure was funded by a soup company that uses large amounts of salt in products. How might funding influence such a study?
- **Choose experts.** When you need information, go to an expert. Consult any of the following: a registered dietitian (RD); licensed dietitian (LD); nutritionist; health care professional; health department; family and consumer sciences teacher; professional organizations, such as the American Dietetic Association; or the nutrition department at a college or university. With reliable resources you have the best chance to get sound advice.

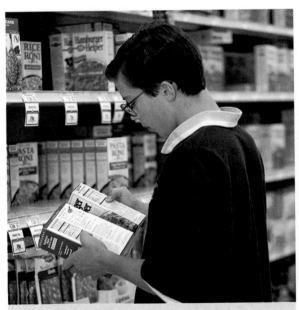

Fig. 10-10 To learn the facts about a product, be analytical. Think, ask questions, and do your research before you believe.

Food Editor

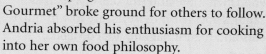

ANDRIA SCOTT HURST: While many adults enjoy visits home to experience the foods of their childhood, Andria Scott Hurst has made a career of it. Andria is senior editor of *All You*, a magazine featuring practical, creative ideas on home and family life. Before that, she spent ten years as food editor for *Southern Living*, the acclaimed magazine of Southern culture and cuisine. Andria's career seems natural since she was inspired by her mother, a talented cook who enjoyed giving parties in their Birmingham, Alabama, home. Yet Andria's career path had different beginnings.

Andria's first career was in retail, but in her words, "My heart kept coming back to food." She traveled and learned about world cuisines. She researched and experimented with ingredients and techniques. This fascination, plus a childhood dream of writing about "romance and adventure," finally changed the course of her career. She returned to school and graduated from the University of Alabama with a degree in English.

Celebrating the South. For Andria early experiences worked to her advantage. When she was finishing school, *Southern Living* needed an assistant food editor. Andria landed the job with personal and professional qualities she had cultivated over the years: a "burning passion for food" and a marketer's eye for interesting stories. A promotion to associate food editor quickly followed.

For a decade Andria guided the *Southern Living* food section, choosing stories, testing and tasting recipes, and approving photos. Travels to discover the history, heritage, and food traditions of the South enabled her to write the Food Finds column. She produced special editions on holiday cooking, summer entertaining, and weddings. On several projects she worked with a longtime favorite personality, celebrity chef Graham Kerr.

In the 1970s, Kerr's popular television show "The Galloping Gourmet" broke ground for others to follow. Andria absorbed his enthusiasm for cooking into her own food philosophy.

A New Adventure. As senior editor of *All You*, Andria is again bringing stories from idea to the printed page. She wants to make food preparation more interesting and rewarding for the everyday cook with articles that meet practical concerns yet fill desires for elegance. Tips for decorating on a budget might be followed by a feature on exotic ingredients for ethnic recipes.

This approach—trying new things and reaching for more in life—is a perfect fit for Andria. After all, she left the security of a good job to begin a new career when retirement could have been on her mind. As a child, Andria may have dreamed of writing about "adventure." As an adult, she is living an adventure. Her secret? "I refuse to recognize any stumbling blocks. If they are there, I just move around them."

On-line Connections

1. To learn more about topics in this article, search the Internet for these key words: *Southern Living* magazine; Southern cooking; Graham Kerr; home entertaining.

2. To learn about related careers, search the Internet for these key words: travel writing; kitchen designer.

Summarize Your Reading

▶ The federal government provides reliable resources for consumers. These include the Dietary Guidelines for Americans, MyPyramid, and Nutrition Facts panels.

▶ Foods with low nutrient density, such as candies and sweet desserts, are low in nutrients and high in fat and added sugars.

▶ To follow eating guidelines correctly, portions of food eaten must be compared to recommended servings.

▶ A Nutrition Facts panel must be displayed on all packaged foods to provide data about the food in the package.

▶ Food myths and advertising might not provide accurate information about nutrients in food and dietary supplements.

▶ All sources of nutrition information should be evaluated to avoid misinformation.

Check Your Knowledge

1. What are the **Dietary Guidelines for Americans**?

2. How are MyPyramid and the USDA Food Guide helpful?

3. Name the basic food groups in the USDA Food Guide.

4. What do foods with high **nutrient density** offer? Give three examples of foods with high nutrient density.

5. What food groups are represented in a taco?

6. Why do people who eat at restaurants often eat more than a recommended serving of food?

7. What methods can you use to judge the portion size of food?

8. What are three basic principles of healthy eating?

9. A friend says she would like to make changes in her eating habits. What can you suggest that will help her be successful?

10. What kind of information is found on a **Nutrition Facts panel**?

11. If a Nutrition Facts panel says the package contains two servings, and you eat the whole package, what do you need to do to make use of the other nutrient information on the panel?

12. Why is it important not to rely on **dietary supplements** to get the nutrients you need?

13. Why do some people take **megadoses** of dietary supplements? In what way can megadoses cause harm?

14. What are **herbals** and how are they used?

15. **CRITICAL THINKING** Why do health experts recommend that people avoid supplements with more than 100 percent of the **Daily Value**?

16. Compare sea salt and regular salt. What is the myth involved?

17. **CRITICAL THINKING** A famous person in a television ad says that a certain supplement improves strength and endurance. What tactic is the advertiser using and how might the information be misleading?

18. How can fraudulent health schemes on the Internet be stopped?

19. What can you do to evaluate health information effectively?

Apply Your Learning

1. **Nutrient Density.** Think of foods with high nutrient density, but that are often prepared and served in ways that reduce nutrient density. Create a class list on the board.

2. **Food Groups.** Find recipes for five dishes that are a mixture of different foods, such as a casserole, pizza, or soup. Study each recipe and list the food groups that are represented.

3. **Web-Site Evaluation.** Develop a checklist to evaluate nutrition Web sites. Then use it to compare two Web sites.

4. **MATH Serving Comparison.** Pour a typical serving of ready-to-eat breakfast cereal into a bowl. Measure the amount and record in a chart. Then measure a recommended serving of 1 ounce. Compare the recommended serving amount to how much you eat. Do this for several foods. What conclusions can you draw?

5. **Menu Analysis.** Using the three principles of healthy eating, analyze a restaurant menu. Would the menu allow people to follow these principles? How could you alter the menu to follow the principles?

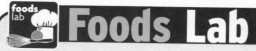

Foods Lab

Food Group Combo

Procedure: Create a salad, sandwich, or other combination as a "model" of the food groups. Use two servings of a grain product as a base, adding other foods from each group. Consider meal appeal as well as nutrition. Plan your creation and make it in the lab or at home.

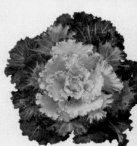

Analyzing Results

❶ What specific nutrients does each food you chose provide?

❷ How did you limit fats and sugars in choosing foods?

❸ How would you improve on this recipe, if at all?

6. **Advertising Analysis.** Find advertisements that illustrate the seven tactics used in food and nutrition advertising. Label and explain each advertisement.

Food Science Experiment

Comparing Fat Content

Objective: To compare amounts of fat in different foods.

Procedure:

1. Rub a small amount of butter into a clean paper towel. Label the spot the butter leaves.

2. Repeat Step 1, using a graham cracker, a snack cracker, a cottage cheese curd, a piece of cheddar cheese, a pretzel, and a piece of caramel-coated popcorn.

3. Observe the spots every 5 minutes for 15 minutes. Record any changes you see.

Analyzing Results

❶ Did any of the spots change? If so, which ones? In what way? Why do you think this occurred?

❷ How do the spots compare to the one left by the butter? What can you conclude from this observation?

Keeping a Healthy Weight

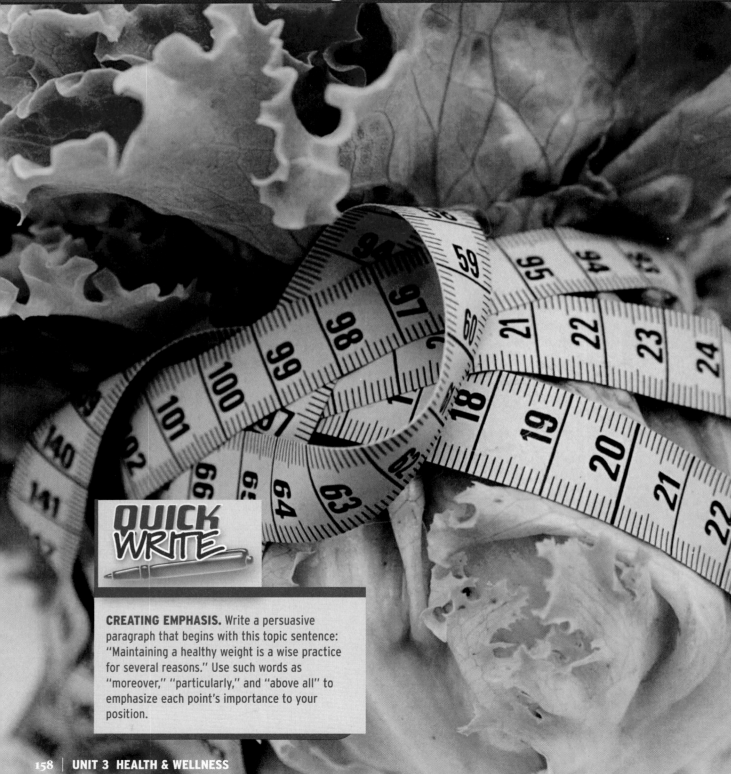

QUICK WRITE

CREATING EMPHASIS. Write a persuasive paragraph that begins with this topic sentence: "Maintaining a healthy weight is a wise practice for several reasons." Use such words as "moreover," "particularly," and "above all" to emphasize each point's importance to your position.

To Guide Your Reading:

Objectives

▶ Explain the impact of unrealistic body images in the media.

▶ Describe causes for the rising number of people who are overweight.

▶ Describe methods for determining a healthy weight.

▶ Give tips for safe, successful weight loss.

▶ Develop an exercise program for weight loss and physical fitness.

▶ Distinguish between fad diets and healthful weight-loss plans.

▶ Describe healthful ways to gain weight.

Terms

aerobic exercise

anaerobic exercise

behavior modification

body fat percentage

body mass index (BMI)

fad diet

I MAGINE THAT AN ALIEN IS VISITING EARTH. Everywhere it looks—in movies, magazines, and newspapers, on television, billboards, and the sides of buses—it sees images of thin, angular women and muscular men. The humans it meets, however, come in a wide range of shapes and weights. The alien is puzzled.

Such confusion is understandable. While the media and fashion industry project images of thinness, many people in society struggle with too much weight. Both of these situations are worth examining, because they affect the well-being of so many people—socially, emotionally, and especially physically. See **Fig. 11-1**.

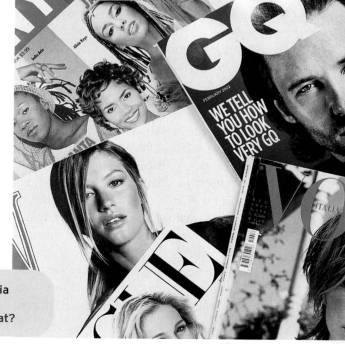

Fig. 11-1 People tend to compare media images of models and celebrities to themselves. What are the dangers in that?

THE IDEAL BODY MYTH

Surveys have found that the average height and weight for a female fashion model is about 5 feet 10 inches and 120 pounds. Compare that to the typical American adult woman at about 5 feet 4 inches and 152 pounds. The average male model stands just over 6 feet and weighs around 155 pounds. His real-life counterpart stands about 5 feet 9 inches, with a weight of about 180 pounds.

People wonder why advertisers and the entertainment media use body images that are so different from how most people look. These images are often viewed as ideals to strive for, which is an impossible goal for most people.

First of all, a person's basic body type is a combination of general body shape and height, which is inherited from biological parents. Genes determine the amount and distribution of fat cells compared to muscle cells, which also strongly influences how easily a person gains or loses weight. These factors cannot be changed.

Also, the slender looks of fashion models and celebrities often result from strict diets and daily workouts. Even then, these "model" figures do not always meet the unrealistic standards. Photos are sometimes touched up to exaggerate good features and gloss over flaws.

On the positive side, some media may finally be inching away from the ultra-thin body images they've been using. Young people today are starting to relate to role models that reflect the diversity and reality they see in themselves.

Health Risks

In their quest for the ideal body, some people diet until they are underweight, depleting the body of both muscle and fat. Muscle loss can lead to fatigue and injury to bones and joints. With too little fat, the body can't store reserves of fat-soluble nutrients. Calcium is lost as supplies of vitamins A and D dwindle. The immune system is weakened. Hormones that regulate normal growth in teens and brain chemicals that stabilize mood and emotions may become imbalanced. Since fat also insulates the body against heat loss, extremely thin people are more stressed by cold weather.

To other people, acquiring the ideal body means adding muscle. They may try high-protein eating plans or protein shakes, bars, and powders. Some people turn to amino acid supplements that promise to build muscle.

Special foods and supplements don't help and may harm. Muscle size is determined by heredity and exercise. Building muscle does take protein, but the body can use only so much at one time. A healthful diet supplies adequate amounts for most people. Extra protein foods can mean extra calories, which may lead to increased fat, not muscle. Moreover, digesting excess protein stresses the kidneys and can promote dehydration.

THE OVERWEIGHT EPIDEMIC

Although starvation is a plight in some parts of the world, overweight is a problem in others, including industrialized nations worldwide. According to the U.S. Department of Health and Human Services, Centers for Disease Control and Prevention, in the United States about 65 percent of all adults are overweight. About 15 percent of children and teens under age eighteen are overweight, a number that has more than doubled in the last 30 years. Some studies suggest even higher numbers.

Carrying excess weight has serious consequences. It puts added strain on bones, muscles, and internal organs. Walking and even breathing take extra effort. Heat and humidity increase the stress, as fat's insulating quality traps body heat. Excessive weight contributes to high blood pressure, heart disease, stroke, diabetes, and certain kinds of cancer. As little as 15 pounds over a healthy weight can raise the chance of early death.

Why Weights Are Rising

One reason for this alarming trend is that modern living makes it easier for people to eat more food than ever, including unhealthful foods. See **Fig. 11-2**. Advertisements and television cooking shows whet the appetite for recipes rich in flavor and calories. Supermarket aisles and vending machines are well stocked with high-fat snacks and sugary soft drinks. People increasingly rely on high-calorie fast foods and highly

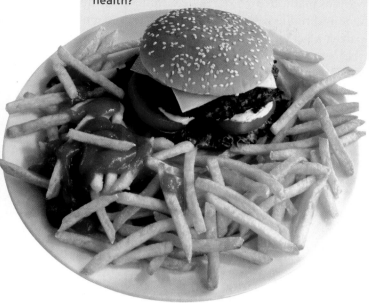

Fig. 11-2 One reason for weight gain is excess calories from foods. If these foods are eaten too frequently, how else can they affect health?

they don't take some factors into account. For instance, everyone has a different skeletal structure, or frame. A person with a heavy frame carries more weight in bone structure than someone of the same height but with a smaller frame.

To assess a person's weight, health professionals use more reliable methods that compare weight to other physical features. These include body mass index and body fat percentage.

Body Mass Index

Body mass index (BMI) uses a ratio of weight to height. The formula for finding BMI is: BMI = weight in pounds × 703 ÷ height in inches, squared (height times itself). Suppose a fifteen-year-old male weighs 137 pounds and stands 5 feet 6 inches (66 inches). His BMI calculations would look like this:

$$137 \times 703 = 96{,}311$$
$$66 \times 66 = 4{,}356$$
$$96{,}311 \div 4{,}356 = 22$$

processed foods, which are available in larger portions. They're eating out more, and restaurant servings may be two or three times the recommended amounts.

At the same time, people are less active. Labor-saving devices and electronic entertainment encourage a "couch potato" lifestyle. Young adults may graduate from a busy school life to a desk job. Unless they eat less or exercise more, weight gain is inevitable. See **Fig. 11-3**.

Also, some people eat for the wrong reasons. Food may be used as a source of comfort or a substitute for love and security. Eating becomes a way to relieve stress, anger, loneliness, and boredom.

Finally, science is learning that some people have a genetic tendency to gain weight more easily than normal. Given the ease with which weight can be gained, this trait is more troublesome today.

WHAT IS A HEALTHY WEIGHT?

An appropriate weight helps people stay healthy throughout life and minimizes the risk of developing diseases. Height and weight charts are widely used to determine a healthy weight, but

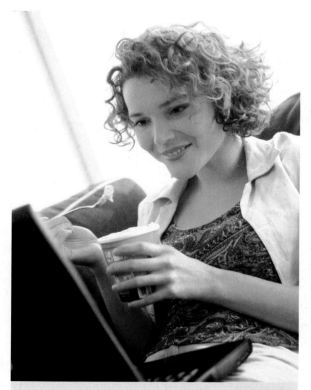

Fig. 11-3 Extra calories, combined with lack of activity, can lead to weight gain. What is the solution?

Charts have been developed to interpret BMI, as shown in **Figs. 11-4**, for teen females, and **11-5**, for teen males. To use a chart, trace your age column until it intersects with your BMI. That point is your percentile. Health professionals consider teens between the 85th and 95th percentile at risk of being overweight. Those with a percentile at or above 95 are overweight. How would you interpret the BMI for the teen described on page 161?

Although it's more accurate than using weight alone, BMI is not a foolproof measure of health or fitness. Athletes and other people with large muscle masses have high BMIs yet are not overweight. A bodybuilder, for example, may have a BMI of 40 or higher. For that reason, some health professionals consider body fat measurements the truer picture of fitness.

Body Fat Percentage

Body fat percentage refers to the amount of body fat a person has in relation to muscle. Various methods are used to determine this ratio. One technique calculates body density by comparing a person's body volume and weight while submerged in a pool. Another method times the speed at which an electrical impulse travels through the body to determine relative amounts of lean and fat tissue.

If interpreted correctly by skilled examiners, tests such as these are accurate to within 2 to 5 percent. Healthy body fat percentages are about 14 to 17 percent for males and 21 to 24 percent for females. People with percentages over these ranges are considered overweight.

Well-conditioned athletes have body fat percentages around 8 percent for males and 18 per-

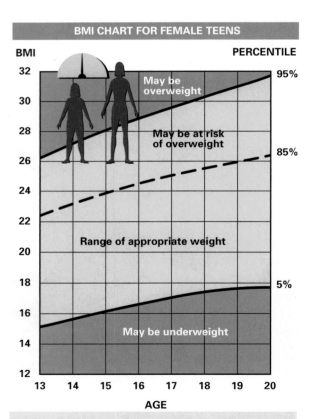

Fig. 11-4 This chart can be used by teen females to interpret body mass index. What is indicated about a female, age eighteen, with a BMI of 24?

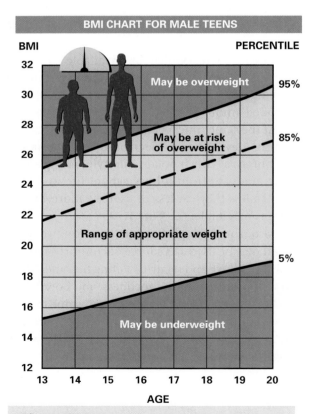

Fig. 11-5 This chart can be used by teen males to interpret body mass index. What is indicated about a male, age sixteen, with a BMI of 24?

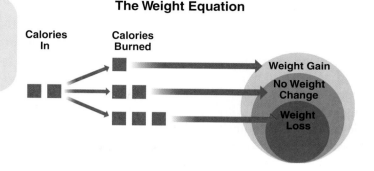

Fig. 11-6 Weight depends on the relationship between calories taken in and calories burned. When these are in balance, what happens? What are the two ways people change that balance?

cent for females. Percentages below these are classed as underweight and may indicate an eating disorder.

A Healthy Weight for You

All the changes teens undergo can complicate life, and that applies to determining a healthy weight. Teens are still growing, but not at a steady pace. For instance, a teen may be overweight just before a growth spurt. Losing weight in this case would be a mistake because once the height increases, it balances out the weight. Maintaining the same weight would be the better goal. Teens mature at individual rates as well, so peers are not reliable predictors of when any one person will experience a sudden growth spurt.

Different growth rates can even occur in the same body. Legs may lengthen and gain muscle before arms do, making the legs look too heavy. Fat cells are redistributed, and females develop more fat deposits. In this case, gaining fat doesn't mean getting fat.

If you're concerned about your weight, comparing yourself to friends or a picture in a magazine won't give you the answer. Instead, talk to a dietitian, a nutritionist, or your health care provider. After learning more about healthy weight, you may discover that you're just fine the way you are.

MANAGING WEIGHT

Identifying a healthy weight is one thing. Achieving that weight is another. Weight management is a kind of budget, a calorie budget. Calories, you'll recall, are units used to measure the energy supplied by food, which fuels the body's life processes and physical activities. Whether you gain, lose, or maintain your weight depends on how many calories you take in and how many you spend. See **Fig. 11-6.**

- If you eat more calories in a day than your body uses, the extra calories are stored as body fat. Over time, you gain weight.
- If your body uses more calories than you get from food, you lose weight.
- If the calories you use during a day equal those you eat, your weight stays the same.

A HEALTHFUL WEIGHT-LOSS PLAN

On a weight-loss diet, you eat fewer calories than you need for activities, forcing your body to use its energy reserves. For example, 1 pound of body fat equals 3,500 calories. Eating 500 fewer calories every day results in a weight loss of 1 pound per week ($500 \times 7 = 3,500$).

The most successful way to achieve and maintain weight loss is through **behavior modification**, making gradual, permanent changes in eating and activity habits. Both limiting calories and increasing activity are essential for lasting weight control.

Any diet should start with a medical exam, to make sure losing weight is necessary and safe. A physician can also make a referral to a dietitian or nutritionist, who can give guidance for cutting calories without neglecting nutrition. This advice is especially important for teens, whose nutritional needs differ from those of adults.

Setting Reasonable Goals

A weight-loss plan is more apt to succeed with realistic goals. Here too a dietitian can help by identifying a healthy weight based on age, height, and gender. Body size and shape must also be considered. See **Fig. 11-7**. For many people, dieting is hard enough without the frustration of trying to reach a clothing size that is unreasonable for their frame.

To focus on a healthy lifestyle, it may be more useful to set goals for positive habits and not just weight loss—to snack on fresh fruit rather than chips, for example. Setting a series of short-range goals, which are also easier to meet, can lead the way to reaching long-range goals.

Health experts suggest 1 to 2 pounds a week as a reasonable weight-loss goal. This rate allows for an eating plan that includes satisfying food choices yet limits calories. The body adjusts more easily to its lower weight when the change comes gradually. Also, the weight is more likely to come from body fat and not muscle.

Changing Eating Habits

The ultimate goal of a healthy weight-loss plan is to develop positive, enjoyable eating habits. Losing weight is just one of its rewards. The fol-lowing suggestions are useful for gaining both of these benefits:

- Eat a variety of foods to avoid monotony and keep the diet enjoyable. Learn to use herbs and spices to flavor foods.
- Choose such foods as fruits, vegetables, whole-grain products, and dry beans. The high fiber content helps you feel full with fewer calories.
- Drink enough liquids each day. Drinking a glass of water before you eat helps decrease your appetite.
- Don't skip meals. If you skip breakfast or lunch, you'll be so hungry that you'll be more likely to snack and overeat later in the day.
- Watch your portion sizes. Each day make sure that you stay within the recommended number of servings for each of the food groups.
- Control emotional eating. If you use food to cheer yourself up, look for other methods. You might take up a hobby, visit with friends, go for a walk, or join a special interest group.
- Eat moderate amounts of healthy fats—polyunsaturated and monounsaturated. Fats are essential nutrients but high in calories.
- Limit your use of high-calorie beverages, such as soft drinks, fruit juice, and fruit drinks.

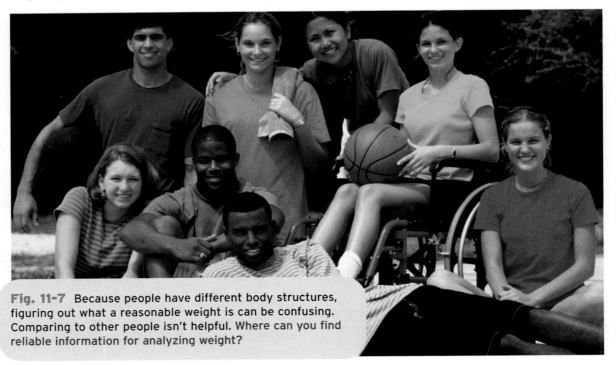

Fig. 11-7 Because people have different body structures, figuring out what a reasonable weight is can be confusing. Comparing to other people isn't helpful. Where can you find reliable information for analyzing weight?

- Cut down on high-calorie, high-fat, and high-sugar foods, such as french fries, chips, cookies, pastries, and candy.
- Don't assume that fat-free and low-fat foods are much lower in calories than the regular products. Compare products by using the calorie information on nutrition labels.

Increasing Physical Activity

For weight loss, some experts believe that physical activity is even more important than cutting calories. First, regular exercise increases "spending" in the calorie budget. Adding activities that use 100 calories a day, for instance, sheds 10 pounds in a year (100 calories × 365 days a year = 36,500 calories ÷ 3,500 = 10.4). **Fig. 11-8** shows how many calories are expended in daily activities and exercise.

Exercise plays an important role in maintaining weight loss. Physical activity speeds metabolism by increasing energy use. It also develops muscle, which takes more energy to maintain than fat does.

Staying active has other benefits as well. It boosts energy and builds endurance. It supports healthy bones, muscles, and joints, to help the skeletal system stay strong and flexible throughout life. By lowering cholesterol and strengthening the heart, regular exercise helps lower the risk of heart disease, high blood pressure, diabetes, and some cancers.

Physical exercise even promotes psychological health by easing stress and anxiety. Studies show that active people have a brighter outlook on life.

Types of Exercise

Any activity that uses one or more muscle groups is a form of exercise. Even some chores, such as cleaning, cooking, and washing the car, fit that description. Exercise of all sorts can be divided into two basic types. A well-rounded exercise program includes both.

Aerobic exercise (auhr-OH-bik) is vigorous activity that increases the heart and breathing rate for at least 20 minutes. Aerobic means "using oxygen." During aerobic exercise, the heart and lungs send more oxygen to the blood, allowing the muscles to work harder for a sustained length of time. The presence of oxygen also permits the body to metabolize fat.

Fig. 11-8

Calories Used in Activities

The number of calories used in an activity depends on age, gender, and weight. Heavier people will use more calories than those who weigh less. The calories listed here are average numbers for someone weighing 150 pounds.

Activity	Calories Used in 30 Minutes	Activity	Calories Used in 30 Minutes
Standing in line	50	Food shopping with a cart	125
Working at a computer	50	Cycling at 5 miles per hour	125
Cooking	90	Vigorous dancing	150
Mowing lawn with power mower	100	Raking leaves	150
Auto repair	100	Rollerblading	160
Playing table tennis	100	Playing tennis	180
Recreational swimming	110	Heavy physical labor	180
Walking 3 miles an hour	120	Playing basketball	180
House cleaning	120	Shoveling snow	200

Aerobic exercises include walking, jogging, climbing stairs, bicycling, aerobic dancing, and swimming. Exercising at a steady, moderately intense pace enables the heart and lungs to supply enough oxygen to the body. Teens should aim for 60 minutes of activity daily.

Anaerobic exercise (a-nuh-ROH-bik) involves short, intense bursts of activity. Anaerobic, as you might guess, means "without oxygen." In anaerobic exercise, the muscles work hard and quickly. They burn glycogen, the form of carbohydrate stored in the cells for immediate use. While this brief exertion doesn't tap fat cells, it does build muscle, raising the metabolic rate. See **Fig. 11-9**.

Running a 100-meter dash is an example of an anaerobic activity. So too is resistance training, which increases muscle strength and endurance. Resistance, or strength, training conditions muscles by requiring them to resist force. The greater the resistance, the stronger the muscles become. Resistance can be provided by weights, machines, or your own body weight, as in push-ups. Resistance training should be done at least twice a week.

Enjoying the Activity Habit

Many people plunge into strenuous activity without preparation. This can do more harm than good. Starting slowly and learning the proper technique for an activity helps prevent injury. Even people who feel healthy should get a medical checkup first.

You're more likely to stick with an activity that holds your interest, one that you can learn easily and do well. It should also fit your lifestyle, schedule, and personality. Games and sports, from bowling to rollerblading, offer chances to meet people and have fun with friends. Many people enjoy dancing or working out to music. Others like to relax with yoga. See **Fig. 11-10**.

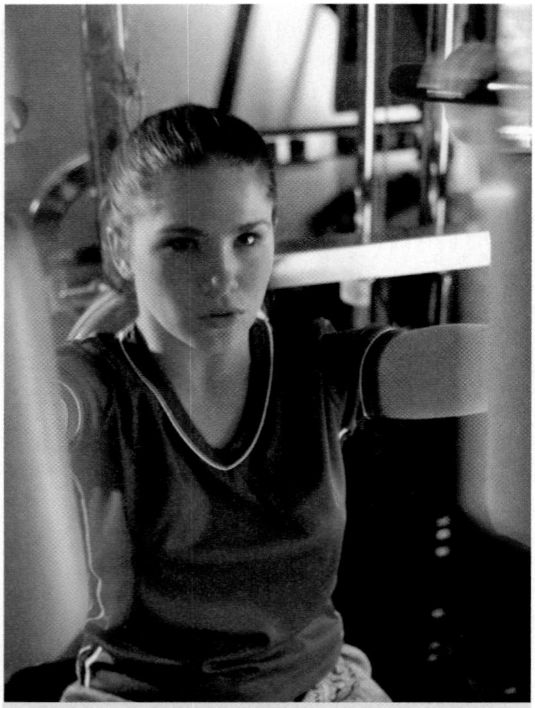

Fig. 11-9 An exercise program should include two types of exercise: aerobic and anaerobic. Which type is this?

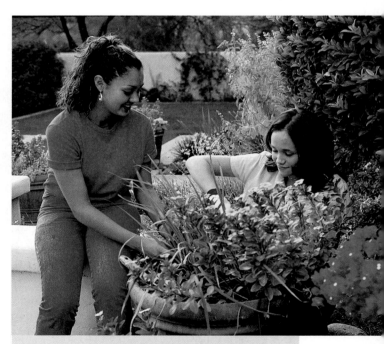

Fig. 11-10 Exercise doesn't always have to be vigorous activity. A hobby like gardening burns calories too. What other activities would be effective?

There is an activity to fit almost every budget. Some equipment can run several thousand dollars. On the other hand, you can start an aerobic program with a sturdy, comfortable pair of walking shoes. Heavy cans make serviceable weights for resistance training.

Setting achievable goals adds challenge and motivation to an exercise routine. Beware of the "no pain, no gain" approach, however. Pain during exercise is a sign that something should be changed—the technique, the equipment, or the activity itself.

Not everyone has 60 minutes to spend on an activity at one time. Studies show that short bouts of exercise throughout the day can have health effects similar to those of longer workouts. Light weight lifting during television commercials perks up the metabolism. Jogging in place between study sessions refreshes the brain and body with oxygen.

As your fitness increases, you may look for other ways to add activity to life. You might look for stairs rather than elevators and find scenic bike routes to the store or a friend's home. You might even take up a new sport.

COMMERCIAL WEIGHT-LOSS PLANS

With so much attention focused on health and appearance, weight loss has become big business. Bookstores, the Internet, and other media are filled with publications and Web sites promoting weight-loss diets, weight-loss centers, weight-loss pills, weight-loss shakes, and prepared meals. See **Fig. 11-11**.

Many of these plans are easily recognized as **fad diets**, popular weight-loss methods that ignore sound nutrition principles. Such diets often "guarantee" dramatic results—lose 10 pounds a week while you sleep, for example. Some allow as little as 800 calories per day. Some require fasting. Other diets drastically reduce basic nutrients or eliminate food groups. They may call for rotating among single foods: cabbage soup one week, citrus fruits the next. Some advocate replacing needed carbohydrates with extra protein foods that are high in fat. To gain dieters'

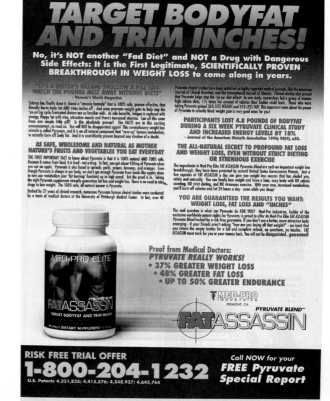

Fig. 11-11 Fad diets and weight-loss products are enticing because they make promises that people want to hear. Unfortunately, the diets are typically difficult to follow long term, and some methods can even be threatening to health.

confidence, many cite scientific-sounding "evidence" to explain how their particular method works.

All of these fad diets have one trait in common: they are temporary plans that do not encourage sound eating habits. Any weight lost is quickly regained as dieters feel the need to return to their old ways. As a result, some people become chronic dieters, jumping from one plan to another, losing and regaining weight.

How can you spot a plan that is based on sound nutrition? Test it with these questions:

- Is the program developed by a qualified health professional, such as a dietitian or nutritionist?
- Does it include nutritional counseling and an individualized eating plan?

- Does it offer a variety of appealing foods from all major food groups?
- Does it supply adequate amounts of needed nutrients?
- Does it make reasonable claims for weight loss?
- Does it teach healthful eating habits?

After finding a trustworthy weight-loss program, more fact finding can show whether it fits on other accounts. What is the initial cost? Are there added expenses, such as dietary supplements or a certain line of prepared meals? How long does the contract last? Can it be cancelled at any time? Does the plan include menus for maintaining weight? Does it provide support in the form of group meetings or on-line chat rooms?

GAINING NEEDED WEIGHT

Gaining weight can be just as challenging as losing weight. People who are concerned about being too thin should discuss the matter with a health professional. They may have a naturally high metabolic rate, or there may be a medical reason for an inability to put on weight.

Here are some hints to help those who need to gain weight:

- Eat three meals a day as well as frequent snacks.
- Eat the higher number of recommended servings from each of the five main food groups.

- Add extra calories to the food you eat. For example, add nonfat dry milk or wheat germ to puddings, mashed potatoes, soups, stews, casseroles, vegetables, and cooked cereals. Spread peanut butter on bagels. Add mayonnaise to sandwiches. Add nuts and cheese to vegetables and salads. See **Fig. 11-12**.
- Drink fluids only between meals or at the end of the meal. Don't drink them just before or with a meal because they can make you feel full.
- Choose calorie-containing fluids, including juice, milk shakes, and smoothies.
- Stay active. Exercise can increase the appetite. It also assures that the weight gained is muscle, not fat.

MAINTAINING A HEALTHY WEIGHT

Remember that maintaining a healthy weight is a balancing act—balancing energy eaten in foods with energy used in physical activity. Changes in body size and composition change basal metabolism. A smaller body runs on fewer calories. More calories are needed to support added weight. New eating and exercise habits must remain part of the daily routine. Understanding the basics of weight maintenance is one of the keys to supplying your body with a lifetime of good nutrition.

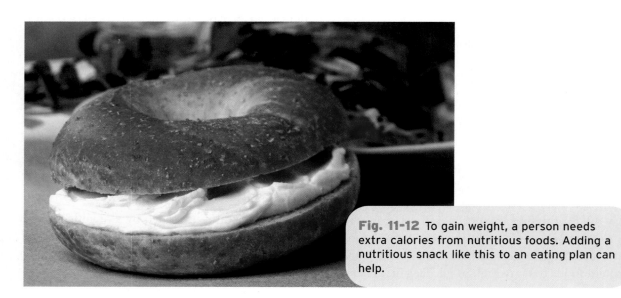

Fig. 11-12 To gain weight, a person needs extra calories from nutritious foods. Adding a nutritious snack like this to an eating plan can help.

Career Pathways

Fitness Consultant

PETER NIELSEN: For a man who lost a year and a half of high school, twelve inches of intestine, and nearly his life to a debilitating disease, Peter Nielsen looks remarkably healthy. Of course, good health is his business—and also his mission.

Peter lives with Crohn's disease, a painful inflammation that prevents the body from fully absorbing nutrients. The ailment hit him full force in his teens, turning a 138-pound high school hockey player into an 86-pound invalid. The emotional impact was devastating. Coming to terms with the disease meant overcoming anger and self-pity. It meant confronting the fear of dying or of living with chronic pain. For Peter, being forced to face these possibilities was a wake-up call. "You realize you could be gone in the blink of an eye or a heartbeat." It inspired a resolution to "maximize" his life.

Rising Above. Part of the process was reclaiming physical health. In his family's small Brooklyn, New York, apartment, Peter found a space to lift weights, amidst the hanging laundry. He turned self-pity to self-challenge. "I loved weightlifting because the sport was me against me." Within three years, Peter earned the Teenage America title in bodybuilding. Three years later he added the American Grand Prix crown, followed by back-to-back wins as Mr. International Universe. His impressive string of victories in competitive bodybuilding continued for ten years.

Meanwhile, Peter built a career as a fitness consultant and therapist. His first training club opened in Farmington Hills, Michigan, in 1985, followed by two more. He has produced books, videos, and countless magazine columns on fitness and nutrition. He promotes "Peter's Principles" of good health on local and national radio and television and on his Web site. Health and bodybuilding magazines have named him a top fitness trainer. In 1996, Peter achieved a sure sign of success in today's society: he became the first bodybuilder in the country with his own collectible trading card.

For all his personal fortitude and talent, Peter is quick to credit success to his education, saying that without it "I would have been doomed." He holds a bachelor's degree in nutrition from Brooklyn College and a master's certification in fitness science from the International Sports Science Association.

The Ongoing Challenge. All the while, the battle with Crohn's disease continues. It required emergency, life-saving surgery in 2000 at the peak of Peter's fitness and success. Today he monitors his diet carefully. His public campaign against the illness includes serving as national spokesman for the Crohn's and Colitis Foundation of America. His goal is to educate but also to motivate. "I want to shout out to the world how fragile our bodies are, how fragile our health is, and how each and every day is a blessing."

On-line Connections

1. To learn more about topics in this article, search the Internet for these key words: Crohn's disease; International Sports Science Association; physical fitness; strength training.

2. To learn about related careers, search the Internet for these key words: physical therapy; sports medicine.

Summarize Your Reading

▶ The body images often promoted in society do not reflect the wide range of shapes and weights found in the general population.

▶ People gain weight when they eat more calories than their bodies can use.

▶ Because everyone has a different skeletal structure, a person's body weight should be assessed by a health professional to determine a healthy weight.

▶ An exercise program should be started slowly and should include interesting activities that fit your budget.

▶ Healthful plans for losing or gaining weight are based on sound nutrition and healthful eating habits.

Check Your Knowledge

1. **CRITICAL THINKING** A friend is determined to lose weight to get the thin, angular look of a fashion model. What would you say to her?

2. What are the risks of dieting until a person is underweight?

3. What are the risks of carrying excess weight?

4. Why are weights rising?

5. **CRITICAL THINKING** Predict consequences in the U.S. if people don't take overweight and obesity seriously.

6. **CRITICAL THINKING** Evaluate the **BMI** of these teens: a sixteen-year-old female who is 5 feet 8 inches and weighs 152 pounds; a seventeen-year-old male who is 5 feet 11 inches and weighs 185.

7. In what way can **body fat percentage** be determined?

8. Why are healthy weights very individual?

9. What two things must a person do to lose weight? Why is each important?

10. Why is **behavior modification** the best way to achieve and maintain weight loss?

11. Why is losing 1 to 2 pounds per week a reasonable goal?

12. How does drinking water before meals help a person lose weight?

13. How does exercise help a person maintain weight loss?

14. Compare **aerobic exercise** and **anaerobic exercise.**

15. What should you do if exercise is causing pain? Why?

16. Why don't **fad diets** work?

17. List qualities of a weight-loss plan that is based on sound nutrition.

18. How can a recipe be calorie enriched for a person who needs to gain weight?

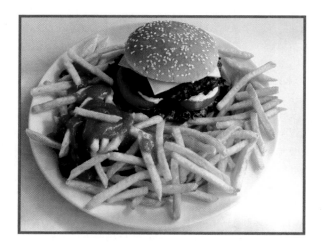

Apply Your Learning

1. **LANGUAGE ARTS** **Weight-Loss Success.** Interview someone who has lost weight and kept it off for a year or more. Report to the class about how the plan worked and why it was successful.

2. **MATH** **Exercise Plan.** Suppose a person plans to lose 5 pounds every month. Part of the plan includes cutting 350 food calories each day. Complete the plan by creating a schedule of weekly exercises that will enable the person to reach the overall monthly weight-loss goal.

3. **Weight-Loss Plans.** Work with a classmate to evaluate two commercial weight-loss plans, using the criteria in the text. How do the plans rate? Suggest changes that would help dieters be more successful.

4. **MATH** **Weight Gain.** How many added calories would a person need to eat to gain 4 pounds? What foods in what amounts could be added to the diet to result in the weight gain over a five-week period?

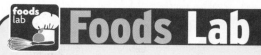

Foods Lab

Weight-Friendly Snacks

Procedure: With your lab team, make a list of simple snacks that would be reasonable to include in an eating plan for people who want to manage their weight. The snacks should be easy to prepare, low in fat and calories, nutritious, and tasty. Choose two snacks to prepare and sample in the foods lab.

Analyzing Results

❶ Why are taste and ease of preparation important considerations when planning snacks?

❷ If someone wants to lose weight, how might snacks cause problems? How might they help?

❸ After sampling the snacks you made, how would you rate them on ease of preparation, fat and calorie content, nutrition, and taste?

Food Science Experiment

Burning Calories

Objective: To demonstrate how chemical processes release the energy in food.

Procedure:

1. Carefully sink the eye of a needle into a cork. Mount a shelled nut on the sharp end of the needle.

2. Remove both ends of a large can and one end of a small can. Punch two holes opposite each other near the open end of the small can.

3. Pour ⅓ cup water into the small can. Record the water's temperature.

4. Run a skewer through the holes in the small can and rest it on the rim of the large can.

5. Following lab safety rules, place the nut and cork on a piece of aluminum foil and light the nut with a match. Set the large can over the nut. Let the nut burn until the flame goes out.

6. Stir the water with the thermometer. Record the water's highest temperature.

Analyzing Results

❶ How much did the water temperature change? What does this change represent?

❷ Supposed you had burned a kernel of air-popped popcorn. Would you expect the temperature change to be greater, smaller, or the same? Explain.

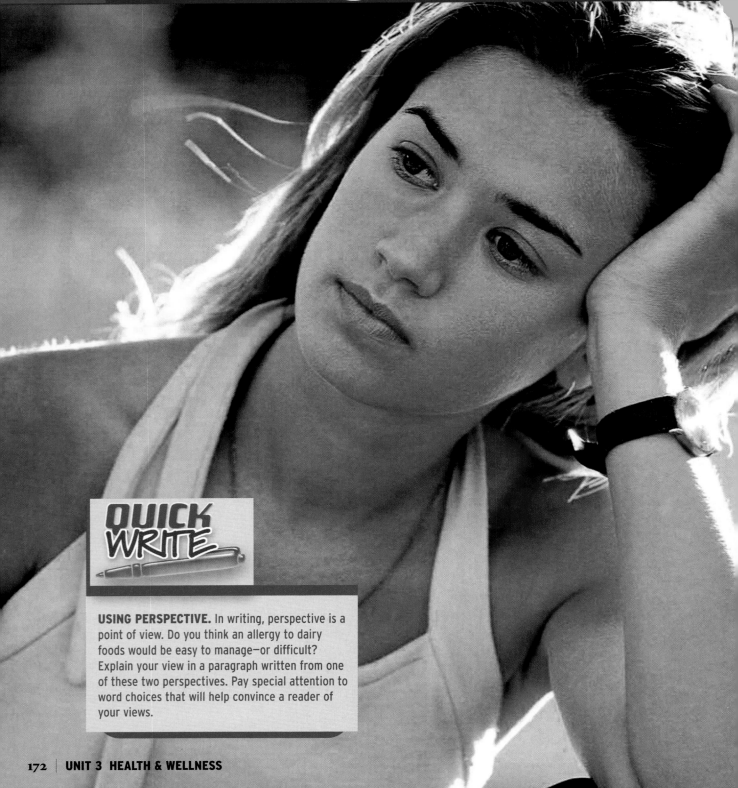

Health Challenges

QUICK WRITE

USING PERSPECTIVE. In writing, perspective is a point of view. Do you think an allergy to dairy foods would be easy to manage—or difficult? Explain your view in a paragraph written from one of these two perspectives. Pay special attention to word choices that will help convince a reader of your views.

Objectives

▶ Explain the relationship between stress and nutrition.

▶ Suggest eating guidelines for stressful times.

▶ Describe various ways to cope with stress.

▶ Explain the role of nutrition in recovery from illness or injury.

▶ Summarize how eating plans can be adapted for people with chronic health conditions.

▶ Describe causes, signs, health effects, treatment, and prevention of eating disorders.

Terms

anorexia nervosa

binge eating disorder

bulimia nervosa

chronic

diabetes

eating disorders

food allergy

food intolerance

HIV/AIDS

stress

W HEN SOME PEOPLE GET A COLD, THEY HEAT a bowl of chicken noodle soup or pour a glass of orange juice to help fight off the illness. That's not a bad idea. Nourishing food and good eating habits can't cure diseases, except for nutrient deficiencies, but they are vital in treating many health challenges. See **Fig. 12-1**.

STRESS

Suppose a friend complains, "What a lousy day! First, I really messed up an exam. Then my folks asked me again what I want to do after high school, and we fought about it. My boss wants me to work late, but I really need to write a paper. Why did I even get out of bed?"

Your friend's troubles have two things in common: first, they happen in the lives of many teens; second, they can all lead to feelings of stress.

Stress is physical or mental tension caused by a person's reaction to a situation. Notice that situations don't cause stress; stress depends on how

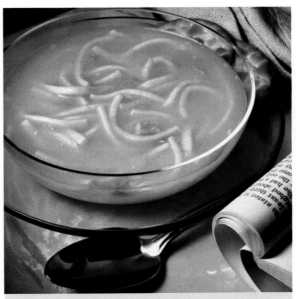

Fig. 12-1 When a cold strikes, people often turn to that age-old remedy, a bowl of chicken noodle soup. The broth provides needed fluid and the warmth is soothing.

people respond to them. That's why different events trigger stress for different people. Some people feel anxious about giving a speech; others enjoy it. A poor grade may frustrate one person, yet it motivates another to do better. Even going on a date, receiving an award, and other positive events can be stressful.

Whatever the situation, stress often upsets the body and the mind alike, with headaches, backaches, insomnia, and irritability. Prolonged stress can weaken the immune system, your body's defense against disease.

Stress and Nutrition

Like many health challenges, stress can have the physical effect of shutting down the appetite. Some people, however, feel an emotional need for calorie-rich, nutrient-low comfort food. Either way, stress can make it harder to eat properly, yet stressful times are just when eating right is most important.

Stress, again like other health challenges, makes physical demands on the muscles and internal organs. Ice cream, chips, and cookies don't supply the sustained energy needed to meet these demands. In fact, digesting the fat they contain taxes the body further. Heavy foods can lead to digestive upsets, which are already more likely in times of stress.

In contrast, eating well strengthens you. Stick to the guidelines for good nutrition. If stress dulls your appetite, be sure to schedule time for nourishing meals. Add appeal by varying food colors, shapes, textures, and temperatures. Avoid filling up on fluids before or during meals. If you tend to snack more when you're stressed, stock up on fruit, yogurt, and other healthful choices. Avoid caffeinated beverages. Caffeine is a stimulant that can aggravate stress.

Coping with Stress

Despite its reputation, stress originally served a valuable purpose. It readied people to take action in the face of danger. Today, the "danger" may be a major school assignment or a troubled friendship, but taking action is still a good way to defuse stress. Start research for the school project. Reach out to heal the friendship. See **Fig. 12-2**.

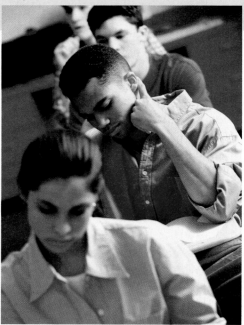

Fig. 12-2 Taking a test is just one stressful situation. If you're someone who feels stress at test time, what could you do to lessen those feelings?

Sometimes, however, stress is energy wasted. You need to learn to recognize these times and to cope positively. In addition to following a nutritious diet, these hints can help:

- Accept what you cannot change. You can't change other people. You can't always change the situation. You can change the way you react to both.
- Develop a sense of humor. Learn to laugh at yourself and your mistakes. Laughter is a good way to relieve body tension. Humor puts things in perspective.
- Take one step at a time. If you worry about all the work you have to do, the task may seem impossible. Break it up into small parts and handle just one at a time. Concentrate on the step before you and don't worry about the others. You'll get more done with less tension.
- Talk over problems with a close friend, relative, health professional, or counselor. Remember, problems feed on worry. Talking often shrinks them down to size.

- Keep physically fit. A fit body copes with life's situations more easily, and physical activity can work off tension. Include exercise on your daily agenda. Wash the car, clean a closet, or do some other useful task.
- Take time for rest and recreation. Getting enough sleep each day helps you handle stress better. Include leisure time too. Spend time on a favorite hobby, visit with a friend, or go to a movie. Relax with a good book or CD. See **Fig. 12-3**.
- Criticize less and praise more. Fault finding can be a habit that leads to anger and self-pity. Instead of criticizing, help someone or work for a solution. Look for something positive in a person or situation, no matter how small, and be grateful for it.
- Don't use drugs to relieve stress, and don't use medications unless advised by your physician. Alcohol, tranquilizers, pep pills, and antacids only ease the symptoms. Their effects wear off and the problems remain. They may even lead to more serious problems.

ILLNESS AND RECOVERY

"Feed a cold; starve a fever." That bit of folk wisdom is only partly right. "Starving" an illness only starves the ill person. A well-nourished body is better equipped to handle any ailment—fever, cold, or broken ankle.

Illness and recovery bring special concerns that are related to nutrition. Some of these are described here:

- **Food-drug interactions.** Certain foods and supplements can alter the effects of certain drugs, and vice versa. A food decrease or increase might affect the absorption of a drug, thereby affecting the level in the body. Calcium binds to some antibiotics, preventing the body from absorbing either one. Some medicines, meanwhile, are better tolerated when taken with a meal. A physician or pharmacist can give detailed instructions for when and how to take medication.
- **Fluids.** Fluids are particularly important when illness strikes, especially a cold or flu. They

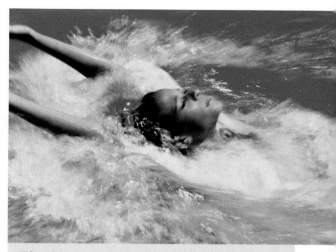

Fig. 12-3 When tension strikes, you can ease the feelings by doing something. Quiet activities can help, but many people find stress relief in energetic activities.

replace water lost to vomiting or perspiration from fever. Cool liquids help control a high temperature. Fluids help moisten nasal and sinus tissue to prevent irritation. Liquid foods are more soothing to sore throats, encouraging the appetite.
- **Calories.** While nutrient needs remain the same, calorie needs may drop if an injury forces a long period of inactivity. Choosing nutrient-dense foods can prevent unwanted weight gain.

CHRONIC HEALTH PROBLEMS

Chronic health problems are long-term or recurring. Managing some of these conditions includes following a special eating plan, or medical nutrition therapy. A dietitian or nutritionist will make specific recommendations, but general guidelines for some major chronic disorders are described here:

- **High cholesterol.** High levels of blood, or serum, cholesterol increase the risk of heart disease and stroke. Medical nutrition therapy includes cutting back on foods high in cholesterol and saturated fat and adding foods high in fiber. Soy proteins are also believed to help control serum cholesterol.

- **High blood pressure.** High blood pressure is also a risk factor for heart disease as well as other medical problems. The most useful diet to reduce blood pressure is low in sodium and saturated fats and rich in calcium, potassium, and magnesium.
- **Diabetes. Diabetes** is a condition in which the body cannot control blood sugar levels. Untreated, it can do serious damage, especially to the kidneys, eyes, and heart. To stabilize blood sugar levels, carbohydrate intake is rationed through regular meals and careful food choices. High-fiber foods may slow carbohydrate digestion and absorption, benefiting blood sugar control.
- **HIV/AIDS. HIV/AIDS** is a disorder that weakens the immune system. HIV-infected people experience nutrition-related problems, including poor appetite, nausea, diarrhea, weight loss, and changes in body composition. Proper nutrition and exercise can help with these problems. In addition, because HIV-infected people are susceptible to foodborne illness, safe food handling is as essential as good nutrition.

Food Sensitivities

Some chronic conditions involve food itself. A **food allergy** is an abnormal response to certain foods by the body's immune system. A trace of the food can trigger symptoms that range from a rash, to stomach cramps and nausea, to trouble breathing. Death occurs in rare cases. Fish, shellfish, eggs, nuts, and peanuts are common triggers for adults. Children are more susceptible to cow's milk, eggs, peanuts, wheat, and soy.

A **food intolerance** is also an adverse physical reaction to food but does not involve the immune system. Reactions are usually less serious digestive problems. For example, some people can't digest lactose, the sugar in cow's milk.

Treating food sensitivities seems simple enough: just avoid the food. People with lactose intolerance can substitute lactose-reduced or soy products. Other times it isn't so simple. A food may be a small or unexpected ingredient in another product—milk proteins in processed meats, for instance. The FDA now requires food allergens to be clearly identified on food labels. For example, to help someone who is allergic to soy, an ingredient list might say "TVP (soy)," or a statement on the label might read "Contains soy."

Eating Plan Strategies

For those with a chronic health condition, following a special eating plan takes a greater awareness of food choices. It means carefully reading food labels and recognizing nutrients and ingredients that must be limited or increased, or looking for fortified products. It means asking restaurant staff about how foods are prepared and requesting special orders if needed.

Eating plans can be opportunities to explore new foods and cooking skills. For instance, a fresh tomato sauce with blended herbs and spices fits a low-fat, low-sodium diet. Many medical centers offer cooking classes for different nutritional needs. See **Fig. 12-4**. Supportive family and friends who try new recipes and share healthful habits also help make the experience positive.

EATING DISORDERS

To people with eating disorders, food is not a physical threat, but a psychological one. **Eating disorders** are conditions marked by extreme emotions, attitudes, and behaviors related to

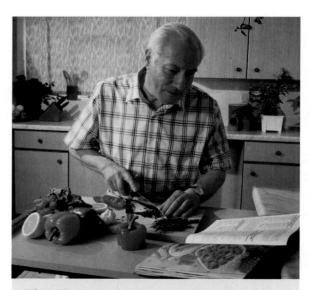

Fig. 12-4 Cookbooks and other references help people with chronic health conditions manage their diet.

food, eating, and weight. These recognized illnesses can damage health and even threaten life. They occur most among teens and young adults, especially females. Anyone can be affected, however, even children as young as eight years old. Numbers are sketchy but suggest that from one to ten percent of all teens have an eating disorder.

Anorexia Nervosa

People with **anorexia nervosa** (a-nuh-REK-see-uh nur-VOH-suh) have an intense fear of gaining weight, although they are extremely thin. Even if dangerously underweight from eating very little, they see themselves as fat.

Food, eating, and dieting become obsessions for people with anorexia. They develop unusual—and often very rigid—eating habits and rituals. They may avoid group meals, eat only a few certain foods, or eat at certain times. Food may be precisely weighed, measured, and arranged on the plate. It may be cut into tiny pieces or extensively chewed. To lose weight, people with anorexia frequently spend hours in strenuous exercise. They may spend less time with friends and give up some activities.

This starvation diet takes a toll. It can lower the heart rate, breathing rate, blood pressure, and body temperature. It can lead to heart problems, osteoporosis, and constipation. It can stunt growth in teens and children and stop menstruation in females past puberty. Anorexia kills about five percent of all those who suffer from it, most commonly by heart attack, electrolyte imbalance, and suicide.

Binge Eating Disorder

People who have a **binge eating disorder** eat abnormally large amounts of food in a short time, called bingeing. During a bingeing episode, they cannot control what or how much they eat— from 3,000 to 5,000 calories in some cases. They may literally eat themselves sick. See **Fig. 12-5**. An eating binge usually occurs when the person is alone and is usually followed by feelings of guilt, disgust, and depression. This disorder leads to excessive weight gain, with related problems of high blood pressure, high cholesterol, heart disease, and diabetes. The unbalanced diet and emotional distress also damage health.

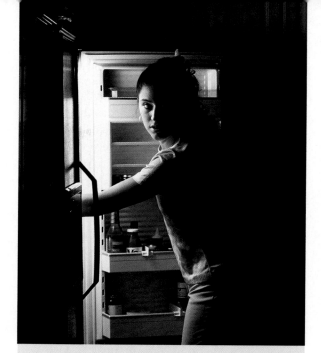

Fig. 12-5 During a binge eating episode, a person with an eating disorder might consume thousands of calories. How does this compare to anorexia nervosa?

Bulimia Nervosa

With **bulimia nervosa** (byoo-LEE-mee-uh), binge eating is followed by purging to rid the body of the food and calories and prevent weight gain. Purging methods include self-induced vomiting; abuse of laxatives, diet pills, and diuretics (water-removal pills); fasting; and excessive exercise. The binge-purge cycle becomes a way of life. Two or more episodes a week are common.

Bulimia hides itself well. Like people with anorexia, bulimics fear getting fat, but usually stay within 10 to 15 pounds of a healthy weight. Signs of the disorder are more subtle—missing food and empty food containers, for example, or the discovery of laxatives or diuretics. Long periods spent in the bathroom after meals may also signal bulimia. Bodily signs include stained, decayed teeth and scarred, blistered hands from self-induced vomiting, and unusual swelling around the jaws from enlarged salivary glands.

Bulimia creates many serious health problems. Vomiting eats away at the teeth, gums, and stomach. It can rupture the esophagus. Many bulimics have constant sore throats. Loss of fluid causes electrolyte imbalance, which can lead to an irregular heartbeat and possibly heart failure.

Causes of Eating Disorders

Eating disorders are as complex as their underlying causes. Genetics and chemical imbalances in the brain may play roles, but emotional and societal pressures are definite contributors. People who have eating disorders struggle with issues of identity and control. They use food to cope with stress, low self-esteem, and fears about the future. Family troubles, loneliness, anger, depression, and being teased about their weight add to the problem.

Quite often, those with eating disorders dislike their appearance intensely. They have accepted unrealistic ideas about body shape and weight. They feel pressured to be something that is not only unreasonable but unreachable as well.

Stopping the Cycle

The earlier an eating disorder is recognized and treated, the better the chance for recovery. Few people can stop these self-destructive behaviors without professional help, yet resistance to treatment is common. People may not see that their eating is disordered or may be ashamed to admit it. It can be frightening to give up eating patterns when they are the "security blanket" that helps a person cope.

Often family and friends who care enough to get involved have to step in and persuade the person to get help. The person may also find a trusted adult to confide in, such as a family member or a school nurse or counselor. A mental health counselor can provide expert help. The Yellow Pages of the telephone directory lists these professionals under "Eating Disorders." See **Fig. 12-6**.

Once accepted, treatment is a team approach. Physicians and nurses deal with the disorder's physical complications. Psychotherapists help uncover and heal its root causes. Behavior therapists and dietitians help the person relearn healthy eating habits. Self-help groups offer reassurance from others who have the disorder.

Career Prep

FCCLA Opportunities

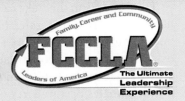
The Ultimate Leadership Experience

FAMILY, CAREER AND COMMUNITY Leaders of America, Inc., (FCCLA) is a national student organization that helps prepare young people for the future. The organization is open to students who are currently taking or have taken courses in family and consumer sciences.

Through various programs, FCCLA helps young men and women become leaders. Students build positive relationship skills and learn conflict management and teamwork. They build skills needed in the home and workplace, including planning, goal setting, problem solving, decision making, and communication. Moreover, as they explore careers, they learn how to be successful on the job. Some FCCLA programs are described here:

- **Families First.** Students plan and carry out projects designed to strengthen their own families, to understand how families function, and to value what families provide for their members and society.

- **Student Body.** Student projects promote healthful choices, including eating right, exer-

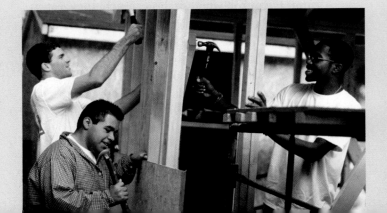

Equally valuable throughout this long, involved process is the support of family and friends.

Preventing Eating Disorders

Preventing any problem saves the physical and emotional wear and tear of treating it. Problem eating behaviors, such as extreme dieting, must be identified early, before they become deeply entrenched. Through education and counseling, people can learn more positive ways to cope with life's challenges.

Moreover, a change in attitude is needed regarding body ideals. The human body comes in diverse shapes and sizes. Society needs to honor and respect that diversity. Insisting that everyone meet any single standard should be recognized for what it is—shallow and insulting.

Progress must start on the individual level. When you value people for what they are and praise their positive accomplishments, you show that you base personal worth on ideals far deeper than body image.

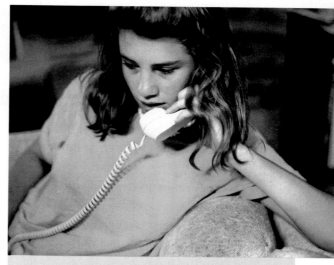

Fig. 12-6 Eating disorders are typically difficult to overcome without help. Health professionals are understanding and skillful in treating such problems.

cising, managing stress, and avoiding harmful substances.

- **Dynamic Leadership.** Students learn about and practice leadership skills, especially as they relate to family, careers, and community life.
- **Community Service.** Students develop, carry out, and evaluate a project that improves the quality of life in the community. It includes an annual Make a Difference Day, in which students can earn cash awards for their charities.
- **Career Connection.** Students complete projects that show how topics in family and consumer sciences courses apply to careers, with an emphasis on relationships between career, family, and community.
- **Leaders at Work.** Students develop leadership skills for a specific career area of family and consumer sciences.
- **Financial Fitness.** Students complete projects that teach other young people about money

management, including earning, saving, and spending money wisely.

- **Power of One.** Working independently, students develop and carry out a project that builds their skills and strengthens family or community life.

Other FCCLA programs are aimed at stopping school and community violence. Some promote safe driving. The organization also sponsors a Japanese exchange program, giving students from Japan and the United States a chance to experience another country's culture firsthand. STAR Events are national competitions for individual and chapter projects.

Career Connection

Career exploration. Choose a career in foods and nutrition that interests you. Develop and carry out an FCCLA project that involves exploring this career.

Summarize Your Reading

▶ Stress often causes people to eat less nourishing foods at times when their bodies need good nutrition.

▶ Not everyone reacts to stress in ways that are the same.

▶ You need to recognize when you're under stress and have a plan for dealing with it.

▶ Eating healthful foods when you're sick or injured can help your body recover more easily.

▶ Special diets can help people manage chronic health problems.

▶ People with food allergies or food intolerances may need to avoid eating certain foods.

▶ Anorexia nervosa, binge eating disorder, and bulimia nervosa are all eating disorders that can affect anyone, but they are especially common among teens and young adults, particularly females.

Check Your Knowledge

1. What is **stress** and what are its symptoms?

2. Why is it important to eat a healthy diet when under stress?

3. What tips for eating are helpful during stressful times?

4. What can you do to cope positively with stress?

5. **CRITICAL THINKING** A teen was stressed about passing an upcoming math test. Instead of her usual run that evening, she went out for ice cream sundaes with a friend to talk about her concerns. After the talk, she decided to study, do her best, and accept the results. What positive and negative actions did the teen take?

6. Why is getting plenty of fluids important when you have a cold or the flu?

7. Why might you need to eat fewer calories if you break your leg?

8. How is a **chronic** health problem different from getting the flu or spraining a toe? Give examples of chronic health problems.

9. What is **diabetes**, and why must someone with diabetes eat high fiber foods?

10. What is **HIV/AIDS**, and why is safe food handling important for a person with this disorder?

11. What are some common symptoms of a **food allergy**?

12. How is a **food intolerance** different from a food allergy?

13. Why are **eating disorders** considered to be illnesses?

14. Describe the possible rituals of a person with **anorexia nervosa.**

15. What is a **binge eating disorder**?

16. How is **bulimia nervosa** different from anorexia nervosa?

17. What are some of the causes of eating disorders?

18. Can a person stop an eating disorder without help? Explain.

19. How can eating disorders be prevented?

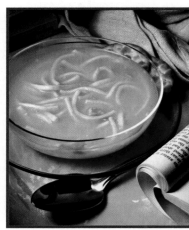

Apply Your Learning

1. Coping Strategies. Develop a list of personal coping strategies to use against stress. Print these onto a bookmark or small card as an everyday reminder.

2. Special Menus. Develop meal plans for three days for these people: a) a child with wheat allergy; b) a person who is lactose intolerant; c) a person who has the flu.

3. Menu Adaptation. Use resources to find meal plans for three days. After studying them explain how you would adapt each one for someone who has a particular chronic health problem. If necessary, research the condition you selected to learn more about eating restrictions.

4. **LANGUAGE ARTS** **Advice Column.** Suppose you write an advice column. Someone writes in, worried about having an eating disorder. People tell her she's too thin, and she is avoiding mealtimes to exercise instead. Write a response.

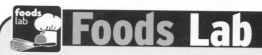

Foods Lab

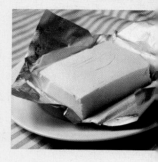

Modified-Diet Recipes

Procedure: Find a recipe that would be suitable for someone on a particular modified diet and that has mostly common ingredients. Prepare and evaluate the recipe.

Analyzing Results

❶ How did the recipe meet the requirements of the particular diet?

❷ How would you rate this recipe in cost and convenience? Could most people prepare the dish? Are the foods readily available?

❸ Would this meal be appealing to people who are not following a special diet? Why or why not?

Food Science Experiment

Comparing Antacids

Objective: To compare the effectiveness of commercial and traditional antacids used to relieve indigestion.

Procedure:

1. Obtain two commercial antacid products that contain different active ingredients. Record the active ingredient in each one.
2. Place 2 cups of red cabbage chunks and 1 cup of water in a blender. Process until the cabbage is finely shredded.
3. Strain the cabbage juice. This liquid will act as an acid indicator. Place 2 Tbsp. of the juice in each of four clear glasses.
4. Into each glass, stir *one* of the following substances: 1 tsp. of baking soda; 1 tsp. of milk; or one dose of each commercial antacid. (Grind tablets to a powder before adding.)

Analyzing Results

❶ What changes, if any, did you notice in each glass? What do you think produced these results?

❷ Which "home remedy" for acid seemed more effective? Which commercial antacid? How did you reach this conclusion?

❸ What is an advantage and disadvantage of using commercial antacids compared to home remedies?

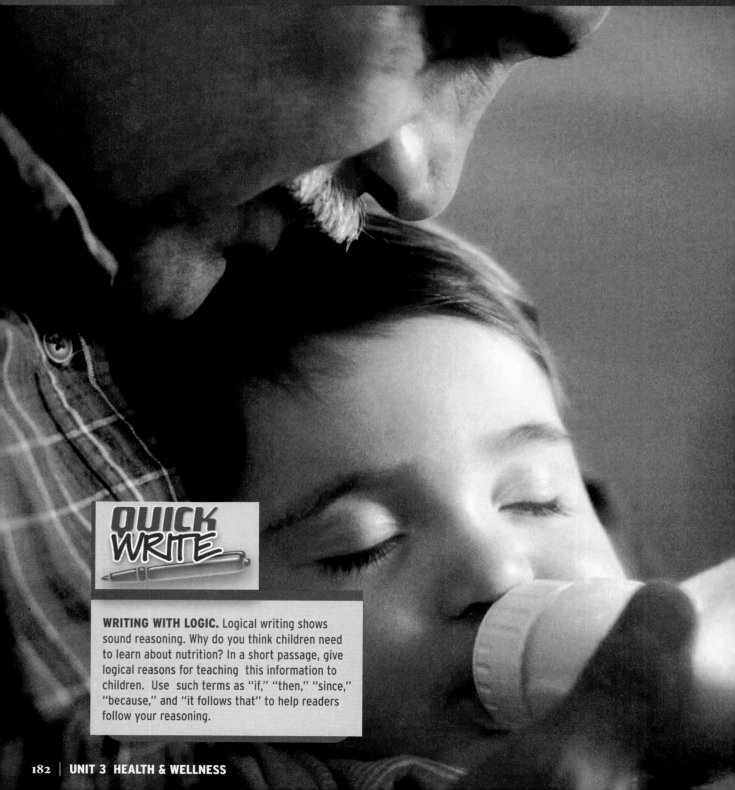

QUICK WRITE

WRITING WITH LOGIC. Logical writing shows sound reasoning. Why do you think children need to learn about nutrition? In a short passage, give logical reasons for teaching this information to children. Use such terms as "if," "then," "since," "because," and "it follows that" to help readers follow your reasoning.

I MAGINE A FAMILY SHARING A SPAGHETTI DIN-ner. The toddler slurps a strand of plain spaghetti from her fingers into her mouth. Her brother, a teen, ladles extra sauce on his serving. Their grandfather sprinkles salt-free seasoning over his smaller portion. One healthful food, enjoyed three different ways to meet the nutrient needs of each life stage—that's the picture of life-span nutrition.

NUTRITION FOR A LIFETIME

Each person in the scene above is in a different phase of the life span. **Life span** refers to the stages of development that people go through from birth through maturity. The human life span includes five such stages: pregnancy, or the prenatal period; infancy; childhood; adolescence; and adulthood. Each stage brings its own growth and nutrition needs and challenges. Meeting these demands promotes good health at each time of life and builds a solid base for the future. See **Fig. 13-1**.

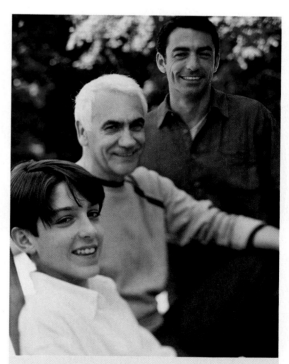

Fig. 13-1 Each stage of life brings different food needs.

PREGNANCY

It's amazing to think how every human being starts as a single cell. During nine months of pregnancy, that cell divides and multiplies a few million times until it develops into a being able to survive in the outside world.

Development in this crucial period depends on getting the right nutrients. Of course, the **fetus** (FEE-tuhs), the unborn baby, cannot control the kinds and amounts of nutrients it receives. The mother alone is responsible for supplying that nutrition through her own food choices. See **Fig. 13-2**.

Ideally, good eating habits are established long before this time. A woman usually doesn't learn she is pregnant until a month or more into the pregnancy. Meanwhile, her diet has been the unborn baby's sole source of nourishment. A woman who is already enjoying healthful foods is more likely to have a healthy baby. Poor eating habits place the baby at risk for serious problems throughout life.

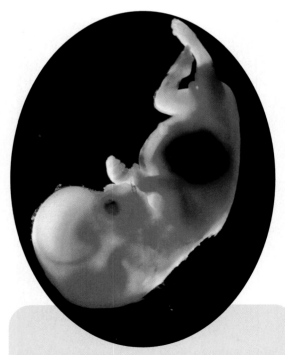

Fig. 13-2 Healthy fetal development requires nutrients. Only the mother-to-be can provide them through the food she eats.

Inadequate nutrition can damage the mother's health as well. Nutrients the baby doesn't get from the woman's diet are drawn from her body tissue, creating a deficiency.

Teen pregnancies are at particular risk because teens need added nutrients for their own growth and development. Poor nutrition increases the chance that the baby will have a low birth weight (under 5½ pounds) as well as physical and learning problems later in life. Because most teens are physically immature, they are also more likely to have difficult pregnancies.

Guidelines for Pregnant Women

As soon as she learns she is pregnant, a woman should see an **obstetrician** (ahb-stuh-TRIH-shun), a physician who specializes in the care of women during pregnancy and childbirth. An obstetrician will recommend specific kinds and amounts of food and possibly supplements of certain nutrients for pregnancy. Most nutrient needs of pregnancy, however, can be met by choosing low-fat, nutrient-dense foods. Pregnant women need the upper range of recommended servings and extra helpings of dairy foods—three to four servings each day, five to six servings for pregnant teens.

Other nutrition concerns of pregnancy include the following:

- Iron needs double during pregnancy. Iron from animal sources is best absorbed by the body. Citrus fruits and other foods rich in vitamin C help absorb iron from plant sources.
- The B vitamin folic acid, or folate, is so valuable to preventing birth defects that federal law requires it to be added to enriched grain products. It's found naturally in fruits and dark green vegetables.
- Contaminants in foods can cause birth defects and **miscarriage**, the spontaneous expulsion of the unborn child. Fish and shellfish, for example, contain various levels of mercury, but large fish, including tuna, mackerel, swordfish, shark, and tilefish, have the greatest amounts. Soft cheeses, such as blue and Queso Fresco, may harbor *Listeria*, the bacteria responsible for listeriosis. Light-colored fish and hard cheeses are safer choices.

- Small amounts of caffeine are thought to be safe during pregnancy. Caffeinated drinks, however, shouldn't replace milk and juices. Drinking at least eight glasses of water a day helps prevent constipation, a common complaint of pregnancy. See **Fig. 13-3**.

Pregnancy and Weight Gain

Women should expect to gain around 25 to 35 pounds during pregnancy.

Underweight women are urged to gain more and overweight women, less. Women carrying twins may be advised to gain as much as 45 pounds.

This added weight comes from the growth of the baby and physical changes of pregnancy. Healthy women need only about 300 calories over their usual intake. These extra calories should come from nutrient-rich foods. Women should not try to gain weight from high-calorie, low-nutrient foods.

Likewise, pregnancy is no time for a weight-loss diet, even for women who are overweight. Limiting food deprives the fetus of vital nutrients. Rather, they can lose weight after delivery by continuing the healthful habits of pregnancy.

INFANCY

During the first year of life, the human body grows and develops more rapidly than at any other time. Good nutrition is critical for keeping this remarkable "construction project" on schedule.

Feeding Newborns

Parents have two choices for feeding a newborn—breast-feeding or bottle-feeding. See **Fig. 13-4**. While both provide all nutrient needs for an infant's first four to six months, experts recommend breast-feeding. Breast milk has the right balance of fat, carbohydrates, and protein for a baby. The protein is better digested and absorbed than the protein in cow's milk.

Breast-feeding also lowers the rate of infections in infants. The mother passes her own immunity to disease through her colostrum. **Colostrum** (kuh-LAHS-trum) is a thick, yellowish fluid that is rich in nutrients and antibodies, proteins that

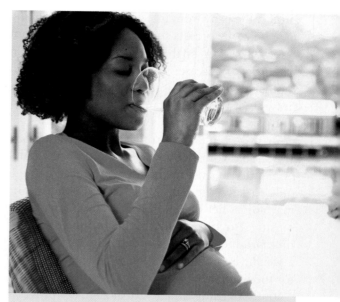

Fig. 13-3 A pregnant woman needs to drink at least eight glasses of water every day. What techniques might help her keep track of her water intake?

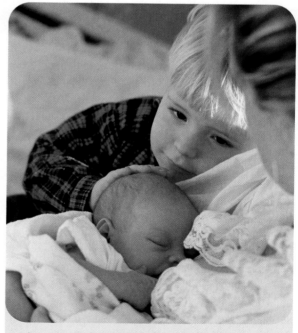

Fig. 13-4 Both breast milk and formula provide an infant with needed nutrients. Why do experts recommend breast-feeding?

protect the baby from infection. Before producing true milk, the breasts supply colostrum for about three days after birth. Since antibodies form in response to diseases in the environment, each mother's colostrum is tailored to fight the illnesses that the infant is most apt to face.

By breast-feeding, a woman continues to nourish her infant from her own nutrient store. She should continue to eat well and drink plenty of liquids to ensure that she produces enough milk to keep the baby well fed and healthy. She may adjust her diet, however, if the infant seems sensitive to certain foods. **Lactation**, or breast milk production, burns added calories that make a weight-loss diet unnecessary as well as unwise for the woman.

Bottle-feeding infant formula also provides good nutrition. In some cases it may be preferred. A mother may need to take certain medications that could be passed to the infant, for example. Infant formula is usually made from cow's milk. Added fatty acids, vegetable oils, and carbohydrates make it more similar to breast milk. Infants who are sensitive to the lactose in cow's milk may be fed a formula containing corn syrup. Other varieties use soy protein rather than dairy protein. Since about one-third of infants who cannot digest dairy protein are also sensitive to soy, a formula with "predigested" protein is also available.

Adding Solid Food

Between four and six months of age, a baby is ready to start the transition to solid food. For easier swallowing and digestion, these "solids" are strained to resemble a mash or gruel. Iron-fortified rice cereal made with breast milk or formula is usually offered first, then vegetables and fruits. Protein foods are usually added at about eight months. New choices should be introduced one at a time. That way, any food that causes a reaction can be easily identified. The child's **pediatrician**, a physician who cares for infants and children, should be notified if a problem persists.

TRENDS in TECHNOLOGY

BIG STEPS IN BABY FOODS

Like babies, the baby food market is expected to grow in the coming years. With technology, baby food makers are making their products more appealing to the tiniest eaters and their caregivers.

Parents want to get their children off to a good start nutritionally. Because newer processing methods reduce cooking time, strained foods retain more nutrients, as well as taste and color. Whole-grain and multi-grain cereals are more available. So too are organic foods, answering parents' concerns about pesticides, preservatives, and other additives.

Caring for babies is a time- and energy-consuming job. To make feeding babies easier, food makers have applied the same technology used in adult foods. Instant rice cereals come in single-serving packets to eliminate the need for measuring. Combination meals for older infants come in lightweight, microwave-safe bowls, which are easy to carry and heat up even away from home.

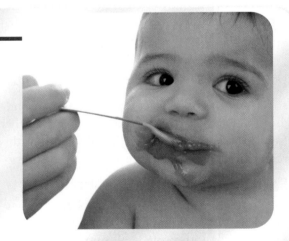

To keep up as their small customers develop eating skills, baby food makers are expanding their lines to include finger food for toddlers. Two-year-olds can feed themselves with bite-size, fruit-filled, whole-wheat squares and graham cracker sticks. This also meets the toddler's need for snacking, while supplying both nutrients and calories for the growing child.

__Think Beyond>> Do you see any possible disadvantages to the trends described? Explain.

At around nine months, infants' eating skills improve. They start to self-feed, picking up and chewing soft "finger foods." Small pieces are easier to handle, and more importantly, guard against the threat of choking. Healthful choices include pieces of peeled fruit, cooked vegetables, and cheese. Small pieces of whole bagels and hard rolls help relieve the irritation as teeth come in.

A one-year-old child usually can eat the same foods as the rest of the family, in smaller amounts, using a child-size spoon. Children under age two have high energy needs, so caregivers should not try to limit fat in their diet.

CHILDHOOD

Young children are active and growing. They need to eat a wide selection of nutritious foods.

Children have small stomachs and short attention spans. Thus they do better on smaller servings and regular snacks throughout the day. Portions at meals might start with 1 tablespoon of food for each year of the child's life—about 3 tablespoons of vegetables for a three-year-old, for example. A child who is still hungry can be given more. Milk, juice, yogurt, pieces of fruit or vegetables, unsweetened cereal, whole-grain crackers, and cooked meat, poultry, and fish all make healthful snacks. High-fat and sugary foods should be avoided.

A child's appetite can vary almost daily. During growth spurts, children may eat more than usual. At other times, they want less. They sometimes go on food jags, insisting on a certain food at every meal. These phases are best humored until they pass.

Encouraging Good Eating Habits

Eating habits and attitudes learned in childhood can last a lifetime. These guidelines help children develop a healthy approach to food and nutrition:

• Serve foods that vary in color and texture. Cut them into imaginative shapes. This adds interest and encourages children to appreciate food's sensory appeal.

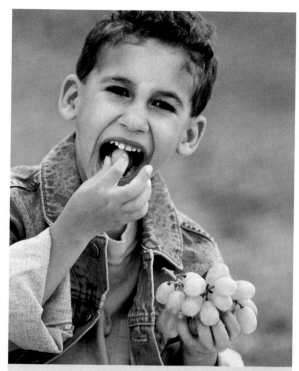

Fig. 13-5 Children follow the examples set for them. If a parent enjoys eating fruits and vegetables as a snack, the child is likely to enjoy them too.

• Share meals with children and make mealtime enjoyable. Model good manners and eating habits. See **Fig. 13-5**.
• Don't use food as a reward or punishment. This practice gives the wrong impression about the purpose of food.
• Don't urge children to clean their plate. Insisting that they finish all their food, even if they're not hungry, can lead to overeating.
• When possible, let children choose meals and snacks from several nutritious options.
• Teach children how to prepare a few simple, healthful foods by themselves, with your supervision. Depending on their age, they might tear lettuce or make sandwiches.
• Make shopping trips with children fun and educational. Help them identify fruits and vegetables. Point out flavorful foods of different cuisines.

- Encourage children to be active, and help them learn to choose healthful snacks. Since overweight and obesity are increasing problems among children, these measures can help.

Nutrition and Special Needs

Meeting the nutrition requirements of children with special needs can bring special concerns. These children have health conditions that impair physical, emotional, or intellectual development. Some of these conditions also have an impact on nutrition. A physical disability can delay self-feeding skills. Metabolic disorders can prevent the body from absorbing nutrients.

Helping a child with special needs live with such challenges takes the combined effort of caregivers, family members, physicians, and dietitians. Caregivers may need to learn how to use a feeding tube or how to respond to disruptive behavior at mealtime. A child with limited mobility may need family support to follow a low-calorie eating plan.

ADOLESCENCE

If people tell you, "I can't believe how you're growing," believe them. Adolescence is the second most rapid growth period of life. At this time dramatic physical changes increase a teen's need for almost all nutrients. Of special importance are iron and calcium for building muscle and bone, a process that continues even after growth stops.

Like children, teens go through growth spurts, when calorie and nutrient needs increase. Every teen's growth rate is different. At any given time, your specific needs may vary from those of your friends. Teens should base food choices on their own body cues, such as hunger and height gain. They may need to resist **peer pressure**, the influence of people in the same age group, to eat more or less than they require.

Nutrition for Teen Athletes

Careful conditioning and sound nutrition are the surest ways to long-lasting, top athletic performance. Daily food choices can make the difference between a good performance and a poor one. See **Fig. 13-6**.

Generally, athletes can meet all their nutrition needs by following the Dietary Guidelines for Americans. As you've read, extra protein from foods or supplements does no good and can be harmful. Likewise, athletes who eat a varied, nutritious diet don't need sports bars or dietary supplements. Two nutrients do play special roles for athletes: carbohydrates and water.

Carbohydrate Needs

You'll recall that during digestion, carbohydrates are broken down into the simple sugar glucose, which is used for energy. Extra carbohydrates are stored in the liver and muscles as glycogen. Glycogen fuels the body during vigorous, extended periods of training and competition,

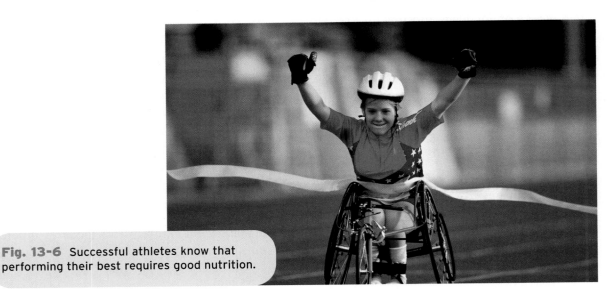

Fig. 13-6 Successful athletes know that performing their best requires good nutrition.

when an athlete may use two or three times as much energy as the average person. When glycogen runs out, so does the energy.

Athletes need to eat plenty of carbohydrates, then, to build their glycogen stores. Teen athletes should get 55 to 60 percent of calories from carbohydrates, with about 20 to 25 percent from fat and 15 to 20 percent from protein.

Water Needs

Did you know that during a strenuous workout an athlete can lose up to 5 quarts of water through perspiration? If water isn't replaced quickly, dehydration can result, which can lead to serious health problems. Athletes should drink water before, during (about every 15 minutes), and after an event, even when they don't feel thirsty. Thirst signals that dehydration has already begun. See **Fig. 13-7**.

One way to gauge the amount of water needed is to weigh in before and after an event. Water loss usually shows up as weight loss. To replace each pound lost, drink two cups of water.

Some athletes drink juices and fruit drinks instead of water. Due to their high sugar content, these beverages can cause stomach cramps, diarrhea, and nausea. They should be diluted with an equal amount of water. Sports drinks that contain carbohydrates and electrolytes are valuable for activities lasting longer than 90 minutes. Salt, potassium, and other minerals lost in shorter events are easily replaced through well-chosen meals and snacks. Caffeinated drinks, which draw water from the body, are not advised.

Even well-hydrated athletes should never exercise in extreme heat and humidity. The result can be heat exhaustion or heat stroke, which require immediate medical attention.

Pre-Event Meals

If you eat just before a competition, the digestive process competes with your muscles for energy. Eating three to four hours before an event allows time for proper digestion.

A good pre-event meal is based on foods that are high in complex carbohydrates. Fats and proteins take longer to digest. Sugary foods can cause a sudden rise—and fall—in blood sugar levels,

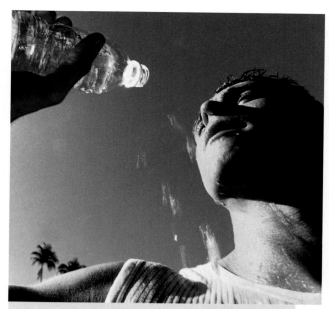

Fig. 13-7 Athletes need to replace the water they lose during an event. Is waiting until you're thirsty advisable?

leaving energy stores empty when they're needed most. Eat familiar foods that you enjoy and drink at least two cups of fluids.

Soon after an athletic event or a hard workout is the best time to refuel the body with nutritious foods and fluids. Studies show that more glycogen can be deposited in the muscles immediately after exercise. Some popular choices include juice and a bagel, a bowl of cereal with fruit and milk, or fruit and yogurt.

ADULTHOOD

Many adults face a nutrition dilemma. They need the same amount of nutrients, but they need fewer calories. The demands of work and family leave less time for exercise and balanced meals. Unless they're careful, adults may find their weight rising, along with the risk of heart disease, various types of cancer, and other assorted health problems.

This problem is definitely easier to prevent than correct. In this case, the prevention and the solution are the same: choosing a variety of healthful, low-calorie foods and making regular physical activity a priority. Your study of foods and nutrition today can help you keep those commitments as an adult.

Older Adults

More and more, research is revealing the role of good nutrition in wellness and disease prevention in older age. Many healthy, active, older people are living proof. See **Fig. 13-8.**

Physical changes of aging do require more care in eating habits, however. Often, calorie needs continue to drop while other nutrition needs increase. To make every calorie count, older people should choose nutrient-dense foods. Due to diseases and effects of aging, the body uses some nutrients less efficiently, notably calcium and vitamins D and B_{12}. Low-fat milk and yogurt are good sources of these nutrients, particularly if dental problems make chewing difficult.

Thirst signals also decline with age. Older people need to make a point of drinking eight cups of water, milk, or juice each day. Moist foods, such as soups and cooked cereals, add fluids and ease chewing problems. Milk-based beverages and homemade smoothies boost nutrition with a minimum of calories. As the sense of taste and smell weaken, older adults can keep meals appealing with flavorful foods and seasonings.

Other circumstances can challenge older adults. Those who live alone or on fixed incomes may not have the desire or the means to prepare nourishing meals. Disabilities can make kitchen tasks painful. The death of loved ones can depress the appetite as well as the spirit.

Career Prep

Interests and Aptitudes

BRITISH AUTHOR KATHERINE Whitehorn once wrote that the best career advice is to "find out what you like doing and get someone to pay you for doing it." Whitehorn understood the value of interests and aptitude in a career plan.

Interests are things that hold your attention, subjects you enjoy studying, and activities you like to do. Aptitude is inborn talent or ease in learning a certain skill. The two often work hand in hand. For example, natural physical ability may lead to an interest in sports. Identifying interests and aptitudes is an early step in career planning.

Some skills and interests are obvious. Others are hidden or scattered among diverse activities. Recognizing these underlying qualities may take personal or professional detective work. You can start by examining your own life, including the following:

- **Values and goals.** What is important to you? Knowing what you value and want to achieve in life can be the key factor in choosing fulfilling work. If giving back to the community is important, for instance, you might want a career in public service.

- **Activities.** Why do you enjoy certain activities? Knowing why you like favorite activities can point you toward work that provides similar satisfactions.

- **Others' observations.** What have other people observed? You may be so familiar with your own qualities that you don't notice them. Ask friends or family members what they think are your strongest positive traits. When and how do these come out?

Social service programs in many communities address all of these needs. At churches and community centers, older people can share good meals and the company of others for a modest price. Volunteer and public agencies put together food baskets and deliver meals. Through nutrition education and screening, they help older adults make good food choices for their individual health needs.

Families and neighbors need to take an active role as well. Grocery shopping for an older relative or inviting an elderly neighbor for a meal satisfies more than a nutrition need. It nourishes the whole person.

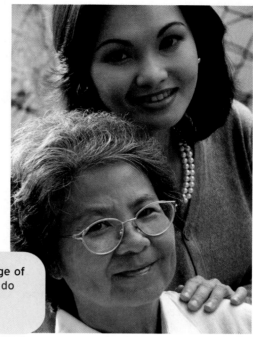

Fig. 13-8 Adulthood covers a wide range of years and changing nutrition needs. How do the needs of people at twenty, forty, and seventy differ?

To match personal qualities to careers, trained counselors have tools that help. One popular tool is an inventory, or survey, of interests or personality traits. One well-known interest inventory uses the proven idea that people in the same line of work often share interests. Called the Strong Interest Inventory, for developer E.J. Strong, it helps discover your interests and identifies those fields where others with similar interests do well.

As with interests, people with certain personal qualities tend to excel in some careers. An inventory like the Myers-Briggs Type Indicator looks for patterns in how you perceive and respond to the world and matches these patterns to personality traits.

As career planning aids, interests and aptitudes have their limits. You may be skilled at something you dislike doing. Also, not every interest translates well in practical terms. Rock climbing may be an exciting hobby, but it might not be the way to earn a living.

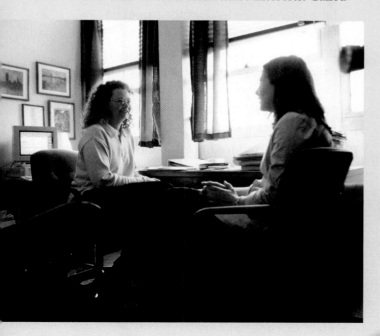

Career Connection

Taking inventory. Locate and complete an interest or personality inventory. Some are available on-line. Do the results surprise you? Are they useful? Share your opinion of the inventory with the class. Share the results only if you like.

Summarize Your Reading

▶ Pregnant women need to make sure they get adequate nutrition for their own health as well as the health of their unborn child.

▶ Women who breast-feed provide nutrients for their child from their own store of nutrients.

▶ Young growing children need plenty of milk and a variety of foods to meet all their nutrition needs.

▶ Children with special needs may require help to get necessary nutrients.

▶ Every teen's growth rate is different, so nutrition requirements differ among teens at any point in time.

▶ Daily food choices for teen athletes can make a difference in their performance.

▶ Older adults who understand and pay attention to their particular nutrition needs increase their chances of living a healthy active life.

Check Your Knowledge

1. Why should a pregnant woman be sure to eat healthfully?

2. How can a woman get the kinds and amounts of nutrients she needs during pregnancy?

3. What vitamins and minerals are particularly important to a pregnant woman, and why?

4. What foods should a pregnant woman avoid, and why?

5. **CRITICAL THINKING** A woman who was expecting twins started a weight-loss diet because she was 5 pounds over the 35-pound weight-gain limit by her eighth month. What would you suggest to her?

6. Why do experts recommend breast-feeding?

7. Why should a woman not go on a weight-loss diet during **lactation**?

8. In what situation is bottle-feeding recommended?

9. When is a baby ready to start eating solid food, and what foods are usually offered first?

10. What is the difference between an **obstetrician** and a **pediatrician**?

11. Why should a child be given smaller servings and regular snacks during the day?

12. **CRITICAL THINKING** A parent offers a young son "trees" of broccoli. The parent puts raisins on an open peanut butter sandwich and lets the boy tear his own lettuce for a sandwich. Why does the parent do these things?

13. What might caregivers do when helping children with special needs manage food challenges?

14. Why are calorie and nutrient needs so important for teens?

15. Why do athletes need to eat plenty of carbohydrates?

16. Why do athletes need to drink lots of water? What beverages should they avoid, and why?

17. What challenges related to eating do older people face?

18. How can families and communities help older citizens get the nutrients they need?

Apply Your Learning

1. **Eating Plan for Pregnancy.** Develop a one-week eating plan that meets nutrition guidelines for a pregnant woman.

2. **Recipe Preparation.** Prepare a recipe featuring foods high in iron or folate for your class. Rate the recipe according to taste, ease of preparation, cost, and nutrition.

3. **Children's Party.** Choose an appropriate theme and plan a children's party that includes healthful foods as refreshments. Carry out the party at a child-care site. Why were the foods you chose healthful?

4. **Pre-Event Meal.** Plan a pre-event meal for a school sports team. Select recipes that fulfill nutrition requirements. Ask permission to prepare the meal for the team.

5. SOCIAL STUDIES **Societal Impacts.** Examine societal factors that may prevent children and the elderly from being well nourished.

Foods Lab

Recipes for Children

Procedure: Prepare a healthful snack or other simple recipe for a five-year-old. Consider visual appeal as well as self-feeding skills and taste preferences of children at this age. If possible, serve the food to children in a preschool, after-school, or kindergarten program.

Analyzing Results

❶ What colors, tastes, textures, or other techniques did you use to make the recipe appealing?

❷ What nutrients does the food supply?

❸ How could a child help prepare the recipe?

❹ How might you change the recipe to serve a ten-year-old?

Food Science Experiment

Adding Milk Protein and Calcium

Objective: To explore how adding powdered milk affects recipes.

Procedure:

1. Prepare the recipes below as assigned by your teacher:

   A. Prepare a recipe for pancakes, using a complete baking mix and adding water as directed. Prepare the recipe a second time, substituting ¼ cup nonfat dry milk for ¼ cup baking mix.

   B. Weigh two, 4-oz. servings of ground beef. Mix 2 Tbsp. powdered milk into one serving. Shape each serving into a patty and cook in a skillet.

   C. Make hot cocoa by blending ¼ cup nondairy powdered creamer, ¼ cup powdered sugar, and 4 tsp. unsweetened cocoa powder. Gradually stir in 1⅓ cups boiling water. Prepare the recipe again with nonfat dry milk instead of creamer.

2. Compare your two recipes on taste, texture, appearance, and ease of preparation.

Analyzing Results

❶ How did adding powdered milk affect each recipe, if at all? What might explain any changes?

❷ What additional modifications would you make when adding powdered milk for extra protein and calcium to a baked good, meat dish, or beverage?

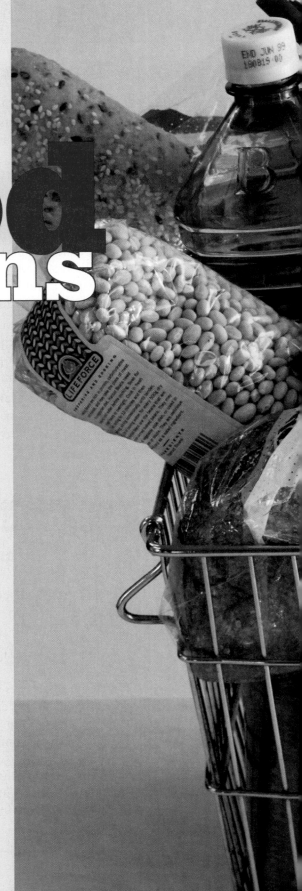

UNIT 4

Food
Decisions

CHAPTER 14 **Eating Patterns**

CHAPTER 15 **Vegetarian Food Choices**

CHAPTER 16 **Meal Planning**

CHAPTER 17 **Shopping for Food**

CHAPTER 18 **Serving Food**

CHAPTER 19 **Etiquette**

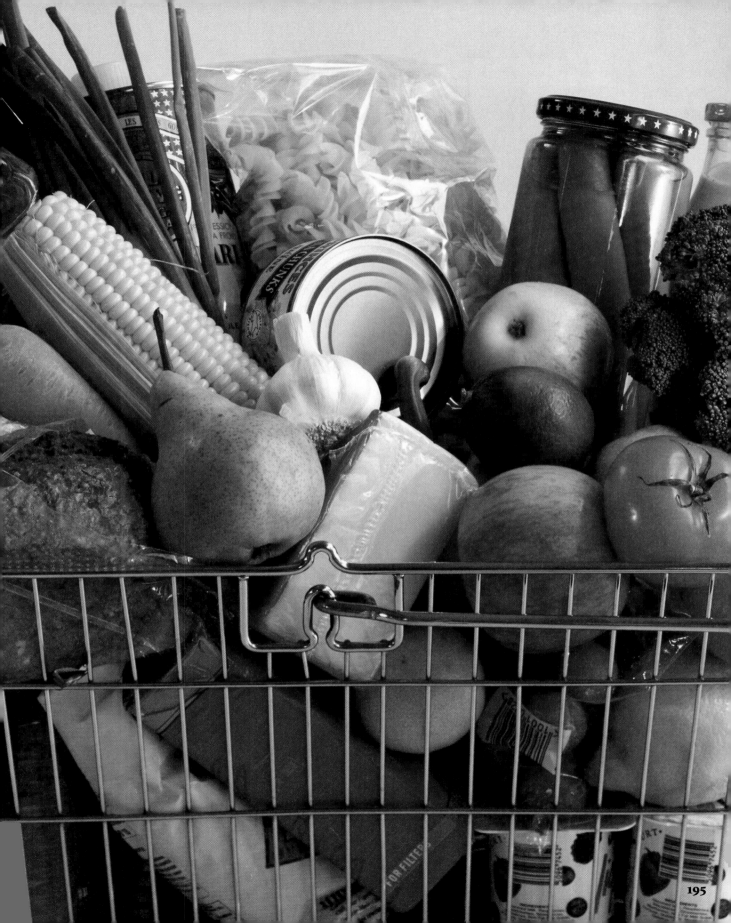

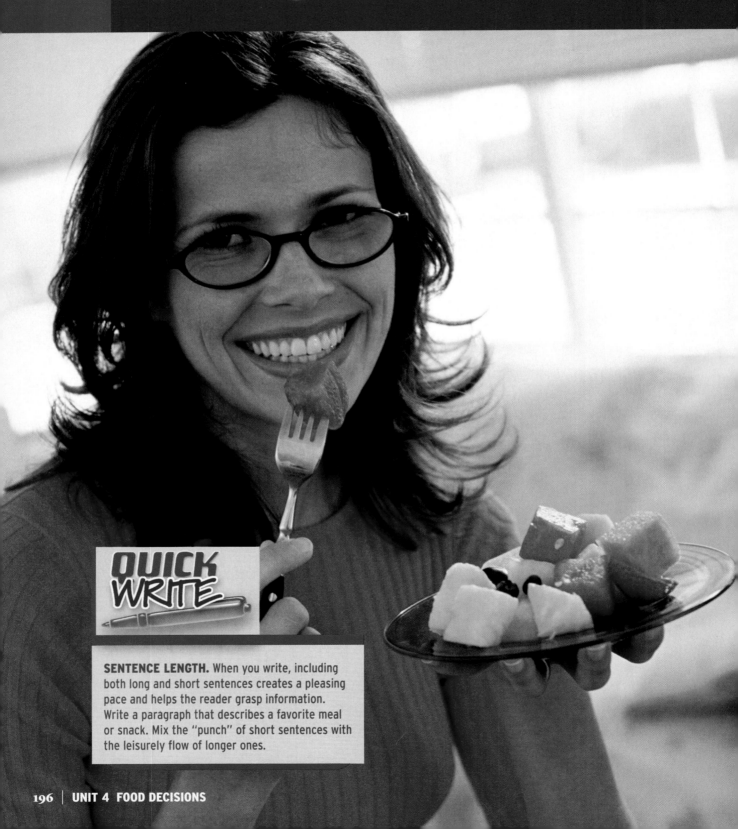

QUICK WRITE

SENTENCE LENGTH. When you write, including both long and short sentences creates a pleasing pace and helps the reader grasp information. Write a paragraph that describes a favorite meal or snack. Mix the "punch" of short sentences with the leisurely flow of longer ones.

THE NEXT TIME YOU'RE GOING THROUGH THE supermarket, notice the shopping carts around you. What do the purchases reveal? Several gallons of milk might indicate a family with small children—or growing teens. Boxed cake mixes might suggest that someone likes to bake but wants convenience.

Social scientists who study the cultural importance of food do research like this. They learn a lot about a society by investigating its food habits and choices. This same kind of study can benefit you too when you choose a meal or snack. Understanding factors that affect what, when, and where you eat can help you make more thoughtful choices.

WHAT INFLUENCES FOOD CHOICES?

Every decision you make is affected by many factors, which carry different weight depending on the situation. Some of the biggest influences, and how they relate to food, are discussed here.

Resources

Resources are people, things, and qualities that can help you reach a goal. This textbook is a resource that helps you learn about food and nutrition. Your own intelligence is another.

Resources affect food choices at a most basic level. Choices increase or decrease with the resources available. The greater your food budget is, for example, the greater your options. A lack of cooking skills reduces options. See **Fig. 14-1**.

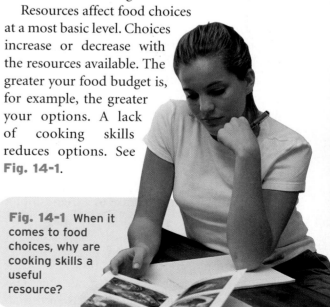

Fig. 14-1 When it comes to food choices, why are cooking skills a useful resource?

No one has an endless supply of every resource, but everyone has some. You can often substitute one resource for another that is in short supply. If you have more time and skills than money, you can still get the same flavor and nutrition with less costly foods.

Family Food Customs

Family may be the single greatest influence on food choices. Children learn food preferences and habits from the example of older family members. Think about your favorite foods. You probably learned to like them because they were served at home.

Families often enjoy special food customs, handed down through generations. Such customs, even simple ones, can create memories and family bonds. In one family, every young adult learns to make the "secret recipe" for cornbread dressing at Thanksgiving.

Food customs can unite families with a sense of pride and identity in their cultural heritage. See **Fig. 14-2**. When Jewish families gather for the Seder meal at Passover, one custom has the youngest child ask the significance of the traditional foods served.

Friends

Food and friendship seem to go together. In fact, the word *companion* comes from the Latin for "with bread." Sharing tastes in food fosters a sense of belonging and identity, especially during the teen years. Thus friends influence each other's food choices.

Given this close connection, it's common to feel pressure to make food choices that please your friends. In the school cafeteria, you might plan on the baked fish and fruit salad—until friends ask for fried chicken and french fries. On the other hand, friends of different cultural backgrounds can share new food choices. What foods have you come to enjoy thanks to a friendship?

The Media

An ad for ice cream and an article on the benefits of oat bran are both examples of how the media can sway your choice of food. They may alert you to food trends, new products, or the latest nutrition advice.

Advertising is designed, at great cost to food makers, to be an especially powerful influence. How often do people buy a snack because it seems "fun" or a cereal because it promises certain health benefits? They may be responding to advertising without being aware of its impact.

Use the same principles you learned in Chapter 10 about evaluating information. These guidelines can help you measure a product's worth with logic rather than emotions.

Personal Influences

Your food choices don't depend entirely on external forces. Influences that you can control also play a part.

Daily Routine

Think of how your daily routine affects your food choices. If you're typically rushed in the morning, you might grab a cereal bar and a glass of orange juice. You'll have a larger meal at lunch when you have more time. If you're an early riser, you might have a full breakfast and pack cheese

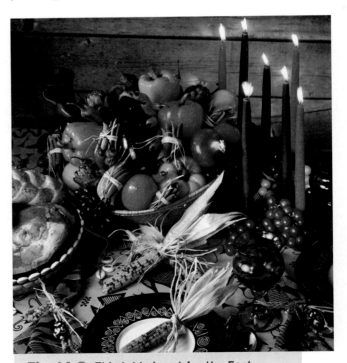

Fig. 14-2 This table is set for the East African harvest festival, Kwanza. Foods that are traditionally served for a family celebration may awaken special feelings throughout a person's life.

and crackers as a midday meal. If you have an after-school job, you may choose different foods on nights that you work than when you eat with the family.

Throughout life, you learn to adapt food habits to different routines. You also have more choices about what, when, and where you eat. If you learn how to plan healthful meals and snacks now, it will be easier to keep the habit as daily routines change.

Values

Values are beliefs and concepts that a person holds as important. People make choices based on their personal values. Someone who believes that supporting local merchants is important might buy at a farmers market.

As a teen, you're developing the critical thinking skills to determine your own values. You have more chances to act on them. Learning about foods, nutrition, and the many related issues can help you make food choices that reflect what's important to you.

Emotions

As you probably know from experience, your emotional state can strongly influence your food choices. People often use comfort foods to cheer them when they're depressed and party food to celebrate an event.

Food often carries strong associations, both pleasant and unpleasant. For one person, corn on the cob may bring back happy memories of summers spent on a grandparent's farm. For another, it may be a reminder of working long hours every summer in a vegetable processing plant.

EATING PATTERNS

Imagine starting the day with a plate of barbecued spareribs and pickled beets. Is that your idea of breakfast? For most people, it isn't typical. **Eating patterns** are a mix of food customs and habits that include when, what, and how much people eat. A typical breakfast for you is just one part of your eating pattern.

Eating patterns vary among different cultures and eras. Any pattern can be healthful, depending on the circumstances.

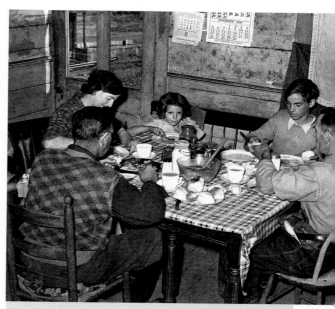

Fig. 14-3 A look at history shows how so many things have changed, even what and how people eat. How were food choices affected in the 1930s and 1940s?

Family Eating Patterns

The history of American family eating patterns mirrors the history of the country itself. Until the Industrial Revolution of the mid-1800s, extended families often lived, worked, and ate together. Sustaining the food supply—by hunting, fishing, or raising crops—was a family effort. Preparing food took the better part of the day for women and older girls.

As families moved to the city, they adopted new food habits. Mealtimes depended on what factory shift family members worked. More foods were available, and waves of immigrants introduced a wide range of cuisines. Diners and lunch counters sprang up, as young men arrived from rural areas in search of work and in need of meals.

Families of the 1930s struggled through the Depression, when a 9-cent loaf of bread was costly. Scraps and leftovers were saved for casseroles, hashes, and other thrifty, filling recipes. See **Fig. 14-3**.

Food shortages continued in the 1940s, when the nation entered World War II. With massive food shipments sent to troops overseas, civilian supplies were rationed. Each family member received a ration book with coupons that specified what food could be bought. Having the coupons, however, was no guarantee of finding the food. Many staples, especially butter, sugar, meat, and canned goods, were scarce or unavailable. Eggs, cheese, and fish, which were too perishable to ship, gained favor as protein foods. Growing and canning vegetables from "victory gardens" kept millions of families from going hungry.

The war had other significant impacts on eating habits. Women became a major part of the labor force, working long shifts in factories and shipyards to keep production rolling. They relied more on convenience foods, such as boxed dessert mixes and macaroni and cheese dinners. Military technology was used to invent instant rice and later, microwave ovens.

At the same time, the federal government was concerned about the number of nutrition-related health problems among its troops. Food guides based on nutrition research were issued to improve national health. In 1943, the Food and Nutrition Board of the National Research Council developed the first recommended daily allowances (RDAs). They specified levels of nutrients needed for almost all healthy people in the United States. Since then, food guides and nutrition have played larger roles in people's food choices.

With relative peace and prosperity in the 1950s, most women gave up their outside jobs. See **Fig. 14-4**. A flood of new appliances encouraged them to prepare interesting, nutritious family meals.

Recent decades have seen continuous changes in society and in family eating patterns. Shifting social and family roles, new nutrition data, and evolving food technology have all strongly influenced today's food habits. What do you think eating patterns will be like in the future?

Stages of Family Life

As with individuals, family eating patterns change with stages of family life. Family members' ages, their activities, and other circumstances create many variations, but eating patterns generally follow predictable trends.

While young children are at home, families tend to eat meals together. If parents are employed, meals prepared outside the home may be common. Choices may include fast foods and supermarket delis. As children become teens with hearty appetites, food costs go up. Teens also have opportunities to eat out on their own, increasing their choices.

When children have grown and left the family home, spending on food and other child-related costs may decrease. With a smaller family, members may have the time and money to eat out more frequently or try new foods. With aging, older adults often become less active and eat lighter meals. Health concerns may play a greater role in food choices.

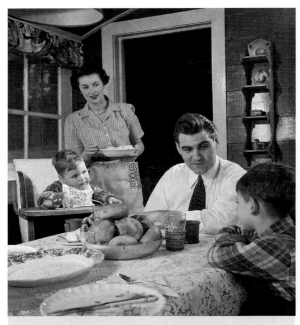

Fig. 14-4 In the 1950s women were typically homemakers. How did this impact family eating patterns?

Daily Meal Patterns

In most cultures relaxing at regular daily meals—breakfast, midday, and evening—shows that a society has the resources to secure a food supply and the stability to enjoy it. Your personal concerns for daily meals are more immediate: nutrition and energy.

Breakfast

You've probably heard breakfast called "the most important meal of the day." A look at the word tells you why. When you get up in the morning, you may have been fasting for 10 or 12 hours. "Breaking" the "fast" with breakfast gives you much-needed energy and helps you feel alert throughout the morning. Not surprisingly, research reveals that students who eat breakfast do better in school than those who go without it. See **Fig. 14-5**.

Not all breakfasts are equal, however. A nutritious combination of carbohydrates, proteins, and a little fat—a whole-grain muffin with milk and a banana, for example—gives long-lasting energy. In contrast, a doughnut and soda are high in calories and added sugars. They will provide a spurt of energy, but it will be exhausted by midmorning—and so will you.

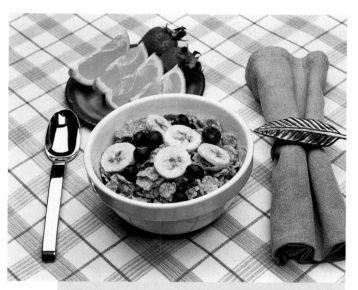

Fig. 14-5 After a full night's sleep, your brain needs a jump start with breakfast. Even nonmorning people can learn ways to incorporate a little breakfast in their routine.

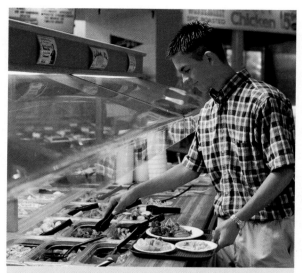

Fig. 14-6 By midday, energy from breakfast is typically used up, and it's time to build up again. Lunch can be simple foods or heartier fare, depending on what works for you.

Midday and Evening Meals

The midday and evening meals go by different names, depending on their size and the area of the country. Most Americans eat a light midday meal, or lunch. The largest meal of the day, traditionally called dinner, is served in the evening, at a time when family members can eat together. In some cultures, people eat the largest meal at midday and a lighter meal, sometimes called supper, in the evening.

Some individuals and families change their usual pattern on weekends or special occasions. On Sunday, for instance, they may eat dinner as their midday meal with a light supper in the evening. Another choice is to have brunch, a late morning meal that combines breakfast and lunch.

Either pattern can be healthful. Some nutritionists recommend you get most of your calories by mid-afternoon and use the evening meal to fill in any nutrition gaps in the day's food choices. Some people find they sleep better if the evening meal is light. As long as the midday meal supplies the energy and nutrients to carry you through the rest of the day, you can follow the pattern that fits your personal preference and schedule. See **Fig. 14-6**.

Grazing

One eating pattern that's gaining popularity is **grazing**, eating five or more small meals throughout the day instead of three large ones. Grazing appeals to people with busy schedules. Someone might have a vegetable salad during a work break, for example, and a sandwich later at home.

Grazing can be as healthful as more conventional meal patterns. Some studies suggest it helps control appetite and calorie intake. Grazing, however, can turn into continuous snacking. Overeating and poor nutrition can result if people lose track of their food choices throughout the day. Healthful grazing takes the same planning as eating three larger meals. By day's end, you should still have needed nutrients and calories from a variety of wholesome foods.

Snacks

As you know, a snack is a small amount of food eaten between meals. Snacking can help meet the increased nutrient and calorie needs of the teen years. Since some snack foods are high in fat and added sugar, choose carefully.

As the definition tells you, size and timing are deciding factors when fitting snacks into your eating plan. Pay attention to size. A cup of tortilla chips is a snack, but when covered with refried beans and cheese, it has the calories of a meal no matter when it's eaten. Watch timing too. If you snack too close to mealtime, you may miss out on needed nutrients from the part of the meal you're unable to eat. Also, limit snacks while watching television. The habit can lead to overeating.

Many people like crunchy snacks, so they often choose chips and cookies, which are high in fat and added sugars. More nutritious choices are apples, carrots, whole-grain cereal or breadsticks, air-popped popcorn, and plain nuts. If you prefer healthful snacks with a smooth, creamy texture, try low-fat yogurt, smoothies, and puddings. Of course, any food you enjoy at a meal can make a good snack if it fits your eating plan for the day. A bowl of soup, a slice of pizza, or leftover pasta salad may be just what you need when hunger strikes.

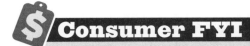

Consumer FYI

Snacking for health. Studies show that about 75 percent of Americans eat at least one snack each day, accounting for about 25 percent of their daily calories. While fruits and nuts are favored for their healthfulness, consumers want nutrition in processed snacks as well. In response, food manufacturers are offering more snacks made with soy products, added fiber, and organic ingredients. They're developing processing methods that use less fat. Instead of submerging foods in oil to cook them, a new technique merely showers them with oil. Health concerns aren't behind every trend, however: Americans bought about $5 million worth of pork rinds in 2000.

CHOICES FOR EATING OUT

Americans keep the food-service industry thriving. They buy about 70 billion meals and snacks from restaurants, caterers, food carts, and other vendors annually. These sales—about $400 million worth—account for almost half the money spent on food.

Three main types of restaurants claim most of the business. These establishments vary in selection and healthfulness of food choices.

- **Full-service restaurants.** Table service is available in these restaurants. Guests are seated and a server takes their order. Some restaurants offer a wide range of choices. Others specialize in seafood, ethnic cuisine, or even meals built on a baked potato.
- **Self-serve restaurants.** These include cafeterias, buffets or food bars, and food courts in malls. Some self-serve restaurants invite diners to return for second and third helpings, which is an invitation to overeat.
- **Fast-food restaurants.** Usually fast-food restaurants offer a limited menu, with many fried foods. Some fast-food chains are adding more healthful choices, such as grilled and roasted foods, salads, low-fat milk, and fruit juice.

Takeouts

As the pace of living increases, so do sales of takeouts, or carryout meals. These are ready-to-eat meals purchased at restaurants and taken elsewhere. See **Fig. 14-7**.

Takeouts have long been a mainstay in food service, where they're known as home meal replacements. Many delicatessens, fast-food chains, and specialized restaurants depend on them. Most full-service restaurants also have take-out menus for delivery or customer pick-up. More supermarkets are adding take-out centers. Resembling restaurant salad bars, these centers feature a variety of items, from salad fixings, to sandwiches, to entire meals.

Take-out Food Safety

To avoid causing illness from harmful bacterial growth, hot food should be served hot and cold food should be cold. That rule deserves special attention when choosing takeout.

Restaurant delivery vehicles are specially equipped to keep food at the right temperature until it reaches your door. Try to time an order so it's delivered when you plan to eat. Food brought into the home but not eaten within an hour should be refrigerated and then reheated to a safe temperature. Take-out food should be eaten within a day of purchase.

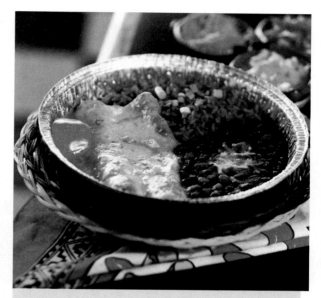

Fig. 14-7 The popularity of carryout foods today is evident. Even many supermarkets have ready-to-eat, hot meals that can be taken home for a quick dinner.

Nutrition Connection

Fast food in school. More schools today include outlets of national fast-food franchises. The practice earns much-needed income for schools, and students like the taste and convenience of fast foods. Parents and educators, however, worry that this encourages less healthful eating. In response, some school districts are creating their own, low-fat recipes for popular fast foods. Others are working with students to find healthful options that teens like.

? **What do you think about having fast-food outlets in schools?**

Eating Out Healthfully

If you eat out only for special occasions, you can indulge in a high-calorie meal without worry about harming your health. On the other hand, if you're a "regular" at local restaurants, choose places that offer an appealing variety of nutritious foods. Most have a limited selection of fruits and vegetables, so keep a supply at home for snacking.

Many restaurants now offer nutrition information for items on their menu. Ask if you don't see the information posted. Some data can be found on restaurant Web sites. You can also spot healthful choices by learning foreign words and phrases that are clues to how the food is prepared. Some are listed in **Fig. 14-8** on page 204.

These additional suggestions can help you make healthful choices:

- Many restaurants serve portions that are larger than recommended. Rather than overeat or waste food, ask for a container to take leftovers home for another meal. You could also share a portion with someone.

- Build your meal around several appetizers or side dishes instead of one large main dish, or **entrée** (AHN-tray). Order fruit appetizers for dessert and juice instead of soda.
- Look for menu descriptions like broiled, poached, steamed, roasted, or au jus. These methods add fewer calories.
- Avoid items described as batter-dipped, fried, creamy, rich, scalloped, au gratin, or crispy. All are high in fat. Alternately, peel off fried batter crusts. They contain most of the fat and calories absorbed during frying.
- Choose salads with care. Chicken, tuna, shrimp, potato, and macaroni salads are usually made

Fig. 14-8

Food Terms to Know

Term	Definition	Term	Definition
à la carte (ah luh CAHRT)	Foods listed and priced individually on the menu. Compare with table d'hôte.	flambé (flahm-BAY)	Served flaming.
à la king	Served in a cream sauce with mushrooms, pimientos, and green peppers.	Florentine (FLAHR-un-teen)	With spinach and Mornay sauce.
à la mode	"In the manner." Usually describes pie served with ice cream.	Fricassee (FRIH-kuh-see)	Poultry stewed with vegetables.
amandine (AH-mahn-deen)	Garnished with almonds.	hors d'oeuvre (awr DURV)	Any food served as an appetizer.
au gratin (oh GRAH-tun)	Topped with buttered crumbs or grated cheese and browned.	jardinière (jahr-duhn-IHR)	Garnished with mixed vegetables.
au jus (oh ZHOO)	Served with its natural juices, such as "beef au jus."	julienne (joo-lee-EHN)	Cut in long thin strips.
au lait (oh LAY)	Served with milk. "Café au lait" is equal parts hot milk and coffee.	Lyonnaise (ly-uh-NAYZ)	Served with cooked onion.
béarnaise (BAY-ahr-nayz)	Rich sauce made with egg yolks, butter, vinegar, wine, and herbs.	meunière (muhn-YEHR)	Floured, then sautéed in butter.
béchamel (bay-shuh-MEL)	Thick, white cream sauce.	Mornay (mawr-NAY)	Cream sauce with cheese.
du jour (doo ZHUR)	Today's specialty, such as "soup du jour," or soup of the day.	mousse (MOOS)	Molded, chilled dessert made with sweetened, flavored whipped cream or egg whites and gelatin.
en brochette (ahn broh-SHET)	Broiled and served on a skewer.	pâté (pah-TAY)	Finely ground mixture of seasoned meat or poultry.
en coquille (ahn koh-KEEL)	Served in a shell.	table d'hôte (tah-buhl DOHT)	Complete meal offered at a fixed price.
en croûte (ahn KROOT)	Prepared with a flaky pastry crust.	vinaigrette. (vih-nih-GREHT)	Dressing of vinegar, oil, and seasonings.

with creamy dressings, which average around 100 calories per tablespoon. Choose salads with fresh vegetables, topped with grilled or baked meat. Ask that dressings be served on the side, or skip the dressing in favor of a seasoned vinegar.

- Choose pasta dishes served with tomato sauces rather than cream sauces. Ask if sauces can be served separately.
- Fish and vegetables are often grilled with oil or butter. Ask that these dishes be prepared without the added fat.

EVALUATING YOUR FOOD CHOICES

If you are like most people, some of your food choices are healthful. Others you make could stand improvement. The first step in improving your choices is to recognize your food habits. Then you can work to replace poor habits and reinforce good ones.

Keeping a Food Record

One way to be more aware of your habits is by keeping a food record. This is a list of everything you eat and drink for a period of time. A food record is not a test that you pass or fail. It's merely a snapshot of your food choices. Whether the picture is a good one or a poor one, you decide how to act on it.

You've already kept a food record to evaluate nutrition. Now use one to learn more about your eating habits. For three days, including a weekend day, record each meal and snack you eat. List specific foods and fluids (water too), the approximate amounts, and the time of day. Add a brief description of the eating situation: the setting, your mood, what you were doing, who you were with, and any other details that could help you understand your food habits. See **Fig. 14-9**.

Using Your Food Record

When your record is completed, look it over. Do you notice any patterns in your food choices? Do certain choices seem linked to certain situations or emotions? You may detect a chain of events. On school days one teen usually skipped lunch, ate a snack later at home, and then left part of her dinner. On the weekend she ate lunch, did not snack, and finished dinner.

Once habits are discovered, look for underlying reasons. Do you skip any meals because you are rushed? Does snacking relieve stress as well as hunger? Some habits result from simple lack of thought. For example, some people always salt their food before tasting it.

Next, decide on specific and realistic actions to correct any problems. For instance, if you skip lunch, you might decide to eat lunch at school or perhaps get up ten minutes earlier to pack a

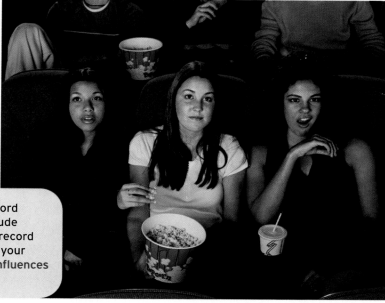

Fig. 14-9 When you keep a food record that examines your eating habits, include descriptions of eating situations. The record will help you examine what influences your food choices. Are there any possible influences at work here?

lunch. Remember that gradual changes are more likely to be permanent.

Also think of ways to support or improve positive food habits. If you already eat plenty of fruits and vegetables, you might add variety to your choices by trying some that you've never eaten before. Pledge to visit the next farmers market or talk to the supermarket produce manager.

As you assess your food choices, remember that eating should be enjoyable, even fun. Choosing healthful foods that you enjoy is one of the best food habits you can develop.

DECISION MAKING

For all the factors that affect your food choices, they are ultimately *your* choices. You decide what, when, and how much to eat. See **Fig. 14-10**.

Like a recipe, a decision is easier to make when you focus on each task involved. When you're faced with a decision, try this seven-step process:

1. **Identify the decision to be made by setting your goals.** Knowing what you want to accomplish makes the decision clearer. Suppose you want to make a snack for a party. Your goals include finding a recipe that other guests will like and then preparing it.

2. **Consider your resources.** Your choice should reflect available resources. If time is short, you might rule out complicated recipes. If a family member offers to help, that too may affect your decision.

3. **Identify your options.** Be realistic, but also creative. If an appealing option seems difficult, try to think of a manageable way to accomplish it. Make a list of the most promising possibilities.

4. **Consider each option.** Imagine the results of each possible choice. If necessary, gather more information. List advantages and disadvantages of each option. How well would each meet the goals you set?

5. **Choose the best option.** After weighing pros and cons, choose the option that seems best. If none of them is acceptable, go back to Step 3 to see whether you missed one.

6. **Carry out your decision.** Make a plan based on your choice. If you decide to bring mini-pizzas to the party, write a grocery list, buy the ingredients, and make the snacks.

7. **Evaluate the results.** If your decision worked out well, take pride in your success. If it didn't, take pride in having done your best. Either way, try to gain from the experience. Maybe you discovered a new resource or learned to recognize workable goals.

With practice, decision making becomes more successful and more satisfying. Your skills will be useful when making food and nutrition decisions and also in many other aspects of life.

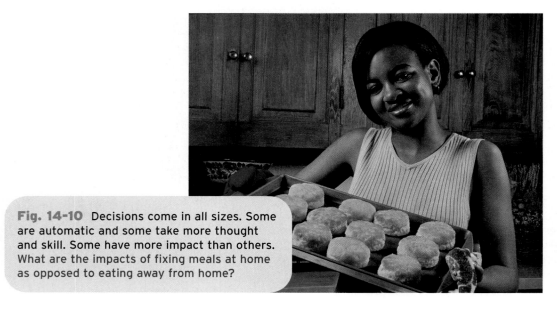

Fig. 14-10 Decisions come in all sizes. Some are automatic and some take more thought and skill. Some have more impact than others. What are the impacts of fixing meals at home as opposed to eating away from home?

Publicist

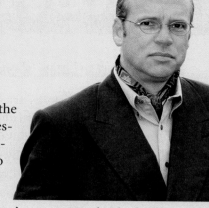

DICK DACE: Talking about food is easy for Dick Dace, a publicist for some of the most popular restaurants in Houston, Texas. Research and persistence, however, make the talk profitable.

Food and Fellowship. The seeds of Dick's career were planted while he traveled throughout Europe as a child with his grandfather. With supermarkets rare at that time, fruits and vegetables were enjoyed only in season. Dick recalls eagerly awaiting the harvest, from strawberries to white asparagus, and the pleasure of preparing meals with, and for, friends. Those days instilled two principles that still guide him: "A bite of something so wonderful you dream about it is more fulfilling than a gallon of anything less" and "Even the simplest meal can be a celebration when shared."

At eighteen, Dick attended one of the oldest cooking schools in Europe. His first job, buying fresh food daily and preparing "feasts" for guests at a small restaurant "was like having a dinner party for ten friends every evening." Later, work as an executive chef and caterer in the upscale tourist city of Vail, Colorado, was not so rewarding. The corporate kitchen, where 50 employees prepared 130 lunches a day, was a far cry from the cozy setting that made cooking meaningful.

Back home in Houston, while getting his degree in business administration, Dick kept up friendships with fellow chefs. One frequent topic was the difficulty of getting the "good press" so vital to drawing customers. They made Dick this proposal: If he could get them reviewed and featured in the local media, they would gladly pay for his service. Dick took up the challenge. With his love for food, experience in the business, and natural people skills, the job of "selling" a restaurant proved a perfect fit.

Finding Something Special. Like any good publicist, Dick starts by knowing the client thoroughly, from the chef's professional accomplishments to whether the restaurant offers a children's menu. He also looks for a distinguishing quality to convince food editors and television show producers that the restaurant deserves a story. Does it serve an unusual "signature" dish? Is it hosting a special event? Follow-up calls to the media, providing them with recipes, photos, and whatever else they may need, helps Dick deliver promised results.

While self-employed, Dick doesn't work alone. He knows he is just one item in a buffet of talent that includes the artistry of both chefs and food writers. Since Dick has dyslexia, part of his success hinged on finding someone with strengths that were not his talents. He is especially grateful for his own long-time editor, who prepares the all-important press releases for publication.

Outside the professional world, Dick hosts international students from local universities. Sharing meals is always a favorite part of the intercultural exchange. "When you break bread with someone," he says, "you become family."

On-line Connections

1. To learn more about topics in this article, search the Internet for these key words: restaurant business; cooking school; publicist.

2. To learn about related careers, search the Internet for these key words: executive chef; food writer.

Summarize Your Reading

▶ Resources, family customs, friends, the media, daily routine, values, and emotions all affect the food choices you make.

▶ Eating patterns are affected by eras, culture, habits, and stages of family life.

▶ Family eating patterns change as American society is affected by industry and the economy.

▶ To distinguish healthful items on a restaurant menu, look for such menu descriptions

as broiled, poached, or steamed, and consider building your meal around appetizers or side dishes instead of one large entrée.

▶ A food record should be kept for three days, including one day on the weekend.

▶ The decision-making process can help you make all kinds of decisions in your life, including many that are food-related.

Check Your Knowledge

1. How do **resources** affect food choices?

2. How do family food customs usually develop?

3. Why is it important to evaluate food advertising?

4. How do emotions affect food choices?

5. What are **eating patterns**?

6. How did the Industrial Revolution affect family eating patterns?

7. How did World War II affect American eating habits?

8. How do adult eating habits change when children grow up and leave home?

9. Why is breakfast an important meal?

10. Why is it important that **grazing** not turn into snacking?

11. **CRITICAL THINKING** Describe your own pattern of eating. How do breakfast and snacks fit into your pattern?

12. **CRITICAL THINKING** Categorize the restaurants in your area according to the three main types named in the chapter. Which ones offer the most healthful meal selections?

13. Why should take-out food that's been in your home for more than an hour be refrigerated and then reheated?

14. Which would probably be the best menu choice for someone who is limiting fat in the diet: en brochette, Mornay, or béarnaise? Why?

15. Why is it sometimes a good idea to take food home with you when you eat out at a restaurant?

16. What descriptive words indicate that foods are high in fat?

17. How can keeping a food record help you?

18. What are the steps in the decision-making process?

19. When making a decision, how do you evaluate options?

20. Why is evaluation a necessary part of decision making?

Apply Your Learning

1. **SOCIAL STUDIES** **Historical Comparison.** Compare influences on a teen's food choices today with those that influenced a teen in colonial America. What similarities and differences can you cite?

2. **Eating Patterns.** Discuss how these situations might impact family eating patterns: a) parents in a family work different shifts; b) teens in a family play school sports; c) a single parent often works late; d) a stay-at-home mother takes a job. What advice might help in each situation?

3. **MATH** **Cost Comparison.** Compare the cost of a take-out meal to a similar meal prepared at home.

4. **Food Record.** Keep a food record for three days, following the procedure described in the chapter. What do you conclude about your own eating habits? What actions, if any, do you need to take?

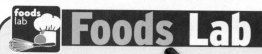
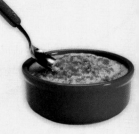

Foods Lab

Quick Breakfasts

Procedure: Evaluate one kind of store-bought, convenience breakfast food, such as frozen waffles, instant oatmeal, or cereal bars. Rate the food on appeal, cost, nutrition, and preparation.

Analyzing Results

❶ Was the food enjoyable? Would you take time to prepare and eat it in the morning?

❷ Could the food be eaten or prepared away from home, as a late breakfast or midday snack? If so, how?

❸ What nutrients does the food provide? In what amounts? How could you make the meal more nutritious?

❹ What is the cost per serving? Could you create a similar recipe from scratch for less money?

Food Science Experiment

Properties of Popcorn

Objective: To identify properties that affect how popcorn pops.

Procedure:

1. Count out three, 50-kernel samples of popcorn, all taken from the same, newly opened container.

2. Seal one sample in a plastic storage bag. Pierce the kernels in the second sample with a pin and seal in a storage bag. Spread another sample on a baking sheet and place it in the oven, which remains off. Leave all samples overnight.

3. The next day, pop each sample separately in an air popper. Compare the number of unpopped kernels and the quality of popped kernels.

Analyzing Results

❶ Which sample left the most unpopped kernels? The fewest?

❷ Which sample produced the largest popped kernels? The smallest?

❸ Popcorn pops when moisture, trapped under pressure inside the kernels, expands rapidly in a heated environment. How does that fact explain the results you noted in questions 1 and 2?

Vegetarian Food Choices

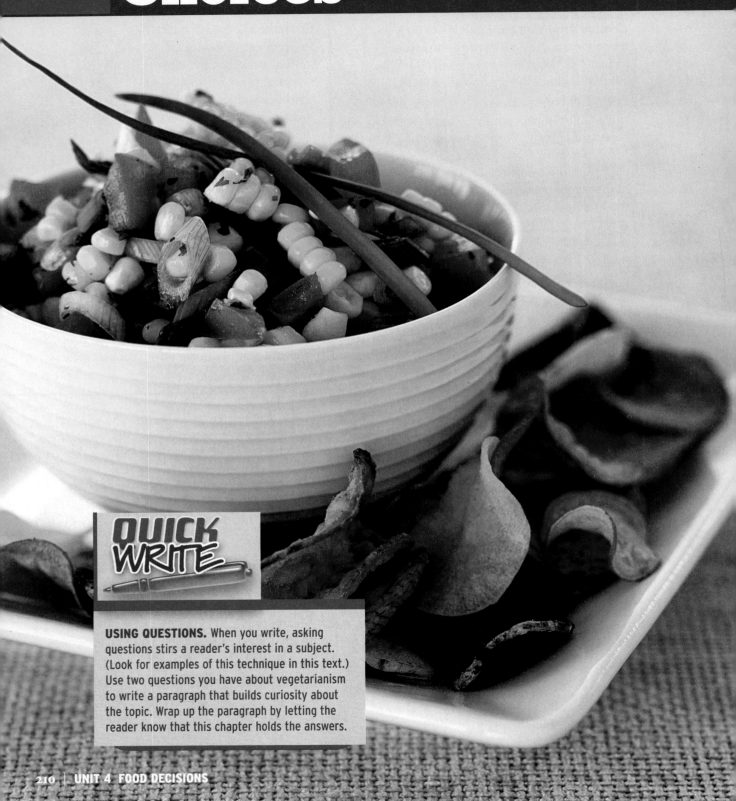

QUICK WRITE

USING QUESTIONS. When you write, asking questions stirs a reader's interest in a subject. (Look for examples of this technique in this text.) Use two questions you have about vegetarianism to write a paragraph that builds curiosity about the topic. Wrap up the paragraph by letting the reader know that this chapter holds the answers.

A**FTER ENJOYING A DELICIOUS BUFFET** dinner at a wedding reception, a guest said, "I didn't even think about it until now, but there was no meat in any of the dishes.

"The bride's a vegetarian," another guest replied. "She said that even people who weren't vegetarian would like the dishes she selected. You know, I think she was right."

What does it mean to be a vegetarian? A **vegetarian** is someone who does not eat meat, poultry, or fish. Vegetarians eat a plant-based diet that is rich in whole grains, fruits, vegetables, legumes, nuts, and seeds. These form the foundation for plenty of delicious dishes enjoyed by many people, and not just vegetarians. See **Fig. 15-1**.

TYPES OF VEGETARIANS

A large percentage of the world's population practices vegetarianism. As individuals, they're not all alike in what they eat. Basically, vegetarians fall into these categories:

• **Vegans.** Vegans (VEE-guhns) eat only foods from plant sources.

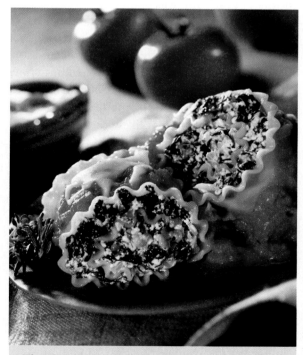

Fig. 15-1 Technically speaking, there is no such thing as a vegetarian food. Anyone can eat the same foods that vegetarians enjoy.

- **Lacto-vegetarians.** People who eat foods from plant sources and dairy products are **lacto-vegetarians**.
- **Ovo-vegetarians.** People who eat foods from plant sources and eggs are **ovo-vegetarians**.
- **Lacto-ovo-vegetarians.** When people eat foods from plant sources, dairy products, and eggs, they are called **lacto-ovo-vegetarians**.

Although the above terms describe basic vegetarians, some people modify these eating patterns to suit them. A **semi-vegetarian** eats no red meat but does eat poultry and fish. Some vegetarians include fish in their diet, but not meat and poultry. Even being a part-time vegetarian is possible. With this choice, people eat vegetarian meals much of the time and choose meat, poultry, and fish occasionally. These variations are sometimes a first step toward becoming another type of vegetarian.

THE VEGETARIAN DECISION

A growing number of Americans are exploring the possibilities of meals without meat. Their reasons for choosing vegetarianism are varied. Health benefits are one attraction. The foods that vegetarians eat are usually high in fiber and low in saturated fats and cholesterol. Studies show that vegetarians have a lower risk of heart disease, high blood pressure, and some forms of cancer. In addition, they are less likely to have digestive disorders, and they have a reduced risk for diabetes and gallstones.

Another reason why many people choose vegetarianism is a concern for animal rights. This concern focuses on the conditions under which animals are raised and slaughtered. Some people oppose the killing of animals entirely. Certain religions, particularly Hindu and Buddhist sects, advocate vegetarianism as part of an ethic of nonviolence and respect for living things.

Some people choose vegetarianism for ecological reasons. They point out that livestock and poultry, on the average, must eat 7 to 8 pounds of grains or soybeans to produce 1 pound of meat. As the global population increases and farmland dwindles, they believe the land and other limited resources could be used more efficiently by raising grains and vegetables for people instead of animals and their feed.

Still another reason cited for a meat-free diet is cost. Vegetarian foods usually cost less than animal foods. For instance, depending on the kind you buy, a pound of ground meat can cost from three to five times as much as a pound of dry beans. When cooked, the meat gives about four 3-ounce servings, while the beans provide about five or six 1-cup servings.

VEGETARIAN NUTRITION

All the reasons for choosing vegetarianism mean little if the eating plan isn't nutritionally sound. Vegetarianism doesn't guarantee good nutrition. Health risks increase, for example, from eating too many high-fat foods, whether the fat comes from meats, dairy products, or fat-laden desserts. Healthful choices make a difference. **Fig. 15-2**.

The foods that vegetarians choose most often will come from three food groups: 1) Bread,

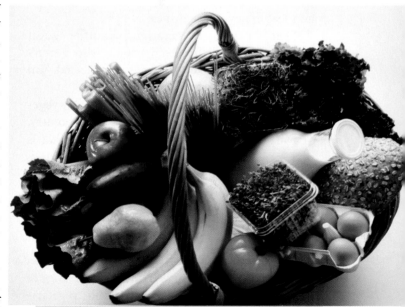

Fig. 15-2 Some people mistakenly think that vegetarians eat only vegetables. Actually they eat foods from other food groups as well. What else is part of a vegetarian eating plan?

Cereal, Rice, and Pasta Group; 2) Vegetable Group; and 3) Fruit Group. Vegetable protein sources are available in the Meat, Poultry, Fish, Dry Beans, Eggs, and Nuts Group. Soy foods, dry beans and peas, peanut butter, and eggs are good options. For servings from the Milk, Yogurt, and Cheese Group, vegetarians who don't eat dairy products can substitute calcium-fortified soy milk and soy yogurt.

Health experts agree that even children can fulfill nutrient needs through vegetarian eating. Food choices, however, should be evaluated by a nutritionist.

Calories are no more or less a problem for vegetarians than for other people. Any adjustments needed to manage weight can be made by changing the amount of food eaten.

Excluding all animal products does pose certain nutrition challenges. Some nutrients that are readily found in meat and dairy foods are less common in plants. Therefore vegans must pay particular attention to choosing foods that provide the nutrients below. They may also benefit from a vitamin-mineral supplement.

- **Zinc.** Although zinc is largely supplied by meat, poultry, and fish, plant sources include whole-grain breads and cereals, dry beans and peas, nuts, and soy foods. See **Fig. 15-3**.
- **Calcium.** Dry beans and peas, nuts, dark green vegetables, fortified grain products, and fortified soy milk products supply calcium. Since

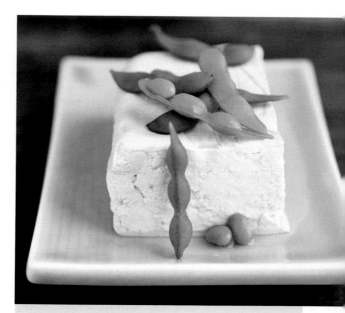

Fig. 15-3 Soy foods add protein and other nutrients to the diet. Blocks of tofu have many uses. Edamame beans are soy beans that cook quickly and can be purchased in or out of the pods.

calcium is so vital for bone development, ovo-vegetarians and vegans need to pay close attention to this need.

- **Iron.** Many of the foods that contain zinc and calcium are also good sources of iron. Eating foods that are high in vitamin C boosts absorption of iron from plants.
- **Vitamins B$_{12}$ and D.** Vegans may find it difficult to get vitamins B$_{12}$ and D, which are found in meat, eggs, and dairy products but not in plant foods. Some cereals and soy foods, especially soy milk, are fortified with both vitamins.

DAILY FOOD CHOICES

As a trip to the supermarket reveals, meatless eating plans need not be boring. The produce department, the cereal section, and the dairy case—all offer a vast and varied selection of foods that are suitable for most vegetarians.

Meat Substitutes

Meat substitutes, or analogs, are made from various blends of selected plant proteins. Thus they can provide quality protein with little or no cholesterol and saturated fat. Spices and flavoring

Nutrition Connection

Linolenic acid. With recent findings on the value of omega-3 fatty acids found in fish, vegetarians who don't eat fish may wonder whether they are denying themselves a heart-healthy nutrient. They might want to add foods that contain linolenic acid to their diet. Linolenic acid is converted to an omega-3 acid in the body, though not efficiently. Walnuts, canola and soybean oils, flax seed, and soy nuts are all good sources.

 How might walnuts and flax seeds be incorporated in an eating plan?

are added to re-create tastes ranging from smoked salmon to Italian sausage. You can find meat substitutes in prepared meals, as deli slices, or in ground form for recipes.

- **Firm tofu.** Firm tofu, or curdled soy milk, is something of a standard in the meat substitute field. Like many soy products, it absorbs flavors from other foods easily, especially if frozen and thawed. It can be cubed for grilling, mashed into patties, or crumbled into chili. See **Fig. 15-4**.
- **Tempeh.** Tempeh (TEHM-pay) is a pressed cake of fermented, cooked soybeans mixed with a grain, usually rice. It's popular in Indonesian cooking. Fermentation gives tempeh a chewy consistency and nutty, yeasty flavor. It is used cubed or shredded. Cooks often marinate and grill tempeh or add it to soups, casseroles, and stir-fries.
- **Seitan.** Wheat gluten is used to make **seitan** (SAY-tahn). It's made by simmering flour in a broth flavored with ginger, garlic, soy sauce, and seaweed. A firm, chewy texture and brown, cooked-meat color earn it the name "wheat meat." Seitan is similar to soy foods in use and in its ability to soak up flavors. It appears in vegetarian dishes in some Chinese restaurants.

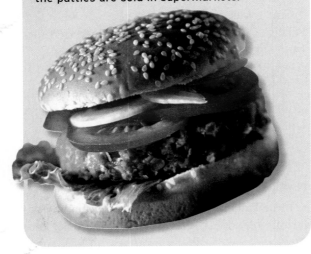

Fig. 15-4 For vegetarians who want a meatlike texture and taste in certain foods, meat substitutes can be used. How about a soyburger? Many restaurants serve them, and the patties are sold in supermarkets.

- **Quorn™.** As a relative newcomer among meat substitutes, **quorn** (KWORN) is made from a fungal protein in the mushroom family and shares a mushroom's meaty texture. The protein is fermented and mixed with egg whites and vegetable oils. Quorn was developed in Great Britain in the 1970s and is popular in Europe. It was introduced in the United States with FDA approval in 2002. A small percentage of people have reported allergic reactions, apparently to the food's fungal component.

Dairy Substitutes

The number of commercial dairy substitutes is small but growing, which is good news for vegans and ovo-vegetarians. Like meat substitutes, many dairy substitutes are soy based.

- **Silken tofu.** Silken tofu covers a variety of recipe needs. Its smooth, custard-like texture makes it a good substitute for cream cheese in dips and desserts. It can also replace eggs in homemade mayonnaise and milk or cream in whipped toppings.
- **Beverages.** Beverages, or milks, are made from various grains. Usually the grain is ground and soaked in water. Enzymes may be added to break down complex carbohydrates for a sweeter, less starchy taste. The liquid is drained, often fortified, and sometimes flavored. Soy and rice milk are the most common types, but almond, oat, and multigrain varieties can sometimes be found.
- **Imitation cheeses.** From cream cheese to nacho-style cheddar, imitation cheeses assume many forms. Yeast extract or vinegar, added to a soy and starch base, creates the characteristic cheese tang.
- **Spreads.** To make spreads, soy products are combined with gums, starches, sugars, and seasonings. The results are dry mixes and prepared spreads in a range of flavors, from butter, to cheese, to ranch dressing.
- **Frozen desserts.** Frozen desserts are often very similar to their dairy equivalent. Soy or rice milk and vegetable oils imitate the richness of cream. Chocolate flavor comes from cocoa powder, not milk chocolate.

"MILKING SOYBEANS"

Vegetarians who use soy products to supply their protein needs might invest in a small appliance to make their own soy milk. The device works something like a coffeemaker. Presoaked soybeans and water are placed in upper compartments. The machine grinds the beans and boils the water, then filters the steaming liquid through the beans and into a carafe (kuh-RAF), a bottle with a flared lip. The process can be adjusted for thicker or thinner milk and for use with rice, nuts, or seeds. The appliance can also be used as a juicer.

Making their own soy milk might inspire some people to make their own tofu. Specialty retailers sell such products as food-grade calcium sulfate and magnesium chloride, which are added to thicken the milk.

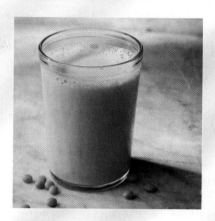

__Think Beyond>> Have you tasted soy milk? Check the labels on different brands to see what soy milk contains. How does it compare nutritionally to milk? Have a taste test in class, using different brands and including chocolate soy milk.

Vegetarian Recipes

While a wide selection of vegetarian cookbooks are available, many vegetarians collect recipes that suit their personal preference. Some are the same recipes used by nonvegetarians. Others become vegetarian through simple modifications. Chunks of sautéed eggplant can add texture as a meat substitute in a pasta sauce. Liquid smoke, rather than bacon, gives a smoky flavor to baked beans. The challenge and satisfaction of successfully reworking a recipe can add to the appreciation of food.

Some ethnic cuisines are based on vegetarian foods. Exploring Asian, Middle Eastern, and Tex-Mex cooking can uncover more meatless recipes and new food ideas.

Eating Out

Eating out for vegetarians takes the same attention to ingredients as grocery shopping. Lacto-vegetarians and lacto-ovo-vegetarians have the widest range of choices, especially since restaurants are offering more meatless dishes; however, foods may be prepared with animal products that don't appear in a menu description. Lard is often used in pastry crusts, for example. Checking with the server is a good precaution.

For vegans, eating out can be more frustrating. "Grazing" at the salad bar, questioning food servers, and asking for a plate of steamed vegetables can get tiresome. They and other vegetarians learn ways to improve their chances of finding acceptable meals. For instance, soups, appetizers, and side dishes often include meatless items that add to their options. A meal of these foods may be more interesting and nutritious than a standard entrée. Also, some ethnic restaurants offer a wider choice of vegetarian meals.

Remember that restaurants are eager to attract and keep customers. Many will honor a request for special preparation of a regular item when possible. Vegetarians who eat out often might

Dining out. It's getting easier for vegetarians to split a pizza or plate of onion rings with nonvegetarian friends. In response to consumer demands and health concerns, some restaurant chains are shifting away from animal-derived products when possible.

Some pizza restaurants make pizza and pasta sauces without meat or beef flavoring. Major fast-food chains that once used beef tallow to fry foods now use only vegetable oils. One Mexican restaurant chain uses all-vegetable oils for refried beans and bean burritos.

Vegans have fewer options. Many salad and slaw dressings contain cheese, eggs, or other dairy products. Even a veggie burger may be off limits if the bun was warmed on the same grill used to broil hamburgers. Vegans may find more choices at sandwich shops, where customers can order specific fillings.

suggest some simple additions to make menus more "vegetarian friendly." A vegetable soup in a tomato base or a zucchini lasagne would satisfy vegans as well as other diners who want lighter, healthful meals.

EXPLORING VEGETARIAN FOODS

As with weight-loss diets, an abrupt switch from a conventional to a vegetarian eating plan may not be successful or wise. As you've seen, it takes planning to supply some nutrients that most people get from meats. Anyone interested in vegetarianism should discuss the options with a dietitian. The following ideas are healthful whether a person eventually becomes a vegetarian or not:

- Identify vegetarian foods you enjoy now. Expand on the staples already in your kitchen. How many different ways can you prepare dried

Career Prep

Goal Setting

"IF YOU DON'T KNOW WHERE YOU'RE going, you may wind up somewhere else." People who don't set goals learn the truth of this saying. Goals give direction to life, including your career path.

GOALS AND CAREERS

As with home and school, work life is filled with both short-term goals, tasks to be done in a few hours or a few days, and long-term goals, which may take several years to reach. A dietitian's short-term goal could be finding low-fat alternatives for the high-fat foods a client likes. A long-term goal might be teaching the client to make healthful food choices.

As a student, you may be at a point where many goals are set for you. As you gain experience, both at work and with goal setting,

you will have more say in the matter. You'll know what needs to be done, and when, and what resources a task requires.

As the example of the dietitian shows, short-term goals can be linked to build long-term goals. That's often how careers are reached. A long-term goal to become a chef, for example, might begin with a series of short-term goals that are tackled first. These become stepping-stones to the career. Short-term goals might include reading about culinary

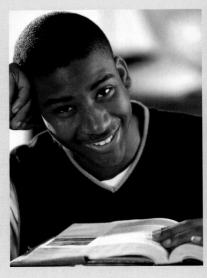

beans? What foods can you add to pasta for complete protein? What main-dish recipes can you find for your favorite vegetables? See **Fig. 15-5**.

- Get creative with substitutions. What can your favorite chili seasoning mix do for chunks of carrots, turnips, and other root vegetables?
- Get familiar with your supermarket. Does your local store carry soy milk? Bok choy? Tahini (a smooth paste of sesame seeds)? Take the time to see what each department holds. You might be surprised at the variety, especially in areas with large ethnic populations.
- Explore new retailers. Farmers markets are a natural stop for vegetarian shopping, of course. Ethnic groceries, health-food shops, and online retailers may carry unusual products, such as tempeh and mesquite-flavored, pumpkin seed snacks. Some items are costly, but they might inspire recipe ideas of your own.

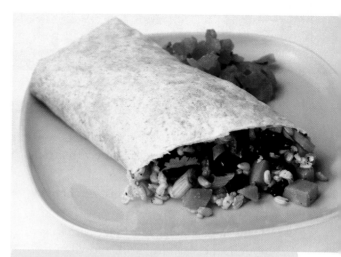

Fig. 15-5 With a little creativity, you can come up with original ideas for vegetarian eating. Such dishes can be part of anyone's eating plan.

schools on the Internet and saving money for training.

As a student, you can link education to career goals by taking classes and finding school experiences that will help prepare you for a job you want. Suppose owning a health food store is someone's career goal. Passing this course and taking part in FCCLA activities are two short-term goals that could be met in high school.

Two characteristics of goals must be considered when setting them. They need to be specific and realistic. Setting a limited time range for reaching a goal also helps.

GOALS AND THE MANAGEMENT PROCESS

Since goals give you things to strive for and keep you on course, it makes sense to learn a process that can help you reach them. The management process outlined below is a plan to use available resources to reach your goals as effectively and efficiently as possible. Planning helps you better predict unwanted results and find ways to handle them. You also reflect on whether the goal is worth the effort and consistent with your values.

1. **Choose a goal.** Choose a goal you genuinely want, not what someone else wants for you.

2. **Make a plan to achieve your goal.** Identify needed resources. Decide how to obtain them.

3. **Carry out your plan.** Allow some flexibility in case you need to substitute resources or alter your time frame.

4. **Evaluate the results in order to learn from the experience.** Did your plan work as expected? Could it be improved?

Career Connection

Goal planning. Choose a foods career that interests you. Assuming that's your long-term goal, list three short-term goals that might help you reach it. Choose one and write a plan for achieving it, including the resources you would use.

Summarize Your Reading

▶ Lacto-vegetarians eat dairy products, and ovo-vegetarians eat eggs. Some vegetarians eat neither of these.

▶ People have different reasons for choosing vegetarianism.

▶ Vegans in particular must take care to get enough zinc, calcium, iron, and vitamins B_{12} and D.

▶ Vegetarians today can choose from a variety of meat and dairy substitutes, such as seitan and milk-free spreads.

▶ Eating out may be challenging for vegetarians, as foods are sometimes prepared with animal products that don't appear in menu descriptions.

▶ Vegetarians can often find unusual but healthful foods at farmers markets, ethnic grocers, health-food shops, and on-line retailers.

Check Your Knowledge

1. What is a **vegetarian**?

2. Which type of vegetarian eats only foods from plant sources?

3. What do **lacto-ovo-vegetarians** eat?

4. What is a **semi-vegetarian**?

5. What health benefits do vegetarians enjoy?

6. How does a concern for animal rights lead some people to become vegetarian?

7. How might vegetarianism help stretch the world's food supply and feed more people?

8. Give an example that shows why some people cite cost as a reason for becoming vegetarian.

9. What must vegetarians do to make sure they get all the nutrients they need?

10. Which foods besides meat, poultry, and fish are sources of zinc?

11. What can a vegetarian do to get enough iron?

12. Compare firm tofu and **tempeh**.

13. Why is **seitan** called "wheat meat"?

14. What is **quorn**?

15. Which foods can be used as dairy substitutes?

16. Explain how pasta sauce and baked beans can be made without meat.

17. What can vegetarians do when making selections in restaurants?

18. **CRITICAL THINKING** One teen said to another, "Why don't we become vegetarians? We can start today. I don't think skipping meat will be that hard, do you?" What might a reasonable reply be?

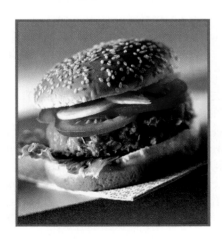

Apply Your Learning

1. **LANGUAGE ARTS Videotaped Interview.** Conduct a mock television interview with someone who is vegetarian. Ask why the person made this choice. Inquire about favorite vegetarian foods. Videotape the interview and show it to your class.

2. **Product Survey.** Survey supermarket shelves to see what's available for vegetarians. Read labels for nutrition and look for specific nutrients that are hard to get in some vegetarian diets. Report to the class.

3. **MATH Cost Comparison.** Compare the cost of a vegetarian meal and a similar non-vegetarian meal. Calculate the cost per serving and the cost per meal. Which is less expensive and why?

4. **Taste Test.** Find a recipe for hummus made with tahini paste. Prepare and serve the hummus with pita chips to the class. How do they like it? When could this dish be used? Find other uses for tahini paste.

5. **Eating Plan.** Create a nutritious three-day eating plan for someone who is a lacto-ovo-vegetarian.

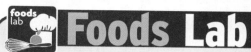 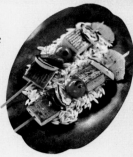

Foods Lab

Using Soy Foods
Procedure: Find and prepare a recipe that uses a soy-based meat or cheese substitute, such as meatless tacos or tofu vegetable dip. Offer samples for tasting and evaluate the finished recipe.

Analyzing Results
❶ How does the recipe's texture, taste, and appearance compare to those of a similar, nonvegetarian dish?

❷ How easy or difficult was the dish to prepare, compared to its nonvegetarian version?

❸ How would you change this recipe, if at all, if you prepare it again?

6. **Different Eating Styles.** Two people are engaged to be married. One is a vegetarian and the other is not. How might their different eating styles affect their life together?

Food Science Experiment

Soaking Beans
Objective: To learn how soaking affects beans.
Procedure:
1. Measure and weigh ¼ cup of the dried bean variety assigned by your teacher. Write down this information.
2. Place the beans in a bowl. Add ¼ cup of water. Cover the bowl and leave it overnight.
3. The next day, drain the beans, reserving the water. Measure and weigh the beans again. Measure the water also. Record your findings.

Analyzing Results
❶ What changes in volume and weight did you discover in the beans?

❷ What caused the changes you noted in question 1? How did you arrive at this answer?

❸ What other changes occurred in the beans as a result of soaking?

❹ Suggest how your findings apply to cooking beans successfully.

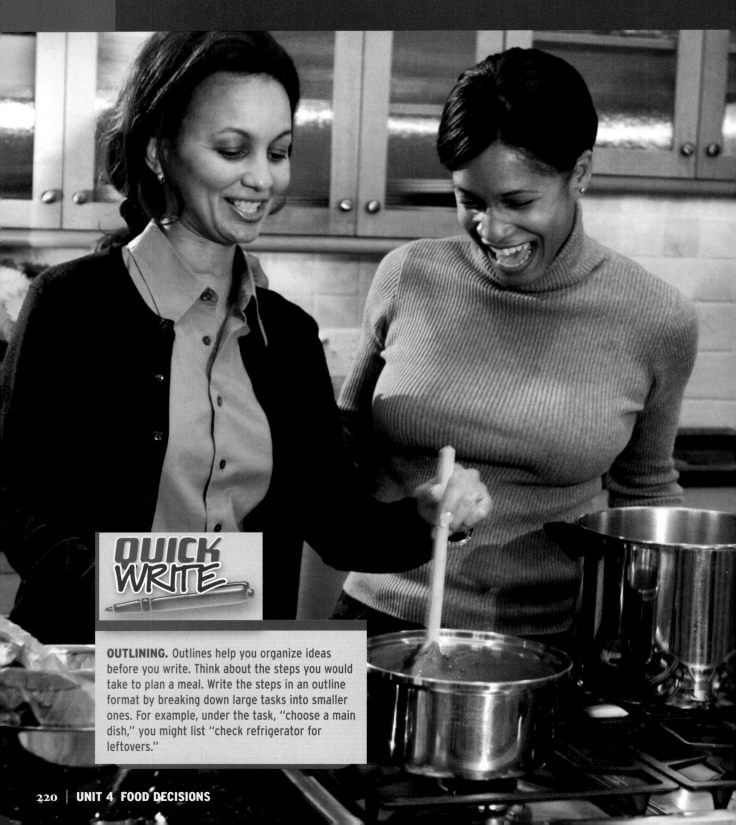

QUICK WRITE

OUTLINING. Outlines help you organize ideas before you write. Think about the steps you would take to plan a meal. Write the steps in an outline format by breaking down large tasks into smaller ones. For example, under the task, "choose a main dish," you might list "check refrigerator for leftovers."

Objectives

▶ Explain the benefits of planning meals.

▶ Explain how to create and manage a food budget.

▶ Describe government food assistance programs.

▶ Summarize ways to incorporate convenience and time savings into meal planning and preparation.

▶ Judge a meal on sensory appeal.

▶ Develop a meal plan for a week.

Terms

budget

bulk foods

commodities

convenience foods

multiple roles

scratch cooking

speed-scratch cooking

staples

HAVE YOU EVER WATCHED A FAMILY breakfast scene from the 1950s or 1960s on television? In the morning, father and the children sit at a neatly laid table, waiting. Mother, perhaps wearing an apron, sets before them the delicious, nourishing breakfast she has prepared. See **Fig. 16-1**.

That scene may seem humorous to many time-pinched families today. Family life has changed considerably, and so have family meals. Nevertheless, family members can still enjoy nutritious, flavorful meals, whether they are all together, or only a few, or even one alone. It just takes planning.

MEAL PLANNING AND REAL LIFE

If you sometimes feel drawn in a half-dozen directions, you're not alone. Most people in society have **multiple roles**. That is, they have specific responsibilities based on their different relationships to others. Certain things are expected of you as a student, a family member, a friend, and possibly a worker or volunteer. Add up the roles of all the people in your family, and you have plenty of demands on people's time and energy.

Planning what to eat—not only for one person for one day, but for a whole family and days in advance—may seem like a lot to ask.

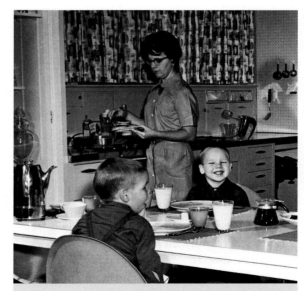

Fig. 16-1 The breakfast scene of today looks different than it did in the 1950s. How has meal planning changed?

It's because lives are so busy that meal planning is important. Meeting even basic demands requires good nutrition. Unfortunately, the more roles you take on, the easier it is to develop poor eating habits. Planning healthful meals is a defense against this tendency. Learning this skill takes time and practice, but it's an investment that will grow in value as you move toward independence.

Like any good plan, a plan for meals starts with identifying available resources. Where food is involved, one of the most important resources is money.

THE FOOD BUDGET

A **budget** is a plan for managing money. When you budget, you decide how much money to spend for food, housing, clothing, transportation, health care, savings, entertainment, and any other expenses.

According to the U.S. Department of Agriculture's Economic Research Service, American families and individuals spend an average of just over 10 percent of their disposable income (after taxes) on food each year. This includes food eaten in and away from the home. The percentage used to be higher but has steadily decreased since the 1960s as incomes have gone up. Families with a lower income typically spend a higher percentage on food than families with a higher income. The challenge for any family is to provide wholesome, enjoyable meals without spending more than the budget allows.

Besides income, other factors determine how much money a family spends on food.

- The number of family members. Logically, it takes more money to feed a larger family than a smaller one.
- The age of family members. It costs more to feed growing teens than elderly adults, for example.
- Time and skills available for food preparation.
- How often family members eat out.
- The amount of food wasted. Food may be wasted if it's not stored or prepared properly. If servings are larger than people can eat, what's left on the plate is usually thrown away.

Setting Up a Food Budget

To set up a food budget, a family first needs to know what is currently spent on food. See **Fig. 16-2**. The simplest way to learn these costs is to record all food purchases for at least two consecutive weeks. Separate records should be kept for foods bought at the store and for those eaten out, including restaurant meals, school lunches, takeouts, and food purchased from vending machines. The receipts for purchases provide the amounts to enter in the record. A small notebook can be used to record items without receipts.

After two weeks, total separately the costs of groceries and of food eaten out. Then add both amounts together. Divide that figure by two to find the average amount spent on food per week.

To find the percentage of income spent on food, divide the weekly average by the family's weekly income. Then multiply that figure by 100. To determine what percentage of food costs went for eating out, first divide the amount spent on food eaten out by the total for all food purchased. Then multiply the result by 100.

At this point, decisions can be made. If current food expenses are acceptable, the record can become a model for the food budget. If costs

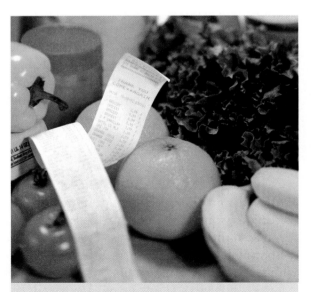

Fig. 16-2 Keeping track of food spending for a period of time helps determine a realistic amount to allow for food in the budget. Receipts provide some of the data needed.

seem too high, the budget can be set slightly lower. Experts suggest a 10 percent reduction to start. If the eating out expense is especially high, cutting there can help save money.

Planning and the Budget

Developing a workable budget often takes time and fine-tuning. Families need to continue tracking food expenses to stay within the guidelines. Weekly spending will vary, of course. It may increase to take advantage of sales or decrease to buy only **staples**, basic items that are used on a regular basis, such as milk, cereal, eggs, and bread. Any money left over can be used for unexpected needs, special occasions, or placed in a savings account.

What if a family regularly spends more than budgeted? If they made only basic purchases, with no expensive items, and didn't eat out, they may need to allow more money for food. They may be able to cut back on other expenses to increase food spending. There are also ways to trim food costs by planning meals with the budget in mind. Cost-cutting strategies include:

- **Preparing simple meals at home more often.** Homemade meals, such as casseroles, hearty soups, stews, and stir-fries, can cost less and taste better than convenience meals and food eaten out. By sharing kitchen tasks, family members can cut preparation time and have fun together.
- **Choosing economical main dishes.** Meat is usually the most expensive item in a food budget. Stretching or replacing animal proteins with high-protein plant foods, such as dry beans and peas and whole grains, can save money. A chili can be made with more beans and less ground meat, for instance.
- **Looking for store advertisements.** Newspaper ads and flyers can point out good prices on many nutritious foods that otherwise might be overlooked.
- **Reducing food waste.** Avoiding waste starts by preparing food properly. Recipes can be reduced for smaller families or appetites. Serving smaller portions also discourages overeating, while safe storage protects leftovers for future meals.

Nutrition Connection

Skimp now, pay later. When setting a food budget, two expressions apply: "an ounce of prevention is worth a pound of cure" and "an apple a day keeps the doctor away." Skimping on the foods you need for good health can cost money over time. A poor diet can lead to health problems that not only require expensive treatment but also prevent people from earning an income. In contrast, eliminating processed foods and snacks saves money in the food budget now and in health problems avoided later.

 A college student said, "I'm really short on money, so I live on popcorn and peanut butter." What advice do you have for the student?

Food Assistance Legislation

The United States has an interest in its people's health. Healthy citizens contribute more productively—to the economy, to their families, and to their community. When people cannot afford food costs due to retirement, illness, or job loss, all of society suffers. To support good health through nutrition, governments supply service agencies with funds and **commodities**, surplus food purchased from farmers and distributed to those in need of food assistance. Many programs are authorized by federal legislation and carried out by state and local authorities. Some of the major programs are described here:

- **National School Lunch Program.** This program grew from the National School Lunch Act of 1946 due to concerns that many low-income students lacked nutritious, balanced meals. It supplies cash and commodities to nonprofit food services in grade schools, high schools, and residential child care centers for serving free or reduced-price meals to children in need. In some areas, the Summer Food Service Program offers breakfast and lunch during summer vacation. See **Fig. 16-3** on page 224.
- **Food Stamp Program.** This national program has undergone many changes since it was created by the Food Stamp Act of 1964. Its major

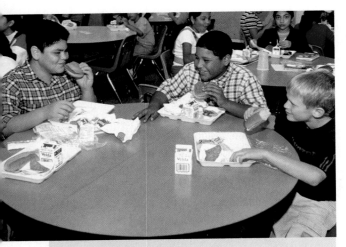

Fig. 16-3 Through the National School Lunch Program, many children get the foods they need for improved nutrition and energy to do well in school.

aim is to improve nutrition among low-income households. Families of a certain size and income qualify for assistance in the form of food stamps or an Electronic Benefits Transfer (EBT) card. These forms of aid are limited to essential food purchases. They cannot be used for nonfood items, tobacco, alcohol, pet food, or restaurant meals.

- **School Breakfast Program.** Created by the Child Nutrition Act of 1966, this federal program ensures that all children have access to a healthy breakfast at school. Nutritionally balanced breakfasts are low-cost or free to eligible students.

- **Child and Adult Care Food Program.** The National School Lunch Act also authorizes this program, which began in 1968 to provide healthful meals and snacks to children in various care settings. It was expanded several times in the 1980s and 1990s to include eligible older adults in adult care centers and families in homeless shelters.

- **Women, Infants, and Children Program (WIC).** First implemented in the early 1970s, this federal program is now under the Healthy Meals for Healthy Americans Act of 1994. The WIC program aims to improve nutrition and health of low-income pregnant and breast-feeding women and of children up to five years

of age. Participants receive vouchers to use at retail food stores for specified, wholesome foods. Supplemental foods, nutrition education, and access to health services are also provided.

- **Elderly Nutrition Program (ENP).** In 1965 the Older Americans Act was passed. The Elderly Nutrition Program was initiated under this federal act in 1972. The program provides grant money and commodities for meals served to aging citizens. Meals are served to the homes of qualifying individuals, community centers, and care facilities for the aging population.

Private organizations and religious groups in many communities run food banks and soup kitchens for people who need meals or food assistance. See **Fig. 16-4**. These programs can almost always use help, and volunteering can be a rewarding experience. Details for those who need help and for those who want to give it are available from local community action centers, public health and social services, and state agencies on aging.

OTHER RESOURCES

Besides money, families use other resources for planning and preparing meals.

- **Available food.** Some foods are more available at certain times of the year or in certain areas. Learning when foods are most plentiful and

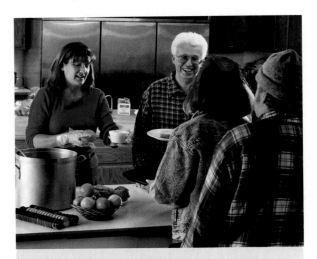

Fig. 16-4 Food assistance programs are operated by private organizations and religious groups. They help people get the food they need.

building meals around them help ensure a high-quality, nutritious diet. Families that learn to preserve foods by canning or freezing get even more value. See **Fig. 16-5**.

- **Time and energy.** Families need to pool the time and energy available to each member. Meal planning and preparation tasks can be assigned based on who can do them most conveniently. Kitchen appliances can help them use time and energy efficiently.
- **Preparation skills.** Successful meal planning takes advantage of each family member's cooking skills. Less experienced cooks can contribute simpler steps, gradually learning more complicated techniques from more skilled family members. They also learn important rules for kitchen safety and cleanliness.
- **Equipment.** Every recipe calls for certain equipment, but sometimes there's more than one right tool for the job. For example, many stir-fries can be prepared in a skillet instead of a wok. Cake recipes often give directions for using different size pans.

PLANNING FOR CONVENIENCE

Here's a time-tested recipe for chicken noodle soup. First, simmer a whole chicken in a pot of water with onions, garlic, celery, carrots, and seasonings for several hours. Meanwhile, cut up more carrots, celery, and onions, shell some fresh peas, and make the noodles. When the chicken is done, strain the broth, remove the meat from the bones, and cut it into bite-size pieces. Finally, add the cooked chicken, noodles, fresh vegetables, and seasonings to the broth. Simmer to blend the flavors, and then serve.

That's the type of recipe that comes to mind when many people think of home cooking, or **scratch cooking**, preparing a dish from basic ingredients. At its best, scratch cooking produces flavorful, economical meals. It uses fresh, quality ingredients, prepared the way you like them.

As the example shows, meals made from scratch can also involve considerable time and energy. Even a practiced cook could easily spend half a day on one recipe and might be too tired afterwards to enjoy it. For many people today,

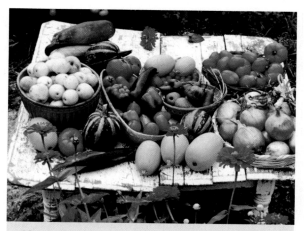

Fig. 16-5 Gardening is a versatile way to accomplish several goals. Not only do families gain inexpensive, nutritious foods, but they also share time, energy, and pride as they work together.

meal plans don't allow for scratch cooking very often. Instead, they turn to time- and energy-saving products and techniques.

Convenience Foods

Convenience foods are foods that have been commercially processed to make them easier and faster to use. They have expanded greatly from the canned soups, frozen dinners, and pudding mixes that have been popular for years. You can find single-serving, microwavable containers of

$ Consumer FYI

Hectic lives versus healthful meals. In one study, consumers cited a lack of time and information as the two biggest obstacles in planning healthful meals. Most respondents believed that meals made from scratch, including children's lunches, were more nutritious than those bought away from home. Many were confused about what a good diet includes and said that busy schedules make it hard to learn about healthful options and prepare them at home. Consumer responses suggested two solutions. People would like to see a greater variety of healthful choices at fast-food restaurants and more sources of information at supermarkets, especially a knowledgeable staff.

foods, ranging from Chinese-style noodles to oatmeal with peaches. Retort packages can be boiled in water for a hot pasta entrée or broccoli in cheese sauce. Chunks of cleaned, peeled fruits are sold in plastic containers, ready for snacks or salads. In the refrigerator case are fresh potatoes, shredded or diced for home recipes.

True to their name, convenience foods slip easily into meal planning. They're valuable for the unplanned as well. Suppose a recipe doesn't turn out or friends drop in near dinnertime. Having a variety of shelf-stable and frozen items on hand can smooth a disappointing or awkward situation.

Convenience foods also have a number of drawbacks.

- **Cost.** Every additional step in processing adds to the price of the food. A ready-to-cook meatloaf purchased at the supermarket may cost twice as much as an equal amount of ground beef. Cut-up chicken pieces usually cost more per serving than a whole chicken.
- **Nutrition.** Newer food technology helps retain quality in convenience foods; however, any processing diminishes some nutrients. Heat destroys vitamin C. Grains lose much of their fiber and nutrients during milling. Convenience foods also tend to be high in fat, sodium, and added sugar.
- **Meal appeal.** Processing affects food flavor, color, and texture. As a result, convenience foods often lack the appeal of those prepared at home.
- **Additives.** Processed foods contain preservatives, coloring agents, and other additives, which many people want to avoid. Some brands offer additive-free varieties.
- **Packaging.** The more convenient a convenience food is, the more packaging it may need. Each ingredient in a casserole kit, for instance, may be sealed in a separate container inside the box. Both producing and disposing of packaging materials, even those that are recyclable, take a toll on the environment. In contrast, you can buy **bulk foods**, which are shelf-stable foods sold loose in covered bins or barrels, in just a single bag or reusable container. Some fresh produce is naturally "packaged" in its own rind or leaves.

Using Convenience Foods

Like restaurant meals, convenience foods can be part of a healthful, balanced diet. Ingredients and directions on the label give clues to how a food might fit into a meal plan. Canned foods may need only heating, but boxed mixes require more preparation and often other ingredients. Some foods give both standard directions and a "light" method that reduces fat and calories. Check the Nutrition Facts panel for the version you plan to use. A package may also include recipes or ideas for using the product. See **Fig. 16-6**.

Speed-Scratch Cooking

A recent trend is giving cooks a satisfying way to blend convenience with scratch cooking. **Speed-scratch cooking** uses a few convenience foods along with basic ingredients for easier meal preparation. With the shortcuts of speed-scratch cooking, recipes that took hours to prepare can be made in 30 minutes or less. As a result, many families are eating at home more often.

For comparison, look at this speed-scratch version of the chicken noodle soup recipe described earlier. Start with boneless, skinless chicken breasts and cut them into pieces. Brown

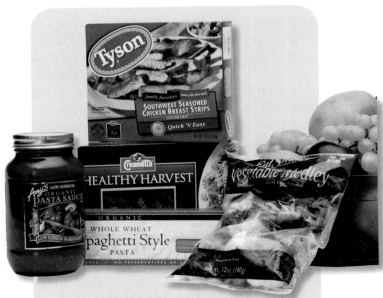

Fig. 16-6 Many people today use convenience foods for help in meal preparation. What are advantages and disadvantages of using convenience foods?

celery, onions, and garlic in olive oil. Then add canned chicken broth along with the chicken and simmer for about 20 minutes. Add packaged noodles, assorted frozen vegetables, and seasonings, and let the soup simmer for 10 more minutes. Meanwhile, you can warm French bread from a bakery in the oven, and toss a salad from a bag of cut greens and shredded carrots.

Speed-scratch cooking is useful for inexpensively adding variety and creativity. You might experiment with an array of store-bought sauces and other condiments. Taco seasoning mix turns cream cheese into a Tex-Mex dip for tortilla chips, while ranch dressing makes a zesty coating for baked chicken. What would a bottled Chinese dipping sauce do for a baked potato?

Time-Saving Techniques

Using convenience foods isn't the only way to simplify meal preparation. These tips can help families enjoy home-cooked meals more often:

- Cut large pieces of meat or whole poultry into smaller portions. Small pieces cook more quickly and can be easier to serve.
- Prepare quick-cooking, one-dish meals. Choose casseroles, hearty salads, and stir-fries that combine vegetables, grain products, and protein foods. If recipes can be made or served in a slow cooker, family members can help themselves when they are ready to eat.
- Serve fish regularly. It's a natural convenience food that is easily prepared and quickly cooked.
- Learn to use a microwave oven to cook food from scratch, as well as to defrost foods and heat leftovers.
- Involve family members in meal planning and preparation when possible. Teens can handle grocery shopping and many cooking tasks. Younger children can set the table. Everyone can help clean up.
- Set aside a weekend day to cook for the freezer. Prepare favorite recipes and freeze them. If family members eat at different times, package dishes in single servings. Include any needed instructions. If a stew is to be served with brown rice, for example, write that on the package. The frozen rice can be thawed at the same time.

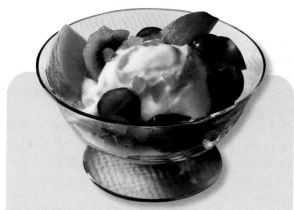

Fig. 16-7 Breakfast doesn't have to be heavy to be helpful. A breakfast that gets your day off to a nutritious start can be as simple as yogurt mixed with fruit.

- Look for recipes that can be used in different ways. A lightly seasoned meat-and-bean mixture can be a base for chili, burritos, and taco salad. Prepare a large amount and freeze it in the quantity needed for each variation.
- If schedules keep family members from eating together at home, find a more convenient location. Parents or teens who work during the dinner hour might meet the family at the meal break for a picnic or a simple supper at the workplace.

Saving Time at Breakfast

Breakfast is the nutritional foundation for the day. Nevertheless, many people don't have much time or appetite in the morning—at least, not for traditional breakfast foods. See **Fig. 16-7**.

Here, too, planning can help. One simple solution is to keep a supply of quick foods on hand, like fresh fruit, yogurt, and instant hot cereal packets that microwave in a minute. Another option is to organize a "breakfast bar." Store assorted cereals, bowls, spoons, and glasses near the refrigerator. Keep milk, juice, and fresh fruit in easy reach on one refrigerator shelf. Also, include breakfast foods when you cook for the freezer. Prepare a whole recipe of pancakes, freeze them individually, and reheat a few in the microwave for a quick pancake breakfast.

Simple breakfasts solve the problem for those people whose appetites don't wake up until mid-morning. A small amount of food can supply enough energy to start the day with very little preparation. It doesn't have to be typical breakfast fare. Any healthful combination of carbohydrates and protein serves the purpose: a handful of raisins and nuts and a glass of milk; a slice of cold pizza and pineapple juice. Later in the morning, a similar snack—yogurt, a small bagel, or cheese cubes, for example—will keep you going until lunch.

PLANNING FOR APPEAL

Suppose that three of your favorite foods were roasted chicken, mashed potatoes, and vanilla pudding with sliced banana. Would you plan a meal of these foods? You might find that the sameness in color and texture makes them less satisfying than when eaten separately. On the other hand, a meal of chili, asparagus, and peanut butter cheesecake isn't an appealing combination either.

Like the musicians in your favorite band, foods in an appetizing meal are not only good but also good together. Foods complement each other—rather than compete against each other—in taste, appearance, and texture.

- **Flavor.** Food flavors should harmonize. Foods in the same meal should keep the taste buds interested, not overwhelmed. Avoid using foods with similar flavors in the same meal. If you serve a fruit salad with the main course, choose a dessert without fruit.
- **Color.** Select foods in a variety of colors. Colorful fruits and vegetables brighten a meal. If the foods you're serving aren't naturally col-

Fig. 16-8

Sample Meal Plan			
	Monday	**Tuesday**	**Wednesday**
Breakfast	Bran cereal Sliced bananas Rye toast Milk/coffee	Fruit smoothie Bran muffin Coffee	Orange juice Bagel with nonfat cream cheese Milk/coffee
Lunch	(Packed) Turkey sandwich on whole-wheat bread Red, yellow, and green pepper sticks Apple Milk or yogurt	(Packed) Peanut butter sandwich on whole-wheat bread Carrots Pear Milk or yogurt	Adults—eat lunch out Jake and Crystal—school lunch
Dinner	Baked fish Coleslaw Broccoli Whole-wheat rolls Milk/coffee	Spaghetti with meatballs Tossed salad Italian bread Milk/coffee	Baked chicken Mashed potatoes Spinach Sliced tomato salad Whole-wheat rolls Milk/coffee
Snacks	Fresh fruits or vegetables Trail mix	Fresh fruits or vegetables Popcorn	Fresh fruits or vegetables Pretzels
Memos	Crystal not home for dinner—swim team banquet.	Everyone home for dinner.	Dad has dinner meeting.

orful, find ways to brighten them. A sprinkle of cinnamon on apple rings, chopped green onion on potatoes, and dill on a catfish fillet add eye appeal as well as a pleasing flavor.

- **Texture.** How a food is prepared affects the way it feels when you chew it. To add crunch, serve carrots raw rather than cooked. Toast Italian bread slices to serve with a creamy tomato soup.
- **Shape and size.** These qualities offer the easiest way to add variety. You can create different effects from a single food. A carrot can be cut into sticks or on the bias. Tomatoes sliced vertically form wedges; sliced horizontally, they show a wagon wheel pattern. A whole ear of corn has different impact from a scoop of corn kernels, although servings may be the same.
- **Temperature.** A food's temperature affects its taste and texture, as well as its safety. Cheese and sausage on a pizza are soft and flavorful when

fresh from the oven. To help keep hot and cold foods at their most appealing temperature, serve them on separate, preheated or chilled plates. Also remember that the outside temperature affects what foods people enjoy. Ice cream stores, after all, are busier in July than in January.

WEEKLY MEAL PLANNING

For some people, deciding what to eat five days from now seems an unnecessary chore. To others, knowing what they'll eat five days from now sounds boring. Planning meals by the week does take some effort. In the long run, however, the effort is rewarded. **Fig. 16-8** shows a sample meal plan. Notice how foods from all the food groups are included so that nutrition needs are met.

Grocery shopping is easier and more economical with a weekly meal plan as a guide. Planning

Thursday	Friday	Saturday	Sunday
Orange juice Oatmeal Whole-wheat toast Milk/coffee	Toaster waffles Strawberries Milk/coffee	Grapefruit Omelet Whole-wheat toast Milk/coffee	French toast with syrup Sliced oranges Milk/coffee
(Packed) Leftover chicken sandwich on whole-wheat bread Carrot and celery sticks Banana Milk or yogurt	(Packed) Leftover chili Cucumber sticks Tortilla chips Mixed fruit cup Milk or yogurt	Hearty vegetable soup Corn muffin Milk/coffee	Pot roast with vegetables Swiss chard Fruit salad Whole-wheat rolls Milk/coffee Angel food cake
Spicy chili with beans Butternut squash Tossed salad Cornbread Milk/coffee	Chinese takeout Milk/coffee	Chicken stir-fry with vegetables Brown rice Whole-wheat roll Milk/coffee Frozen yogurt with chocolate syrup	Sandwiches on assorted breads Tomato-cucumber salad Milk/coffee
Fresh fruits or vegetables Popcorn	Fresh fruits and vegetables with yogurt	Popcorn Flavored yogurt Mixed fruit juice	Fresh fruits or vegetables Rice cakes
Jake's basketball game— eat early. Plan next week's meals.	Mom working late shift. Dad will pick up Chinese takeout on way home from work.	Shop for food. Rob and Cindy coming for dinner.	Aunt Clara coming for dinner.

meals also helps you plan preparation; some tasks can be done earlier if it's more convenient. Choosing foods in advance actually helps keep meals interesting. It's harder to think about variety and meal appeal when you're hungry or tired.

Planning a week's worth of meals is much like planning daily menus, except on a larger scale. Some families set aside a regular time and place for meal planning. This helps with organization and lets family members share scheduling issues that may affect the menus and recipes chosen. Shopping, cooking, and clean-up tasks can be assigned or rotated.

To avoid wasting food, meal planning should include a check of the refrigerator, freezer, and fruit bowl for leftovers and fresh produce so these perishable foods can be used up. At the same time, it's wise to develop a few emergency meals based on nutritious convenience foods. Once developed, basic meal plans can be used over again, like a pattern.

PLANNING FOR ONE

Meal planning is just as essential for single people as for families, and maybe more so. Planning menus, shopping for food, and cooking may not seem worth the effort for just one person. Without definite plans, single adults may slip into poor eating habits, relying on frozen meals or takeouts, or substituting snacks for regular meals. See **Fig. 16-9**

Meal planning for one does pose challenges. Foods are often packaged to serve a group, and some foods, once opened, must be used quickly. Smaller sizes, if available, usually cost more per serving. To avoid meal plans based on "what needs to be eaten," many singles buy large food packages to share with a friend or to freeze in single-serving packages. Bulk foods can solve some problems, since they can be bought just as needed. Also, while prepared salads from a supermarket deli cost more than the fresh ingredients, they can save money by reducing food waste.

Career Prep

Education and Training

ONE ADVANTAGE IN THE FIELDS OF foods and nutrition is that jobs exist for every level of education. You can find work while still in high school. Many other jobs reward years of study and experience.

- **Entry-level jobs.** First jobs in foods and nutrition are often entry level, which require little experience. In these jobs, such as wait staff and dishwasher, pay tends to be low and authority is limited. Such positions, however, instill good work habits and help you plan further possible steps on your career path. You can survey the workplace overall to decide whether you would enjoy the environment.

- **Technical jobs.** Jobs that require a degree from a community college or technical school are also available. A dietetic technician, for instance, has an associate's degree in science.

A chef may earn a certificate from a culinary arts school.

- **Professional jobs.** A four-year degree or higher opens the door to a world of professional possibilities. Dietitians, food scientists, and family and consumer sciences teachers all hold at least a bachelor's degree; many have a master's degree, and some, a Ph.D.

BEYOND THE CLASSROOM

In some careers, on-the-job training supplements formal studies. A budding pastry cook might combine class work with hands-on experience in an apprenticeship. College-level studies in microbiology are useful for a health inspector, who also completes a supervised certification program. A college graduate who is accepted in a company's executive training program learns all areas of the business, from

Recipe selection may take more thought also. Most recipes serve six or more people. Some recipes can be creatively "downsized." For instance, the stuffing for a roast chicken can be as easily used with chicken breasts, or even pork chops, as with a whole bird. When reducing ingredients is not practical, cooking for the freezer comes in handy. By choosing recipes that freeze well, a single person can prepare enough individual servings for five more meals.

Like grocery items, larger recipes can also be shared. Singles who enjoy eating with others can meet regularly and take turns cooking for each other. Some clubs have a weekly or monthly potluck, with each member bringing a dish.

Meals alone aren't necessarily lonely, however. Enjoying flavorful, healthful foods, accompanied by your favorite music, can be a soothing end to a busy day.

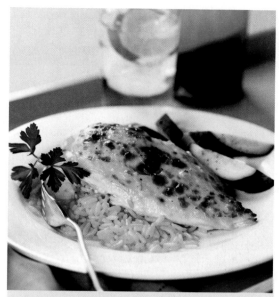

Fig. 16-9 Meals for one shouldn't be neglected or eaten on the run. With a little planning, downsizing to single-serving meals is not that difficult.

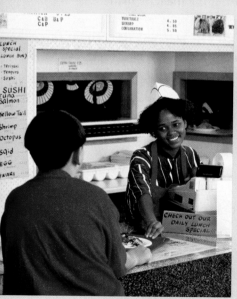

assembly line to marketing.

Continuing education is also valuable, and sometimes required, in certain professions. Teachers in family and consumer sciences, for instance, attend conferences and seminars to learn the latest ideas in education as well as foods and nutrition.

One often-overlooked option for foods and nutrition training is military service, which offers unusual tests of culinary skills—cooking in a moving truck, for example.

Before enrolling in any program, do some research. Learn about graduation and placement rates. Ask graduates whether they were prepared for the job they wanted.

Make sure the program is accredited, meaning it meets the educational standards of a recognized authority. Some types of tuition aid can be used only at accredited schools. Some professional groups have accrediting councils. For example, nutrition and dietetic programs should be accredited by the American Dietetic Association. An accrediting body for cooking schools is the American Culinary Federation, Inc.

Career Connection

On-line education. More and more schools offer degrees on-line. Investigate one such program that would be useful to a foods and nutrition career, such as an associate's degree in business or hotel management. How is the degree earned? How long does it take? What costs are involved? Is the program accredited? With classmates, compile your findings into a class resource.

Summarize Your Reading

▶ Planning helps people in families of all sizes, including individuals who are alone, enjoy nutritious, flavorful meals.

▶ Learning to manage within a food budget involves making nutritious food choices without overspending.

▶ Several federal food assistance programs help low-income children, families, and older adults eat nutritious meals.

▶ Families can eat healthful meals and yet save time by incorporating convenience foods and time-saving techniques.

▶ A meal should have sensory appeal through appetizing combinations of foods that have varied shapes and sizes, colors, flavors, textures, and temperatures.

▶ A written weekly meal plan lists what a family intends to eat for breakfast, lunch, dinner, and snacks on each day of the week.

Check Your Knowledge

1. Why is meal planning so important?

2. What factors determine how much money a family spends on food?

3. **CRITICAL THINKING** Develop a series of numbered steps that show how to set up a food budget.

4. If a family needs to reduce the amount spent on food, what might the family do?

5. What are **commodities**?

6. Compare the National School Lunch Program and the School Breakfast Program.

7. Describe the Women, Infants, and Children Program (WIC).

8. What federal program serves meals to aging citizens?

9. How can families make the most of their resources for planning and preparing meals?

10. What's the difference between **scratch cooking** and **speed-scratch cooking**?

11. What are some of the drawbacks of **convenience foods**?

12. How can you simplify meal preparation without using convenience foods?

13. How can families serve breakfast quickly without going to too much trouble?

14. What makes a meal appealing?

15. **CRITICAL THINKING** A teen prepared this meal: white fish, rice, cabbage, and applesauce. How could the meal be made more appealing?

16. **CRITICAL THINKING** How might meal appeal affect the quantity and the kinds of foods people eat? When might this be a help and a hindrance?

17. Why is it important to develop a weekly meal plan?

18. Why should families check to find what foods they already have before planning the week's meals?

19. How can single people plan healthful meals?

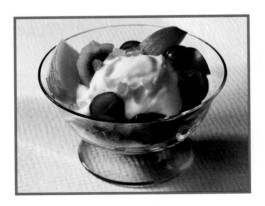

Apply Your Learning

1. **MATH** **Food Spending.** Suppose two families of four each spend $360 on food every month. One family has a net monthly income of $3,000 and the other, $1,900. What percentage of income does each family spend on food? Compare how the overall budgets for the two families may be affected.

2. **MATH** **Food Budget.** Develop a full week of meals for a family of four (two adults; one male, age seventeen; and one female, age twelve). List all foods to buy, excluding staples. Estimate food costs by checking supermarkets and advertisements. As you plan, stay within the food budget amount assigned by your teacher.

3. **State and Local Programs.** Investigate what programs, other than federal, help people with food and nutrition needs in your area. How do programs work and where are they located? Who is eligible to participate?

Foods Lab

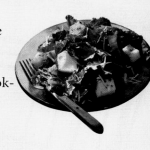

Using Dry Mixes

Procedure: Create a recipe that uses a commercial dry mix, as for baking or salad dressing. Look through cookbooks for ideas on ingredients and proportions, if needed. Prepare the recipe and evaluate the results.

Analyzing Results

❶ How did you add flavor, color, and texture to the recipe?

❷ How did using the mix shorten preparation time?

❸ How do you think the mix affected the dish's nutritional value, as compared with the same recipe made from scratch?

❹ Do you think you could create a similar mix at home? Why or why not?

Food Science Experiment

Effects of Freezing

Objective: To compare how freezing affects ingredients in leftovers.

Procedure:

1. Cut a carrot into $\frac{1}{2}$-inch slices. Measure two, $\frac{1}{4}$-cup samples.

2. Cook each sample in a small amount of water in a saucepan. Cook one sample until tender; cook the other sample until slightly firm.

3. When the samples are cool enough to handle, place them in separate, rigid, freezer containers. Label and place the containers in the freezer.

4. Repeat Steps 2 and 3, using $\frac{1}{4}$-cup samples of uncooked rice and the package directions.

5. Remove the samples the next day and reheat them. Evaluate them on appearance, texture, and taste.

Analyzing Results

❶ Which sample of each food was more pleasing? Why?

❷ What factors do you think affected the quality of each sample?

❸ Based on your findings, how would you prepare a casserole that you planned to freeze?

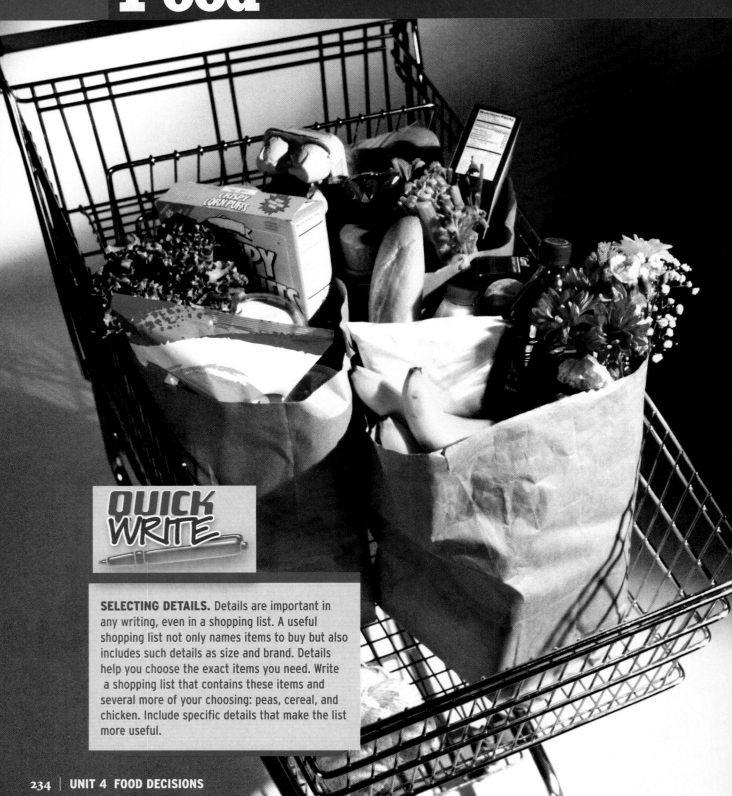

Shopping for Food

QUICK WRITE

SELECTING DETAILS. Details are important in any writing, even in a shopping list. A useful shopping list not only names items to buy but also includes such details as size and brand. Details help you choose the exact items you need. Write a shopping list that contains these items and several more of your choosing: peas, cereal, and chicken. Include specific details that make the list more useful.

To Guide Your Reading:

Objectives

▶ Compare different types of food stores.

▶ Evaluate a food store for quality and cleanliness.

▶ Develop a useful, well-organized grocery list.

▶ Explain how label information helps in making food purchases.

▶ Describe how to get quality and save money when shopping for food.

Terms

code dating

comparison shopping

food cooperative

impulse buying

natural foods

open dating

organic foods

perishable foods

rebate

sell-by date

store brands

unit price

universal product code (UPC)

use-by date

S HOPPING FOR FOOD MAY SEEM LIKE A FAIRLY simple task. Like any activity, however, having certain skills and knowledge helps you get the most from it. Mixing butter, sugar, and eggs does not guarantee a delicious cake. Likewise, spending money in a supermarket doesn't guarantee a satisfied shopper.

Food shopping, like cooking, is a process. Learning the proper technique for each step, from choosing a store to checking out, improves your chances of success.

WHERE TO SHOP

Stores that sell food go by many names: groceries, food marts, mini-marts, pantries, and more. Whatever they are called, they generally can be categorized based on their size, prices, and services.

Supermarkets

As the name implies, supermarkets offer shopping on a large scale. Most are part of a regional or nationwide chain, which gives them the buying power to offer a vast selection of foods at competitive prices. They typically stock about 15,000 different food items—"superstores" may carry twice that number—as well as paper products, cleaning supplies, and health and beauty aids. Many supermarkets have their own bakeries, butcher shops, and take-out food departments. Local banks may operate a small banking center inside.

Over the years, the basic supermarket has developed variations that emphasize price or convenience.

- Supercenters are huge stores that combine a supermarket with other types of shops in one building. They may include a full-service pharmacy, a hair salon, a vision center, or an entire department store.

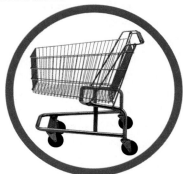

- Warehouse stores are so called for their "no-frills" approach. Prices are low because the store spends less on labor, decoration, and customer services. Basic food items are displayed in cardboard shipping boxes. Shoppers bag or box their own groceries when checking out, using their own bags or spare store boxes. Larger "super warehouse" stores have separate food departments.
- Health food supermarkets carry only **natural foods,** those that have been minimally processed and contain no artificial ingredients or added color. Thus they are sometimes called natural food stores. Here you will find many vegetarian foods, unusual grains, and even natural sodas. A store may specialize in **organic foods**, which are produced without the use of pesticides, artificial fertilizers, growth hormones, or antibiotics. Organic foods are not genetically modified or irradiated. Some stores sponsor cooking classes and lectures on health and nutrition.
- Warehouse clubs, or wholesale clubs, require an annual membership fee. Members can buy a large variety of food items at low prices, but usually in extra-large quantities only—four-pound bags of tortilla chips and one-gallon jugs of salsa, for example. Some stores carry gourmet items, along with clothing, housewares, and small appliances.

Other Store Types

Supermarkets are popular, all-purpose stores. They account for about 75 percent of all grocery sales. Other types of stores fill other, specific needs.

- **Independent grocers.** While they may be as large as supermarkets, these stores are owned by individuals. Prices may be higher as a result, but independent grocers have more freedom to reflect the "local flavor." They can stock more regional favorites and locally produced foods.
- **Specialty stores.** These small, independent stores limit their stock to a specific type of food, such as gourmet, fish, cheese, or baked goods. They are noted for high-quality, fresh food and unusual items. Ethnic grocers are an excellent

source for hard-to-find staples of different cuisines. Prices are generally higher than those in supermarkets.

- **Food cooperatives.** A **food cooperative**, or co-op, is a food distribution business mutually owned and operated by its members. To keep down costs, the cooperative buys food in quantity and members do much of the work. They also receive a discount based on hours worked. This hands-on approach gives members more control over the quality and type of food in their store. Many cooperatives emphasize fresh or natural foods. Some are licensed to sell to the public.
- **Convenience stores.** These include service station food marts and drugstores. Like convenience foods, they're quick and easy to use. Some stores never close. Their line of groceries is limited and based on staples and snacks. Shoppers pay for the convenience: food prices are generally higher than in most other types of stores.
- **Farmers markets.** These markets, where area farmers sell their produce during the growing season, are popular in cities, large and small. Locally grown fruits and vegetables are often fresher and less expensive than those in super-

$ Consumer FYI

Farmers markets. Farmers markets are a vital resource, even in urban areas. Produce growers are usually experts on storing and preparing the foods they sell. Some offer pamphlets with nutritional facts and recipes.

Most of the 3,000 markets in the United States take part in the federal government's Farmers Market Nutrition Program, which provides coupons for fresh foods to low-income families and older adults. Some contribute unsold produce to food banks and other social service agencies.

Farmers markets bring a social element to shopping. In discussing food, farming, and news of the day, buyers and growers get a better appreciation for each other. They strengthen their sense of community.

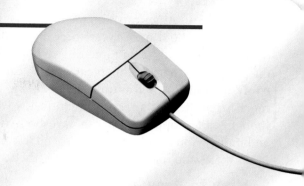
GROCERIES IN YOUR COMPUTER

With the popularity of on-line shopping, it was just a matter of time before supermarkets used this technology. In some areas today, you can order groceries by mouse click for next-day delivery. The process is much like using an on-line catalog. You create an account at a supermarket's Web site or lease software from a food supplier.

The goal of on-line food sellers is to combine at-home convenience with in-store advantages. To make ordering easier, you can save a list of frequently purchased items for future visits. You can also "browse the aisles" or do a key-word search as well as compare prices. Some grocers allow you to choose food in specific forms, such as husked corn on the cob or quarter-inch-thick pork chops, and note what substitutions, if any, you'll accept. They may provide close-ups of items, including the Nutrition Facts panel, and personal pages, with coupons that appeal to each shopper's buying habits and past purchases.

To schedule delivery, you choose a convenient time slot from those available. Delivery vehicles equipped with refrigeration and freezer units ensure the quality and condition of perishable foods.

__Think Beyond>> On-line shopping has advantages. What might be some disadvantages?

---

markets. You may also find homemade preserves, baked goods, and seasoning mixes.

- **Internet.** A variety of food sellers operate partly or entirely on-line. Some supermarket chains allow shoppers to order groceries through the store Web site. They prepare orders for pick-up or deliver them for a fee. The site may provide coupons, recipes, and cooking tips and even plan menus and prepare shopping lists. Specialty retailers offer foods ranging from gourmet chocolates to organic oats.

Choosing a Store

If you listen to advertisements, you know stores pride themselves on offering "friendly service," "low prices," "convenient locations," and "an unbeatable selection." How do you identify these qualities when you walk through the store doors? Ask yourself the following questions:

- How do the store's regular and sale prices compare with those of other stores? Are prices well marked, either on the products or on the shelves?

- Are the employees courteous and helpful? Is there an information center to answer your questions?

- If the store is large, do overhead signs identify the food in each aisle for easy navigation?

- Is the store, including shelves, cases, and bulk bins, clean and neat? Are food packages in good condition? Does the store smell clean? Foul odors may indicate leaking food packages or temperatures that are too high to maintain quality.

- Are shelves and cases well stocked with a variety of brands and sizes?

- Does the produce department feel cool? Do fresh fruits and vegetables look fresh? Are greens kept moist and berries dry?

- Are the meat and dairy cases cold enough to keep the foods at a safe temperature?

PLAN YOUR SHOPPING

The typical American shopper goes to the supermarket about once every three days. Some of these trips result from forgetting to buy items on the previous trip. "Emergency runs" can be costly, in money as well as time, if you have to pay more for an item as a result. In contrast, a well-thought-out shopping trip can save both time and money. You avoid extra trips, spend less time in the store, and manage your spending better.

Getting to Know a Store

Some stores are so big you may feel like you need a map—and some stores provide one. At the store entrance, look for a directory sheet showing which items are found in each aisle.

Whatever the size, most food stores follow the same general layout. Once you understand how they are organized, you can navigate them easily. If time is a priority, you may want to do most of your shopping at one store. That way, you can become familiar with the location of the items.

If a store were a city, its "downtown" would be the rows of shelves stocked with packaged, shelf-stable foods, as well as household goods and health and beauty aids. These are arranged according to type—rice and pasta, canned fruits and juices, and cereals, for example.

Usually nearer the "suburbs," or store walls, you find coolers and cases for **perishable foods**. Such foods can spoil or decay, which occurs faster without proper storage. Many must be refrigerated or frozen to maintain quality. Here's where you will find perishable foods:

- A produce department for fresh fruits and vegetables.
- A refrigerated meat, poultry, and fish department.
- Refrigerated sections for dairy products, eggs, cured luncheon meats and sausages, and fresh pasta.
- A freezer section for all frozen foods, including many convenience foods.

Bulk foods may be sold in a separate department or with other foods of the same type. Bins of nuts would be found in the produce depart-

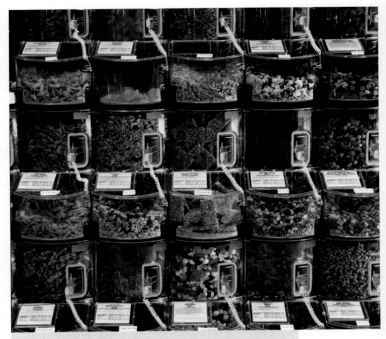

Fig. 17-1 Bulk food bins are usually marked with a number. After filling the bag, you write the bin number on a tag or sticker. When the code number is entered during checkout and the product is weighed, the correct price is determined.

ment and barrels of flour with baking supplies. To buy bulk foods, you fill a container, usually a bag, with the desired amount of food. You mark the container by writing the food's identification number on a tag or sticker, which lets the checkout clerk identify the contents. See **Fig. 17-1**.

To save time and stress, find out the store's busiest hours—then try to avoid them. Typically, a supermarket is most crowded between 4:30 p.m. and 6:30 p.m. Weekends are also busy. If you can shop during less congested hours, you may feel less rushed and make better choices.

Writing a Shopping List

If you plan a shopping trip, you'll probably be buying more than a few items. A shopping list helps you remember them all. It can also help prevent **impulse buying**, or buying items you didn't plan to purchase and don't really need. Impulse buying can ruin any food budget.

You can start to prepare a shopping list during weekly meal planning. Do you need to buy anything for the menus and recipes? List these items in the amounts needed, increasing the quantities if necessary to cook for the freezer. Before finalizing menus, check the store ads for any sale items that might be used in meals.

Next, check your supply of staples, as well as food you keep on hand for emergencies, such as frozen dinners and shelf-stable foods. Don't forget paper products and cleaning supplies.

The store layout is a useful guide for writing your shopping list. You can write down items in the order they're found in the store. You can group items that are in the same department, as in the sample shown in **Fig. 17-2**.

Many families keep a shopping reminder list handy in the kitchen for jotting down items that are running low. Some people keep copies of a basic shopping list of things they usually buy. Each week, they circle the items they need and add any others. Many store the list in their computer. When they finish the week's menus, they add the needed foods to the basic list and print out the final one.

To make a list even more useful, take a pen or pencil to cross off items as you find them. That way, you won't overlook anything.

USING FOOD LABELS

Thirty years ago, shoppers didn't expect to learn much more from a food label than the product name, its price, and directions for use. In contrast, wrappers on today's packages are packed with details about the food inside. Like advertisements, food labels are part promotional and part informational. Interpreting them is part of becoming a shrewd shopper.

Basic Information

As you recall, the Nutrition Facts panel is your source of valuable facts on calories, nutrients, number of servings, and portion size. Make a habit of turning to the panel on every food you consider buying.

Other information on food labels is becoming more complete, accurate, and useful to consumers. This is due to the FDA's exacting requirements, which even include placement and lettering size.

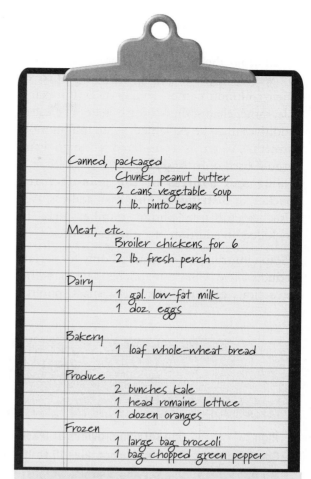

Fig. 17-2 A well-organized shopping list makes it easier to find needed items once you get to the store. Why are frozen foods likely to be found last in a store?

- **Kind of food.** The basic kind of food is identified, such as chicken pot pie or peaches packed in syrup. Manufactured foods are not called by the name of the food they replace. Soy "sausages" may be labeled "breakfast links." The food's form is shown or stated if more than one form is commonly available. Canned tomatoes might be described as diced or whole.
- **Amount of food.** The amount is given in both customary and metric measurements. It may be stated in volume, such as 2 liters, or as net weight. Net weight is the weight of the food and any added liquid but excludes the packaging.

- **List of ingredients.** Any food that contains more than one ingredient has these listed in order from the largest to the smallest amount by weight. Ingredients must be identified by their common name—baking soda, for example, rather than sodium bicarbonate. The use of additives must be explained, as "to inhibit mold growth." Water is considered an ingredient, even if used only for packing.
- **Name and address of the manufacturer, packer, or distributor.** An e-mail address, Web site, or toll-free phone number may be included, in addition to a physical address.

Some information is required only for certain products. The USDA mandates safe handling instructions on packages of raw meat, poultry, and eggs. Beverages that contain fruit juice must list the percentage of juices.

Most labels include a picture of the product and directions for use. If the product is not shown exactly as it's found in the package, the photo must be labeled "serving suggestion." Storage methods that are recommended to maintain quality or safety are noted, such as "Refrigerate after opening."

Claims on Labels

Inspired by consumers' growing interest in nutrition, food makers may point out a product's nutritional advantages on the label. Certain widely used terms are also precisely defined by the FDA, including those listed in **Fig. 17-3**.

Fig. 17-3

Decoding the Food Label	
Term	**Description of Food**
High	One serving provides at least 20 percent of Daily Value for specified nutrient.
Good source	One serving contains 10 to 19 percent of Daily Value for particular nutrient.
More	One serving contains at least 10 percent more of Daily Value for nutrient than food to which it's compared.
Free	Used for fat, saturated fat, cholesterol, sodium, sugar, and calories. Has no significant amount of nutrient or ingredient in question. May be percentage, such as "97 percent fat-free." "Nonfat" sometimes used for dairy foods.
Low	Can be eaten frequently without exceeding recommended amount of fat, saturated fat, cholesterol, sodium, and calories.
Reduced	Has at least 25 percent less of nutrient or calories than food to which it's compared. "Reduced" compares nutritionally altered product to regular version. Regular cottage cheese might be labeled "35% less fat than sour cream." Reduced-fat cottage cheese could claim "25% less fat than regular cottage cheese."
Lean	Meat or poultry product with less than 10 g fat, 4.5 g or less saturated fat, and less than 95 mg cholesterol per serving.
Extra lean	Meat or poultry product with less than 5 g fat, less than 2 g saturated fat, and less than 95 mg cholesterol per serving.
Healthy	Low in fat and saturated fat and contains limited amounts of sodium and cholesterol. Single-item food provides at least 10 percent of the Daily Value of vitamins A or C, iron, calcium, protein, or fiber.
Fresh	Raw, preservative-free, and has not been heated or frozen.
Fresh frozen	Frozen while still fresh.

The FDA also allows a growing number of claims about the health benefits of foods that meet certain definitions. These statements have strict guidelines. First, the claim must be supported by science and research. The food must meet specific nutrient levels that are set by the government. It must be carefully worded to explain clearly the relationship between the food or nutrient and a particular disease or health condition. Also, it must state that eating the food is only part of managing the condition. A box of oat bran, which qualifies as high in fiber, might carry this claim: "Studies show that a diet high in fiber helps reduce the risk of heart disease."

The Organic Seal

The USDA uses approved state and private agencies to inspect farms and companies and to certify them as organic food producers. Their products are labeled with "Certified organic by" followed by the name of the certifying agent. Foods that contain only certified organic ingredients can also be marked "100 percent organic." Those that are 95 percent or more certified organic ingredients can be called "organic." Both classes of food can display the USDA organic seal, shown in **Fig. 17-4**.

Processed products that contain at least 70 percent organic ingredients cannot carry the seal but may be labeled "Made with organic ingredients." If the product has less than 70 percent organic ingredients, the word "organic" can appear only in the ingredients list. Note that the term "natural" is not legally defined and is not the same as organic.

Product Dating

Some packages are stamped with a date to help ensure product freshness. **Open dating**, which uses a calendar date, is found mainly on perishable foods, such as meat and dairy products. The product and the wording determine the date's meaning for the consumer.

- **Sell-by date.** The last day the product should remain on the store shelf is the **sell-by date**. It allows for a reasonable amount of time for home storage and use after the date. The package may state "Sell by" or "Best if purchased by." Although intended for the retailer, the sell-by date is useful to consumers. See **Fig. 17-5**.
- **Use-by date.** The **use-by date** suggests the last date the product can be used with high quality. "Quality assurance date" means the same. If a date appears without wording on baked goods, it is usually a use-by date.

Open dating does not guarantee quality. That also depends on how the product is processed and handled. It is a tool that helps food makers, sellers, and buyers exercise quality control. Foods are still safe to eat after the date, although nutrition and flavor may suffer. State laws vary, but nationally, open dating is required only on infant formula and baby foods.

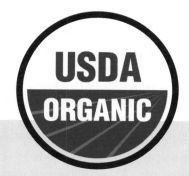

Fig. 17-4 This USDA seal indicates that a food was organically grown. What foods qualify to carry the seal?

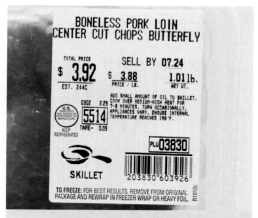

Fig. 17-5 The sell-by date helps the seller tell when a product should no longer be on the shelf. How does it differ from the use-by date?

Code dating refers to a series of numbers or letters that indicate where and when the product was packaged. Processors use it to identify shelf-stable products. If a recall is necessary, the products can be tracked quickly and removed from the shelves. Federal law requires code dating on most canned food.

Universal Product Code

That series of black bars on almost every food package is the **universal product code (UPC)**. This is a bar code that can be read by a scanner. It's probably best known to shoppers for making checkout faster and more accurate. An electronic scanner identifies the product, enters the correct price on a screen for the customer to see, and adds it to the receipt. At the same time, the store computer automatically deducts the item from inventory. See **Fig. 17-6**.

Below the UPC black bars are the equivalent numbers in the code. These serve as a backup if the bar code cannot be read. Although several UPCs exist, the one you see often on foods has 12 digits. The first digit, on the far left, identifies the code. The next five digits, grouped together, identify the manufacturer. The following five digits, also grouped, identify the product. The last digit, to the far right, checks whether the number scanned correctly.

A similar code to UPC is European Article Numbers (EAN), used in other countries. Scanning equipment in the U.S. will eventually have to recognize these codes as well.

Fig. 17-6 At the checkout counter, the scanner reads the UPC. What information is recorded this way?

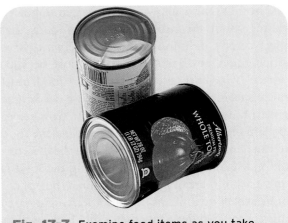

Fig. 17-7 Examine food items as you take them from the supermarket shelf. What signs tell you that these foods should not be purchased?

GETTING QUALITY

Successful shopping is not a simple matter of finding the food on your list and buying it. You want to get the best value for your money. That doesn't always mean buying the cheapest foods. It means learning to balance food price with food quality. Quality foods are fresh and nutritious, and they maintain that condition longer. Poor quality food is no bargain, no matter how low the price. It may even be unsafe to eat.

Checking product date is one way to help ensure quality in foods you buy. Here are others:

- If you combine your shopping trip with other errands, do those tasks first. That way, you can bring the food directly home and store it properly. Allowing perishable food to warm to room temperature invites harmful bacteria growth.
- Plan your route through the store. The freezer section; the meat, poultry, and seafood departments; and the produce department should be your last stops.
- Avoid packages that are dirty, rusty, leaking, or otherwise damaged. See **Fig. 17-7**. Harmful bacteria may have contaminated the food. Put meat, poultry, and fish packages in plastic bags so they won't drip on other foods in your cart or shopping bag. These juices can also harbor bacteria and unpleasant odors.
- When buying frozen foods, avoid packages that are frosted with ice. Frost means the package

may have started to thaw and then refrozen, which can damage food.

- Place fragile items on top of heavier ones when adding food to a cart or bag.

GETTING YOUR MONEY'S WORTH

The other half of the formula for value is paying a fair price. You may not be able to control what stores charge for food, but you do have options for how much you pay.

What Affects Food Prices?

You might expect to pay more for fresh peaches in the spring than in late summer. Produce is more plentiful and thus less expensive during its growing season, yet why would the price of your favorite cereal jump seemingly overnight? Forces that raise and lower food prices often develop over time.

- **Marketing costs.** You'll recall the pipeline that food travels from producer to consumer. Costs incurred at every stage, from the price of seed to the cashier's wages, add to the price of food. These expenses are dependent on other factors. A rise in oil prices can add to the cost of operating farm machinery, processing plants, and delivery trucks.
- **Supply and demand.** The price of seasonal produce is one example of supply and demand. As supply increases, prices tend to go down. A good or poor growing season can magnify the impact. Peaches will be more expensive, for example, if a late freeze destroys part of the crop. Consumer demand also affects food prices. High demand increases prices, and vice versa. For example, if a bakery notices people are buying less bread, they might cut their prices to encourage sales.
- **Consumer carelessness.** Careless consumers sometimes damage food when they shop. Some damaged goods are sold at a discount. Most are thrown out. In addition, shoplifting and grocery cart theft are widespread. Stores are compelled to raise prices to make up for their losses.
- **Government policies.** Governments may buy crops or foods for their commodities programs or reimburse growers for farming-related

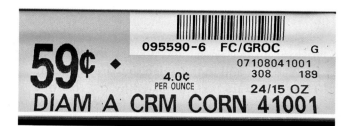

Fig. 17-8 Unit pricing helps you get the best buy without having to do the math in your head. How does it work?

expenses. These practices are meant to stabilize food prices by helping more farmers stay in business and ensuring them a buyer for their products. Government price supports for corn are one factor that keeps colas and baked goods made with corn syrup affordable. International trade deals can also affect the price of both domestic and imported foods.

Comparison Shopping

When faced with so many different products, brands, and sizes, how can you choose the best buy? Comparison shopping can be of help. **Comparison shopping** means matching prices and characteristics of similar items to determine which offers the best value. Two pieces of information can help you make this decision: unit price and cost per serving.

Unit Price

Unit pricing gives you a quick and easy way to compare prices. The **unit price** is an item's price per ounce, quart, pound, or other unit. It's shown in the store on the shelf tab below the item, next to the total price. See **Fig. 17-8**.

If no unit price is given, you can find it by dividing the item's total price by the number of units. Suppose a 12-ounce jar of spaghetti sauce costs $1.32, while a 16-ounce jar costs $1.52. The small jar of spaghetti costs 11 cents per ounce ($1.32 ÷ 12). The larger jar costs 9.5 cents per ounce ($1.52 ÷ 16).

Periodically check the unit price of items you buy often. Instead of raising a food's price, manufacturers often reduce the size of the package.

Cost Per Serving

Unit price is not always the best basis for comparison. In fresh meat and poultry, for example, bone and fat add to the weight but are not eaten. These foods are best compared by the cost of a serving.

To find the cost per serving, determine how many servings a certain amount of food contains. Divide the price of that amount by the number of servings. The result is cost per serving.

As an example, look at **Fig. 17-9**. Suppose fish fillets are on sale at $1.80 per pound, and a whole broiling chicken is $1.06 per pound. At first, the chicken might seem to be a better buy. The chicken includes bones and fat, however, so there is less meat. A pound of fish makes four servings, while a pound of chicken makes only two. The cost per serving for a pound of the fillets is 45 cents ($1.80 ÷ 4 servings). The cost per serving for a pound of chicken is 53 cents ($1.06 ÷ 2 servings).

You can use this math to find the cost per serving of prepared foods also, by dividing the item's price by the number of servings shown on the label. To estimate the cost per serving of a homemade recipe, add the cost of the ingredients. Divide the sum by the number of servings the recipe makes.

Remember that cost is not the only factor in determining value. A larger size may have a lower unit price, but if a food loses quality before you finish it, you lose money and food. Personal preference matters too. You might buy your favorite cereal even if the price has gone up because you know you'll eat it all—and enjoy it.

Using Coupons

Coupons offer savings on the price of a specified product. You can find them in newspapers, magazines, product packages, mailed advertisements, and on the Internet. In some stores, the checkout computer prints out coupons for future use based on the buys you just made. See **Fig. 17-10**.

Coupons are of two basic types. A cents-off coupon offers a reduced price on a certain item. You present the coupon to the cashier when you check out. The face value is subtracted from your bill before you pay.

A second type of coupon is a **rebate**, a partial refund from the maker of a purchased item. You pay the full price at the store. Later you fill out the rebate coupon and mail it, along with the required proof of purchase, to the address given. The proof of purchase might be part of the package, a cash register receipt, or both. The maker sends you a check for the coupon's face value.

Clipping and sorting coupons takes time. For some people, the money saved is well worth the effort. Some families and friends save and swap

Fig. 17-9

Servings per Pound of Meat, Poultry, and Fish	
Food	**Servings Per Pound**
Meat	
Lean, boneless, or ground	3 to 4
Some bone or fat	2 to 3
Large amount of bone or fat	1 to 2
Poultry	
Boneless or ground	4
With bones	2
Fish	
Fillets or steaks	4

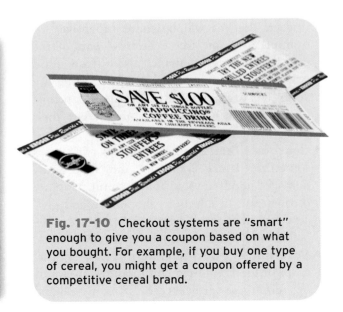

Fig. 17-10 Checkout systems are "smart" enough to give you a coupon based on what you bought. For example, if you buy one type of cereal, you might get a coupon offered by a competitive cereal brand.

coupons they can't use for ones they need. Others find they save just as much money through careful shopping.

If you collect coupons, be selective. Focus on items you usually buy or want to try. Avoid the temptation to buy an item just because you have a coupon. Read coupons closely to be sure they are useful. Some are good only on one size of a product or at a certain store. Most coupons have an expiration date printed on them. Stores cannot accept them after that time.

Other Money-Saving Strategies

Do you recall that people who skip a meal tend to be so hungry that they overeat at the next one? Hunger has the same effect on food shopping. Studies show that people spend up to 15 percent more on food when they shop while hungry, due to impulse buys. The lesson: eat before you shop.

Other ideas to help control supermarket spending include:

- Take only enough money to cover planned purchases, plus a little extra. Take a small calculator to keep track of your spending.
- Resist impulse spending "traps." Stores may offer free samples, product promotions, and discount bins. Candy, magazines, and other small, high-profit items are placed at checkout lanes. Foods that are often served together may be displayed side by side. Seeing packages of shortcake next to the strawberries might entice you to buy them both.
- Use your shopping list but be flexible. Stores often have unadvertised specials. Look for sale items that you can substitute for the ones on your list.
- Consider **store brands**, also called "private labels." These items are produced and packaged for the store, sometimes by the makers of name-brand goods. Thus they are generally equal in quality and lower in price compared with name brands.
- Meat, poultry, and produce may be packaged in larger amounts than you can safely store or use. Ask if a clerk can repackage it for you.
- Join a store's discount club, which gives customers an identification card that entitles them to reduced prices on certain items.

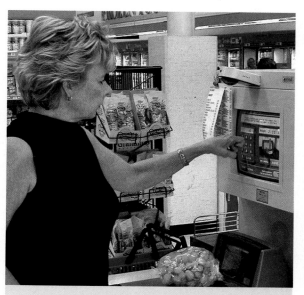

Fig. 17-11 Self-checkouts are in many supermarkets today. Why do you think stores use them?

CHECKING OUT

Your final stop is the checkout lane. Have ready any coupons or store discount cards you plan to use. You may be able to use an express lane if you have a limited number of items or if you're paying cash. Some stores offer a self-checkout counter where customers can check out their purchases themselves to save time. See **Fig. 17-11.**

Be aware of the store's policy regarding forms of payment. To pay by check, you may need a store check-cashing card. Most supermarkets accept credit cards and automated banking cards; however, don't let the ease of using credit tempt you to go over your food budget.

Watch the checkout screen as items are listed to make sure the prices are correct. Review the register tape before leaving the store to see that any discounts and coupons have been included. If a charge seems incorrect, ask the cashier to check it for you.

Take your purchases home right away and store them properly. Store frozen foods immediately, quickly followed by refrigerated foods, and finally shelf-stable ones. Repackage bulk foods in airtight, durable containers.

RESPONSIBLE SHOPPING

While shopping isn't primarily a social outing, courtesy makes the trip more pleasant. Apply the rules of the road to grocery store aisles. Push your cart at a safe speed, keeping to the right-hand side. If you bump another shopper or want to pass someone, excuse yourself. Avoid blocking aisles or other busy areas when you "park" to look for specific items.

Handling food carefully helps maintain its quality for other shoppers. Return a product to its proper place if you choose not to buy it. If you find food that is past its expiration date, notify a store clerk. Use the scoop or tongs provided for bulk foods, rather than your hands, and close the bin when done. Remember that comparison shopping does not include opening packages or sampling the contents. Damage and theft are costly for sellers, and costs are passed along to all consumers.

If you take a shopping cart to the car for unloading, return the cart to the proper area to keep it out of traffic lanes. Scratched and dented car doors should not be part of the cost of shopping.

RESOLVING PURCHASING PROBLEMS

Suppose you slice open a fresh head of cabbage and find the inside soft and slimy. If you're not satisfied with a food purchase, return it to the store with your receipt, the sooner the better. If your complaint is valid, the manager or someone in customer service should replace the product or refund your money.

Career Prep

Managing Resources

WHAT DOES YOUR FOODS AND

nutrition teacher have in common with a help-wanted ad? Both can be resources for launching a career.

A resource is anything you can use to accomplish a goal. Resources fall into three broad categories.

- **Human resources.** These are people, along with their qualities, skills, knowledge, and experience. When a co-worker shows you an easier way to finish a task, you benefit from the co-worker's skill at the job and your own ability to learn the skill.

- **Material resources.** Physical things make up material resources. For a caterer, material resources range from huge ovens and hundreds of foods to cook, to the skewers in fruit kebabs.

- **Community resources.** Public properties and organizations are community resources. Many provide services at little or no cost. Libraries, trade organizations, and chambers of commerce are useful community resources for finding jobs and careers.

MANAGEMENT STRATEGIES

Accomplishing a task is easier when you have all the resources you need; however, they aren't always readily available. With management skills, you find ways to increase resources, and you use them wisely to get the most from them.

The first step to managing resources is identifying them. Often you have more resources than you realize. The more you look, the more options you may find. Seeing beyond the obvious takes creativity and sometimes help from others. One teen didn't notice her skills as a mediator until a friend pointed them out to her.

Sharing resources extends your supply. Not only do you wind up with more resources, but you help someone else at the same time. Substituting resources may work for ends that

You may want to comment or complain to a food processor. You can write to the address on the label, send an e-mail, or call a toll-free consumer service number. If no number is given, try calling toll-free directory assistance. If you write or e-mail, follow these guidelines:

- Be brief but include all facts. Give the product name, size, and the product code from the package. Mention the date of purchase and the store name and address.
- Express your problem or comments clearly. Explain what action, if any, you want the company to take.
- Include your name, address, and phone number.

If you find foreign particles in packaged foods, report to the consumer complaint coordinator at your area's FDA district office. For a meat or poultry problem, call the USDA. Phone numbers and addresses are listed in the telephone book under "U.S. Government" or "U.S. Department of Heath and Human Services."

As a consumer, you are entitled to protections. You have these rights: to safe products; to be truthfully informed; to choose from a variety of reasonably priced goods and services; to have your opinions about legislation and decisions heard; to redress, that is, have problems corrected; and to have helpful consumer facts. These basic rights have been written into protective laws.

can be achieved in more than one way. Suppose you don't have a car to get to work. Public transportation or riding a bike may be a practical option.

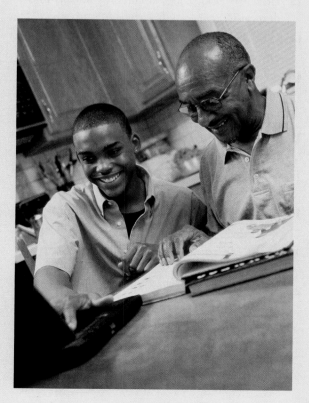

Matching resources to needs is one way to get the most from them. For instance, time and money may be better spent by enrolling in a class rather than trying to learn something on your own. Also, time is usually better spent gaining an education than on a job that earns money. That's because education and training typically pay off many times over—in a higher salary and greater job satisfaction. Although money is a resource too, making do with less for a while can have long-range benefits. Think carefully about costs and rewards, now and in the future, when a choice between resources must be made.

Career Connection

Identifying resources. Join with a few other students to create three separate lists of resources for each of these: finding a job, keeping a job, and advancing in a career. Compare lists with those of other groups. Which resources were mentioned most? Which seem most useful for all three goals?

Summarize Your Reading

▶ Large food stores can offer a huge selection of foods at lower prices, while other types of stores fulfill specific needs.

▶ A good food store offers fresh, healthy foods in a clean, safe environment.

▶ A well-organized grocery list can make grocery shopping trips easier and quicker.

▶ Labels provide information on the kind of food, amount of food, ingredients, and name and address of the manufacturer, packer, or distributor.

▶ Quality foods are worth the extra cost because poor-quality foods don't keep long and may even be unsafe to eat.

▶ Responsible consumers are considerate of others when they shop, and they express complaints appropriately.

Check Your Knowledge

1. Compare the following terms as related to supermarkets: supercenters, warehouse stores, health food supermarkets, and warehouse clubs.

2. What is a **food cooperative**?

3. **CRITICAL THINKING** Why do you think food prices are generally higher in convenience stores?

4. How would you determine that a certain food store or market is not a place where you want to shop?

5. Why should shoppers avoid emergency runs to the supermarket?

6. What are **perishable foods** and where are they found in supermarkets?

7. What tips can help you make a weekly shopping list?

8. **CRITICAL THINKING** The ingredient list on a bottle of juice says "orange juice." Another bottle of the same size lists sugar, orange juice from concentrate, and water. Which bottle contains more juice, and why?

9. How do you know that a food you're buying is organic?

10. Compare **open dating** and **code dating**. Name two types of open dating.

11. What is the purpose of the **universal product code (UPC)**?

12. What can you do besides check the product date on foods to help ensure quality in the foods you buy?

13. How are food prices affected by supply and demand?

14. Why does the government sometimes buy crops or foods from growers?

15. Why is the cost per serving sometimes a better way to find the lowest food price than checking the **unit price**?

16. Identify one positive and two negative aspects of using coupons.

17. What steps should you follow to take advantage of a **rebate**?

18. What can you do to avoid overspending when you shop for food?

19. What can you do to protect the quality of the foods you buy when you get home?

20. When shopping for food, how can consumers be responsible?

21. What can you do if you want to complain about a food you purchased?

Apply Your Learning

1. **Store Evaluation.** Develop a checklist for evaluating a food store's services, quality, and cleanliness. Visit and evaluate two food stores in your area, using your checklist.

2. **Supermarket Map.** Draw a map of a supermarket where your family shops, including merchandise placement and customer services. Prepare a well-organized shopping list to use in the store.

3. **MATH** **Unit Cost.** Calculate the unit cost of a batch of homemade cookies and compare to the unit cost of similar cookies purchased in a bakery. Which is more expensive? When and why might you use the more expensive cookies?

4. **LANGUAGE ARTS** **Skits.** With other students, write and present a skit on one of these topics: a) resolving a purchase problem; b) courteous versus rude food shopping; c) how consumer carelessness and theft affect prices; d) how to use self-checkout counters.

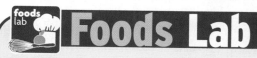
Foods Lab

Using Package Directions
Procedure: Prepare a convenience food that offers two preparation methods, such as heating on the cooktop and in the microwave. Use the variation assigned by your teacher, following the directions exactly. Evaluate the results.

Analyzing Results
❶ Were the directions clear and complete? What would you add or change?
❷ What other information or instructions on the package were helpful?
❸ Overall, were you satisfied with the outcome? What might have caused any disappointing results? How would you solve the problem? Would you buy the product again?

Food Science Experiment

Storing Foods

Objective: To compare how storage conditions affect different foods.

Procedure:

1. Place one lettuce leaf in each of two plastic storage bags. Seal tightly, forcing out as much air as possible. Place one bag in the refrigerator and the other bag in the freezer.
2. Repeat Step 1, using a slice of processed cheese. Repeat again, using a slice of bread.
3. Remove the foods after two days. Thaw the frozen samples. Observe and record each food's texture, appearance, and taste.

Analyzing Results
❶ Which foods kept better in the freezer? In the refrigerator? Explain.
❷ How did the storage conditions affect the water in the foods? How did it react to refrigeration? To freezing?
❸ Based on these results, predict the results of freezing the following foods: gelatin dessert; Parmesan cheese; strawberries; shelled nuts.

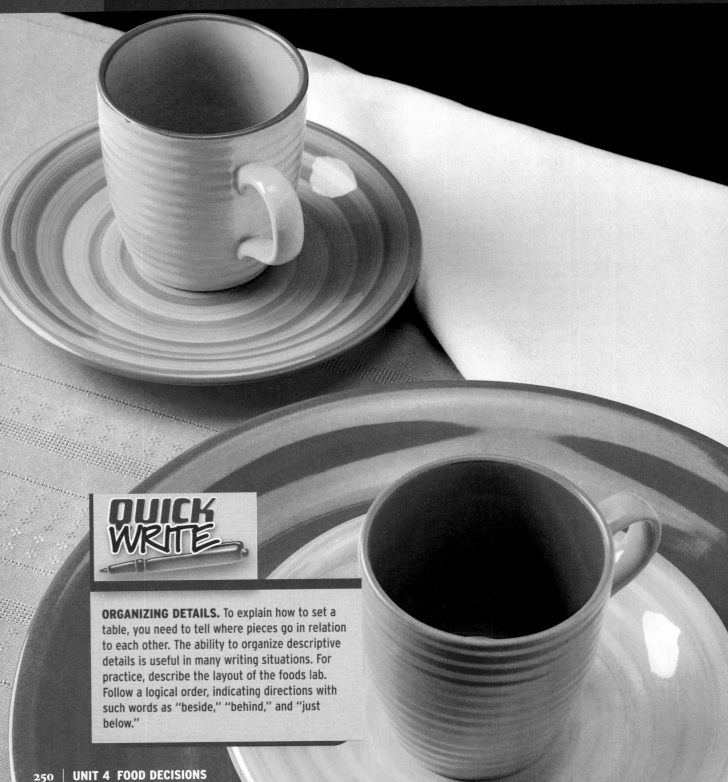

QUICK WRITE

ORGANIZING DETAILS. To explain how to set a table, you need to tell where pieces go in relation to each other. The ability to organize descriptive details is useful in many writing situations. For practice, describe the layout of the foods lab. Follow a logical order, indicating directions with such words as "beside," "behind," and "just below."

For many people, serving a feast on a table set with "the good dishes" is part of what makes a special event special. For some busy families, sitting down to a meal together is a special event that calls for a more casual "celebration." Whatever the event, or even without one, any meal can feel more satisfying when the table setting, serving style, and food suit the occasion. That could mean fine china on a linen tablecloth or a favorite soup mug on a plastic placemat.

TABLEWARE

You can probably think of meals that you have eaten entirely out of hand—a hamburger and milk from a fast-food place, perhaps, or a piece of cold pizza and a can of apple juice. To serve even simple meals like those, however, you need tableware. **Tableware** refers to any item used for serving and eating food. You set out a plate, a glass, and typically a knife, fork, and spoon—in other words, a **place setting**, which is the tableware needed by one person to eat a meal. See **Fig. 18-1**.

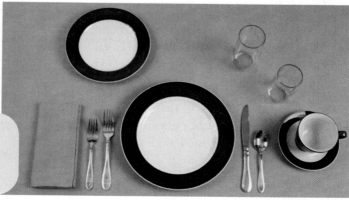

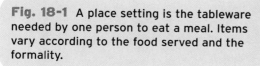

Fig. 18-1 A place setting is the tableware needed by one person to eat a meal. Items vary according to the food served and the formality.

Formal meals require more, and more varied, tableware. A place setting might include several pieces of dinnerware, flatware, and glassware.

- **Dinnerware.** This is what most people mean by "dishes." Dinnerware includes the largest pieces in a place setting—the dinner plate, salad plate, cup, and saucer—as well as numerous serving vessels. It's made from a range of materials. To produce fine china, earthenware, ironstone, and stoneware, different blends of clay are baked at high temperatures and coated with a liquid glass glaze. These materials are all fragile. Newer technologies have produced plastic dinnerware that is attractive and break-resistant.
- **Flatware.** Knives, forks, and spoons, plus larger utensils, such as gravy ladles and cake servers, are all examples of **flatware**. These pieces can be crafted from sterling silver, silver plate, or stainless steel. By law, sterling silver must contain 92.5 percent silver. Copper is added for strength. Silver plate has only a thin coat of silver over a base metal, making it much less expensive than sterling. Whether pure or plated, silver tarnishes unless polished regularly. Stainless steel resembles silver but is more durable and needs no polishing. Regardless of composition, all flatware should be comfortable to grip.
- **Glassware.** To serve beverages, the choices are stemware and tumblers. Stemware has a thin stem between the bowl and the base, which lends an elegant, graceful appearance. A tumbler is flat-bottomed with no stem. See **Fig. 18-2**. Some people find them easier to hold. **Crystal** indicates the glass contains lead, which gives it clarity and sparkle. Plastic glasses are a sturdier option.
- **Holloware.** The name **holloware** is given to serving containers made of silver, silver plate, or stainless steel. A silver cake tray is considered holloware, for instance. A glass cake tray is not.

Tableware is typically priced and sold by the place setting, in boxed sets that serve a certain number of people. Some brands are also available as **open stock**, meaning each piece can be bought separately. This is an advantage if a piece needs to be replaced. Serving utensils also may be sold in sets or individually.

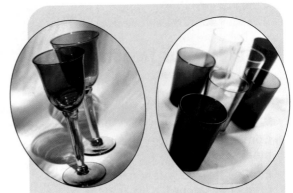

Fig. 18-2 The basic difference in glassware is that some have stems and some are flat-based tumblers.

Tableware is available in many different patterns, from elegant to dramatic. You can buy a complete set of one pattern. Some people create an interesting effect by combining several patterns that complement each other.

Prices also vary widely, depending on the material used, the quality, and the brand name. Fine china, sterling silver flatware, and crystal glassware are the most expensive choices. They also require more care when handling and washing. People who have these tend to use them more for special occasions. For everyday use, tableware

Nutrition Connection

Lead precautions. Lead has long been recognized as a health hazard, although it is no longer used in lead paints. Small amounts of lead can be found, however, in lead crystal glassware and in cookware made from improperly glazed ceramic pottery. Lead is a toxic metal that can travel from container to food, especially acidic ones. In most cases, the risk is small. For safety, however, avoid storing beverages in lead crystal for more than a few hours, especially fruit juices. Limiting the use of lead crystal is another precaution.

 Why shouldn't fruit juices be stored in lead crystal?

that is safe for the microwave and dishwasher is practical. Some dinnerware is also oven-safe and can be used for both cooking and serving. Pieces that stack easily are convenient to store.

Table Linens

Table linens not only protect the dining table and the diner during a meal, but they also add beauty and interest.

- **Tablecloths.** Whole table coverings can be formal or fun. They look most attractive if they hang at least 6 inches below the tabletop.
- **Runners.** You can "run" these long, narrow cloths down the center of the table or on the sides.
- **Place mats.** Place mats are less formal but convenient for covering a table under each place setting. They can be made of fabric, straw, or plastic.
- **Napkins.** Napkins come in different sizes. They should be large enough to be useful for diners but small enough to handle comfortably.

Given the high risk of staining, table linens that require the least amount of care are understandably popular choices. Those that have a stain-resistant and permanent-press finish are easy to wash and don't need ironing. Linens made with lace or delicate fabrics may require special care, including dry cleaning.

Like dinnerware, table linens are sometimes sold in sets. For eye-catching table settings, you can also mix and match designs, using contrast to add color and texture.

TABLE-SETTING BASICS

Just as a painting must be finished before it is shown, a table should be set before people sit down to eat.

A clean, uncluttered table is your blank canvas. Start by creating a background. After cleaning the table, put your choice of linens in place. Add a simple decoration—a single flower in a vase, a small houseplant, or perhaps a grouping of interesting seashells.

In this portrait the place settings are the subjects. The arrangement of a place setting is called

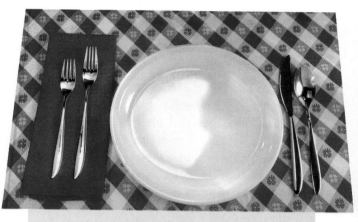

Fig. 18-3 A cover is the arrangement of a place setting. The cover for a more formal dinner might have additional flatware. Where would you put a beverage glass in this cover?

a **cover**, as shown in **Fig. 18-3**. The placement of pieces in a cover is based on both tradition and function. One rule, for example, is to allow at least 20 inches in width for each cover. This prevents crowding pieces, which is unattractive, and crowding diners, which is uncomfortable.

For each place setting, center the plate on the cover, about 1 inch from the edge of the table. In some serving styles, diners do not fill their own plates at the table. In that case, leave a space for the plate on the cover.

Flatware is arranged in the order in which it is used, starting at the outside and working toward the plate.

- Place knives to the right of the plate with blades facing the plate.
- Place spoons to the right of the knives. If you have both a soupspoon and a teaspoon, the soupspoon will probably be used first. It goes to the right of the teaspoon.
- Place forks to the left of the plate, tines up. If dessert forks are needed, bring them to the table when dessert is served, after the plates and other dinnerware have been cleared.

The beverage glass sits just above the tip of the dinner knife. If a water glass is used, it takes that position, and the beverage glass is set to its right.

A cup and saucer for coffee or tea would go to the right of the spoons but are often brought to the table after the meal.

If a bread-and-butter plate is used, place it above the forks. You might not use this plate at family meals, but guests may appreciate the convenience. Place the salad plate or bowl either to the left of the forks or above them, depending on the space available. Finally, place the folded napkin to the left of the forks. You can also arrange it on the dinner plate or tuck it into a glass.

SERVING MEALS AT HOME

Imagine a teen asking family members, "Should we serve dinner using family or plate service tonight?" The question might be met with surprise. Typically, families set up for a daily meal with little thought. At times, however, they want to change the routine. A look at different serving styles can show when each one might work best. Sometimes combining styles gives the best results.

Family Service

In **family service**, the cover is set with the necessary tableware. Foods are placed in serving dishes and passed around the table—all in the same direction, usually to the right, to avoid confusion. People help themselves to as much or as little as they want.

Family service is popular for everyday meals at home. Some restaurants also use this style. Its main advantage is that diners can serve themselves. Many people prefer this, especially those who are following restricted diets.

The method also has its drawbacks. Hot food left on the table in serving dishes may quickly cool to room temperature, allowing harmful bacteria to grow. Family service doesn't promote portion control, which can encourage overeating. It may also waste food and money, since servings left on a plate must usually be thrown away.

Plate Service

In **plate service**, the table is set with a space left on each cover for the plate. Food is portioned out on individual plates in the kitchen and brought to the table. See **Fig. 18-4**. This process is faster if family members help.

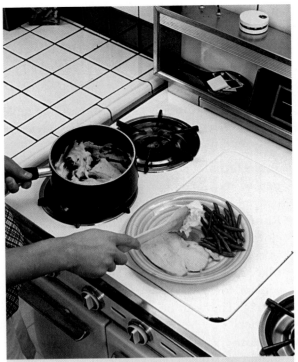

Fig. 18-4 Plate service works well for busy families. What are the advantages?

The advantages of plate service make it the preferred method for many families. The food remaining in pans can be kept hot on the range or in the oven. Portion control is easier. Cleaning up takes less time and effort because serving dishes are not used.

Modified English Service

Modified English service is a more formal way of serving a meal for a small group. Foods for the main course are brought to the table in serving dishes. They are placed in front of the host, along with a stack of dinner plates. The host carves the meat, if necessary, and then places the entrée and vegetables on a dinner plate. The first plate is passed to the right, down to the person at the end of the table. When all the people on the right have received their plate, those on the left are served.

The salad may be served in the same way. It may also be placed on individual plates in the kitchen and set on each cover before guests are seated. Rolls, butter, salad dressings, and other accompaniments are usually passed at the table so people can serve themselves. Dessert is served after the table has been cleared.

Buffet

At a family reunion or neighborhood get-together, there may be more people than can comfortably sit at a dining table. A practical, easy solution is to serve a **buffet**, where people help themselves to food set out on a table. See **Fig. 18-5**.

A buffet can be as informal as a sit-down meal. Prepared foods can be placed in serving dishes and arranged on a kitchen counter, a large table, or furniture draped in tablecloths. Plan the set-up to allow a smooth traffic flow and easy access for diners. You can add serving space vertically, if needed, by creating tiers. Set clean, cloth-covered boxes or overturned bowls and flowerpots on the table and place serving dishes on top. Guests can sit at small tables or hold plates of food on their laps. In nice weather, extra seating might be found outside.

When setting up the buffet, stack the plates where you want the guests to start serving themselves. After the plates, set the main dish, followed by vegetables, salad, rolls, and butter. Place napkins and flatware last. Rolling flatware into a napkin makes a bundle that is easy to pick up.

A buffet menu should be neat to serve and to eat. Foods that don't require cutting are good choices, such as casseroles, stir-fries, sandwiches, and salads. You may want to serve beverages after guests are seated.

Keeping foods at safe temperatures is a special concern at buffets. Use an electric skillet, slow cooker, chafing dish, or electric warming tray for hot foods. Keep cold food on ice or in insulated containers.

SERVICE FOR LARGE GROUPS

Serving styles that work well for families don't often translate to large affairs. Methods must be adapted when the guest list numbers several dozen people or more. As a foods and nutrition professional or as a guest, you may be part of an

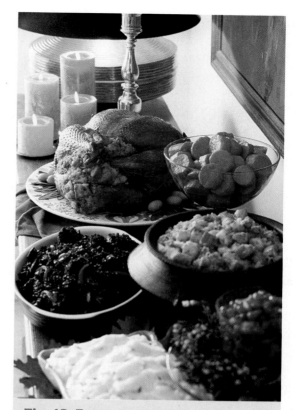

Fig. 18-5 When passing foods at the table would be difficult, the buffet style of food service works well. For a very large meal, similar dishes can be grouped together, even on separate tables.

event that calls for feeding large groups skillfully and with style.

Receptions

A **reception** is a social gathering usually held to honor a person or to celebrate an event. See **Fig. 18-6** on page 256. Receptions often follow weddings and graduations. A club may have a reception to introduce newly installed officers.

Receptions are meant as much for meeting as for eating. Buffet service is often chosen to encourage mingling. To accommodate a crowd, foods are placed on a large table. The same foods are served along both sides, allowing people to move in two lines instead of one. Coffee is poured at one end of the table and tea at the other. Fruit punch may be served as well.

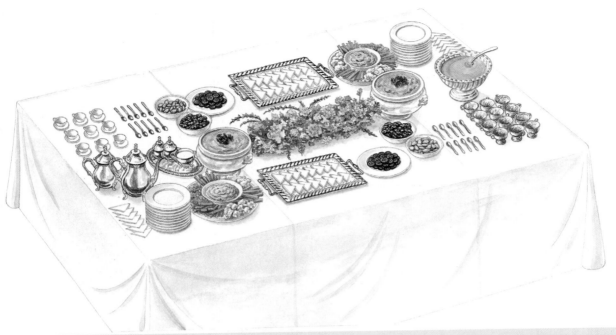

Fig. 18-6 A reception table should be organized for the convenience of both servers and guests. This table set-up will accommodate two lines of people.

The menu is usually light and often imaginative. Modest events may offer nuts, candies, small sandwiches, and fruit-and-cheese kebabs. Formal receptions feature **hors d'oeuvres** (awr DURVS), small morsels of hot or cold food usually eaten in one or two bites. Mushroom caps may be wrapped in bacon, for example, or dates stuffed with cream cheese. Also popular are **canapés** (KA-nuh-pays), which are small pieces of bread cut in decorative shapes with a flavorful topping. See **Fig. 18-7**. Crackers and pastry are sometimes used. Small cream puffs may be filled with a seafood spread. Toasted bread triangles might be topped with melted cheese and olive slices.

Formal Service

Formal service is the most elaborate style of serving. Because it requires hired help, it's often used for banquets held in restaurants or hotels. See **Fig. 18-8**.

For formal service, the cover is set with glassware and flatware. Every course requires its own flatware, so a place setting with half a dozen forks, spoons, and knives is not uncommon. Instead of

a dinner plate, the cover includes a **service plate**. This large, beautifully decorated plate is used only for the first course, the appetizer. An **appetizer** is

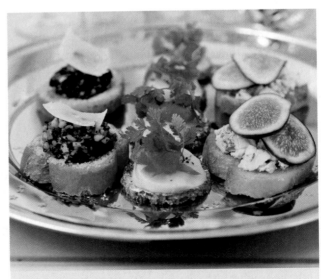

Fig. 18-7 Canapés make a delicious, and eye-catching, finger food for special occasions. You can use your creativity to make them.

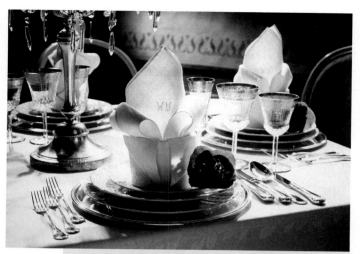

Fig. 18-8 If you attend a formal dinner, you may have more flatware and other items than you regularly use. If you're not sure what they're for, watch the host for cues.

a small portion of food served at the beginning of a meal to whet the appetite, such as a cup of soup or a small fruit salad. It is served on a separate plate, which is placed on the service plate. After the first course, the service plate is removed. Each course that follows—and there are several—arrives on its own plate.

ENJOYABLE FAMILY MEALS

A family meal is a chance for everyone to relax, to enjoy food and each other's company, and to catch up on family news. It should be free of television and other distractions. Conversation may be light and cheerful or lively and intense, but problems and disputes should be dealt with at another time.

Table settings for meals at home can be as basic or detailed as a family likes, and simple is quite common. Most meals need only a dinner plate, fork, knife, teaspoon, and beverage glass. A more formal place setting would include separate forks for the salad and main dish. Add a cup and saucer or a mug for a hot beverage, if needed, and a soup or salad bowl if either food is on the menu.

For many teens, eating meals with the family is a scheduling challenge. The effort is certainly worthwhile. Studies show that teens who share dinner with parents at least four or five times a week are twice as likely to get top grades as their peers who eat with parents less often. They are less likely to use alcohol, tobacco, and other harmful drugs and more likely to practice good nutrition.

Why do you think family meals can have such a positive impact? You might recall from earlier chapters that families greatly influence food choices. Food is central to many family customs and memories. Meals, like any time spent together, can be opportunities for teens and parents to give and get advice and encouragement. In a sense, sharing family meals is a healthful habit.

Creating Atmosphere

Are there some eating places where you go to enjoy the atmosphere at least as much as the food? It might be a friendly, family-run lunch counter with mismatched dishes and handwritten daily specials clipped inside plastic-coated menus. Maybe it's a café with a sunny patio where you can talk with friends or watch birds feast on bread crusts.

You can create an atmosphere—in fact, different atmospheres—when serving meals at home, whether you eat at the kitchen table, a card table, or in the dining room. Look for items around the house or find inexpensive additions to bring a sense of beauty, serenity, or curiosity, as the mood strikes. Here are a few ideas:

- Add a decorative touch of nature to the table by filling a small basket with real or artificial flowers, fresh fruit, colorful gourds, or clean leaves and nuts.
- For an elegant air, tuck a fresh or silk flower into every napkin. Arrange a centerpiece, using tall candles in candleholders, or float small candles in glass dishes of colored water. Play soft music.
- Shop garage and rummage sales for cartoon character glasses, souvenir salt and pepper shakers, and other novel tableware. Use these to add fun to mealtime.

PACKING A LUNCH

For some grade-school children, trading lunches is the best part of lunchtime. Often, a classmate's lunch seems better than the one from home.

As a teen, you're able to pack a lunch that you appreciate for its taste and healthfulness, not its "market value." Packing a nutritious, delicious, portable lunch can be just as rewarding as trading for one. It has economic rewards too. Each meal brought from home can save dollars over one you buy. See **Fig. 18-9.**

Lunch-Packing Pointers

Imagine three or four family members rushing around the kitchen trying to pack their lunches at the same time. This is not a picture of likely success.

A little organization can help. Take turns being the family's "designated lunch packer" for a day or a week, or just two people might work together. Set aside a section in the freezer, refrigerator, and nearby cabinet for lunch foods and packing supplies. Plastic wraps and bags, aluminum foil, and wax paper all work well as wrapping materials.

To save money and avoid waste, save an assortment of clean, empty margarine tubs, cottage cheese cartons, and other reusable containers. Make sure caps and covers seal securely to help keep liquids from leaking out and moisture from leaking in. Likewise, tuck a wet washcloth in a plastic bag for cleaning hands and wiping up spills, rather than packing paper napkins or premoistened wipes.

When possible, start packing the night before. If pasta salad from dinner is to be someone's lunch, scoop out a portion and set it aside in a single-serving bowl. In the morning, apply assembly-line techniques—for example, make all the sandwiches, wrap all the sandwiches, and add all the utensils.

For safety and enjoyment, foods must stay at the right temperature. For such hot dishes as soup, stew, chili, and stir-fries, use a wide-mouth vacuum bottle. A **vacuum bottle** is made of plastic or metal with a glass lining and a vacuum space between the outer container and the inner lining. Preheat the bottle before filling it with hot food. Fill it with hot tap water and let it stand a minute or two. Empty the water, fill the bottle with the piping hot food, and close tightly. If the food is still steaming at lunchtime, you know the bottle is doing its job.

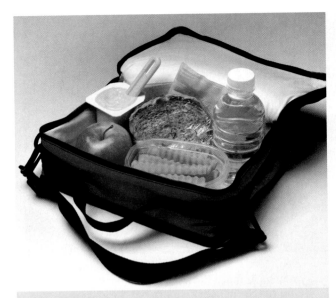

Fig. 18-9 A well-packed lunch offers healthful eating at an economical cost. An insulated container helps keep your lunch cold. How could you ensure that the foods stay cold?

A vacuum bottle works just as well for cold food, from milk to pudding. Chill the bottle first by filling it with cold water. A reusable frozen gel pack is another option. You can make edible freezer packs by freezing sandwiches and juice boxes. They will thaw by lunchtime, keeping other foods cold in the meantime. Double bagging also provides insulation. Whatever the method, keep the food in the refrigerator or freezer as long as possible. For added insurance, pack hot and cold foods in an insulated lunch bag, but not together.

Even eating a packed lunch can have a homelike feel with the addition of a few select items. Pack "real" utensils and brightly colored plastic plates. Drop in a foil-covered candy. For others, add a cheerful note, cartoon, or inspiring thought from a page-a-day calendar.

Food Choices

Any nutritious food can make a tasty lunch. Choose those that are also good travelers. Sliced chicken or meatloaf on a sturdy whole-wheat roll stands up well. A moist egg salad on sliced white bread can turn drippy and be hard to handle. Bean spread sticks to a tortilla, while whole beans tend to fall out. See **Fig. 18-10.**

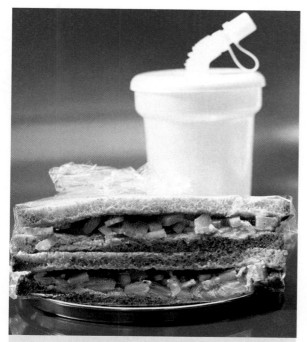

Fig. 18-10 Some foods hold up better than others when packed for lunch. How will this sandwich fare in a packed lunch?

Some foods are best if assembled just before eating. Lettuce leaves stay crisper if packed separately and added to a sandwich at lunchtime. For a salad, keep the dressing and croutons in individual containers and toss with the greens when you sit down to eat.

SERVING MEALS OUTDOORS

For a change of pace, many people enjoy eating outdoors. Interestingly, as indoor cooking grows easier and more sophisticated, outdoor cooking and eating grow more popular.

Outdoor Grilling

Cooking food outdoors is big business. Whether it's called grilling, barbecuing, or just cooking out, people enjoy preparing and eating foods cooked outdoors over an open flame. Americans spend around $4 billion a year on grills, cookware, and other accessories, yet a backyard cookout doesn't require expensive extras. It doesn't even require a backyard. An open deck will work, and tabletop grills are available for balcony grilling.

A few items do make cooking outdoors safer and more convenient. Large trays are useful for carrying foods and utensils in and out. Long-handled tongs, spatulas, and heavy mitts allow careful turning and removal of foods from grill to plate. If you also plan to eat outdoors, burn citrus candles to keep bugs away. Nest bowls of chilled foods in bowls of ice. Families that grill foods regularly might invest in a set of reusable plastic dishes and utensils.

Many foods can be prepared on the grill, with little extra cookware. You can make vegetable kebabs by stringing whole cherry tomatoes and chunks of green pepper and onion on wooden or metal skewers. Grill fish in a long-handled basket. Other foods can be placed directly on the grill: large pieces of meat and poultry and some shellfish; corn on the cob, still in the husk; and sliced bread or eggplant. Even homemade pizza can be baked on the grill. See **Fig. 18-11**.

When planning to barbecue, remember that grilling is less controllable than range-top or oven cooking, so cooking times are less predictable.

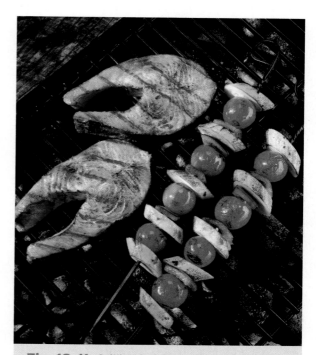

Fig. 18-11 Grilling is fair-weather fun in many households. What foods besides these would be good for kebabs?

Start early enough to have food ready on time. Set the grill a safe distance from trees and buildings, but with easy access to the kitchen.

Picnics

For some families, food tastes better in "the great outdoors." Many state and city parks provide picnic areas with grills and running water. If you venture into more remote areas, you can experience some truly amazing scenery and fascinating wildlife.

Since you may be traveling miles from home, planning for a picnic is essential. Make a list of each food you want to take, plus the tableware and tools it requires, such as a can or bottle opener, a paring knife, and a cover to protect it from pests. Don't forget cleanup supplies, for the picnic site and the picnickers: washcloths, trash bags, and extra plastic bags for dirty utensils. As you pack each item, check it off your list.

The same food safety rules for packing a lunch apply to picnics. Pack nonperishable items in a basket or other container. Use an insulated cooler and frozen gel packs for perishable food. See **Fig. 18-12**. Try to bring only as much food as you think you will need. Leftovers may not be safe to eat after the trip home. If possible, use a different cooler for cold beverages to avoid frequently opening the cooler that holds the perishables. Keep frozen foods in the freezer until you're ready to go.

Hot foods should be taken only if you know they will be eaten within two hours. Transport them in a separate insulated container. If you're taking raw meat or poultry to cook at the picnic site, pack it in its own cooler to prevent juices from contaminating ready-to-eat foods. Partially cooking foods at home and then finishing them at the picnic is a dangerous practice. Harmful bacteria may grow in the half-cooked food. A safer option may be to take cold, cooked food and warm it up, if desired, when you arrive.

To pack for a picnic, think backwards. Foods should stay in the cooler until they're needed. Therefore pack the items you will need last on the bottom, so the ones you need first will be on top. This order eliminates the need to open and repack the cooler every time you want something.

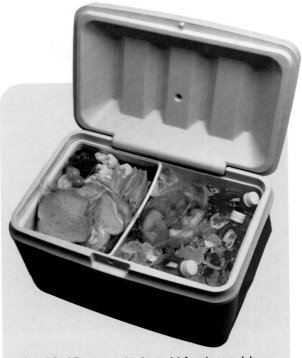

Fig. 18-12 On a picnic, cold foods must be kept cold and hot foods kept hot so that they are safe to eat.

Dessert goes in first, followed by main and side dishes. Put fragile foods in crush-resistant plastic containers.

When you are traveling, keep the cooler in the air-conditioned interior of the car, not in a hot trunk. Keep it closed at all times. At the picnic site, keep the cooler in a cool, shady spot. Even an insulated cooler won't stay cool sitting in the sun, a hot car, or a car trunk.

Before you leave, clean up the picnic site. If no containers are provided to dispose of trash, take it home with you. Leave the site in good, usable condition for the next group to enjoy.

ENTERTAINING

What's a good reason to have a party? Honoring an anniversary, playing the last game of the season, and getting a promotion at work—any of these events can be worth a gathering of friends and family. Special occasions may call for a sit-down dinner. Soup and salad might fit a more casual get-together. For impromptu parties, those arranged on short notice, you might need only a selection of snacks and beverages.

Whatever the event or the size of the celebration, careful planning goes a long way. With preparation and organization, entertaining can be as much fun for the host as it is for the guests.

If you want to plan a party, the first step is to check with the adults in your home. Make sure the time and type of event fits in with their schedule. Also check your budget. How much money is available for food and decorations? How will you spend it?

Next, decide on the type of party you want to give. Think about your entertaining skills. Inexperienced hosts may want to start with a simple, informal event, which lends itself to buffet service rather than a sit-down meal.

For inspiration in planning a party, consider a theme, or a unifying idea that is reflected in the menu, decorations, and activities. Carrying out a theme for a party is like creating an atmosphere for a meal, but in greater detail. See **Fig. 18-13**.

Holidays, birthdays, and graduations provide ready-made themes. If no occasion presents itself, be creative in inventing one. Choose an interest you and your guests share, such as sports or old movies. Surprise friends with the unexpected. Invite them to an indoor beach party in the middle of winter, for example.

Invitations

Decide whom you will invite to the party. For an impromptu gathering, you can probably just ask friends in person or by phone. If you're planning a party for a larger group, written invitations help guests avoid mix-ups on time and date and help you plan details.

Invitations should be sent ten days to two weeks before the party. Be sure to include the date, location, starting and ending time of the event, and your name. Mention the theme or occasion, if there is one. Also include the letters R.S.V.P. This abbreviation stands for the French phrase "Répondez, s'il vous plaît" (ray-pon-DAY seal voo play), or "Please reply." It is followed by your phone number and a date by which guests are to reply. The number of expected guests tells you how much food to buy.

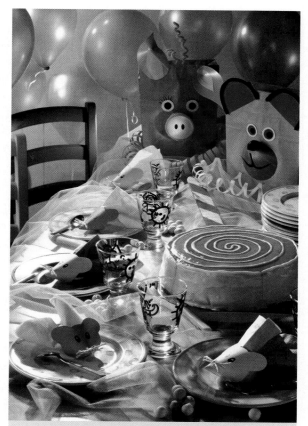

Fig. 18-13 A festive table adds to the pleasure of a party. Choosing a party theme makes decorating easier. What theme might you select for a child's birthday party or one for a friend?

Food for Entertaining

Before planning your menu, learn whether any guests have special food needs or preferences. Look for recipes that can be prepared ahead of time with a minimum of last-minute preparation. Think of creative ways to connect foods to your theme, perhaps by color or ingredient. For a simple dessert for an Italian theme party, represent the colors of the Italian flag with red and green apple wedges and a white cream cheese dip. Aim for variety, to ensure that every guest finds foods to enjoy.

Knowing how much food to prepare can be a challenge. You want to prepare enough food so guests don't feel self-conscious about how much they take. Consider how popular a food is and

Fig. 18-14

Try This! **Recipe**

Fruit Punch

Yield	Nutrition Analysis
About 32 servings	**Per Serving:** 60 calories, 0 g total fat, 5 mg sodium, 14 g total carbohydrate, 0 g dietary fiber, 14 g sugars, 0 g protein **Percent Daily Value:** vitamin A 0%, vitamin C 30%, calcium 0%, iron 2%

Ingredients

6 oz. frozen lemonade concentrate, thawed

6 oz. frozen orange juice concentrate, thawed

32 oz. cranberry juice cocktail, chilled

2 qt. ginger ale or lemon-lime soda, chilled

Directions

1. Combine thawed juice concentrates and cranberry juice cocktail in pitcher.
2. Pour juice mixture into a punch bowl.
3. Add ginger ale or lemon-lime soda and stir the mixture gently.
4. Serve chilled, garnished with citrus fruit slices or an ice ring, if desired.

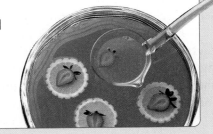

how many different foods you plan to serve. Consult food packages and recipes to learn how many servings they yield, and prepare a little more than you think you'll need. Try to have suitable emergency foods on hand—frozen egg rolls for a buffet, for example, or canned chili that you can stir into the homemade recipe.

In every budget and skill level, there's room for nutritious, interesting choices. Sliced cheese with crackers and raw vegetables with a low-fat dip are popular, easy-to-prepare combinations for buffets. Look into prepared foods, such as frozen cocktail meatballs and chicken nuggets. Use speed-scratch recipes by buying ready-made tart shells and filling them with fresh fruit. For a more substantial meal, try chili, casseroles, and other one-dish recipes. You can make the meal part of the entertainment. Have guests build their own pizza, tortilla, or ice cream sundae. For a special addition, you could make a punch, like the one in **Fig. 18-14**.

Making a Schedule

To keep even simple party plans on track, a time schedule is useful. Start by listing everything that needs to be done. Include food shopping and preparation, decorating, setting the table, and cleanup. Next to each task, write the day it must be done.

From this list, make up two new lists. On one, write those things that must done before the day of the party. On the other, write jobs to do the day of the party, including the time each should be done. List the tasks in order, beginning with the one that needs to be done first. Check the lists regularly to make sure you are on schedule. As you take care of each item, cross it off. When your guests arrive, you'll be able to focus on enjoying their company.

Remember that planning doesn't guarantee that nothing will go wrong. You could spill the punch or run out of ice. If you maintain a positive attitude and show you're not upset, your guests are likely to follow your example. That is what really makes an event a success.

Career Pathways

Professor

BILL QUAIN: Physically, Bill Quain's vision is very limited. A disease that is known as macular degeneration has left him essentially blind. Personally and professionally, Bill's vision is boundless. Throughout his life, it seems, the less he saw of the physical world, the more clearly he saw the possibilities.

Bill landed his first restaurant job at age fifteen, just as his eyesight started to fail. He owned and ran his own hotel and restaurant before turning twenty-one. After earning bachelor's and master's degrees in hotel administration, he taught as an assistant professor at universities in New Orleans, Louisiana, and Las Vegas, Nevada. Besides training future leaders of the restaurant and tourism trade, he was also a consultant to hotel chains and convention centers.

In addition, Bill has written a dozen books and countless articles. Today, with a Ph.D. in education administration, he is professor of hospitality management at Florida International University. He's also in demand as a motivational speaker, giving presentations on "Winning with a Positive Attitude" and "Creating Excellence."

Tapping Unseen Assets. How has Bill overcome blindness? He tackles the problem as any skilled manager would, by tapping his resources and thinking creatively. He canoes to work, for example, since he is unable to drive. That theme underlies his philosophy: the qualities needed for professional success also lead to personal fulfillment. When Bill lectures on effective management, he's teaching effective self-management too. Lessons on increasing profits are lessons on optimism.

One message you won't hear is "nice guys finish last." To Bill, building personal relationships is as essential to success as nuts-and-bolts knowledge of food preparation and accounting. Success means more than reaching your own goals. It's also helping others reach theirs: "Help them identify their dreams and show them how to acquire them."

Perhaps the best illustration of Bill's spirit is a television series he once hosted. "Cooking without Looking" was the first show designed to help visually impaired people work in the kitchen. Bill demonstrated some of the strategies he had learned as a professional chef, while a voice-over described the action. Topics ranged from serious—kitchen safety—to humorous—eating ribs in public.

Fun and Profit. As you might expect, Bill finds his greatest reward in motivational speaking, in "meeting new people and inspiring them to solve their own problems." He mixes shrewd business advice with personal stories and a generous dose of humor, a combination that earned him several Professor-of-the-Year awards. A discussion on tracking customer trends is called "The Chickens Don't Order Dessert." "Let Me Introduce You to 200 of My Closest Friends" gives tips on providing personalized service. If he ever teaches a course called "Seeing Opportunities," Bill Quain will be his own best visual aid.

On-line Connections

1. To learn more about topics in this article, search the Internet for these key words: hospitality industry; motivational speaking; employee management.

2. To learn about related careers, search the Internet for these key words: education administration; food service manager.

Summarize Your Reading

▶ Table settings vary according to how formal a meal will be. Most families serve meals using either family service or plate service. A buffet might be chosen for a family get-together but may also be used for large receptions.

▶ Insulated lunch bags, double bagging, and freezing foods before packing can help ensure the safety of foods packed for lunch.

▶ When packing for a picnic, a list is a guide for bringing everything you need to make the picnic safe and enjoyable.

▶ Parties can be anything from a selection of snacks and beverages to a sit-down dinner.

▶ Having a theme for a party helps create an enjoyable atmosphere.

Check Your Knowledge

1. Name and give examples of four different kinds of **tableware**.

2. When buying tableware, why is **open stock** an advantage?

3. Compare these table linens: tablecloths, runners, and place mats.

4. How should **flatware** be arranged on a **cover**?

5. Compare **family service** with **plate service** when serving meals.

6. How is **modified English service** different from other methods of serving food?

7. How should a **buffet** be organized?

8. What is the relationship between a buffet and a **reception**?

9. Compare **hors d'oeuvres** with **canapés**.

10. Describe **formal service**.

11. What is the function of a **service plate**?

12. What are the advantages of families sharing meals together?

13. How can you create a pleasing atmosphere when eating with family and friends at home?

14. How can using a **vacuum bottle** ensure safety when packing a lunch?

15. **CRITICAL THINKING** How might you effectively pack an egg salad sandwich with lettuce for lunch?

16. What items help make grilling a safer experience?

17. What safety rules should you follow when bringing hot and cold foods to a picnic?

18. Why should a dessert in a sturdy container be packed at the bottom of the cooler?

19. List some things to consider when planning a menu for a party.

20. How are lists useful when planning a party?

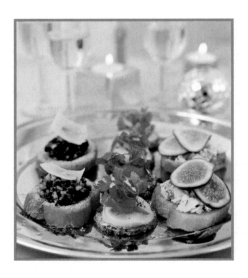

Apply Your Learning

1. **Place Settings.** Draw and label typical place settings for a variety of meal services.

2. **Table Design.** Make a poster that shows your design for a dinner or buffet table for a special occasion. Use drawings, fabric scraps, old catalog or magazine photos, and any other useful materials to convey your ideas.

3. **Table Setting.** Set a table appropriate for a specific occasion.

4. **Packed Lunches.** Plan bag lunches for a week. Use the following guidelines: no microwave oven or refrigerator is available; lunches should be nutritious; to make lunches interesting, foods should not be repeated exactly; and foods must be safe.

5. **Food Event.** Plan and carry out food service for a specific occasion. Ideas are a class picnic, a cookout, or an event that recognizes an achievement of some kind. Work in groups with other students to determine recipes, preparation, tools and equipment, food safety, and set-up at the site. Afterwards, evaluate the foods and procedures.

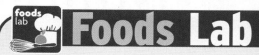 **Foods Lab**

Serving Something Special

Procedure: Create a simple recipe for an hors d'oeuvre or canapé. You might use variations of recipes in cookbooks or develop an original recipe. Design an attractive presentation for the dish. Prepare and share dishes buffet style in class. Evaluate the finished product.

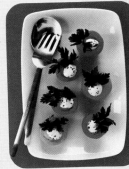

Analyzing Results

❶ Was the dish convenient to make, serve, and eat? Why or why not?
❷ How did the dish rate on appeal and nutrition?
❸ How would you change this recipe to improve its convenience, nutritional value, or other qualities?

 Food Science Experiment

Properties of Insulation

Objective: To identify qualities that contribute to good insulation.

Procedure:

1. Gather three, equal-size Styrofoam cups and two larger, equal-size Styrofoam cups. Line the inside of two of the smaller cups completely with aluminum foil.

2. Bring 2 cups of water to a boil. Carefully divide the water equally among the three smaller cups. Cover the cups tightly with aluminum foil. Poke a small hole in the center of the foil and insert a food thermometer into each cup.

3. Set the small, unlined Styrofoam® cup and one of the lined cups inside the larger cups.

4. Record the water temperature after 5 minutes, 10 minutes, and 20 minutes.

Analyzing Results

❶ Which container was most effective in retaining heat? Least effective?
❷ How do you explain the results you noted in question 1?
❸ Do you think the results would be similar for a cold liquid? Why or why not?

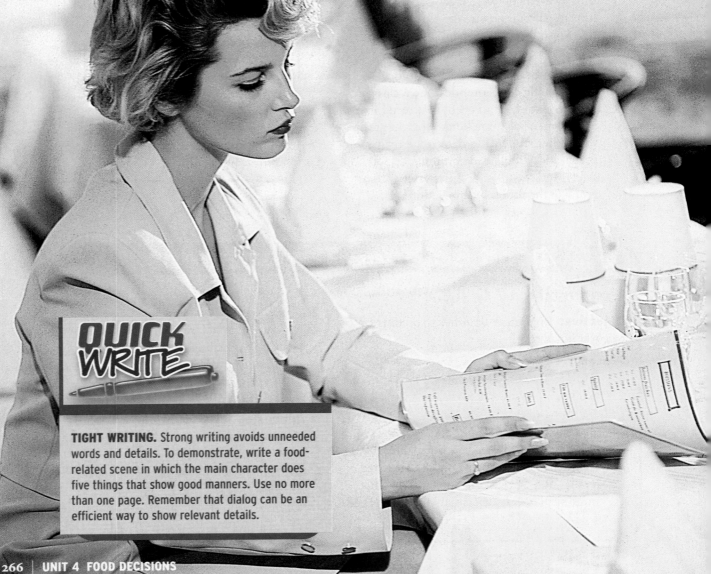

QUICK WRITE

TIGHT WRITING. Strong writing avoids unneeded words and details. To demonstrate, write a food-related scene in which the main character does five things that show good manners. Use no more than one page. Remember that dialog can be an efficient way to show relevant details.

To Guide Your Reading:

Objectives
▶ Demonstrate basic table etiquette guidelines.
▶ Describe a respectful attitude toward cultural differences in table etiquette.
▶ Explain rules of etiquette for eating in someone else's home.
▶ Explain rules of etiquette for eating at restaurants.

Terms
à la carte
gratuity
reservation
table etiquette

WHAT COMES TO MIND WHEN YOU THINK of table etiquette? Using the correct forks for the main course, salad, and dessert? Saying "Thanks" when a classmate offers you a snack? These actions are part of **table etiquette**, which is the courtesy shown by using good manners when eating. Like other types of good manners, table etiquette consists of rules of social conduct that are based on consideration and respect for others. Table etiquette guidelines are meant to put you at ease in social situations by helping you know how to act. Besides feeling more comfortable, you gain respect from others as well. See **Fig. 19-1**.

Knowing table etiquette can be an asset in the working world. When applicants are interviewed for a job, a restaurant meal is often part of the selection process. How people handle themselves in a social setting can show an interviewer whether they would make a capable, positive representative for the company. For example, many business deals are finalized at the business lunch. People who order an entrée with confidence and treat servers with consideration show good qualities for dealing with larger matters.

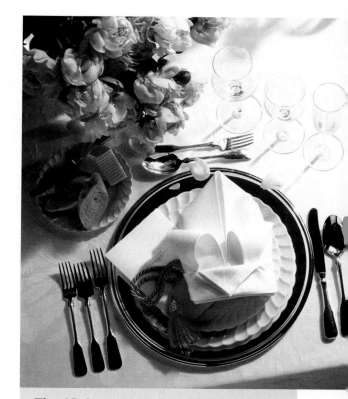

Fig. 19-1 When you know the guidelines for table etiquette, you're less likely to wonder what to do in social situations.

TABLE ETIQUETTE BASICS

As with setting a table, a few basic etiquette skills cover most dining situations. You're probably familiar with many such rules—chew with your mouth closed, for example, and swallow food before speaking. Here are some other general guidelines:

- Unfold your napkin on your lap before you start eating. If you sit properly, tucking it into your belt or shirt collar is unnecessary as well as incorrect.
- Sit up straight when you eat. Bring the food to your mouth rather than bending toward the food. You may lean slightly forward so any food that drops will land on the plate. Avoid resting your elbows on the table.
- Dip the soup spoon away from you in the soup bowl. Sip soup from the side of the spoon without making a slurping sound.
- If you feel a cough or sneeze coming on, cover your mouth and nose with a handkerchief or a napkin and turn away from the table. If the coughing continues, excuse yourself and leave the table.
- Cut each food into manageable pieces as you eat it, rather than all at once. Break bread and rolls into smaller pieces before buttering.
- You may reach for serving dishes as long as you don't have to lean across your neighbor. If you can't reach the food easily, politely ask the person nearest the food to pass it to you.
- After stirring a beverage with a spoon, place the spoon on the saucer. A spoon sticking out of a cup may be hit accidentally, knocking over the cup. See **Fig. 19-2**.
- If you have trouble getting peas or other food onto your fork, push it on with a piece of bread or the tip of your dinner knife.
- For removing an inedible part of food from the mouth, remove it as discreetly as possible. If a spoonful of cherries contains a pit, quietly work it to the front of your mouth and then onto the tip of the spoon. Then place the pit to one side of your plate. The same applies to a piece of fatty meat on a fork. Fish bones are an exception. Because they are so small, they may be removed with the fingers.

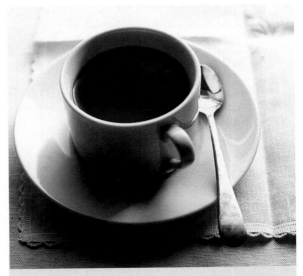

Fig. 19-2 When not in use, the spoon used to stir a beverage should be placed on the saucer beside the cup.

- When you have finished eating, place your fork and knife across your plate, side by side, pointing toward the center. Fold your napkin and place it to the left of the plate.
- Use a toothpick in privacy.
- Never comb your hair or apply makeup at the table.
- Wait for others to finish before leaving the table. Excuse yourself if you must leave.

Respecting Cultural Differences

If you were eating a meal in China, no one would mind if you held your rice bowl up to your mouth and pushed the food in with your chopsticks. In Morocco, meanwhile, you would be careful to eat using only the thumb and first two fingers of the right hand. Using four or more fingers is the same as gobbling your food, and the left hand must be kept clean for passing dishes to other diners. In a traditional Ethiopian meal, you would be given a large, round flat bread to scoop up your stew.

In traditional Japanese etiquette, slurping noodles shows appreciation for the meal. In Thailand, the practice is thought rude. Americans apologize for burping. In Indonesia, a loud burp at the end of the meal is a compliment to the cook.

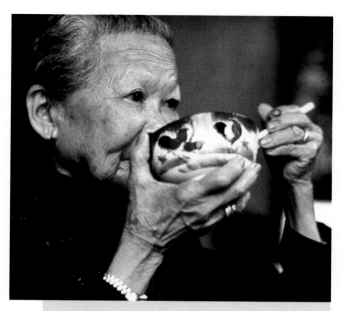

Fig. 19-3 Sipping soup from the side of a bowl is appropriate in some cultures. How can you benefit by knowing about variations in cultural etiquette?

As you can see, table etiquette varies among cultures. These differences should be respected. See **Fig. 19-3**. If you were to investigate, you would see how rules for eating and serving food develop in response to each culture's customs and heritage. Chopsticks came into use during a time of great social upheaval in China, for example, because knives and forks too closely resembled weapons of war.

Etiquette for Guests

Being invited to a meal in someone's home is a privilege. Guests should show their appreciation by acting courteously. If you are asked to reply to an invitation, follow through by phone, e-mail, or a brief note in the mail. If you have significant diet restrictions, politely mention them.

Be sure to arrive at the time specified. When a guest is late, food gets cold or overcooked. The host and other guests become displeased or concerned. Call if a delay is unavoidable so the host can decide whether to hold the meal for your arrival. On the other hand, don't arrive early unless you have been asked to help. Last-minute preparations for a party or dinner can be hectic. An early arrival only adds complications.

When you arrive, greet everyone, including the adults present. Bringing a small gift of food is a thoughtful gesture, especially if it's homemade. Remember that the menu is already planned. Choose something the family can enjoy later, such as a quick bread or preserves. See **Fig. 19-4**. If a special request is made, cooperate graciously. Keeping music low might be a request, for example, if an ill child is sleeping.

If food is served buffet style, don't touch food unless you intend to eat it. Ask the host if you have questions about a food's ingredients, rather than picking it up and returning it to the serving plate. Likewise, if a dip is served, dip a piece of food into the mixture just once. Germs spread when people bite off a piece of food and then put the remainder into the dip again. If you need more dip after taking a bite, use a serving spoon and put some on your plate.

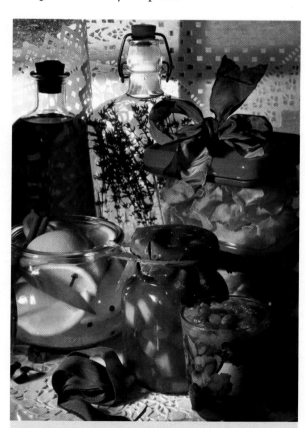

Fig. 19-4 When a host or hostess invites you for a meal, you can show appreciation by giving a small gift when you arrive. Here you see some ideas. Can you think of others?

Offer to help the host when you see the opportunity. Remove empty soda bottles as they accumulate. If food falls on the floor, pick it up before someone steps on it. Immediately wipe up any spills on the floor or furniture.

For a sit-down meal, follow these additional guidelines:

- If there are six or fewer people at the table, wait until everyone is served before you begin to eat. If there are more, wait until two or three have been served.
- If you're not sure how to eat a food or which flatware to use, follow the lead of your host.
- Try to eat at the same pace as your companions. Participating in conversation as you eat can help pace your eating.
- If for any reason you cannot eat a food that is being passed at the table, don't make an issue of it. Simply pass it on. If it's a matter of personal preference, you might try a small serving out of politeness.
- Before taking the last serving of a food, ask whether anyone else would like it.
- If you spill anything, mop it up quickly with your napkin. If it's a major accident, ask the host what you can do to help.
- Don't feed pets from the table.

RESTAURANT ETIQUETTE

Is it okay to eat fried chicken with your fingers? That depends. Feel free to do so at home, at a picnic, or in a fast-food restaurant. In fine restaurants, eating all meat, except crisp bacon, calls for a knife and fork. On the other hand, some foods are normally eaten with the fingers in any setting—bread, celery, olives, carrot sticks, pickles, corn on the cob, and most sandwiches, for instance.

This example shows one way that etiquette for restaurants differs from the rules for eating at home. The same good manners apply in both cases. Additional guidelines apply to situations found only when eating out. See **Fig. 19-5**.

Sit-Down Restaurants

If you plan to go to a formal restaurant, it's wise to make a **reservation**. This is an arrange-

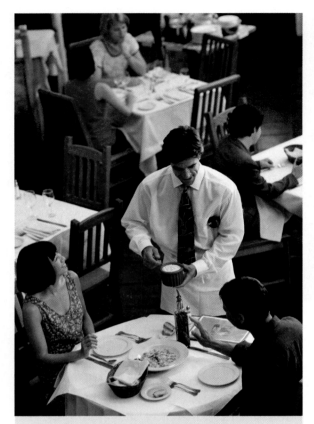

Fig. 19-5 Your comfort level goes up when you're prepared for a new situation. How can a person who hasn't had the opportunity to dine in fine restaurants prepare for the opportunity?

ment made ahead of time by telephone for a table at a restaurant. Give your name, the number of people in your group, and the time you plan to arrive. If you find that you will be late or decide not to go, call to change or cancel the reservation.

When You Arrive

If you're eating with others, wait for them before being seated. Never seat yourself unless a sign states otherwise. A restaurant employee will direct you to a table.

Near the entrance, you may see a checkroom. If you do, leave coats, umbrellas, packages, books, and briefcases with the attendant. Otherwise, set personal belongings beside your chair or under the table, never on top.

Before ordering, read the menu carefully so you understand what a meal consists of and how items are priced. Sometimes the price of the entrée includes side dishes, such as vegetables and salad. À la carte means items are listed and priced individually. Knowing the difference can prevent an embarrassing situation. Don't be afraid to ask servers about an item. They understand menu terms and know how foods are prepared.

On occasion, each person in a group will want to pay for his or her own meal. Most restaurants permit separate checks for smaller parties if requested when ordering. If this is not an option, you might ask the server to list each person's order separately.

During the Meal

When eating out, keep in mind that other diners want to enjoy their meal as much as you do. Avoid disturbing others with loud talk and laughter. If you carry a cell phone, avoid using it. If you must use the phone, go out into the lobby.

Remember that servers are there to help you. If you drop a utensil, tell a server and ask for a clean one. Also call a server if you drop or spill food, so it can be cleaned up as soon as possible.

Also remember that servers are working hard to please you and a number of other people at the same time. Be considerate and patient, especially during busy times. To call your server, calmly raise your hand. If necessary, ask another member of the wait staff to get your server. Calling out or snapping your fingers disturbs other diners and is rude to the server.

Paying the Check

At the meal's end, the server will bring the check. Look it over carefully and add up the items. If there's a mistake, quietly point it out to the server, who should correct any mistake or explain why the amount is right.

When paying the bill, it's customary to leave a tip, or **gratuity** (gruh-TOO-uh-tee). See **Fig. 19-6**. This is extra money given to the server in appreciation for good service. Servers rely on tips as an important part of their income. A standard tip is 15 percent of the pretax food bill, 18 percent if you request separate checks. **Fig. 19-7** shows a more detailed list for different types of restaurants and circumstances.

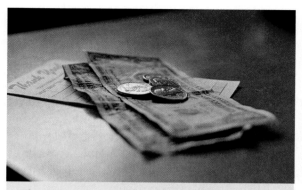

Fig. 19-6 You can calculate a tip in your head. On the pretax bill ($19.75), move the decimal one position to the left to get 10 percent ($1.97, or $2). Divide the result in half ($1) and add the two together to get 15 percent ($3), or double the 10 percent figure to get 20 percent ($4). Rounding numbers helps.

In some restaurants, you pay the server for the meal. In others you take the check to the cashier. If you're not sure what to do, watch what others do or ask the server. When paying in cash, place the money, including the tip, on the table or in the tray on which the check was presented. Some people wait until the server takes the money to be sure it is received. If you pay the cashier, leave the tip on the table.

Fig. 19-7

How Much to Tip	
Type of Restaurant	**Amount to Tip**
Fancy	20 percent
Family	15 percent; more for exceptional service
Coffee shops	Beverage only: at least 25 cents
	Food order: 15 percent or at least 50 cents, whichever is higher
Buffets	10 percent if server filled water glasses, brought beverages, and cleared table
Fast-food	None

If you use a credit card, the server or cashier will process the card and hand you the credit card slip. Again, go over the math to be sure the totals are correct. The slip has a space for a tip. Fill in the amount, add the final total, sign the slip, and hand it back to the server or cashier. Be sure to get your copy of the slip for your records and don't forget your credit card. Pick up any belongings left in the checkroom. The attendant also receives a tip, based on the number of items. Fifty cents to a dollar per garment is typical.

Fast-Food Restaurants

Even in the informal setting of a fast-food restaurant, certain manners are appreciated. Make any special requests as you order each item. Understand that policy often requires restaurants to charge for some added ingredients. This is not the employee's or the manager's choice. When paying, hand the money to the cashier. It's easier than picking it off the counter. Try to pay for small orders with small bills.

Supplies cost restaurants money, even packets of ketchup and paper napkins. Refilling supplies means extra work for employees. Take only as much as you need. See **Fig. 19-8.** Clear your table after eating. Dispose of trash and stack your tray in the place provided. Tell an employee if a trash container is full.

The drive-through is the "express lane" of a fast-food restaurant. Go inside to place large orders. If possible, know what you want to order before you pull up. Have your money ready when you pick up your food.

Complaints and Compliments

It is not poor etiquette to complain to the staff about a poor restaurant experience. Restaurants

Locating Job Opportunities

FROM THE SUPERMARKET BULLETIN board to the Internet, sources for job openings are more plentiful than ever. Tips for using some of the most common resources are given below.

- **Counselor's office.** Often businesses in an area contact high schools to look for students who want work. The school counselor and teachers in career technical education classes may have leads. Counseling offices in junior colleges are a resource for the future, as are placement services at universities.

- **Newspaper want ads.** The classified section of a local newspaper is a good source of jobs in your area. The ads also give you an idea of "what's out there" in terms of jobs, wages, and skills needed.

- **Networking.** Networking is the practice of using personal and professional contacts as sources of help and information. Mention that you're looking for a job to friends, family members, teachers, and employers and employees at the type of business where you want to work.

- **Visiting businesses.** Asking whether a business is hiring is the most direct approach to finding a job. Although asking takes some boldness and the willingness to hear "no" more often than "yes," even employers who aren't currently hiring may be impressed with your initiative. You can ask to fill out an application or leave your name and phone number.

- **Employment agencies.** For a fee, an employment agency tries to find the type of job you describe—part-time or clerical, for example. The fee may be a percentage of your salary. It may be split between you and the employer or fall to you alone. You might owe the fee even if you quit or lose the job. One advantage of this

genuinely want to please customers. Politely discussing a problem that you had helps them to serve others better. Make complaints about the food to the server. Make complaints about the service to the manager.

Be equally ready to express your appreciation to both the server and management for excellent food and service. Compliments are just as helpful as complaints. They encourage servers to continue doing their best and may alert management to a hard-working employee who deserves a raise or a promotion.

Remember that underlying all the rules, the ultimate principle of etiquette is showing kindness and helping people feel comfortable in social situations. If you don't know the "right" thing to do in a certain situation, ask yourself what you would want someone to do for you.

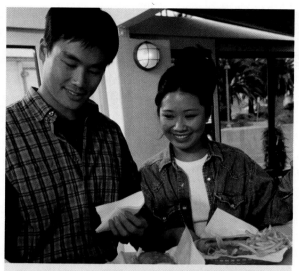

Fig. 19-8 Etiquette applies when eating anywhere, including fast-food restaurants. Why should customers take only the supplies they need for the meal? What may happen if people waste supplies?

option is that an agency can consider qualities and talents that may not be listed on a job application. An agency may also have many contacts that streamline the process.

- **"Temp" agencies.** This type of employment agency, which specializes in supplying temporary work, is growing in popularity. Some agencies work with food service and hospitality companies. Employers pay the agency to find them workers as needed. You sign up with the agency, which sends you to different employers on a short-term basis. A temporary job may lead to full-time employment later, although you need to discuss how the agency handles such situations.

- **On-line job listings.** Numerous on-line job banks enable you to search for openings according to job type, salary level, location, and other criteria. Some sites specialize in jobs for students and teens. On-line newsletters and trade magazines often have industry-related links and a classified section, although these are aimed at older, more experienced workers.

- **Job fairs.** Job fairs may be offered by schools, conference organizers, or local agencies. Employers in a certain field or region supply information about themselves and the industry.

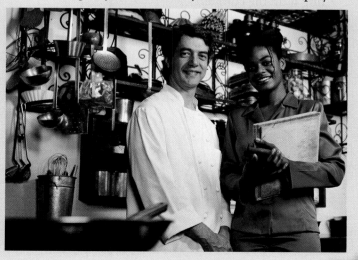

Career Connection

Comparing sources. Try to locate a certain job in foods and nutrition, using one of the sources listed. Discuss the results in class. Compare advantages and disadvantages and give tips for using each option.

19 Review & Activities

Summarize Your Reading

▶ Table etiquette guides diners in knowing how to use good manners while eating.

▶ Table etiquette varies among cultures, and these differences should be respected.

▶ Guests can show their appreciation by bringing a small gift for the host.

▶ Some etiquette guidelines for eating at home differ from those to follow in restaurants.

▶ Restaurant etiquette includes not disturbing others with loud talk and cell phones.

▶ The ultimate principle of etiquette is showing respect for others and treating people with kindness.

Check Your Knowledge

1. Why is practicing **table etiquette** a useful skill?

2. What should you do if you feel a cough or sneeze coming on at the dinner table?

3. What should you do when eating if you have trouble getting peas or other food onto your fork?

4. A diner got a cherry pit in his mouth while eating. What should he do?

5. Why is it considered rude to use all five fingers or to eat with your left hand when in Morocco?

6. **CRITICAL THINKING** Why should people show respect for cultural differences, such as varied ways of eating?

7. Why shouldn't you arrive early or late when invited to someone's home for dinner?

8. When eating buffet style, why is it rude to dip a piece of food into a mixture such as guacamole more than once?

9. What should you do if you're not sure how to eat a certain food, such as crab legs?

10. **CRITICAL THINKING** When eating at a friend's house, a teen passed on eating the hot dogs, saying they make her sick. Then she dropped a spoon of potato salad on the floor and left it. Evaluate her actions.

11. When is it okay to eat fried chicken with your fingers?

12. What information do you need when you call a restaurant for a **reservation**?

13. How can you tell whether a salad and vegetable come with your meal in a restaurant?

14. What should you do if you drop a utensil when eating at a restaurant?

15. Describe a **gratuity** and explain why this custom is practiced at restaurants.

16. Do you pay the server or take the money to the cashier when paying in a restaurant? Explain.

17. In a fast-food restaurant, why should you hand the money to a cashier instead of setting it on the counter?

18. What rules of etiquette should you follow when you order at the drive-through window of a fast-food restaurant?

19. Why is it okay to complain to restaurant staff about a poor experience?

Apply Your Learning

1. **Table Etiquette.** Demonstrate appropriate table etiquette for the following: cutting meat, buttering bread, eating spaghetti, eating peas, removing a cherry pit from your mouth, and eating soup.

2. **Etiquette Situations.** Plan and present a skit that shows proper etiquette in one of the following situations: a) ordering from a menu; b) eating in a nice restaurant; c) paying the check; d) eating at a friend's home.

3. **SOCIAL STUDIES World Etiquette.** Invite an exchange student to visit your class to describe eating patterns and table etiquette in the person's home country. Find out what you would need to know to eat politely in that country.

4. **LANGUAGE ARTS Polite Complaints.** With another student, demonstrate how to make a complaint to the server or the restaurant manager. What would you keep in mind when making the complaint?

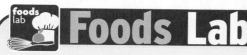

Foods Lab

Demonstrating Etiquette

Procedure: With your lab team, role-play a scene that shows etiquette in a dining situation, such as asking about menu items at a restaurant, eating a challenging food, or having unexpected guests at dinnertime. Don't rehearse the scene; instead, improvise realistically, using etiquette guidelines. Introduce likely problems or difficulties. Have the rest of the class critique your performance.

Analyzing Results
❶ How did each person contribute to the comfort and ease of the dining experience?
❷ What personal qualities were helpful for dealing with difficulties or unexpected events?

Food Science Experiment

Melting Rates

Objective: To compare the melting rates of various bread spreads.

Procedure:
1. Place 1 Tbsp. each of butter, regular margarine, and reduced fat margarine on separate plates. Note the shape and consistency.
2. Observe and evaluate each sample after 5 minutes, 15 minutes, and 30 minutes. Record your observations.

Analyzing Results
❶ How did the samples' appearance and consistency compare at each interval?
❷ Read the ingredients list on the package of each sample tested. How did their composition affect their melting rates?
❸ Besides neatness, give another reason why a serving of bread spread is placed on the bread plate rather than the dinner plate.
❹ How might a meal preparer slow or delay this reaction?

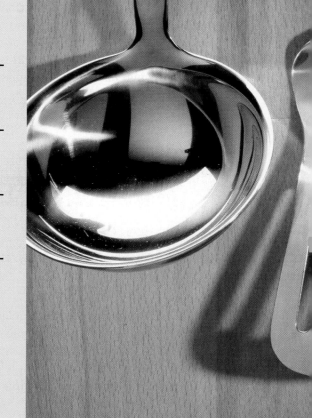

UNIT 5
Kitchen Basics

CHAPTER 20 **Food Safety & Storage**

CHAPTER 21 **Preventing Kitchen Accidents**

CHAPTER 22 **Equipping the Kitchen**

CHAPTER 23 **Conserving Resources**

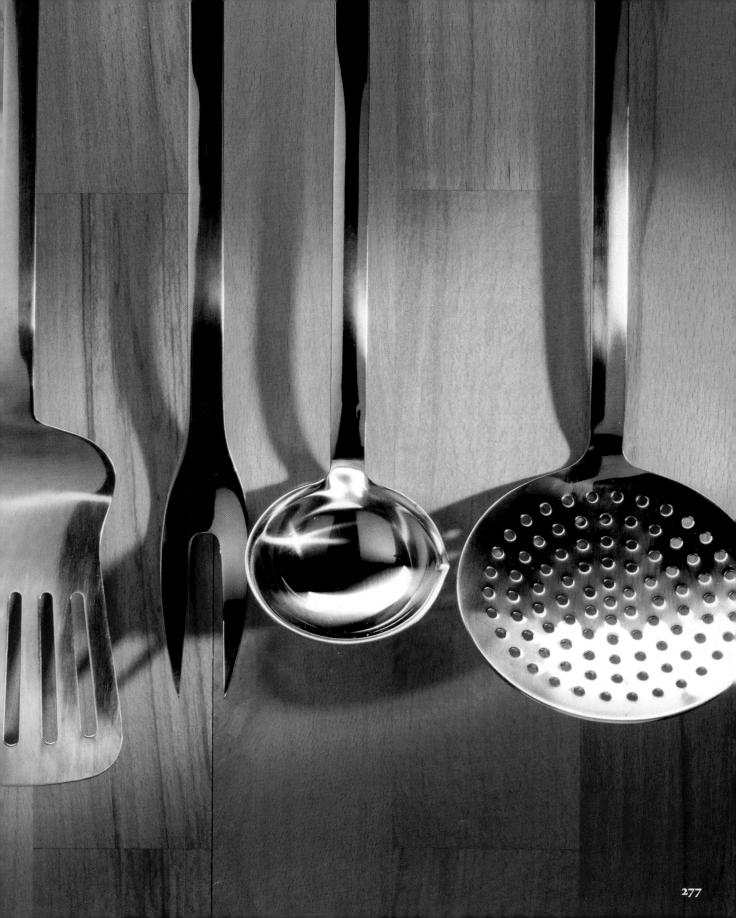

Food Safety & Storage

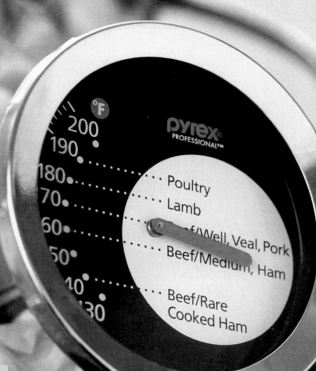

°F
200
190
180
70
60
50
40
130

pyrex
PROFESSIONAL™

Poultry
Lamb
ef/Well, Veal, Pork
Beef/Medium, Ham

Beef/Rare
Cooked Ham

QUICK WRITE

RHYTHM AND RHYME. A list of safety rules can be hard to remember. Write a fresh, appealing slogan or short verse based on one of these food safety guidelines: wash your hands before preparing foods; keep pets away from food; refrigerate perishable foods. Focus on the rhythm and rhyme of your words.

W HEN YOU SIT DOWN TO A MEAL, HOW often do you wonder whether the food is safe to eat? Most people take food safety for granted. They might not think about **contaminants**, substances that make food unfit for use. Certain chemicals and organisms in the environment are contaminants that can pass into food, making it unsafe for eating. Fortunately, many steps are taken to help ensure that food won't harm you. You can take some steps yourself.

FOODBORNE ILLNESS

When people have an upset stomach, they often blame "a flu bug." Actually, they may have been poisoned—by food. Fever, headache, and digestive troubles are symptoms of **foodborne illness**, sickness caused by eating food that contains a harmful substance.

Foodborne illness strikes about 75 million Americans every year. Children, pregnant women, older adults, and chronically ill people are most at risk. Most cases are mild, lasting just a day or two; however, more than 300,000 victims require hospitalization. About 5,000 people die annually from complications caused by food poisoning.

Roots of Foodborne Illness

Most cases of foodborne illness can be traced to **microorganisms**, living creatures that are visible only through a microscope. See **Fig. 20-1**.

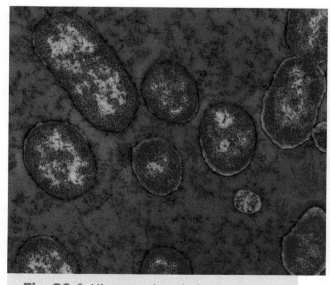

Fig. 20-1 Microorganisms in food can cause foodborne illness. Here you see magnified *Salmonella* cells.

Microorganisms include single-celled organisms called bacteria. Thousands of bacteria types are naturally present in the environment and the human body. Many are harmless. Some, like those that aid in food digestion, are essential for health.

Other bacteria are the most dangerous microorganisms in the food supply. They produce **toxins**, or poisons, that can cause illness. Some bacteria also produce **spores**, which are protected cells that develop into bacteria under the right conditions. Those conditions include the combination of food, warmth, and moisture—as might be found in a potato salad left out at a picnic. **Fig. 20-2** lists some of the bacteria that cause foodborne illness and where they might be found.

Bacteria cannot travel far by themselves. They are carried on people, animals, insects, and objects. Harmful bacteria may occur naturally in food when you buy it; however, most arrive through careless handling when food is prepared and served. Once established, bacteria reproduce at an amazing rate. In just a few hours, one bacterium can multiply into thousands, yet the food may look, taste, and smell completely safe to eat.

A healthy human body can tolerate limited amounts of harmful bacteria. As their numbers multiply beyond a certain level, however, they create a health hazard.

The preventive to foodborne illness is food safety. **Food safety** means keeping food safe to eat by following proper food handling and cooking practices. These include the following:

- Keep yourself and your kitchen clean.
- Don't cross-contaminate.
- Cook food thoroughly.
- Refrigerate food promptly.

Fig. 20-2

Some Bacteria That Cause Foodborne Illness

Bacteria and Disease	Common Sources
Campylobacter jejuni (disease: campylobacteriosis)	Contaminated water; unpasteurized milk; undercooked meat, poultry, and seafood.
Clostridium botulinum (disease: botulism, which can be fatal)	Improperly processed, home-canned and commercially canned foods; garlic in oils; vacuum-packed or tightly wrapped food.
Clostridium perfringens (disease: perfringens food poisoning)	Environments where there is little or no oxygen. Sometimes called the "cafeteria germ" because it is often found in food served in quantity and left for long periods on a steam table or at room temperature.
E. coli (disease: hemorrhagic colitis)	Unchlorinated water; raw or rare ground beef; raw alfalfa sprouts; unwashed produce; unpasteurized milk or apple cider.
Listeria monocytogenes (disease: listeriosis)	Raw or undercooked meat, poultry, or fish; unwashed produce; soft cheeses; unpasteurized milk; ready-to-eat foods, such as hot dogs, cold cuts, dry sausages, and deli-style meats and poultry.
Salmonella (disease: salmonellosis)	Raw or undercooked poultry, eggs, meat, and seafood; unpasteurized milk.
Staphylococcus aureus (disease: staphylococcal food poisoning)	Prepared foods left too long at room temperature. Typical sources are meat, poultry, egg products, and such mixtures as tuna, chicken, potato, and egg salad; cream-filled pastries.

CLEANLINESS IN THE KITCHEN

A clean kitchen isn't only a point of pride for the cook. It is the starting point of **sanitation**, the prevention of illness through cleanliness, and of food safety as well.

Personal Hygiene

You probably don't think about preventing foodborne illness when you shower, bathe, or wash your hair—until you think that for bacteria, it's a short trip from your body to work surfaces, utensils, and food. By practicing **personal hygiene**, you keep yourself clean to avoid transferring harmful bacteria when handling food.

Because your hands come in close contact with food, keeping them clean is the single most effective way to prevent bacterial transfer. A proven technique is the **20-second scrub**. See **Fig. 20-3**. Using soap and warm water, scrub your hands for 20 seconds. Use a brush to clean your fingernails. Keep them trimmed and remove chipped polish.

Do a 20-second scrub before working in the kitchen. Also scrub your hands right after handling raw meat, poultry, fish, shellfish, and eggs. Scrub your hands immediately after you use the toilet, blow your nose, handle pets, or touch your face, hair, or any other part of your body while working with food.

Bacteria travel from food handlers to food by other routes as well. Sneezing or coughing into food is one obvious example. Bacteria can grow

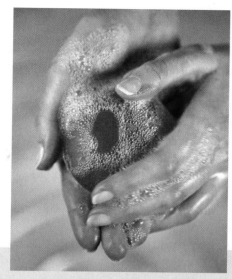

Fig. 20-3 To wash hands properly, use soap and warm water. Rub vigorously for 20 seconds before rinsing and drying well.

even in spots and stains, so wear clean clothes covered with a clean apron. Remove dangling jewelry and roll up long sleeves. Tie back long hair. Open wounds on the hands should be covered with rubber or plastic gloves, and gloved hands washed as often as bare ones.

A Clean Kitchen

A clean cook is backed up by a clean kitchen. Follow these guidelines to limit bacteria in the kitchen environment:

- Keep pets out of the kitchen. Pet hairs float through the air, carrying bacteria with them.
- Wash work surfaces and utensils in hot, sudsy water before you prepare food.
- Wash the tops of cans before opening them.
- If you use a spoon to taste food during cooking, wash the spoon before using it again.
- Change dishtowels often. Use separate towels for wiping hands, wiping dishes, and any other purposes.
- At the end of the day, put the dishcloth in the laundry and replace with a clean one. Wash sponges by hand or in a dishwasher and let them air-dry overnight.

SAFETY ALERT

Eating out. To protect yourself from foodborne illness when eating out, choose restaurants that look clean and are well maintained, both inside and out. Clean tables, walls, floors, and restrooms offer clues. Servers should look clean and follow rules of safe food handling. Hot and cold foods should be served that way. Although restaurants are inspected by state health departments, you can be watchful too in case a slip occurs.

Pest Control

Insects bring harmful bacteria into the kitchen. To keep pests away, don't leave crumbs or food spills on floors, counters, and tables. Make sure garbage is taken to an outside, covered can at least once a day, more often if needed. Wash garbage cans regularly. See **Fig. 20-4**.

Chemical insecticides are effective in controlling bugs, but they can be hazardous to people and the environment. Before resorting to insecticides, repair holes in walls and screens where pests get in. Caulk cracks and crevices. Sprinkle chili powder, paprika, or dried peppermint across ant trails. If you must use a commercial insecticide, follow the label directions carefully, and don't let the spray get onto dishes, counter tops, or food.

Cleanup Time

Dirty dishes are not only unappealing but they can also harbor disease-causing bacteria. The campaign for cleanliness continues after a meal has been prepared, served, and eaten.

If the kitchen is equipped with a food waste disposal and a dishwasher, follow the instructions in the owner's manual for their use. To wash dishes efficiently by hand, try this system. First, scrape and rinse soiled dishes and place them to one side of the sink. Group like items, arranged in this order: glasses first, then flatware, plates and bowls, kitchen tools, serving pieces and containers, and cookware. Keep sharp knives separate. If food is stuck to cookware, presoak the pan. Pour in a little detergent, add hot water, and let it stand while you wash the other dishes.

Next, fill a dishpan or sink with sudsy water that is hot enough to remove grease but does not burn your hands. Using a sponge or dishcloth, wash the dishes in the order you arranged, glasses first and greasy cookware last. Refill the sink or dishpan with clean, hot, soapy water as needed.

Rinse dishes thoroughly in hot water, especially the insides of containers. To quickly rinse the outsides, put the washed dishes in a dish rack, place the rack in the sink, and let hot water run over them. Let the dishes air-dry in the rack, or dry them with a clean, dry towel. Wash knives after the other dishes, handling with care, and towel them dry.

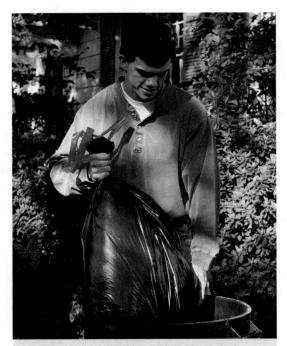

Fig. 20-4 For pest control, kitchen garbage must be regularly removed to an outside garbage can.

Wash all work areas and appliances that were used, from the can opener blade to the cutting board. As you work, rinse the dishcloth often in hot, sudsy water.

Mop up any spills on the floor. Wash the sink to remove grease and bits of food. If the sink has a disposal, run it one last time. Finally, put any garbage in a plastic bag and close tightly.

DON'T CROSS-CONTAMINATE

Cross-contamination occurs when harmful bacteria spread from one food to another. It can occur with any food, cooked or uncooked, but the juices from raw meat, poultry, and seafood are noted bacteria carriers. Don't let them drip on other foods in your shopping cart and grocery bags. Store them in the refrigerator in sealed containers or plastic bags.

When you prepare raw meat, poultry, or seafood, wash every surface the food touched with hot, soapy water. That includes plates, tools, and utensils, as well as your hands. Always put cooked food on a clean plate, not a plate that held the raw food.

Cleanliness When Serving Food

Cross-contamination threatens prepared foods also. Wash the dining table before and after eating. Always handle cooked foods with clean utensils, never by hand. Place a serving utensil in every serving dish. Don't refill a serving dish of food that has been sitting out for a while. Instead, get a clean dish. Hold cups and flatware by their handles and glassware by the lower third. When you carry more than one plate of food, don't overlap them.

Cutting Boards

Cutting boards are a common source of cross-contamination. If possible, have two cutting boards and always use the same one for meat, poultry, and seafood.

According to the USDA, microorganisms are easier to wash from plastic than from wood. To keep any cutting board clean, wash it in hot, sudsy water after each use. Rinse and air-dry or dry with a clean towel. Some plastic boards can be washed in a dishwasher. All cutting boards eventually wear out or develop hard-to-clean cuts and grooves. Discard them and replace with new ones.

COOK FOOD THOROUGHLY

Food temperature affects bacterial growth. Take a close look at **Fig. 20-5**. What happens to bacteria as temperatures get hotter or colder? As you can see, bacteria grow fastest within a range that includes room temperatures. The less time food spends at room temperature, the less chance of harmful bacterial growth. During cooking, high food temperatures normally kill most bacteria, although spores and some toxins can survive. With cold refrigerator temperatures, bacteria grow more slowly, yet remain alive. Freezing stops bacteria from growing, but also without killing them. When frozen food thaws, the bacteria start to grow again.

Since you need high temperatures to kill bacteria, how do you know when meat and poultry have been cooked thoroughly enough? You can't tell by looking. The surest way to test doneness is to use a food thermometer to check the **internal temperature**. This temperature, registered at the

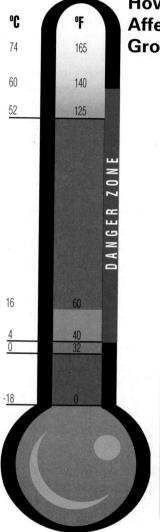

How Temperature Affects Bacterial Growth

Fig. 20-5
Temperature has strong impact on bacterial growth in foods. Bacteria die when foods are thoroughly cooked at high temperatures. Do bacteria die when food is frozen?

center of the thickest part of the food, must be high enough to kill harmful bacteria. That usually takes at least 160°F. Upcoming chapters give safe internal temperatures for specific foods.

Based on how temperatures impact bacteria, several guidelines should be followed when you cook foods.

- Taste foods containing ingredients from animal sources only after they are fully cooked, not when raw or while cooking.
- Never partially cook food and then wait to finish the cooking later. Cook the food completely at one time.

- Some foods cook unevenly in a microwave oven. Cool spots may remain where bacteria can survive. For even cooking, cover the food and stir or rotate it. Allow the recommended standing time so the heat can circulate throughout.
- When reheating food that has been refrigerated, bring it to an internal temperature of 165°F or higher to kill any bacteria. Keep in mind that if the food has been improperly stored, reheating won't make it safe.

Serving Food Safely

Temperature concerns continue even after a food has been cooked. When serving food, remember three rules. First, keep hot foods hot, at a temperature higher than 140°F. Extra quantities of food can be kept hot on the range, on a warming tray, or in an electrical serving dish. Second, keep cold foods cold. Refrigerate them until serving time. Third, follow the two-hour rule. Perishable foods that contain meat, poultry, fish, eggs, or dairy products should not sit at room temperature longer than two hours. If the air temperature is higher than 90°F, the limit is one hour.

REFRIGERATE FOOD PROMPTLY

Since bacteria thrive at room temperatures, you'll want to refrigerate food promptly. Any perishable food that is not in use should be in the refrigerator or freezer, whether it's ground turkey just home from the store or cheese slices used to prepare a snack.

Leftovers require special care. They should be refrigerated or frozen immediately, before cooling to room temperature. To ensure quick, thorough chilling, cut large pieces of meat into smaller ones. Store leftovers in shallow containers, tightly closed and labeled with the current date. These foods should either be eaten within three or four days or frozen for longer storage. You may want to keep all leftovers on the same shelf so none gets overlooked.

It may seem wasteful, but perishable food that has been left at room temperature for too long should be thrown out. The cost of the food is trivial compared to the cost of a foodborne illness.

Thawing Food

Concerns about temperature also apply to thawing frozen food. Never defrost food at room temperature. By the time the inside is thawed, millions of bacteria will have grown on the outside.

To thaw food safely for later cooking, place it in a container in the refrigerator. The container prevents leakage onto other foods. The cold temperature slows bacterial growth.

For faster thawing, you can place the food in a watertight plastic bag and submerge it in a bowl or sink filled with cold water. Change the water every 30 minutes to keep it cold. See **Fig. 20-6**.

You can also defrost food in the microwave according to the manufacturer's directions. Since defrosting in the microwave starts the cooking process, use this method only if you plan to cook the food right away. Another method is to thaw food as part of the cooking process by cooking it longer. Make sure the food reaches the proper internal temperature.

STORING FOOD

Have you ever bitten into a soft, stale cracker that was on the shelf too long? Who hasn't opened a container from the refrigerator only to

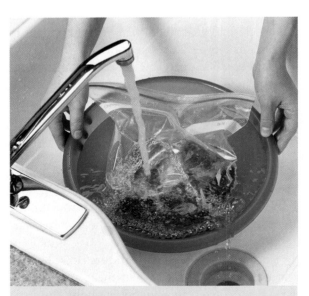

Fig. 20-6 You can thaw frozen food in cold water. How can you do this safely?

find mold covering the unrecognizable food? If food is improperly stored or stored too long, it loses quality and nutrients and eventually spoils. When bad flavors and odors develop, the food must be thrown out. Some types of spoilage even cause foodborne illness. You can minimize these problems with proper storage techniques.

Spoiled Food

What makes food spoil? Many foods are affected by light, heat, air, and other elements. As you've seen, dirt, heat, and moisture promote the growth of harmful bacteria, yeasts, and molds. Heat also speeds the action of enzymes in food, which trigger chemical changes that diminish food quality. A lack of moisture wilts some fresh foods and causes staleness in others. Air and light can destroy nutrients.

While proper storage protects food quality, improper storage hastens spoilage. Fortunately, spoilage often shows. Fresh produce may look wilted, wrinkled, bruised, or brown. Meats may become slimy. Spots of mold and a foul taste or smell are also sure signs that food has gone bad. See **Fig. 20-7**.

Food packages can also warn of spoiled contents. Be alert to damaged packaging, which

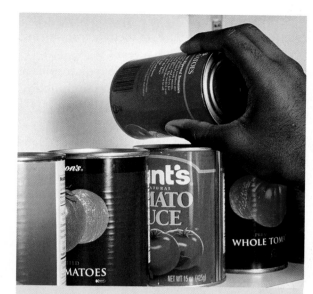

Fig. 20-8 Why is it a good idea to put newly purchased food items behind similar ones that are already on the shelf?

makes spoilage more likely. Bulging cans, liquids that spurt when you open a container, and cloudy fluids that should be clear all indicate bacterial action.

Spoiled food should not be tasted and must be discarded completely. Moldy foods require special handling to avoid spreading spores. Very gently wrap or place the food in a bag before discarding. Examine other foods that may have been in contact with the moldy item and wash the container that held it. If you suspect the mold is spreading to other foods, wash out the refrigerator.

How to Store Food

Proper storage controls the factors that affect freshness and spoilage. It helps preserve a food's nutrients, flavor, texture, and appearance. While different foods need different types of storage, these guidelines help protect quality in all types of stored food:

• Buy only what you need.
• Follow package directions for storing an item.
• Follow the principle of "first in, first out." Storing newly purchased food behind older food of the same kind reminds you to use the older items first. See **Fig. 20-8**.

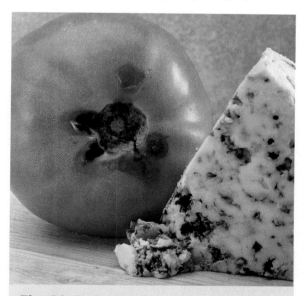

Fig. 20-7 Blue cheese gets its flavor from a special type of mold that can be eaten. Most molds on foods, however, mean that the food must be discarded.

- If containers have no sell-by or use-by dates, write the purchase date on them before storing. Use canned food within a year.
- Clean storage areas regularly. Wipe up spills as they occur. Wash and dry surfaces thoroughly.

Room Temperature Storage

Room temperature—generally below 85°F and above freezing, 32°F—is suitable for storing shelf-stable foods. These foods include unopened canned foods, dry beans and peas, oils and shortening, and many grain products, except whole grains. Kitchen cabinets are most often used. Cabinets should be clean and dry, with doors to keep out light and dirt. They should not be near or above heat sources, such as a range, radiator, or toaster. Remember that refrigerators also give off heat. Avoid using cabinets under the sink and in other areas that tend to be damp.

Areas used to store household cleaners or chemicals are also poor choices. The risk of contamination is too great. In addition, keep household cleaners and chemicals in their original packages, never in empty food packages or other food storage containers. In a clear plastic container, dry milk powder and plant fertilizer granules look too much alike.

After you open shelf-stable foods, the storage requirements change. Some foods, including most canned foods, must be refrigerated. Others, such as a bag of dry beans or a box of cereal, can remain at room temperature. If possible, reseal the package to keep out dirt and insects. Otherwise, transfer the contents to a storage container with a tight-fitting cover. Do the same with bulk foods.

Refrigerator Storage

The temperature inside your refrigerator should be no higher than 40°F. The owner's manual gives recommendations for setting the temperature control, but it's a good idea to keep a thermometer in the refrigerator to monitor the temperature. Avoid overloading the refrigerator, so that cold air circulates to all areas. If you see frost or ice forming, the temperature is too low. This wastes energy and can damage foods.

Because storage areas on the door are exposed to more warm air, save that space for soft drinks and other less perishable items.

Be sure that foods are tightly covered. This keeps them from drying out or picking up odors from other foods. Transfer opened canned foods to a glass or plastic container with a tight lid.

Foods that need refrigeration include:

- Foods that were refrigerated in the store, including dairy products, eggs, and delicatessen items.
- Most fresh fruits and vegetables. Exceptions are onions, garlic, potatoes, and sweet potatoes, which should be kept in a cool, dry place. Wash produce before storing only if dirt must be removed. Use a clean towel to dry hard-skinned fruits and vegetables. Let others drain well before storing.
- Whole-grain products, seeds, and nuts. Their high oil content makes them prone to **rancidity** (ran-SIH-duh-tee), or spoilage due to the breakdown of fats. Rancidity gives foods a stale flavor.
- Baked products with fruit or cream fillings.
- Any foods that, according to label directions, must be refrigerated after opening.

Freezer Storage

Freezing is used for long-term storage. At temperatures of 0°F or below, foods keep from one month to a year, depending on the type of food and its packaging. **Figs. 20-9** and **20-10** give a general timetable for storing perishable foods in the freezer. Refrigeration limits are also shown.

In contrast to a refrigerator, a fairly full freezer functions best. Frozen items act like ice blocks, keeping each other cold.

Unless you plan immediate use, foods purchased frozen should be promptly placed in the freezer. Other foods can be frozen to lengthen their shelf life. These include meat, poultry, and seafood; baked products; and home-prepared meals and leftovers.

Some foods don't freeze well. Those with high water content are especially vulnerable. Most fresh fruits and vegetables get soft and limp.

Fig. 20-9

Cold Temperature Storage of Meats, Poultry, and Fish

Food	Refrigerator Storage 40°F	Freezer Storage 0°F
Uncooked		
Beef, lamb, pork, or veal chops; steaks; roast	3-5 days	4-12 mos.
Chicken or turkey, whole	1-2 days	1 yr.
Chicken or turkey, pieces	1-2 days	9 mos.
Ground meats or poultry	1-2 days	3-4 mos.
Lean fish (cod)	1-2 days	6 mos.
Fatty fish (salmon)	1-2 days	2-3 mos.
Shellfish (shrimp)	1-2 days	3-6 mos.
Cooked/Leftover		
Cooked meats; meat dishes	3-4 days	2-3 mos.
Fried chicken	3-4 days	4 mos.
Poultry, in broth	3-4 days	6 mos.
Fish stews, soups (not creamed)	3-4 days	4-6 mos.
Cured Meats		
Hot dogs, opened	1 wk.	1-2 mos.
Lunch meats, opened	3-5 days	1-2 mos.
Hot dogs, lunch meats, unopened	2 wks.	1-2 mos.
Bacon	7 days	1 mo.
Smoked sausage (beef, pork, turkey)	7 days	1-2 mos.
Hard sausage (pepperoni)	2-3 wks.	1-2 mos.
Ham, canned, unopened	6-9 mos.	*
Ham, fully cooked, whole	7 days	1-2 mos.
Ham, fully cooked, half or slices	3-5 days	1-2 mos.

*Food should not be stored here.

Fig. 20-10

Cold Temperature Storage of Dairy Products and Miscellaneous Foods

Food	Refrigerator Storage 40°F	Freezer Storage 0°F
Dairy Products		
Fresh milk, cream	7 days	3 mos.
Butter, margarine	1-3 mos.	6-9 mos.
Buttermilk	2 wks.	3 mos.
Sour cream	1-3 wks.	*
Yogurt, plain or flavored	1-2 wks.	1-12 mos.
Cottage cheese	1 wk.	*
Hard cheese, opened (cheddar)	3-4 wks.	6 mos.
Hard cheese, unopened	6 mos.	6 mos.
Ice cream, sherbet	*	2-4 mos.
Miscellaneous Foods		
Bread	7-14 days	3 mos.
Cakes; pies (not cream-filled)	7 days	2-3 mos.
Cream pies	1-2 days	*
Fresh eggs, in shell	3 wks.	*
Raw yolks, whites	2-4 days	1 yr.
Hard-cooked eggs	1 wk.	*
Egg substitutes, opened	3 days	*
Egg substitutes, unopened	10 days	*
Mayonnaise, opened	2 mos.	*
Salad dressing, opened	3 mos.	*
Salsa, opened	3 mos.	*
Cookies	2 mos.	8-12 mos.

*Food should not be stored here.

Freeze them only if you plan to cook them. Thickened sauces, gravies, and fillings tend to separate, as do yogurt and sour cream. Custards and cream fillings, meat and poultry stuffing, and raw or cooked whole eggs also fare poorly.

Packaging Foods for Freezing

Foods that are purchased frozen are specially packaged to preserve quality. Those frozen at home, however, need added protection to avoid freezer burn. **Freezer burn** is moisture loss caused when food is improperly packaged or stored in the freezer too long. Cold air penetrates the package, damaging the food's quality. Food with freezer burn may have tough, grayish-brown spots and a stale taste and aroma.

Packaging materials for freezing must be vapor- and moisture-resistant as well as airtight. Good choices include plastic containers with tight-fitting lids, heavy-duty plastic freezer bags, and heavy-duty foil and freezer wrap. Regular refrigerator storage bags and plastic margarine or yogurt tubs don't give enough protection. The lightweight store wrap on fresh meat, poultry, and seafood also needs added layers for freezing.

When wrapping such solid foods as meat, aim for a tight fit. Squeeze out as much air as possible. Seal packages with freezer tape. When filling a container, leave enough space for food to expand as it freezes, about 1 inch of space in a quart container. Then seal the container tightly. Label all items with the contents, amount or number of servings, the date frozen, and any special instructions.

For best quality, freeze food quickly. Spread packages out in one layer so they all touch the cooling coils or sides of the freezer. Leave enough space between packages for air to circulate. Give the food at least 24 hours to freeze, and then stack like items together.

Keep an inventory of the food in the freezer. List the food, date frozen, and quantity. Update the inventory as you use food so that you know how much is left.

When the Power Goes Off

If the power goes off or the refrigerator-freezer breaks down, food inside is in danger of spoiling.

Transfer the food to another working appliance, if available. Carry the frozen foods to the new location in coolers or heavily wrapped in paper or plastic. If you can't move the food, keep the freezer or refrigerator door closed as much as possible to help keep cold temperatures.

Frozen Foods

After losing power, a full freezer should keep food frozen for about two days. A half-full freezer may keep the food only half as long. If the freezer is not full, quickly stack packages closely together so they will stay cold. Separate frozen raw meat, poultry, and seafood from other foods to avoid cross-contamination if they start to thaw.

If the power will be off longer than two days, you can nest foods in the freezer in bags of ice cubes from the store. You can also use dry ice (frozen carbon dioxide), but be very careful. Never touch dry ice with bare hands or breathe its vapors in an enclosed area. Carbon dioxide gas in high concentration is poisonous. See **Fig. 20-11**. A blanket or layers of newspaper on the outside of the freezer can insulate and also delay thawing.

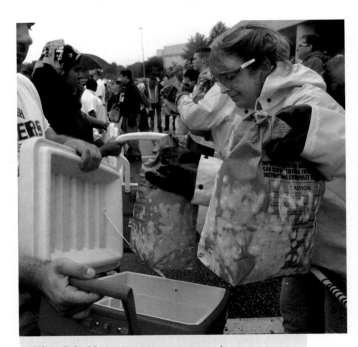

Fig. 20-11 If the power goes out, refrigerated foods must be kept cold or discarded. Here dry ice is distributed to people who have lost electricity during a hurricane.

Once the freezer is back in service, use the lowest setting to quickly refreeze any salvageable items. A food is safe to refreeze if ice crystals are still visible, though it may lose quality. Mark these foods to be used as soon as possible. Food that has thawed but is still cold can be refrigerated and used within the recommended time. Raw meat, poultry, and seafood can be refrozen after cooking. Throw out any food that has a strange odor.

Refrigerated Foods

Food will usually keep in a nonworking refrigerator for four to six hours, depending on the temperature of the room and how often you open the door. If the power will be out for a long time, try to keep foods cold by placing a large bag of purchased ice cubes in the refrigerator.

Foods that are still chilled can remain refrigerated when the power returns. Check all foods for signs of spoilage, especially butter, margarine, and fresh produce.

Once the refrigerator and freezer are working again, clean up any food spills and wipe surfaces dry. If odors remain, wash again with a solution of 2 tablespoons of baking soda dissolved in 1 quart of warm water. An open box of baking soda left inside will continue to absorb odors.

SAFEGUARDING THE FOOD SUPPLY

If you think ensuring the safety of your personal food supply takes diligence, imagine protecting the food supply for an entire nation. That responsibility means ensuring that foods are handled properly from farm to marketplace. It includes testing ingredients, testing new processing technologies, and guarding against contamination.

A job this big takes cooperation among governmental groups, led by those at the national level. Each of the federal agencies described here has distinct but interrelated duties.

Food and Drug Administration

The Food and Drug Administration (FDA), a division of the Department of Health and Human Services, is charged with the overall safety of the food supply. It has an impact on every food and beverage you buy.

Food Additives

A scan of food package ingredient lists shows that most foods contain preservatives, dyes, or other additives. See **Fig. 20-12**. Each of these ingredients has been approved by the FDA. After conducting public hearings and reviewing test results, the FDA determines how the additive may be used and in what amount. It also decides how the ingredient should be listed on the food label.

Not all additives are subject to this intense scrutiny. Those with a long history of safe use are classified by the FDA as "Generally Recognized as Safe" (GRAS). Items on the **GRAS list**, which range from sugar to seaweed, can be used by food processors for specified uses without further testing.

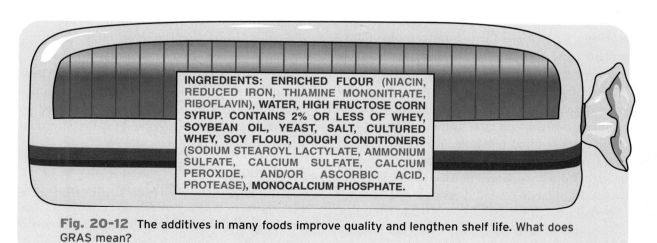

INGREDIENTS: ENRICHED FLOUR (NIACIN, REDUCED IRON, THIAMINE MONONITRATE, RIBOFLAVIN), WATER, HIGH FRUCTOSE CORN SYRUP. CONTAINS 2% OR LESS OF WHEY, SOYBEAN OIL, YEAST, SALT, CULTURED WHEY, SOY FLOUR, DOUGH CONDITIONERS (SODIUM STEAROYL LACTYLATE, AMMONIUM SULFATE, CALCIUM SULFATE, CALCIUM PEROXIDE, AND/OR ASCORBIC ACID, PROTEASE), MONOCALCIUM PHOSPHATE.

Fig. 20-12 The additives in many foods improve quality and lengthen shelf life. What does GRAS mean?

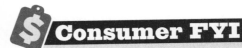
Policing the food supply. As of 2004, all companies that process, package, or hold food for sale in the United States are required to register with the FDA. The measure helps health officials track sources of tainted food in case of an outbreak of foodborne illness. It's a response to concerns that certain groups might use contaminated foods as "biological weapons."

The rule applies to makers and distributors of fresh and processed items, even chewing gum and animal foods, whether they are located in the United States or overseas. A few types of businesses are excluded, farms, restaurants, and supermarkets among them. Meat, egg, and poultry producers, which are regulated by the USDA, are also exempt.

No additive, even a GRAS item, is approved permanently. The FDA may require retesting, and possibly revoke approval, when scientific evidence casts doubts on an additive's safety.

Fat Replacers

Have you noticed the many fat-free and reduced-fat products on the market today? Many processed foods are now made with substitutes for fat. Fat replacers mimic the smoothness and creaminess of fat, without the less healthful qualities. The many processed foods made with fat replacers help people manage their fat intake. To ensure safety, the FDA oversees the use of fat replacers.

Food manufacturers use three types of fat replacers. They make them from carbohydrates, proteins, and fats. Sometimes a combination is used.

Carbohydrates have long been used as thickeners and stabilizers in foods. Modified food starch, cellulose, dextrin, and guar gum are a few of the carbohydrates in fat replacers. Since fat replacers based on carbohydrates withstand only limited heat, they don't work well in fried foods. They do work well in fat-free salad dressings.

Protein-based fat replacers are made from egg whites and fat-free milk. They are often used in frozen and refrigerated products. Like carbohy-drates, they can withstand some heat, but not enough to be used in fried foods. Low-fat cheese, ice cream, baked products, and cream soups contain protein-based fat replacers.

Fat-based replacers are made from chemically altered fats. They are stable in heat and very versatile, making them suitable for baked foods, cake mixes, frostings, dairy foods, and some fried foods. Olestra (oh-LESS-truh) is a fat-based replacer that passes through the body without being digested or absorbed. Thus fat-soluble vitamins may not be fully absorbed. For this reason, foods made with olestra are fortified with vitamins A, D, E, and K. Olestra may cause mild digestive problems for some people. Salatrim is another fat-based replacer found in baked goods, dairy products, and sweet products.

Most fat replacers have fewer calories than the fat replaced. A food, however, might still be high in calories from other ingredients. Check the Nutrition Facts panel for the amount of fat and calories in a food serving.

Hazard Analysis and Critical Control Point

Some outbreaks of foodborne illness have been traced to contamination during processing. To avoid such occurrences, the FDA requires some processors to use a system called Hazard Analysis and Critical Control Point (HACCP, pronounced "hassip"). HACCP is designed to predict and prevent threats to food safety at various points in food processing and service. See **Fig. 20-13.** Specific potential dangers are identified at each stage and steps are taken to avoid them. For instance, bacterial contamination is a common threat during meat grinding. Sanitizing machinery is a preventive measure.

HACCP includes record keeping and other documentation to show whether the program is working. HACCP procedures are promoted by international food agencies and followed by manufacturers worldwide.

Irradiation

The FDA also judges the safety of a processing technique itself. One well-known example is irradiation. **Irradiation** is the process of exposing food to high-intensity energy waves to increase its

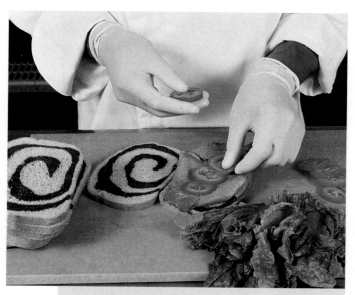

Fig. 20-13 The HACCP system helps make sure products are kept safe in the food industry. What food safety precaution do you see here?

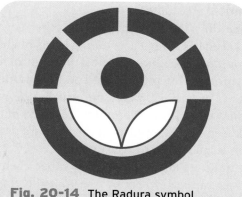

Fig. 20-14 The Radura symbol shows that a food has been irradiated. It appears either on the food label or on a sign nearby.

shelf life and kill harmful microorganisms. Irradiation does not make foods radioactive. Like other processing methods, it can slightly affect flavor, texture, and vitamin levels.

The FDA first approved the use of irradiation for spices and wheat flour in 1963. The process proved successful, with no known negative health effects. Approval was gradually extended to include produce, poultry, ground beef, and seafood. Irradiated foods must be identified with the symbol shown in **Fig. 20-14**.

Like food additives, irradiation has met with mixed response. Supporters point to its potential to reduce cases of foodborne illness and control pests without poisons. Critics claim the process creates harmful byproducts that can lead to cancer and birth defects. They fear that the radioactive elements used in irradiation plants endanger workers and communities.

Recalls

What happens if a manufacturer or the FDA learns that a food on the market is unsafe? Most often, a food maker issues a **recall**, the immediate removal of a product from store shelves. The brand name and package code numbers are publicized through the media. Consumers who have purchased the food are urged to return it to the store. If the company does not voluntarily recall an item, the FDA may take legal action, seeking a recall and penalties for the manufacturer.

Environmental Protection Agency

The environmental impact of food production is one concern of the Environmental Protection Agency (EPA). The EPA regulates the disposal of wastes generated by processing. It enforces laws that protect the nation's water supply.

The agency's primary role in food safety involves pesticides. Just as the FDA controls additives, the EPA decides when, how, and in what amounts pesticides can be used in growing food. See **Fig. 20-15**.

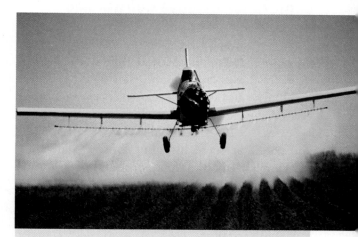

Fig. 20-15 The EPA regulates how pesticides can be used in growing food.

Chemical Residues

One duty the EPA shares with other government agencies is regularly testing levels of chemical residues. Residues are substances left in food as byproducts of processing. The EPA monitors traces of pesticides, which are usually the main residues in grains and produce. Pesticide in livestock feed can accumulate in the animal's tissues, which is later eaten by consumers.

A build-up of pesticides and other chemical residues can lead to serious health problems, in people and other inhabitants of an ecosystem. For every pesticide, the EPA establishes a **tolerance**, or a maximum safe level for a certain chemical in the human body. A tolerance represents a legal limit on pesticide use.

Food Safety and Inspection Service

The Food Safety and Inspection Service (FSIS), a branch of the USDA, is responsible for the wholesomeness of meat, poultry, and eggs. FSIS inspectors check the sanitation of packing plants and storage facilities. They test food products for residues of hormones, antibiotics, and other drugs used to improve an animal's condition. They keep diseased animals out of the food supply. FSIS officials work with foreign governments to ensure that imported animal products meet U.S. safety standards. Like the FDA, the FSIS can request a recall if it believes a meat, poultry, or egg product poses a health risk. See **Fig. 20-16**.

Centers for Disease Control and Prevention

The Centers for Disease Control and Prevention (CDC) is the lead federal agency for protecting the health and safety of people. Foodborne and waterborne diseases are one concern of the CDC's National Center for Infectious Diseases (NCID). This agency works with private and public partners, including those at state and local levels, to monitor foodborne and waterborne diseases, train people to identify them, research causes, and promote prevention and control.

Bioterrorism

Recent world events have brought attention to the threat of **bioterrorism**. This is the intentional

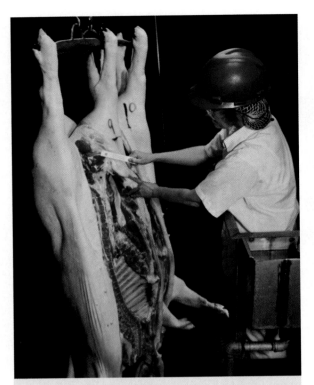

Fig. 20-16 The Food Safety and Inspection Service (FSIS) is a branch of the USDA. What foods are inspected?

use of biological agents—bacteria, viruses, and toxins—to harm people, animals, or plants. One example of bioterrorism is deliberately contaminating some part of the food supply to cause illness and make the food unfit for use.

Current safety practices go a long way to prevent such an occurrence; however, government groups recognize the need for greater precautions. Both the FDA and the FSIS have added offices of food security. They and other agencies have focused on improving communication and coordination to increase security throughout food production.

Likewise, the basic safety measures described in this chapter offer a defense against contamination. Stay alert to signs of tampering when you shop and report any to the store manager. If you suspect a case of food poisoning, notify the local health department. Your actions could save many people from the unpleasant effects of foodborne illness.

Home Economist

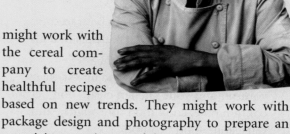

CHARLA DRAPER: Can you make up recipes that use a boxed cake mix or a can of cream soup? Charla Draper gets paid to do that—and a lot more. For the founder and owner of the food marketing firm, It's Food Biz!, recipe development is only part of a day's work.

Nothing in Charla's childhood in Chicago, Illinois, suggested a career in home economics. Her interest in foods began with a class she took in college. "I enjoyed the foods course more than any other, and that's how I became a home ec major." She later added a degree in marketing communications.

The Advertising Biz. Based on her education, Charla has made a career of blending consumer education and food marketing. As a home economist for Kraft Foods, she guided recipe development. While at Campbell's Soup Company, she worked with marketing managers, helping to create public relations campaigns for soup brands. She promoted products through press releases and appearances at special events. If families bought any Campbell's or Kraft product, from chicken noodle soup to Cheez-Whiz®, Charla may have had a hand in influencing their decision.

Stepping into the publishing industry, Charla spent two years as food editor of *Ebony* magazine. Her eye for trends and consumer appeal shaped the magazine's food coverage and helped increase advertising income from food advertisers by 50 percent. Her articles in other publications shared her own food heritage—soul food and Southern cooking.

Charla's Biz. In 1989, Kraft Foods was purchased by another company, and Charla was out of a job. Sensing an opportunity, she launched her own firm. It's Food Biz! is "one-stop shopping" for marketing services that promote food products. Does a cereal maker want to update the image of its cornflakes? Charla and her staff

might work with the cereal company to create healthful recipes based on new trends. They might work with package design and photography to prepare an appetizing new image of the product for package labels or for television or magazine ads. This multi-pronged approach has worked for projects with several clients, including the Pillsbury Company and McDonald's.

Charla's work calls for a lot of personal resources: knowledge of food science, interpersonal and communication skills, and a good measure of creativity. It takes flexibility too, for as Charla says, "no two days are alike."

Heart and Soul. Charla's on-line column, *A Dash of Soul*, explores her family's food heritage. The column includes traditional soul food recipes, revised to focus on more healthful preparation in keeping with today's health concerns. Though *A Dash of Soul* includes such popular favorites as pork chops, collard greens, and sweet potatoes, one recipe missing from the collection in the column is her family's favorite lemon pound cake. That rich dessert defies the "light" treatment. Besides, it's her mother's secret, so you won't see it on a box of cake mix either!

On-line Connections

1. To learn more about topics in this article, search the Internet for these key words: brand placement; food advertising; soul food.

2. To learn about related careers, search the Internet for these key words: public relations specialist; consumer psychologist.

Summarize Your Reading

▶ Most foodborne illness can be traced to microorganisms, living creatures that are visible only through a microscope.

▶ In order to avoid foodborne illness, keep yourself and your kitchen clean, don't cross-contaminate, cook food thoroughly, and refrigerate food promptly.

▶ Safe food handling practices include storing food at appropriate temperatures in the proper containers in either a refrigerator or freezer.

▶ The Food and Drug Administration (FDA) is a division of the Department of Health and Human Services and is charged with the overall safety of the U.S. food supply.

Check Your Knowledge

1. What are symptoms of **foodborne illness**?

2. What conditions encourage the production of **toxins** and **spores**?

3. When is a **20-second scrub** needed for food safety?

4. Describe how to wash dishes by hand.

5. What situation often causes **cross-contamination** to occur?

6. What can you do to prevent cross-contamination from occurring?

7. How does temperature affect bacterial growth?

8. How can you be sure that meat and poultry have been thoroughly cooked?

9. What are three rules for serving food safely?

10. Why should you never defrost food at room temperature?

11. What signs in a food or package indicate spoilage?

12. What guidelines help protect quality in stored foods?

13. Where would you store each of the following, at room temperature or in the refrigerator: unopened cans, box of cereal, eggs, onions, whole-grain products, and a custard dessert?

14. Why is it best not to freeze thickened sauces, gravies, and fillings?

15. How can you tell that a food has **freezer burn**?

16. **CRITICAL THINKING** Returning from a three-day trip, a family learns the power was out for 46 hours and restored two hours ago. What should the family members do about the food in their full refrigerator and freezer?

17. What does **GRAS** mean, and why are some foods classified by the FDA as GRAS?

18. What are fat replacers and how are they made?

19. What does the HACCP program do?

20. What is **irradiation**?

21. What happens when a manufacturer or the FDA learns that a food on the market is unsafe?

22. What are chemical residues, and why does the EPA establish a **tolerance** level?

23. What is the responsibility of the Food Safety and Inspection Service (FSIS) and how do they accomplish it?

Apply Your Learning

1. **Hand Washing.** Have someone time you in hand washing. How close to 20 seconds did you come? Time 20 second's worth of lines from a favorite song so you can sing the lines to yourself as you scrub.

2. **LANGUAGE ARTS** **PSA.** Develop and record a 30-second public service announcement about food safety. Air it on the school's public address system.

3. **LANGUAGE ARTS** **Puzzle Creation.** Develop a crossword puzzle on food safety, using an Internet puzzle-creation site. Exchange puzzles with a classmate and complete them.

4. **Demonstrations.** Demonstrate one of these topics: a) cross-contamination prevention; b) personal hygiene when handling food; c) proper dishwashing procedure; d) serving food safely; e) defrosting techniques; f) action during a power failure.

5. **SCIENCE** **Freezing Food.** Conduct an experiment on the effectiveness of different wraps and packaging when freezing food. Summarize your results in a chart.

Foods Lab

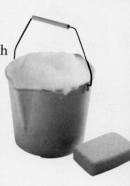

Food Safety Observation

Procedure: Prepare a dish with your lab team, as assigned by your teacher. One student on the team should observe and note safe and unsafe food handling practices. (An alternative is to have two observers, one focused on safe practices and the other on unsafe.) Follow up by discussing the observations.

Analyzing Results

❶ What safe practices were observed?
❷ What unsafe practices were observed? Why did these occur? Why are they dangerous?
❸ How might food safety techniques be improved?

6. **SOCIAL STUDIES** **State and Local Codes.** Choose a state or county and investigate their food codes. Report on two topics in the code.

Food Science Experiment

Testing for Contaminants

Objective: To test the foods lab environment for airborne microorganisms.

Procedure:

1. Cut a slice of bread in half. Place each half on a small plate.
2. Cover one plate tightly with plastic wrap. Leave both plates in the same place in the foods lab. Label them clearly "Do not eat."
3. Observe the pieces of bread after two, four, and six days. Record your findings.

Analyzing Results

❶ Describe the appearance of each piece of bread after six days. What process were you observing?
❷ Based on your answers from question 1, what can you conclude about the presence of spoilage microbes in the foods lab? Does this conclusion surprise you? Why or why not?
❸ From what sources might spoilage microbes be brought into a foods lab or home kitchen? What does this experiment tell you about the value of practicing good sanitation?

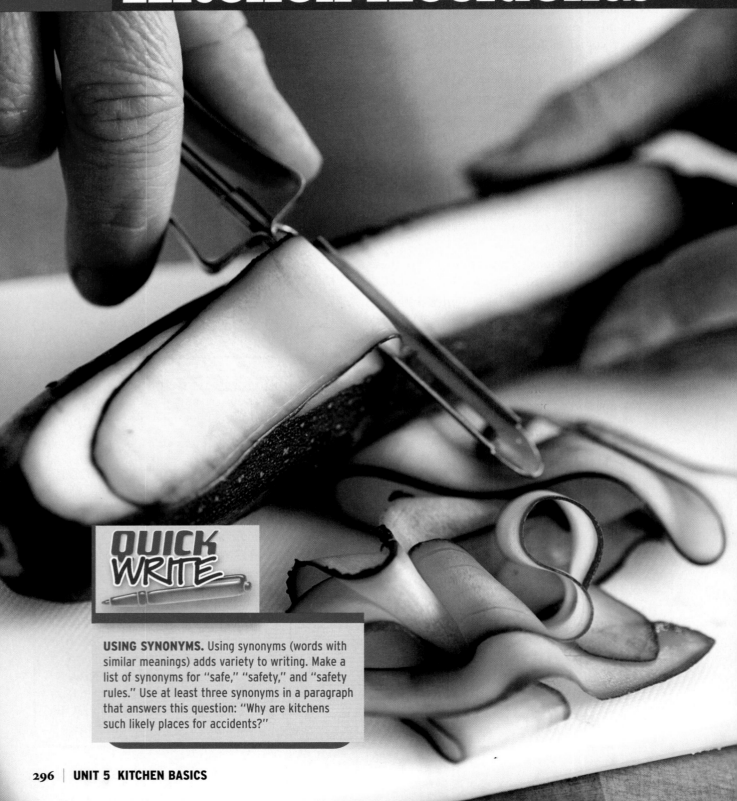

Preventing Kitchen Accidents

QUICK WRITE

USING SYNONYMS. Using synonyms (words with similar meanings) adds variety to writing. Make a list of synonyms for "safe," "safety," and "safety rules." Use at least three synonyms in a paragraph that answers this question: "Why are kitchens such likely places for accidents?"

To Guide Your Reading:

Objectives

▶ Compare safe and unsafe kitchen work habits.

▶ Describe how to cook safely outdoors.

▶ Summarize ways to make kitchens safe for children and people with physical challenges.

▶ Explain how to prepare for, and respond to, accidents or emergencies in the kitchen.

Terms

carbon monoxide

cardiopulmonary resuscitation (CPR)

Heimlich maneuver

polarized plugs

"We had an accident in the foods lab today," one teen said. "What happened?" his concerned parent asked. "Our cake sunk in the middle," the teen replied. A failed cake is disappointing, but kitchen accidents that cause injury are far worse. Smart and careful work habits can help you prevent them.

KITCHEN SAFETY BASICS

Whether you're an experienced cook or just learning to boil water, a review of basic safety guidelines is a good idea.

- Focus on what you're doing. The most routine tasks can be dangerous if your mind wanders.
- Dress for safety. Wear short or snug sleeves. Tie back long hair and apron strings. Dangling pieces of jewelry and other items can tangle in appliances or catch fire.
- Practice safe use of all tools and equipment. Use the right tool for the job. A butter knife is handy for spreading homemade jam, but it takes a can opener to pry off the jar lid.
- Close drawers and doors completely. Otherwise, a serious bump, bruise, or cut on the head could result.

- Store large pots and other heavy or bulky items on low shelves, within easy reach.
- Control clutter. Put items back where they belong as soon as you finish using them. Wash and dry dishes and empty the drying rack as needed.

PREVENTING FALLS

Whatever the fashion, snug shoes with no trailing shoelaces are always "in" for preventing falls. Skirts and pants should be a length that doesn't cause tripping.

Eliminating hazards in the environment can also reduce slips and trips. Keep the floor clear of clutter. Wipe up spills, spatters, and peelings. If you spray oil on baking pans, hold the pan over the sink. Otherwise, drifting oil can create slick spots on the floor. Secure slippery throw rugs with tacking or tape, or replace them with non-skid mats. Damaged or worn flooring should be repaired.

To reach higher shelves, use a sturdy stepstool. A chair or box can be unbalanced by trying to stand on it.

HANDLING SHARP EDGES

Which is more dangerous, a sharp knife or a dull one? If you've ever sawed a loaf of bread with a dull blade, you know the force it takes. Under that much pressure, a knife can easily slip. A sharp blade, in contrast, cuts through with less effort. Although it's actually safer, a mishandled sharp blade can produce a serious cut too.

All knives deserve respect. Store them in a divided drawer, knife block, or knife rack so you can pick them up by the handle. Knives come in different types; learn when and how to use each one. Always use a cutting board. For added security, create a nonskid backing by placing the board on a damp dishcloth.

Knives are not the only sharp edges in a kitchen. Graters, peelers, chopping tools, mixers, and can lids require the same caution. Keep fingers away from rough surfaces, slicing edges, and rotating beaters. Keep other tools away from a running mixer as well. If a cake recipe says "Scrape the bowl while beating," for instance, stop the mixer before using the scraper.

Cleaning sharp-edged tools takes extra care too. Don't soak them in a sink or dishpan, where suds or other dishes can hide them from view. Wipe knives carefully, with the blade pointed away from you. Air-dry other cutting blades. If a sharp-edged tool starts to fall, resist the impulse to catch it. Step back and pick it up when it comes to a complete rest.

Unintended sharp edges are another kitchen hazard. Wet dishes can slip from hands. A hot beverage can crack delicate glassware. Sweep up dangerously broken items at once with a broom or whisk broom and dustpan. See **Fig. 21-1**. If you need to pick up pieces by hand, use a wet paper towel instead of bare fingers. Seal broken bits or pieces in a bag and place it in the wastebasket. Take out the trash as soon as possible.

PREVENTING FIRES AND BURNS

The range is the mostly likely place for fires and burns to occur. Be careful, however, around any appliance that provides heat.

Fire and burn prevention starts with cleanliness. Grease and bits of food that build up in

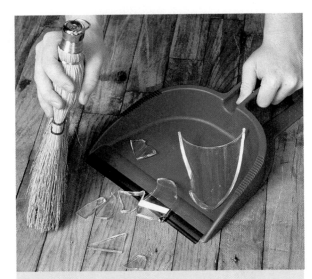

Fig. 21-1 If you break a glass, carefully sweep up all the pieces. A broom and dustpan can pick up most pieces, but if glass shatters into fine particles, what should you do?

burners, ovens, range hoods, and toasters can catch fire. Also check that cookware is in good condition. A pan with a warped bottom is easily upset. Those with loose handles can behave unpredictably. A glass baking dish with a hairline crack can fracture coming out of a hot oven. If any hot food or liquid gets on you, the consequences can be painful.

Cooktop Safety

On a cooktop, pots and pans can get hotter than the food inside. Always handle them with dry potholders or oven mitts. Wet fabrics carry heat.

When placing a pan over heat, turn the handle toward the back or center of the range top, where it's less likely to be hit and the pan knocked over. To remove a lid, lift the far edge first so the steam rises away from you. Steam can deliver a worse burn than hot metal or boiling water. The same applies to removing tops from microwave cookware. Make sure unused heating units are turned off before reaching over them.

Foods may not be the only fire and burn hazard on or near a cooktop. Curtains, kitchen linens, paper goods, and potholders can catch on fire just sitting close to a hot burner. A draft could cause them to touch. Plastic utensils used on the cooktop, such as turners for nonstick pans, should be heatproof. Other plastics are highly flammable and give off poisonous fumes when they burn. Aerosol cans should be stored away from heat.

Oven Safety

How hot is a hot oven? For comparison, safety experts recommend that home water heaters be set no higher than 120°F to prevent skin burns, yet recipes call for oven temperatures of 325°F and upwards.

To avoid contact with these hazardously high temperatures, arrange oven racks as needed before you turn on the oven. You risk being burned if you have to reposition them once the oven is hot. To remove baking pans, stand to one side when you open the oven door, away from the heat rushing out. Pull out the rack, using a potholder or an oven mitt, rather than reaching into the hot chamber. See **Fig. 21-2**. Be sure the oven and broiler are turned off after using them. Clean up spills and crumbs after the oven has cooled. Otherwise, they might catch on fire the next time the oven is used.

Gas ranges carry risks from the gas and the open flame. If you smell gas, check to see whether any pilot lights have gone out. If so, light a match first; then turn on the burner and light it. If you turn on the burner first, gas will accumulate and could explode when you strike the match.

If all the pilot lights are on, turn off all range controls and open the windows for ventilation. Don't try to find the source of the gas leak yourself. Alert others and get outside immediately. Call the gas company from another location.

If a Fire Starts

Like any hazard, a fire caught early is easier to contain. Smoke detectors are literally lifesavers. Test them every six months, and check the inside for cobwebs. A working fire extinguisher should be standard equipment in every kitchen, and using one is a skill to learn. See **Fig. 21-3**.

Quick action can also keep a fire from getting out of hand. If you see flames in an electric skillet or pan on the cooktop, turn off the heat. Smother the fire with a lid, another pan, or with salt or baking soda. Don't use baking powder or flour, as

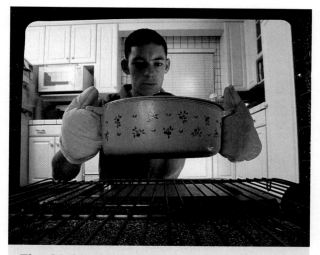

Fig. 21-2 Oven mitts protect your hands completely when reaching into a hot oven.

they can explode. Never use water. It makes grease spatter, spreading the flames and possibly inflicting a severe burn. Likewise, never carry the pan to the sink or outside, as you could hurt yourself and start a bigger fire when air fans the flames. Flames on clothes should be smothered too. Remember the advice to stay calm and "stop, drop, and roll."

If a fire is in the oven, broiler, microwave, or toaster oven, turn off or disconnect the appliance. Keep the oven door closed until the fire dies out.

If you can't put a fire out quickly, alert others and leave at once. Call the fire department from another location.

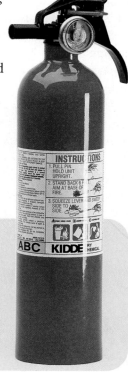

Fig. 21-3 Letters and drawings on fire extinguishers show use. This extinguisher works on ordinary combustibles like wood and paper (A), flammable liquids like grease (B), and electrical fires (C).

USING ELECTRICITY SAFELY

Although electric appliances save both time and work in the kitchen, they can also be the source of shocks, burns, and other injuries. Before using an electric appliance, read the owner's manual carefully. Refer to it as needed for directions on use and care.

Once plugged in, a cord is a river of electrical current. Check it for damage before each use. Even a single exposed wire is a fire or shock risk. Keep cords away from hot surfaces. Don't try to staple or nail them in place, but also avoid letting them hang off the counter. They could be snagged and the appliance pulled off. To disconnect an appliance, grasp the plug at the electrical outlet rather than tugging on the cord.

Limit the number of cords in an electrical outlet. An overloaded circuit can start a fire. See **Fig. 21-4**. Avoid regularly using extension cords, however. Choose a heavy-duty cord designed for appliances if one is needed.

To reduce the risk of shock, newer appliances have **polarized plugs**, which are made with one blade wider than the other and designed to fit in a matching outlet. These may not fit in older outlets. Trying to force or reshape the plug to make it fit is unsafe. Hardware stores have adapters.

Turn off small appliances as soon as you are through with them. Never put your fingers or a kitchen tool inside an appliance that is plugged in. Besides getting a painful shock, you can hurt yourself if you accidentally hit the "on" button. For example, unplug a mixer before removing the beaters. Also unplug an appliance immediately if it starts to overheat or gives a shock. Have it repaired before using it again.

Because water conducts electricity, the two can be a deadly mix—keep them apart. Never use an electric appliance with wet hands or while standing on a wet floor. Don't even run the cord around the sink. If an electric appliance falls into water or gets wet, unplug it immediately before touching the appliance itself. If the owner's manual permits cleaning a small appliance with water, unplug the machine first.

HAZARDOUS HOUSEHOLD CHEMICALS

In your home do you keep poisonous chemicals that can burn and make it hard to breathe? You do if you use oven cleaners, lighter fluid, drain cleaners, pesticides, or polishes. In many homes, these potential hazards are right under the kitchen sink.

Properly used, these products are helpful and sometimes necessary; however, simple, less toxic substitutes may also be effective in some cases. Baking soda and boiling water dissolve some sink clogs. Borax sprinkled outside the door discourages ants. Diluted vinegar cleans glass.

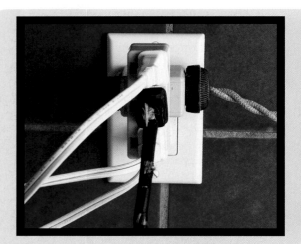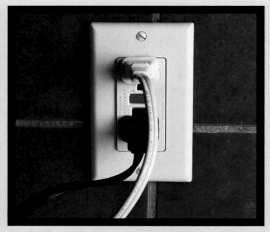

Fig. 21-4 Putting too many cords into one outlet can overload the circuit and cause a fire. Required wattage is printed on appliances. Most home outlets can support 1,500 watts, and some, 2,000.

If you decide to use household chemicals, read the label before buying. Does it give exact instructions for use? What directions are given about proper ventilation, protection for people and pets, and disposal of any unused product? What should you do if the substance is accidentally swallowed or inhaled? Keep hazardous products in their original containers so you can refer to the directions each time you use them.

Never mix cleaning products, such as bleaches, chlorine, ammonia, toilet bowl cleaners, and rust removers. Chemicals in the mixtures may interact and release poisonous gases. When spraying a product, make sure the nozzle is pointed in the right direction, not toward people. Use such products in a well-ventilated area.

Store hazardous chemical products away from food. Flammable products, including kerosene, lighter fluid, and aerosol sprays, must be stored away from any source of heat. In households with children, all hazardous household chemicals belong in a locked cabinet.

COOKING OUTDOORS SAFELY

Burning coals can generate temperatures up to 1,000°F. To deal with that kind of heat, follow these grilling guidelines:

- Start with a clean grill. Baked-on food and grease can cause flames to flare up when you light the charcoal. Clean the grill with a hard-bristle brush after each use. Wipe and wash the grate in hot, soapy water.
- Set the grill on a level, paved surface where it won't tip over, away from buildings, shrubs, trash containers, or anything else that could catch fire. Keep a fire extinguisher on hand as an added precaution.
- Never use a charcoal grill or hibachi inside the home or garage. Burning charcoal gives off large amounts of **carbon monoxide**, an odorless, highly poisonous gas. It can build in an enclosed area, causing drowsiness, headaches, nausea, and eventually death.
- If you use charcoal starter fluid, apply enough before striking the match. Adding fluid to lighted coals could trigger an explosion. The same is true of gasoline and kerosene.

- Use fireproof gloves and heavy-duty grilling tools with long handles. With long-handled tongs, turners, and basting brushes, you can reach food yet stay a safe distance from the heat.
- Fat and meat juices dripping on coals can cause flare-ups. If that happens, put out the fire carefully by raising the grate, covering the grill, or spreading the coals with a long-handled tool. You can also use a pump-spray bottle filled with water to mist the flare-up. Water poured directly on burning charcoal creates a dangerous cloud of steam.
- When you're finished grilling, let the coals burn down to ashes. Douse the ashes with water and put them in a metal trash can. Don't dump hot coals or ashes on the ground. They can burn grass and people and may even start a fire.

PROTECTING FAMILY MEMBERS

Anything you do to prevent accidents benefits the entire family. Ensuring the safety of certain family members may need added consideration.

$ Consumer FYI

Childproofing the kitchen. Watchful adults, trying to keep children safe in the kitchen, might find help in a variety of protective gadgets.

A stove guard reduces risks around the range. This clear plastic rectangle attaches to the edge of the cooktop, angling up and outward, to block heating units from a child's reach. Rounded plastic covers fit over knobs to make them harder for small hands to grip. Knob locks are discs that fit under the knob to stop it from turning.

Other devices help check children's natural curiosity. A dishwasher safety belt stretches over the control panel to keep a child from pushing buttons or opening the door, which may be full of sharp utensils. A two-piece freezer lock that attaches with strong adhesive can also secure refrigerators and dryers. Magnetic locks seal cabinet doors from inside. The attraction is broken by holding a magnetic "key" to the outside of the door.

Children

"What are you doing? Can I help?" If young children are in your home, you've probably heard these words. Small children like to be with older family members, especially in the kitchen. Time spent in the kitchen can be fun and educational for children if certain precautions are taken.

- Never leave young children alone in the kitchen, even for a few seconds.
- Protect toddlers by using safety latches on drawers and cabinet doors.
- If children want to help you work, set up a child-size table or a safe stepstool. Provide small utensils that they can handle for simple tasks, such as mixing and mashing. Don't let young children use knives or work near the range. Supervise them at all times.
- Model safe work habits. Teach by example.

People with Physical Challenges

Some changes in tools or workspaces make it easier for people with poor eyesight, arthritis,

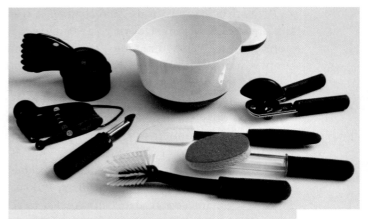

Fig. 21-5 Many kitchen tools are made to be comfortably used by anyone, but for those with arthritis, ease of use is essential.

and other physical challenges to use the kitchen safely. Even simple changes help. See **Fig. 21-5**.

- Add more or better lighting.
- Use unbreakable dishes and glassware.
- Store frequently used tools and foods in easy-to-reach places.

Career Prep

Choosing Entrepreneurship

DO YOU EARN MONEY WATCHING children? Walking dogs? Then you know some of the risks and rewards of entrepreneurship, owning and operating your own business. Entrepreneurship is vital to the American economy and can be an exciting way to earn a living. Entrepreneurship favors people with certain characteristics. Successful, happy entrepreneurs are likely to have the following characteristics:

- **Experienced.** Even if your skills are already professional, working for someone else before taking off on your own can acquaint you with other aspects of business, such as budgeting, advertising, and insurance.
- **Self-motivated.** An entrepreneur makes all business decisions and is ultimately responsi-

ble for carrying them out. From learning tax law to dusting window displays, the entrepreneur's motto is, "If it is to be, it's up to me."

- **Organized.** Paperwork and record keeping take a lot of time and space in running a business. Setting and maintaining a schedule is a challenge, especially when it must be balanced with family, community, and personal life.
- **Resourceful.** Things don't "fall in your lap" when you're an entrepreneur. From financing to floor space, meeting business needs may take creative thinking.
- **Confident.** Success may come slowly—or not at all. You must believe in yourself and your business through lean or discouraging times.

- Keep a magnifying glass in the kitchen for reading small print. Re-label items in larger letters with stick-on labels and a marking pen.
- Supply round, rubber jar openers for gripping appliance knobs.
- Put mixing bowls on a damp dishcloth or round, rubber jar opener to secure them on the countertop during mixing.

IN CASE OF ACCIDENT

Despite all precautions, you can't prevent every kitchen accident; however, you can be prepared. Keep emergency numbers next to the phone and a first-aid kit in a handy location. Remember the 911 number. If you aren't trained in first aid, ask the American Red Cross about classes.

Two first aid measures in particular can be lifesavers. One is the **Heimlich maneuver**, a procedure for dislodging an object from the throat of a person who is choking. The Heimlich maneuver uses a series of upward thrusts on the abdomen. Equally valuable is **cardiopulmonary resuscita-**

SAFETY ALERT

Choking. Choking incidents are frightening but may be avoided. Chew food slowly and thoroughly before swallowing. Also, try not to talk or laugh with food in your mouth. For small children, cut foods like grapes into little pieces. While pieces of a well-cooked carrot can be eaten easily, don't give raw pieces that can get stuck. Hot dogs are a definite choking hazard.

tion (CPR) (cahr-dee-oh-PUL-muh-ner-ee ri-suh-suh-TAY-shun), a technique used to revive a person whose breathing and heartbeat have stopped. In CPR, alternating chest compressions and assisted breathing get oxygen into the blood to keep the heart and lungs working.

If an accident does occur, stay calm. Panic only keeps you from thinking clearly. If necessary, take a few deep breaths to get yourself under control.

Never hesitate to call for help, whether for yourself or someone else.

- **Risk takers.** So many things, both within and beyond your control, must go right for your enterprise to thrive. Suppose operating costs rise or the economy weakens. You need a high tolerance for such uncertainties.

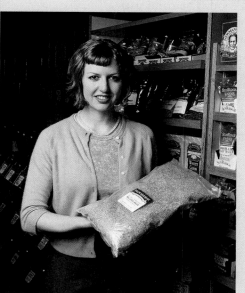

For adventurous types who have the qualities just described, opportunities abound in foods and nutrition. You might create a product or sell someone else's. You could provide a service—skills as a personal chef, for instance, or knowledge as a fitness consultant.

To avoid some risks, you might buy a chain restaurant or health food store franchise. A franchise is the legal right to sell a company's goods and services, using its name, logo, and concepts. In exchange, the buyer, or franchisee, agrees to operate the business according to corporate rules and standards. This arrangement offers the satisfaction of running a business, although technically not your own, with the security of an established name and management practices.

Career Connection

From fun to profit. Outline a plan for a business based on one of your interests or skills. What service or product will you offer? How will you make or distribute it? What supplies and other resources will you need? What expenses and profits do you anticipate? Present your research in a report or brochure.

Summarize Your Reading

▶ To work safely in a kitchen, you should become familiar with a number of guidelines. Besides learning basic guidelines, you need to form safe work habits that deal with preventing falls, handling sharp edges, preventing fires and burns, using electricity, and dealing with hazardous household chemicals.

▶ Specific guidelines can help you grill safely outdoors.

▶ Children enjoy time spent in the kitchen, but their presence requires special safety precautions.

▶ Kitchen modifications can help people with physical challenges work effectively and safely.

▶ If an accident occurs, staying calm helps a person think clearly.

Check Your Knowledge

1. What are six basic safety guidelines for working in the kitchen?

2. What safety precautions can be taken to prevent falls in the kitchen?

3. How does keeping a knife sharpened make it a safer tool?

4. How should knives be stored?

5. What precautions should be taken when washing sharp utensils?

6. Why does prevention of fire and burns start with cleanliness?

7. How should you handle these cooktop situations: a) direction of pot handles; b) lifting a lid; c) use of fabric and paper items; d) plastic utensils; e) aerosol cans?

8. What can you do to avoid burns when working with a hot oven?

9. When igniting a pilot light, do you light the match first or turn on the gas? Why?

10. What should you do if you see flames in an electric skillet or pan on the cooktop?

11. What are **polarized plugs**, and how do they enhance safety?

12. What rules should be followed regarding water and electric appliances?

13. Name some poisonous chemicals that are often found in homes.

14. What guidelines should be followed when grilling?

15. How does a stove guard help childproof a kitchen?

16. **CRITICAL THINKING** A five-year-old child stands on a chair at the counter, helping her parent fix food. The child uses a small steak knife to make bread cubes while the parent steps away to stir something on the range. Evaluate this situation for safety.

17. **CRITICAL THINKING** Why should people who aren't parents also be aware of child safety guidelines?

18. What is the **Heimlich maneuver**?

19. When might you need to perform **cardiopulmonary resuscitation**?

20. Why should foods like grapes be cut into little pieces for children?

Apply Your Learning

1. **Safety Cartoon.** Draw a cartoon with at least three panels that highlight a kitchen safety rule.

2. **Demonstration Videos.** Produce a demonstration video on one of these kitchen safety topics: a) storing and cleaning knives; b) smoke detectors; c) how to use a fire extinguisher; d) handling a fire in the kitchen; e) electrical safety.

3. **LANGUAGE ARTS** **A-Z Safety Lists.** Make an A-Z list of safety rules for the kitchen. For example, the first one might be "Appliances should be unplugged when not in use."

4. **Accessibility.** Evaluate your classroom kitchen or family kitchen on convenience and safety for people with physical challenges. What changes would be helpful?

5. **First Aid.** Investigate first-aid procedures, including the Heimlich maneuver and CPR. (A first-aid teacher might demonstrate.) Find out where you can take a CPR class.

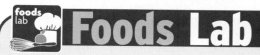

Foods Lab

Safety Demonstration

Procedure: Demonstrate a simple kitchen task, such as chopping vegetables or heating soup, pointing out the necessary safety precautions. Have the class critique your demonstration.

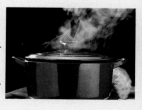

Analyzing Results

❶ Did you gain your audience's interest early and maintain it throughout?

❷ Did you balance demonstration with explanation when needed?

❸ How could you improve on your presentation in the future?

6. **First-Aid Kit.** Check the first-aid supplies in your lab. What is included and why?

Food Science Experiment

Smothering Flames

Objective: To learn ways to smother flames in a kitchen fire. In this experiment, follow safety precautions for working with a flame.

Procedure:
1. Place a small tea candle on a heatproof surface, such as a glass plate or aluminum foil. Light the candle. Carefully turn a sturdy, clear drinking glass upside down over the candle. Time how long it takes for the flame to go out.
2. Light the candle again. Drop about ½ teaspoon of salt over the flame and observe what happens.

3. Repeat Step 2, but use baking soda. Be sure you use baking soda because baking powder can explode.

Analyzing Results

❶ How effective was each method in putting out the flame?

❷ Why did the candle go out when under the glass?

❸ Which method would you most likely use in a kitchen fire? What circumstances might change your reaction?

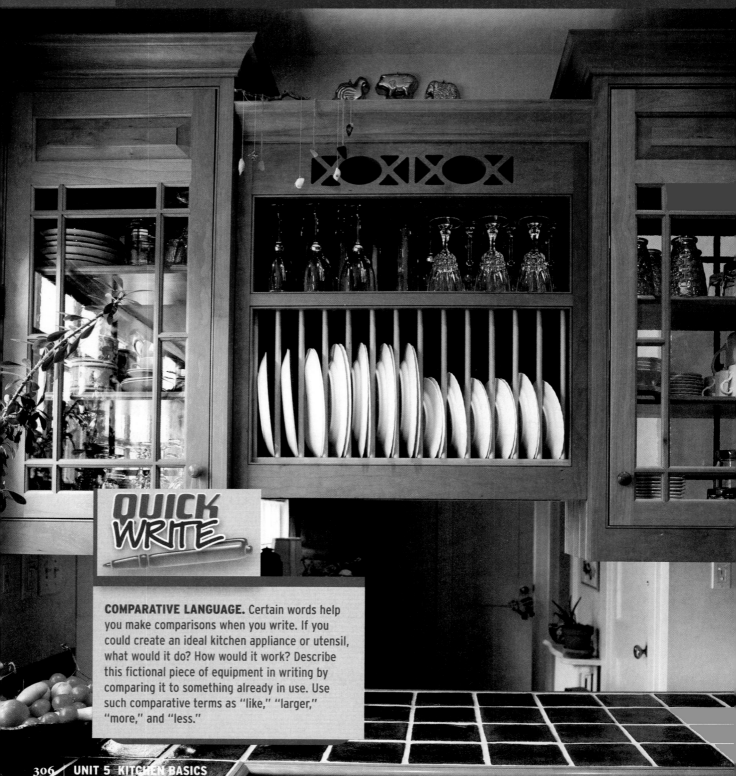

Equipping the Kitchen

QUICK WRITE

COMPARATIVE LANGUAGE. Certain words help you make comparisons when you write. If you could create an ideal kitchen appliance or utensil, what would it do? How would it work? Describe this fictional piece of equipment in writing by comparing it to something already in use. Use such comparative terms as "like," "larger," "more," and "less."

To Guide Your Reading:

Objectives

▶ Evaluate kitchen designs for convenience of work centers and work triangles.

▶ Describe factors to consider when choosing kitchen components.

▶ Explain what you need to know to be a smart shopper.

▶ Compare different models of ranges, refrigerators, and other appliances.

▶ Explain the use and care of kitchen tools and equipment.

Terms

annual percentage rate (APR)

bakeware

convection oven

cookware

credit

down payment

EnergyGuide label

finance charge

grounding

heating units

interest

island

peninsula

principal

service contract

task lighting

universal design

warranty

work center

work flow

work triangle

S OME PEOPLE SPARE NO EXPENSE IN DESIGING and furnishing a kitchen. Others adapt to a simple kitchen and outfit it with a few essentials. At each extreme and points in between, equipping a kitchen successfully takes an understanding of basic kitchen plans and the tools most useful for preparing foods. With this knowledge, you can organize your kitchen to make the best use of the space you have. See **Fig. 22-1**.

KITCHEN DESIGN BASICS

Efficiency may not sound like an exciting quality. If you spend much time working in a kitchen, however, you appreciate having things handy. An efficient kitchen starts with a well-designed floor plan that promotes the work flow. **Work flow** is a pattern of activity that begins with removing food from storage and continues with washing the food if necessary, preparation, and serving.

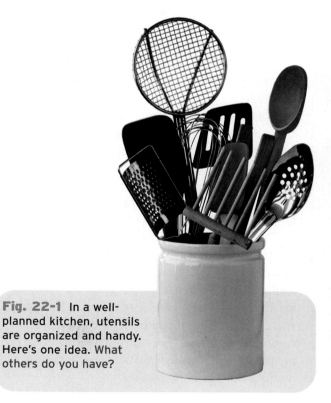

Fig. 22-1 In a well-planned kitchen, utensils are organized and handy. Here's one idea. What others do you have?

Work Centers

Kitchen floor plans are based on work centers. A **work center** is an area designed for performing specific kitchen tasks. A well-designed center has the needed equipment plus convenient and adequate storage and work space. A kitchen has three major work centers, based around the refrigerator-freezer, the sink, and the range.

- **Cold-storage center.** This center includes the refrigerator-freezer. Items stored here might include plastic storage bags, food wraps, and containers for leftovers.
- **Sink center.** This is the site for tasks that require a sink and water, including cleaning fresh fruits and vegetables, draining foods, and washing dishes. Dishpans and other cleanup supplies should be stored in this area. A garbage disposal and dishwasher would also be found here.
- **Cooking center.** This center includes the range, small cooking appliances, and related items. Storage is needed for pots and pans, cooking tools, and possibly canned and packaged foods.

Some kitchens have additional work centers. Foods may be mixed and prepared in a mixing center. Here you would find measuring cups, mixing spoons, and related appliances, along with such ingredients as flour and spices. Small kitchens might combine this center with one of the others.

More and more, the kitchen is a multipurpose room. For many families, it's a social area where guests enjoy both visiting and dining. Some kitchens make room for a small office, complete with computer. Others include a play or study area for children. Large kitchens might use some space for a laundry center with a washer and dryer.

The arrangement of the three main work centers forms the **work triangle**, or the primary path of work flow. Each center is one point in the triangle. For an efficient work flow, the distance between the three centers should total between 12 and 26 feet. To avoid confusion and accidents, the work triangle should limit through-traffic, that is, people walking through the kitchen work area to go from one room to another.

When one person works in the kitchen alone, the work triangle can be compact. If people share kitchen tasks, additional work space and duplicate work centers are useful. For example, a second sink lets one person scrub vegetables while another washes dishes. This arrangement might create adjacent or overlapping work triangles.

Basic Kitchen Plans

Kitchen plans determine the work triangle. The four most common plans are shown in **Fig. 22-2** and described here:

- **One-wall.** All three work centers are on one wall. These kitchens tend to be small, with limited storage and counter space.
- **L-shaped.** Work centers are on two connecting walls. This layout reduces the problem of through-traffic interrupting the work flow.
- **Corridor.** Work centers are located on two parallel walls. This design can be convenient for one cook. If doorways are located at opposite ends of the kitchen, however, through-traffic can be disruptive.
- **U-shaped.** Work centers are on three connecting walls, forming a U shape. This can be a very efficient arrangement.

These basic kitchen plans may be modified by adding a peninsula or an island. A **peninsula** is a countertop extension, open on two sides and one end. An **island** is a freestanding counter, open on all sides and often in the center of the kitchen. Both can include storage space below the countertop. They can be equipped with a sink or cooktop or may serve as an eating area.

Universal Design

To make kitchen space usable for everyone, regardless of age or physical ability, designers and appliance makers incorporate **universal design**. See **Fig. 22-3.** Universal design, also called lifespan design, allows wider doorways and work areas to accommodate wheelchairs and walkers. Work surfaces at various heights allow tasks to be done sitting or standing. Open shelves and drawer spaces are more accessible than closed cabinets.

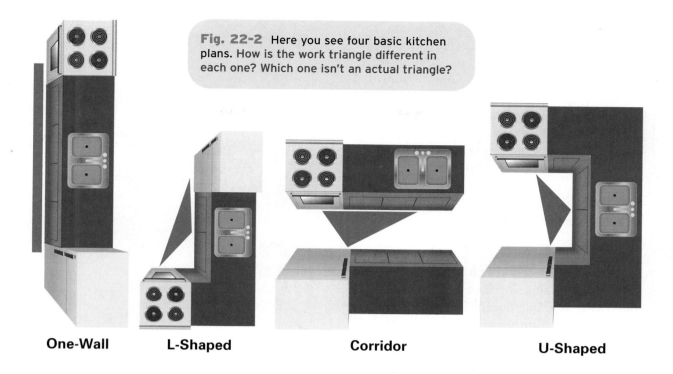

Fig. 22-2 Here you see four basic kitchen plans. How is the work triangle different in each one? Which one isn't an actual triangle?

One-Wall   **L-Shaped**   **Corridor**   **U-Shaped**

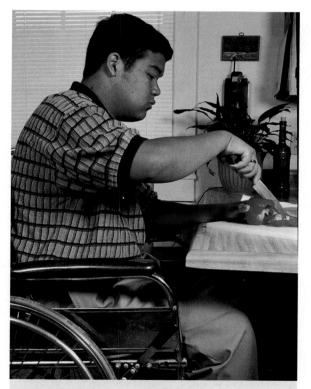

Fig. 22-3 Through universal design, kitchens can be easily used by everyone, regardless of differing physical abilities.

Existing kitchens may need adaptation for specific needs. Easy-to-grasp handles can replace cabinet knobs. Appliance controls can be marked in braille. A cart with wheels helps move food and equipment. Tongs or grippers grab items that would otherwise be out of reach. Stools or tall chairs make working at counters more comfortable.

KITCHEN COMPONENTS

Cabinets, countertops, flooring, and other essential components complete a well-thought-out kitchen design. The materials used for these must withstand the impact of food, heat, and moisture. This combination is unique to kitchens. It can cause accidents and invite harmful bacteria, insects, and other pests unless the area is kept dry and clean. Therefore everything in the kitchen, from floors, to lighting fixtures, to accessories, should be as follows:

- **Washable.** Materials that hold dirt or require special care may defeat your best efforts at cleanliness.
- **Moisture-proof.** Furnishings should be either naturally moisture resistant or treated with a

moisture-proof finish. Good ventilation, from windows, exhaust fans, and exhaust hoods over the range, speeds evaporation of moisture. An exhaust fan system can also limit the spread of mold spores and airborne particles of grease.

- **Heatproof.** Highly flammable materials don't belong in the kitchen. Use only heatproof objects near any appliances that produce heat, such as a range or toaster oven.

Cabinets

Kitchen cabinets that rest on the floor under a countertop are called base cabinets. Their standard size is 24 inches deep and 36 inches high, although heights vary if drawers are added. Wall cabinets of various sizes attach to the wall above the countertop. Tall, floor-to-ceiling cabinets are called pantries. Pantries may include a shelf for a microwave oven.

Cabinets are made of solid wood or stainless steel, popular for their natural beauty and durability; however, most people choose plastic laminates. Laminates are layers of paper, compressed and bonded with liquid plastic. They resemble more costly materials but need less care. Cabinet sides are often compressed wood that is chemically treated to resist water.

Many options add convenience to cabinets. Roll-out shelves bring items to you. Pop-up shelves hold mixers, and vertical dividers organize baking sheets and trays. Pull-out, ventilated baskets provide cool, dry storage for produce. Storage aids, such as door racks and shelves, stackable bins, and turntables, are sold in store housewares departments. For convenient and frequent cleaning, shelf lining is specially made to wipe off easily. See **Fig. 22-4**.

Storage Strategies

"A place for everything and everything in its place" applies to kitchen storage. If a utensil is used in several locations, store it where you would use it most often. When space is limited, store seldom-used items outside the kitchen.

The place for large, heavy equipment is in low cabinets, where they're easy to reach and lift. Stack glass items as little as possible, with heavier

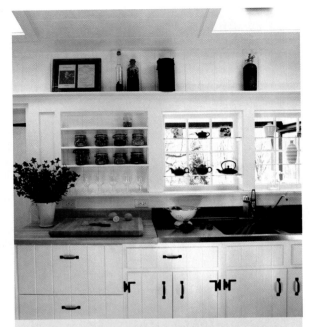

Fig. 22-4 Kitchens should suit the people who use them. How might a kitchen for a single person be different from the one a large family prefers?

ones on the bottom and limited stacking heights. Keep tools with sharp or pointed parts in drawers where you can see and access them easily.

Countertops

Countertops come in varied materials—from wood, to concrete, to marble. Some kitchens use several different materials, based on the advantages and disadvantages of each. Counters near sinks might use moisture-resistant, glazed tile. Heat-resistant granite works well near the range. Price and care needs also affect choices.

Since countertops are valued as work space, people often wish they had more. Work space can be added in the form of a cart, a table, or a portable base cabinet. Flip-down shelves, pull-out breadboards, and adjustable cutting boards that fit over the sink also increase work space.

Floors and Walls

Like countertops, floors take wear. Thus both surfaces use similar materials. Comfort is an added factor in flooring. To be easy on the feet, floors should be resilient, springing back under pressure. Vinyl and linoleum share this quality. Neither one needs waxing or polishing; however, both can be nicked by sharp objects. Stone floors are hard to damage but also hard to stand on. The impact can be eased with mats or throw rugs. Hardwood adds warmth but requires more care to maintain appeal.

Easy cleaning may be the most important quality in kitchen wall coverings, or treatments, especially near the sink and range. Wallpaper and paint are both practical. Vinyl-coated wallpaper can be wiped with a sponge, while paper backing adds strength. In paints, semigloss is best at releasing dirt. Ceramic tile holds many creative possibilities but is more expensive.

The Electrical System

Safe and sufficient are words that describe an effective electrical system. Make sure you have enough power coming into the kitchen, sufficient outlets, and a grounded electrical system.

Grounding minimizes the risk of electric shock by providing a path for the current to travel back through the electrical system, rather than through your body. The National Electric Code requires grounded wires in new homes. Outlets with three holes usually indicate the wiring is grounded; however, check with an electrician to be certain. Grounded outlets accept three-pronged plugs from grounded appliances. See **Fig. 22-5**.

If appliances work slowly or poorly or lights dim or go out when you use an appliance, the wiring does not provide enough power to meet your needs. Have a qualified electrician check out the electrical system.

Lighting

Good lighting is essential for both comfort and safety. A ceiling light or lighted panels can provide adequate general lighting. Close work takes **task lighting**, bright, shadow-free light over specific work areas. For instance, lighting fixtures may be mounted beneath overhead cabinets to light countertops. Recessed spotlights or track lights on the ceiling can be positioned to highlight specific locations. Adjust brightness with dimmer switches.

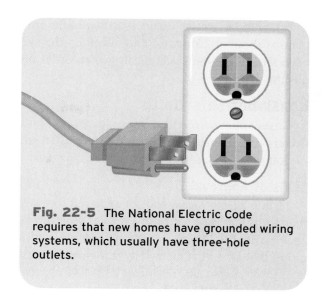

Fig. 22-5 The National Electric Code requires that new homes have grounded wiring systems, which usually have three-hole outlets.

BUYING FOR THE KITCHEN

Kitchen purchases range from a mixing spoon to a refrigerator-freezer. The size of the investment affects the forethought and research that go into the decision.

Before You Buy

Before setting foot in a store, think about whether you need an item. Can equipment you already own perform the same tasks? If you're updating a model of something you already have, will the improvement justify the cost? How much can you afford to spend? How will you pay?

Next, identify the most important features, based on your needs and wants. If you're buying a freezer, write down the measurements of the space where it must fit. Note whether dishes must be microwave-safe. Because items in your price range might not have all the features you want, rank your wants from most to least important.

Finally, gather information about the product. Look for advertisements and articles in magazines and newspapers. Some consumer magazines conduct unbiased tests to compare brands of similar items. Most appliance manufacturers have Web sites with up-to-date information on products.

Dealer reliability is also important, especially for major purchases. If you shop by catalog or on the Internet, make sure the seller is reputable.

Check with the Better Business Bureau for complaints about a company and whether they've been settled. Use only secure sites when ordering on-line.

Consumer Safeguards

Government agencies, manufacturers, and dealers help ensure that consumers are satisfied. As you shop, look for these consumer safeguards.

Seals of Approval

Testing agencies give seals of approval to show that a product meets certain safety and performance standards. A seal is only as reliable as the group that issues it. One widely recognized group is Underwriters Laboratories (UL). On electric appliances, the UL mark certifies that the appliance design is reasonably free from risk of fire, electric shock, and other hazards. The American Gas Association (AGA) seal attests to the design, performance, and reliability of gas appliances. See **Fig. 22-6**.

EnergyGuide Label

The **EnergyGuide label** is a tool for estimating an appliance's energy costs. A dollar figure gives the average yearly cost of operating a model so

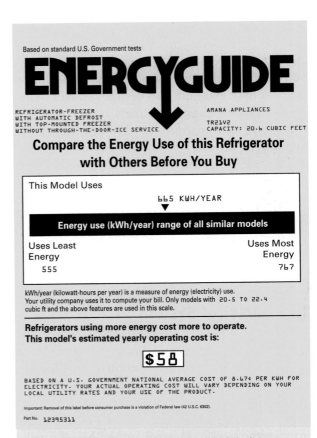

Based on standard U.S. Government tests

ENERGYGUIDE

REFRIGERATOR-FREEZER
WITH AUTOMATIC DEFROST
WITH TOP-MOUNTED FREEZER
WITHOUT THROUGH-THE-DOOR-ICE SERVICE

AMANA APPLIANCES
TR21V2
CAPACITY: 20.6 CUBIC FEET

Compare the Energy Use of this Refrigerator with Others Before You Buy

This Model Uses

665 KWH/YEAR
▼

Energy use (kWh/year) range of all similar models

Uses Least
Energy
555

Uses Most
Energy
767

kWh/year (kilowatt-hours per year) is a measure of energy (electricity) use. Your utility company uses it to compute your bill. Only models with 20.5 TO 22.4 cubic ft and the above features are used in this scale.

Refrigerators using more energy cost more to operate. This model's estimated yearly operating cost is:

$58

BASED ON A U.S. GOVERNMENT NATIONAL AVERAGE COST OF 8.67¢ PER KWH FOR ELECTRICITY. YOUR ACTUAL OPERATING COST WILL VARY DEPENDING ON YOUR LOCAL UTILITY RATES AND YOUR USE OF THE PRODUCT.

Important: Removal of this label before consumer purchase is a violation of Federal law (42 U.S.C. 6302).

Part No. 12395311

Fig. 22-7 With the EnergyGuide label, you can compare energy efficiency of different appliance models. What might it cost to run this appliance for a year? How does its energy use compare to other models?

you can compare costs among different models. You can also estimate your own energy expenses based on the cost of gas or electricity in your area. EnergyGuide labels are required on refrigerators, freezers, and dishwashers. See **Fig. 22-7**.

Warranties

A **warranty** is a manufacturer's guarantee that a product will perform as advertised. If you have problems with the product, the manufacturer promises replacement or repair. Warranties have time limits and coverage is usually conditional. For example, most don't pay for damage resulting from use that the owner's manual warns against. Some manufacturers sell extended warranties that offer additional coverage for a longer time period.

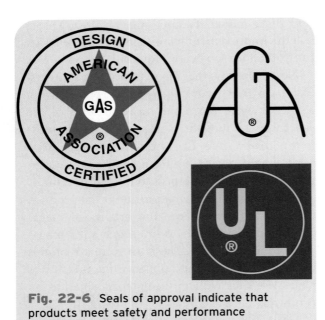

Fig. 22-6 Seals of approval indicate that products meet safety and performance standards. What types of products might carry the seals shown here?

Service Contracts

A **service contract** is repair and maintenance insurance purchased to cover a product for a specific length of time. It is usually offered by the dealer who sold you the product, not the manufacturer. Service contracts are often expensive. Frequently, they don't cover the total cost of repairs and parts and may duplicate protections received free with the warranty.

Be a Critical Shopper

The same comparative shopping skills that help keep a food budget balanced can help with larger buys as well. Depending on the size of the purchase, you may want to take some or all of these steps:

- Keep written notes as you shop. To help you make a final decision, list your likes and dislikes for each product.
- Consider accident prevention. Check carefully for potential hazards as well as features that guard against them—a heatproof handle on a waffle iron, for instance.
- Handle tools, cookware, and appliances. Do they seem well made and comfortable to use?
- Look at the owner's manual. Will the item be easy to use and care for? What does the warranty cover?
- Compare prices. More features and better quality usually come at a higher price. You pay for the reputation of well-known brands, yet a less familiar name doesn't always mean inferior quality.
- Ask the dealer about additional costs, such as delivery and installation charges.

Paying for Your Purchase

Most people pay cash for small items. Some save money to pay cash for larger purchases as well. Nonetheless, many major purchases are bought with credit. **Credit** is a financial arrangement that delays payment for an item. Using credit is more expensive than paying cash, but you can use the product while you pay. See **Fig. 22-8**.

Like cooking, credit has a language of its own. When you buy on credit, you may have to make a **down payment**, a portion of the purchase price paid right away. This is deducted from the total purchase price, leaving the amount to be financed, or the **principal**. You borrow this amount from a lender—a credit card company, bank, or finance company. The lender charges you **interest**, a fee for the loan, expressed as a percentage of the amount borrowed. Interest rates can vary greatly. By law, lenders must state the **annual percentage rate** (**APR**), or the yearly rate.

Besides interest, the lender may add other costs of doing business, such as a service charge or insurance premiums. These fees, along with

Fig. 22-8 A monthly billing statement tells what is owed on a credit purchase.

ABEL'S APPLIANCES
"Where Customer Satisfaction Counts"
1221 Sixth Avenue
Middland City, IL 00000
(000) 555.7076

STATEMENT
DATE: February 29, ___

To:
Gregory Ledsma
782 Pinehurst Way
Middland City, IL 00000
Acct #: 5809-2333-66

NEW BALANCE	PREVIOUS BALANCE	CLOSING DATE	AMT DUE	PAYMT DUE DATE	PLAN TYPE
$581.12	$622.25	02/17/__	$72.50	03/20/__	C-349

ITEMS PURCHASED	PURCHASE DATE	ORIGINAL PURCHASE PRICE
Deluxe Refrigerator/Freezer w/ ice-maker, adj. shlv, clim ctrl, cubic cap EE: K133-95	11/14/__	$799.48

		CREDIT HISTORY				
Billing Cycle 31 days	Balance Subj. to Finance Chg	Daily Periodic Rate **V** = Variable **F** = Fixed	Corresp. Annual Percentage Rate	Finance Charges	**BALANCE SUMMARY**	
	$0.00	**V** 0.0504110%	18.40%	$0.00	Previous Balance	$622.25
	Balance Calc Code (see reverse side)				Payment Rec'd	-$72.50
					Interest Charges	$31.37
					Late Fee (if applc'bl)	$0.00
					FINANCE CHARGE	$0.00
					NEW BALANCE	$581.12

interest, make up the **finance charge**, the total amount you pay for borrowing, shown as a dollar figure. Monthly payments usually equal the total cost (principal plus finance charges) divided by the number of months agreed to pay off the account.

Shop for credit as carefully as for a purchase. To find the lowest cost of borrowing, compare APRs and other fees. Don't be lured into spending more than you can afford. Failing to make payments on time can cause serious problems. You can lose the purchased item and may have trouble getting credit in the future.

Protecting Your Purchase

With your purchase you bring home some important papers: the warranty, owner's manual, and sales receipt. Keep these documents together in a safe place where you can easily find them. If you need to use the warranty, the receipt proves date of purchase. Fill out and send in any warranty registration card. This validates the warranty if you lose the receipt. Also, the manufacturer can send product information or notify you if a danger or defect is discovered.

Read the owner's manual before using the product. Then test it to make sure it works. If it doesn't, return the item to the store or call the dealer.

MAJOR APPLIANCES

A major appliance is a large device powered by electricity or gas. Except for the microwave oven, cooks have typically relied on the same major appliances for the last fifty years: the range, the refrigerator-freezer, and the dishwasher. Of course, designs have changed considerably. Yesterday's cook might be amazed at what today's appliances can do.

The Range

The conventional range is a single, freestanding unit consisting of a cooktop, an oven, and a broiler. Cooking heat is generated by **heating units**, which are energy sources in the range. Most ranges are either gas or electric. Dual-fuel ranges use both fuels: electricity for the oven, gas for the cooktop.

On the cooktop, heat is controlled with dials, buttons, or touchpads that are numbered or marked with temperature settings. Oven controls are thermostatic, allowing more precise temperatures. Settings vary from "warm," below 200°F, to "broil," about 500°F. The broiler cooks foods by direct heat from a heating unit in the top of the compartment.

Ovens are available with a number of features. Adjustable self-cleaning cycles use intense heat to burn off spatters and spills. Digital displays used to program cooking instructions are becoming common. Warnings appear in the display panel to identify a malfunction. Some ovens have "half racks" that allow lower racks to hold oversize pans. Pull-out warming drawers create a slightly humid environment that helps to raise yeast breads or to hold cooked foods safely without drying them out.

Gas Range

The heating units in a gas range are called burners. Burners heat with a visible, easily regulated flame that is quickly raised or lowered. In newer ranges, gas flows through and is ignited by an electronic spark when a burner is turned on. Older models have pilot lights, small flames that burn continuously. When the burner is turned on, the pilot light ignites the gas.

Some gas ranges have sealed burners that are easy to clean. Others have one continuous grate so cookware can slide from one burner to

---

SAFETY ALERT

Pilot lights. Natural gas requires oxygen to burn completely. Incomplete burning creates carbon monoxide. Signs of this include a pilot light that burns yellow and a buildup of soot near the range. To ensure a good air supply to a gas range, take care to keep air vents open. Don't line the burner bowls with foil. If a burner lights only partially, try clearing the holes with a metal wire or paper clip. Don't use toothpicks, which can break and plug the holes.

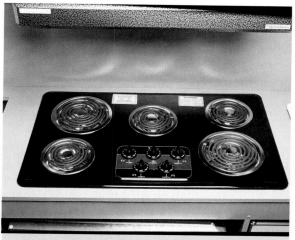

Fig. 22-9 The heating elements in one type of electric range are exposed metal coils. How is this different from a gas range?

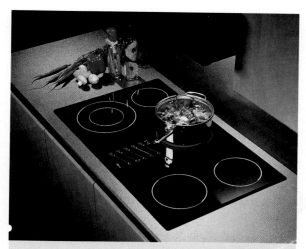

Fig. 22-10 Some electric ranges have a glass-ceramic smoothtop. The heating elements are underneath the top. What advantage does this offer?

another. The oven and broiler in a gas range are in separate compartments, with the broiler generally below the oven.

Electric Range

The heating units in electric ranges are called elements. Because elements retain heat longer than gas burners, many ranges have a warning indicator that stays on until the cooktop is safely cooled.

Two basic cooktops are available in electric ranges. Exposed, metal, coil elements turn red when the heating unit is on. These spiral-shaped coils vary in size to fit small and large cookware. See **Fig. 22-9**. A second option is a glass-ceramic smoothtop that covers "ribbon" heating elements, making cleanup easier. See **Fig. 22-10**. Some smoothtops have a bridge to connect several elements into a single surface for oblong pots and pans. Others have a low-heat, warming zone to keep food hot without burning.

Baking and broiling in an electric range occur in the oven. A heating element at the bottom of the oven bakes food. An element on the top comes on for broiling.

Convection Oven

Both conventional and convection ovens use convection currents, created by rising air as it warms. A **convection oven** also has a fan that circulates heated air to equalize temperatures throughout the oven. The result is faster and more even cooking and browning. See **Fig. 22-11**.

Some ranges combine convection and microwave cooking, offering the advantages of each. These powerful, top-of-the-line models are similar to those used in professional kitchens. Cooking times are half those of conventional

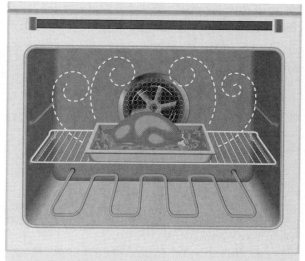

Fig. 22-11 Convection ovens have a fan in the back, which forces air to circulate around the food. How is cooking speed affected?

cooking, which helps foods retain moisture and flavor. Conversion programs adapt a conventional recipe's time and temperature to the oven's combination cooking methods.

Built-In Units

Rather than a freestanding range, some kitchens have separate cooktop and oven units. Each component can be located where most convenient. Ovens are built into walls, with added insulation to protect adjacent areas. Cooktops are set in cabinets. Some have modules for grills and griddles. A downdraft exhaust system draws heated air into a duct below the cooktop.

Microwave Oven

In a microwave oven, a magnetron (MAG-nuh-trahn) tube converts electricity into microwaves, a form of energy that travels through space like radio waves. A fanlike device called a stirrer blade distributes these waves throughout the oven, where they bounce off the walls and floor. Microwaves pass unaffected through paper, glass, and plastic. They are absorbed by the molecules in food, however, causing the molecules to vibrate against each other and produce friction. This friction produces heat that cooks the food in as little as one-fourth the conventional time. See Fig. 22-12.

Microwave ovens vary in size from about ½ cubic foot to 2 cubic feet. Large models convert more electricity than small ones, producing more microwaves and cooking foods more quickly. An oven's power rating indicates the amount of electricity it uses, as measured in units called watts. A compact oven might generate 600 watts of electricity. Large versions produce up to 1,100 watts.

Some microwave ovens are countertop models. Others can be built into a wall or mounted over a range. Turntables that rotate foods for more even cooking and racks that increase

oven capacity are common features. Many models have recipe programs to cook food automatically at a preset time and temperature. Some have sensors that adjust cooking conditions based on the amount of moisture left in a food.

Refrigerator-Freezer

Refrigerator-freezers create cold storage by means of a chemical blend called a refrigerant. The refrigerant circulates in the refrigerator walls, compressing into a liquid and expanding into a gas. As it expands, it absorbs heat, which escapes through coils outside the unit.

Full-size refrigerator-freezers range in size from 10 to 30 cubic feet. Most have two outer doors, one each for the refrigerator and freezer. The freezer may be at the top, bottom, or alongside. It maintains a temperature of 0°F, so it can freeze fresh foods as well as store those already frozen. Small, single-door models have a frozen food compartment at the top of the interior, behind a lightweight inner door. With a temperature of 15°F, this section is only cold enough to store already frozen foods for about two weeks.

Added options make refrigerator-freezers more convenient. Small, slide-in shelves can be adjusted to customize refrigerator space. A freezer

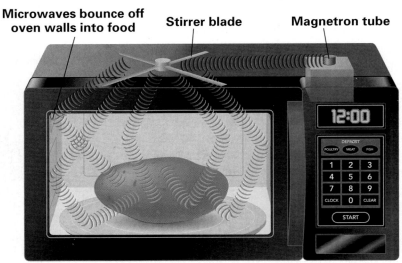

Microwaves bounce off oven walls into food   **Stirrer blade**   **Magnetron tube**

Microwave Oven

Fig. 22-12 In a microwave oven, the stirrer blade distributes the microwaves produced by a magnetron tube. **What happens if the food is sitting in a glass or plastic container?**

light lets you see what's inside. A pull-out freezer drawer brings food into view. "Freezerless" refrigerator modules fit into cabinets.

Dishwasher

People who use dishwashers have ever-increasing choices. The standard, built-in model fits under the countertop and attaches to a hot water line, drain, and standard outlet. Portable units on wheels connect to the sink faucet and drain into the sink. You can also buy a small, in-sink dishwasher. As part of a double sink, it converts quickly into a dishwasher for small loads.

Depending on the model, a dishwasher can be set for various wash cycles, from a rinse to a sanitizing cycle that heats the water to above 140°F. Typical features include adjustable racks for varied tableware, a food disposer to keep food from resettling on clean dishes, and insulation for quiet operation. With the delayed-start feature, you can run the dishwasher when convenient.

SMALL APPLIANCES

Some kitchen jobs are easier with the right small appliance, a small, electric, household device that performs a simple task. These machines can save time over doing tasks by hand. They save money and energy when substituted for larger equipment.

While you can find a device for almost any kitchen task, accumulating appliances can create clutter. Before buying, think about whether the appliance will be helpful enough to justify the cost and space required or just gather dust in the back of a cabinet. These are some basic small appliances (see **Fig. 22-13**):

- **Blender.** Chops, blends, and liquefies foods. Various speeds are used for different food preparation tasks.
- **Food processor.** Performs tasks similar to a blender but is more powerful and versatile. Assorted blades and discs do specialized jobs, such as extracting juice from fruit.
- **Electric mixer.** Blends, beats, and whips ingredients. Hand-held models are convenient for small jobs. Stand mixers are heavy-duty models that can handle kneading bread and pasta doughs.
- **Toaster.** Browns bread and pastries on both sides at the same time. Two- and four-slice models are available.
- **Toaster oven.** Mostly heats or bakes small amounts of food. Some can broil.
- **Electric skillet.** Fries, roasts, steams, and bakes. The skillet has a thermostatic temperature control.
- **Slow cooker.** Cooks food slowly for hours. The deep pot has a heating element in the base and conveniently cooks one-dish meals.
- **Broiler/grill.** Grills food indoors and is portable and electric.
- **Rice cooker/steamer.** Cooks large amounts of rice and steams vegetables.

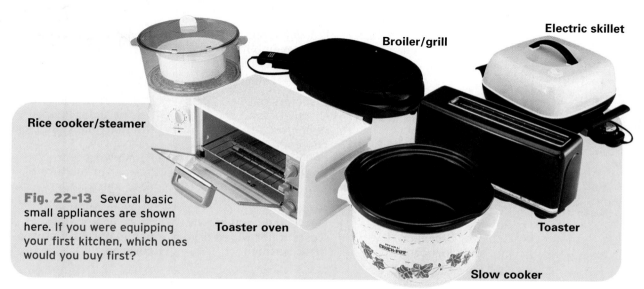

Fig. 22-13 Several basic small appliances are shown here. If you were equipping your first kitchen, which ones would you buy first?

Rice cooker/steamer

Broiler/grill

Electric skillet

Toaster oven

Toaster

Slow cooker

COOKWARE AND BAKEWARE

Cookware is equipment for cooking food on top of the range. **Bakeware** is equipment for cooking food in an oven. Both are available in a variety of materials, which are sometimes combined. Each material has advantages, disadvantages, and recommendations for use and care, as shown in **Fig. 22-14**.

Fig. 22-14

Cookware and Bakeware Materials			
Material	**Advantages**	**Disadvantages**	**Use and Care**
Aluminum	• Conducts heat quickly and evenly if heavy. • Lightweight and durable. • Comes in a variety of finishes. • Comparatively inexpensive. • May be clad (covered) with stainless steel for benefits of both.	• Warps, dents, and scratches easily. • Darkens and stains, especially in dishwasher. • Pits if salty or acid foods used.	• Wash by hand, not in dishwasher. • Cool before washing to prevent warping. • Avoid sharp tools like knives and beaters. • Do not use to store salty or acid foods.
Anodized aluminum (coated with a hard protective finish)	• Maintains even, consistent cooking temperature. • Durable. • Will never peel, chip, or crack. • Resists sticking and scratching.	• Heavy. • Can be expensive. • Less reactive to salty or acid foods than non-anodized aluminum.	• Wash by hand, not in dishwasher. • Use nonabrasive cleaners and nylon scrubbers. • Anodizing makes aluminum easier to clean.
Stainless steel	• Durable, tough, hard. • Lightweight. • Will not dent easily. • Can withstand use of metal utensils. • Attractive; keeps bright shine. • Moderately priced.	• Conducts heat unevenly; thick aluminum or copper core bottom helps. • Stains when overheated or from starchy foods. • Can develop hot spots. • Pits if salty or acid foods used.	• Use nonabrasive cleaners and nylon scrubbers. • Use stainless steel cleaner to remove stains. • Do not use to store salty or acid foods.
Copper	• Excellent heat conductor. • Heats quickly and evenly and cools quickly. • Attractive.	• Discolors easily. • Discolors food and may create toxic compounds, so must be lined with tin, silver, or stainless steel. • Expensive.	• Dry after washing. • Do not scour inside—the thin lining can be worn away. • Polish with copper cleaner or mixture of flour and vinegar.
Cast iron	• Distributes heat evenly. • Retains heat well. • Good for browning, frying, and slow cooking.	• Heavy. • Heats and cools slowly. • Rusts if not wiped dry after washing.	• Store in dry place. • Store lid separately—pan may rust if stored covered.

Whether bought as sets or individual pieces, cookware and bakeware are major investments that many cooks keep for years. The materials and finishes in high-quality items are durable enough to withstand daily use. Metals are heavy to resist warping. Handles are heat-resistant. Construction is seamless and balanced, with smooth edges, flat bottoms, and secure lids.

Fig. 22-14 (continued)

Cookware and Bakeware Materials

Material	Advantages	Disadvantages	Use and Care
Glass	• Attractive. • Can be used for cooking and serving. • Easy to clean.	• Breaks easily, especially if exposed to extreme temperature changes. • Some can be used only on the cooktop, others only in the oven. • Holds heat, but does not conduct heat well.	• May need a wire grid if used on an electric cooktop. • Use nonabrasive cleaners and nylon scrubbers. • Do not plunge hot pan into cold water or put into the refrigerator.
Glass-ceramic	• Goes from freezer to oven or cooktop. • Durable, attractive, heat-resistant. • Used for roasting, broiling, and baking in conventional or microwave ovens.	• May break if dropped. • May heat unevenly. • Holds heat well—reduce oven temperatures by 25°F for baked goods. • May develop hot spots.	• Use nonabrasive cleaners and nylon scrubbers. • Dishwasher-safe. • Use manufacturer's care instructions.
Stoneware	• Attractive. • Can be used for cooking and serving. • Retains heat.	• Breaks easily.	• Dishwasher-safe. • Use nonabrasive cleaners and nylon scrubbers.
Enamel (glass fused to a base metal)	• Attractive. • Can be used to cook and serve.	• Chips easily.	• Dishwasher-safe. • Use nonabrasive cleaners and nylon scrubbers.
Microwave-safe plastic	• Durable. • Stain-resistant. • Easy to clean.	• Some cannot be used in conventional ovens. • Can be scratched by sharp kitchen tools.	• Dishwasher-safe. • Use nonabrasive cleaners and nylon scrubbers.
Nonstick finishes (many types used inside and outside varied items)	• Keeps food from sticking—fat may not be necessary for browning, sautéing, or frying. • Easy to clean.	• Easily scratched by metal kitchen tools or abrasive cleaners. • High heat may stain finish or warp pan.	• Follow manufacturer's directions. Some cannot be washed in dishwasher. • Use nonmetal tools to prevent scratching.

Cookware

Most people use the words pots and pans interchangeably, but there's a difference. These and other cookware items are described here and shown in **Fig. 22-15**:

- **Saucepans.** Have one long handle and sometimes a small handle on the opposite side. Many come with a lid. Saucepans are usually made of metal or heatproof glass. Sizes range from ½ quart to 4 quarts.
- **Pots.** Larger and heavier than saucepans. Pots range in size from 3 to 20 quarts and have two small handles, one on each side, for easier lifting. Most come with lids.
- **Skillets.** Used for browning and frying foods. Skillets are also called frying pans. They vary in size and often have matching lids. A griddle is a skillet without sides.
- **Double boiler.** Consists of a small saucepan that fits into a larger one, plus a lid. Simmering water in the bottom pan gently heats food in the pan above. Used for foods that scorch easily (chocolate, sauces, cereals).

- **Dutch oven.** Heavy pot with a close-fitting lid. Dutch ovens are suitable for range or oven. Some have a rack to keep meat and poultry from sticking to the bottom.
- **Steamer.** Covered saucepan with an insert that holds food over a small amount of boiling water. Holes in the insert allow steam to pass through and cook the food. Metal and bamboo steamers are available, as are steamer inserts that fit in a covered saucepan.
- **Pressure cooker.** Heavy pot with a locked-on lid and steam gauge. Steam builds inside the pot, creating very high temperatures that cook food quickly.

Bakeware

Bakeware consists of baking pans of various shapes, sizes, and materials. Each of these qualities affects the texture and appearance of the finished product. Baking times and temperatures in recipes may have to be adjusted to the pan you use. Basic bakeware includes the following (see **Fig. 22-16**):

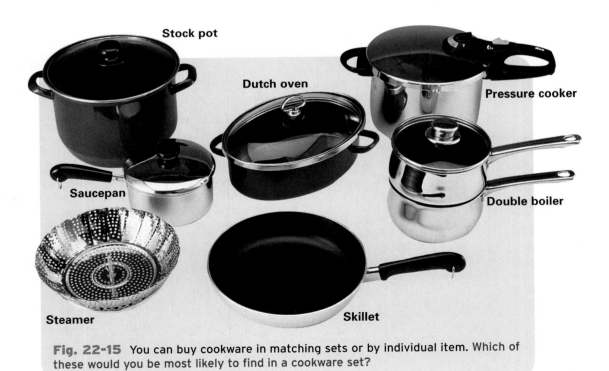

Fig. 22-15 You can buy cookware in matching sets or by individual item. Which of these would you be most likely to find in a cookware set?

Clay-pot cooking. The clay pot, an early-model slow cooker, is standard equipment in many cuisines. Clay roasters and casseroles come in assorted shapes and sizes and are made of unglazed terra cotta, which absorbs moisture through its pores and releases it when heated. With a tight-fitting lid, the pot becomes a steam chamber that adds moisture to meat and grain dishes and blends flavors in casseroles.

Creating this effect takes time and effort. The pot must be soaked in warm water before use. Cooking begins in a cold oven to prevent cracking the unglazed clay. The pores absorb oils and strong flavors such as garlic, transferring them between recipes. Some experts recommend separate pots for fish, pasta sauce, and other potent dishes. The pots also absorb soap and must be cleaned by scrubbing with very hot water and baking soda.

- **Loaf pan.** Deep, narrow, rectangular pan for baking loaves of bread or meat.
- **Cookie sheet.** Flat, rectangular pan with two or three open sides. Used for cookies and biscuits.
- **Baking sheet.** Similar to a cookie sheet, but four sides are about 1 inch deep. Used for sheet cakes, pizza, chicken pieces, and fish.
- **Cake pans.** Usually round or square, from 8 to 10 inches in diameter. Novelty shapes range from horseshoe to cartoon characters.
- **Tube pan.** Deep, one- or two-piece cake pan with a center tube. Used for angel food and sponge cakes.
- **Springform pan.** Round pan with a removable bottom. The side is latched but opens to remove cheesecake or other dessert.
- **Pie pans.** Shallow, round pans with slanted sides. Tart pans are similar in shape but smaller.
- **Muffin pans.** Also called tins. Different sizes hold 6 to 12 muffins, rolls, or cupcakes at a time.
- **Roasting pans.** Large, heavy, oval or rectangular pans. Used for roasting meats and whole poultry.

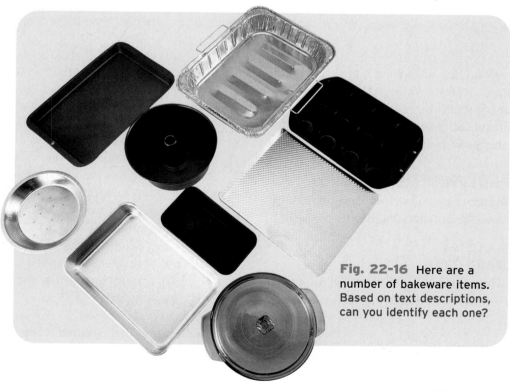

Fig. 22-16 Here are a number of bakeware items. Based on text descriptions, can you identify each one?

NONSTICK FINISHES

Have you ever wondered how a nonstick coating sticks to a pan since nothing sticks to the coating? This complex process uses both mechanics and chemistry, but it's something like painting a wall.

To prepare a wall for painting, you apply an undercoat of primer. Besides hiding the old color, primer gives a slightly rough texture so the new paint sticks better. Likewise, aluminum cookware is first coated with a film that contains microscopic grains of ceramic and sometimes titanium, a sturdy element that resists heat and corrosion. This mixture is liquefied at very high temperatures and then sprayed with incredible force. The heat and the impact create pits in the softer aluminum, with tiny ceramic bumps. An adhesive layer is applied next, which also helps hold the top, nonstick surface coat. The whole thing is baked at 800 degrees for about five minutes, melding the layers.

Though common, nonstick finish is impressive technology. This material is the most slippery substance known, certainly the ideal surface for "food release." The thin coat on cookware and

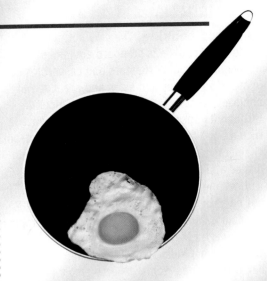

bakeware is prone to scratching by metal utensils, yet in other applications, this substance is rugged enough to insulate space suits and the Statue of Liberty.

__Think Beyond>> The popular nonstick material Teflon® was discovered by accident. What qualities in the scientists might have helped them make this discovery? How were they similar to cooks developing a new recipe?

- **Casseroles.** Used for baking and serving main dishes and desserts. Various sizes are available, with or without lids.
- **Aluminum foil pans.** Lightweight, disposable, recyclable pans. Helpful for single-use needs.

FOOD PREPARATION TOOLS

Like other crafts, food preparation requires simple but efficient handheld tools for specific tasks.

Measuring Tools

Following certain recipes would be impossible without some of the following measuring tools (see **Fig. 22-17**):

- **Dry measuring cups.** Come in a set of several sizes, usually $\frac{1}{4}$ cup, $\frac{1}{3}$ cup, $\frac{1}{2}$ cup, and 1 cup. A

metric set includes 50-mL, 125-mL, and 250-mL measures.
- **Liquid measuring cups.** Transparent cups with measurements marked on the side. They are typically marked in fluid ounces as well as fractions of a cup and milliliters. A headspace of about $\frac{1}{4}$ inch helps prevent spills when moving a filled cup. A spout helps with pouring. Common sizes are 1 and 2 cups.
- **Measuring spoons.** Generally come in sets of four or five. Standard sets include four sizes: $\frac{1}{4}$ teaspoon, $\frac{1}{2}$ teaspoon, 1 teaspoon, and 1 tablespoon. Metric sets include five measures: 1 mL, 2 mL, 5 mL, 15 mL, and 25 mL.
- **Kitchen scales.** Used to measure food by weight rather than volume. They can be spring or digital.

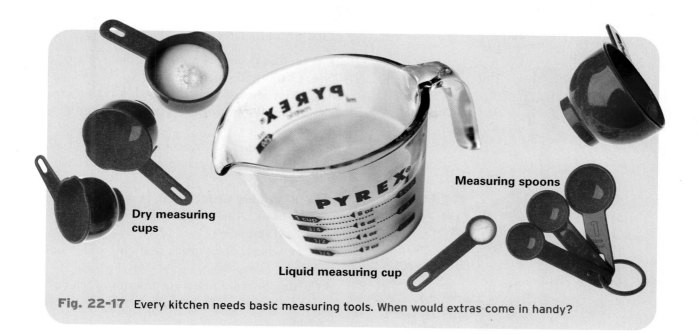

Dry measuring cups

Liquid measuring cup

Measuring spoons

Fig. 22-17 Every kitchen needs basic measuring tools. When would extras come in handy?

Cutting Tools

Many cutting tasks require a knife. Quality knives have a sturdy handle firmly attached to the blade by at least two and sometimes three rivets, or bolts with heads. As shown in **Fig. 22-18**, basic knives and their uses are as follows:

- **Bread knife.** Has a serrated or saw-tooth blade for slicing breads.
- **Slicing knife.** Large knife used for such foods as meat and poultry.

- **Chef's knife.** Also called a French knife. Its large, triangular blade is ideal for slicing, chopping, and dicing.
- **Utility knife.** Similar to a slicing knife but smaller. It cuts small foods, such as tomatoes and apples.
- **Boning knife.** Has a thin, angled blade, well suited for removing bones.
- **Paring knife.** Removes a thin layer or peel from fruits and vegetables.

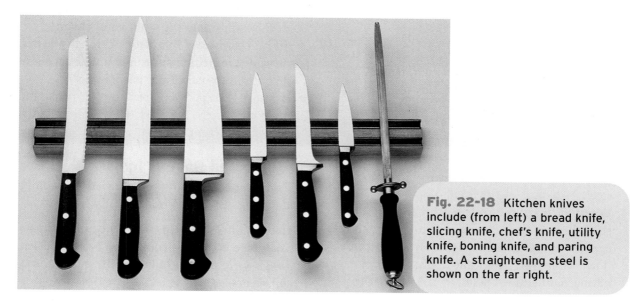

Fig. 22-18 Kitchen knives include (from left) a bread knife, slicing knife, chef's knife, utility knife, boning knife, and paring knife. A straightening steel is shown on the far right.

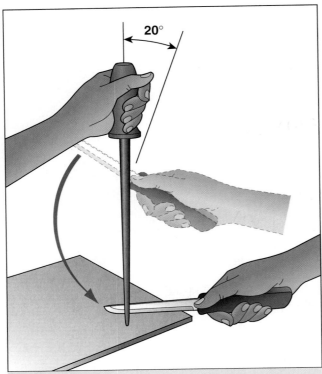

Fig. 22-19 Use gentle pressure when straightening a knife blade, as described below.

Knife blades are sharpened periodically with a sharpening appliance or a special stone, called a whetstone. In between sharpenings, blades can be straightened with a steel, a long rod with a handle. See **Fig. 22-19**. Use the steel regularly, following these directions (reverse if you are left-handed):

1. Hold the handle of the steel in your left hand. Place the point straight down, very firmly, on a secure cutting board. In your right hand, hold the knife by the handle, blade down.
2. Hold the knife blade at a 20-degree angle against the right side of the steel. The knife blade and steel should touch near the handles.
3. Gently draw the blade down the steel and toward you, keeping a 20-degree angle to the steel.
4. When the tip of the knife reaches the tip of the steel, repeat the process, holding the knife against the steel on the left. Draw the blade down along the steel four or five times, alternating right and left sides.

Other tools fill more cutting needs. Have you used any of these?

- **Vegetable peeler.** Has a swivel blade. Used to pare fruits and vegetables.
- **Kitchen shears.** Scissors used for snipping, trimming, or cutting dried fruit, fresh herbs, or pastry.
- **Food chopper.** Ranges in size from small, handheld nut chopper to a large model with several blades.
- **Food grinder.** Grinds meat, poultry, nuts, and other foods. Also used for finely cutting, grating, and shredding.
- **Pizza wheel.** Slices pizza and cuts rolled-out dough.
- **Cutting board.** Protects countertop when cutting. Plastic resists bacteria better than soft woods.

Mixing Tools

Unlike many items, basic mixing tool designs haven't changed much from your grandparents' day. Besides multisized mixing spoons and bowls, a number of specialized inventions are still useful. See **Fig. 22-20**.

- **Wire whisk.** Usually a balloon-shaped instrument made of wire loops that are held together by a handle. Used for stirring, beating, and whipping.
- **Rotary beater.** Mixes and whips food more quickly and easily than a spoon or whisk. Very good for whipping egg whites and cream.
- **Sifter.** A canister with a blade or ring inside that forces dry ingredients through a wire screen at the bottom to make finer particles.
- **Scrapers.** Scrape food from bowls, pans, and other containers. Also used for light mixing. Come in different sizes.

Cooking and Baking Tools

Some tools are useful for a variety of cooking and baking tasks. See **Fig. 22-21**.

- **Turner.** Lifts and turns flat foods, such as pancakes on a griddle or cookies on a cookie sheet.
- **Tongs.** Grip and lift bulky foods, such as broccoli spears.

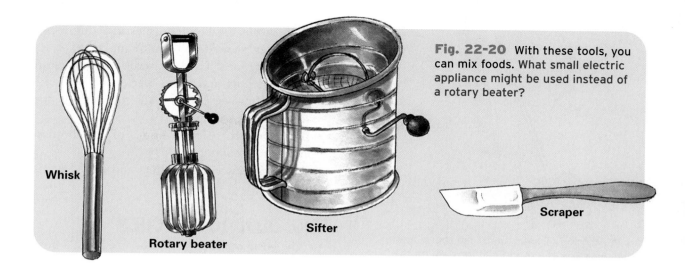

Fig. 22-20 With these tools, you can mix foods. What small electric appliance might be used instead of a rotary beater?

Whisk

Rotary beater

Sifter

Scraper

- **Baster.** Long tube with a bulb on the end. Suctions up meat juices or syrups for basting.
- **Ladle.** Small bowl on a long handle for dipping hot liquids from a pan.
- **Pastry brush.** For brushing a sauce on hot foods or a glaze on pastry.
- **Rolling pin.** For rolling out dough for biscuits, cookies, and pies.
- **Wire cooling rack.** Holds baked products until cool or hot pans removed from the oven.
- **Potholders and oven mitts.** Thick cloth pads that are used to protect hands while handling hot containers.

Food Thermometers

In cooking, safety and success sometimes depend on knowing a food's exact temperature. Some thermometers measure internal temperature, the surest sign that meats, poultry, egg dishes, and leftovers are safely cooked or heated.

- **Oven-safe.** Large dial or other indicator on a probe stuck into roasts or whole poultry and left in during cooking. Cannot be used with small pieces of food. Thermometers specifically for microwave ovens are available.

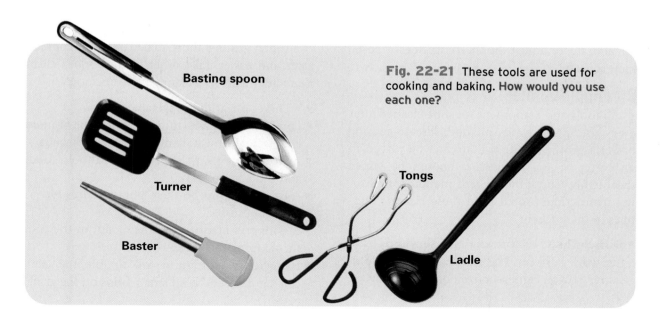

Fig. 22-21 These tools are used for cooking and baking. How would you use each one?

Basting spoon

Turner

Baster

Tongs

Ladle

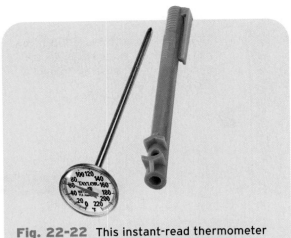

Fig. 22-22 This instant-read thermometer has a case and a round dial for reading the temperature.

- **Instant-read.** Probe with a dial or digital display used to check internal temperatures instantly. See **Fig. 22-22**.
- **Disposable indicator.** Sensor that changes color when food reaches the proper internal temperature. It is used one time only.
- **Pop-up.** Sensor sometimes inserted in turkey or roasting chickens by food processors. It pops up when food reaches the proper internal temperature.

Other thermometers are needed for particular cooking methods. A candy thermometer clips to the side of a pan to measure the temperature of syrup as it cooks. A frying thermometer records the temperature of oil in a deep-fat fryer. All thermometers should be easy to read. A mechanism to calibrate, or adjust the thermometer for accuracy, is useful.

Cleanup Supplies

All tools and equipment must be cleaned after every use. Even in bits of food, disease-causing bacteria grow. Any item that can't be placed in dishwater or the dishwasher should be wiped thoroughly. Check the owner's manual for cleaning instructions. You'll need these cleanup supplies in the kitchen:

- **Dishcloths.** Used for washing dishes and cleaning work surfaces. Have at least a dozen plus spares, so you can use a fresh one every day.
- **Dishtowels.** Used to dry dishes and equipment. Have plenty and keep them clean.
- **Scouring pads.** Used to scrub hard-to-clean spots on pots and pans. Steel wool pads are highly abrasive. Nylon pads are needed for some metals and finishes.
- **Bottle brush.** Cleans insides of jars, bottles, and similar containers.
- **Dish drainer.** Holds washed and rinsed items to air-dry.

THE OUTDOOR KITCHEN

The basic outdoor grill has a fire bowl, a box- or bowl-shaped metal container that holds the burning charcoal. A metal grate fits over the fire bowl to hold food over hot coals. This design has many variations, from a portable hibachi to a 6-foot stretch grill. Kettle grills stand on long metal legs. Other models are set into a cart-like base with a work table attached. Some have domed lids to help maintain even temperatures.

Gas grills use propane gas, supplied in a heavy tank that attaches to the base. Gas grills are more expensive than charcoal grills with similar features. A smoker is a covered grill that burns aromatic wood chips, flavoring food as it cooks.

The combination of high heat and outdoor elements makes stability and durability important qualities in grills. Legs should be level and the fire bowl balanced evenly on them. All parts should be securely attached. Heavy, stainless steel construction withstands rust, wear, and tear.

Proper grilling tools make outdoor cooking safer and easier. Like other kitchen tools, clean them after each use. Handy items include:

- A basket for grilling vegetables.
- Long metal skewers, thin rods with one pointed end, to make meat, fruit, or vegetable kebabs.
- A work table near the grill to hold tools, food, and other supplies.
- A baster or spray bottle to put out flare-ups.
- Fireproof mitts.
- A wire grill brush, which has a slot in the end, for scraping the grate.
- Heavy-duty aluminum foil to line the grill, catch grease, and hold small foods on the grate.

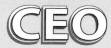

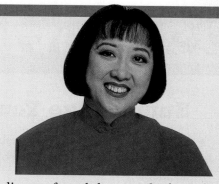

HELEN CHEN: As a chef of Chinese descent, Helen Chen makes use of traditions that span 3,000 years. As an entrepreneur, her goal is to keep those traditions alive in today's kitchen.

Cooking is part of Helen's family heritage, as well as her culture. Her parents ran two successful restaurants in Cambridge, Massachusetts, after emigrating from China in 1949. Helen grew up in the business, packing takeouts, washing dishes, and waiting tables. Her mother Joyce, a culinary innovator and recognized authority on the foods of her native Northern China, also wrote cookbooks and had a television show.

Joyce Chen taught her daughter the finer points of Asian cooking, and more. Helen recalls: "She was always thinking about how to do things better. She never took no for an answer, and this stubbornness and belief in herself made her a pioneer in her field. It was this delight in her work and her boundless creative energy that influenced me most."

East Meets West. One thing that could be better, Joyce Chen decided, was the Chinese cookware available to American cooks, herself included. The quest for quality cooking tools led to buying trips to the Far East, and in the 1960s, to the founding of Joyce Chen Products, Asian houseware suppliers with the motto "Eastern cookware for the Western kitchen."

As in the restaurants, Helen was a "Jill-of-all-trades" in her mother's business: bookkeeper, office manager, assistant buyer, and product developer. Helen learned from other experts as well, which proved invaluable to her growing responsibilities. "Surround yourself with smart people," she advises. "Don't be afraid of constructive criticism, but learn from it."

In the early 1980s, when Helen was the national sales manager and spokesperson for Joyce Chen Products, Alzheimer's disease forced her mother's early retirement. Helen took over as president and CEO (chief operating officer). She expanded the company's catalog, offering more elements of authentic Asian cuisine—from original-design teapots honoring each animal of the Chinese zodiac to a line of stir-fry marinades, oils, and sauces. Maintaining its reputation for excellence, she helped the company grow into the largest supplier of Asian cookware in the United States.

New Directions. In 2003 Helen and her husband sold the company, freeing her to focus on other projects. She consults on marketing and design for other cookware makers, teaches cooking classes at schools from California to Connecticut, and tests recipes for her latest cookbook. She gives cooking tours of Boston's Chinatown neighborhood.

The schedule is demanding, but Helen is energized by the diversity that each day brings. She tackles the roles with the qualities that have marked her career and her life: "passion and dedication, and good old, roll-up-your-sleeves hard work."

On-line Connections

1. To learn more about topics in this article, search the Internet for these key words: Northern Chinese cuisine; Asian cookware; cooking tours.

2. To learn about related careers, search the Internet for these key words: restaurant owner; cooking instructor.

Summarize Your Reading

▶ The work centers in a kitchen should be organized efficiently to avoid confusion and accidents.

▶ Because people often share kitchen tasks, additional work space and duplicate work centers are useful.

▶ Kitchen components include cabinets for storage, countertops for work space, floors, walls, a grounded electrical system, and good lighting.

▶ When making kitchen purchases, you'll make better decisions if you understand seals, labels, warranties, and financial terms.

▶ Equipping a kitchen means choosing from major appliances, small appliances, tools, and various equipment. Comparing models and functions helps you choose effectively.

▶ Proper care of appliances, tools, and equipment promotes food safety.

Check Your Knowledge

1. What does each of the basic **work centers** in a kitchen contain?

2. What are signs of an effective **work triangle**?

3. Describe four common kitchen plans.

4. What is the advantage of **universal design**?

5. What qualities do kitchen components need?

6. What strategies are recommended when storing items in cabinets?

7. Why should electrical outlets be **grounded**?

8. Why is **task lighting** useful in the kitchen?

9. List three helpful actions to take before buying an item.

10. What is the Underwriters Laboratories (UL) seal?

11. What does an **EnergyGuide label** provide?

12. Why is the **warranty** on an appliance useful?

13. Describe the **credit** process, using five vocabulary terms from the chapter.

14. Compare **convection** and conventional ovens.

15. Which small appliance would you use for the following: a) making a fruit smoothie; b) toasting a large bagel; c) cooking beef for sandwiches to eat right after work; d) mixing cake batter; e) cooking broccoli?

16. What's the difference between **cookware** and **bakeware**?

17. What cookware or bakeware would you use for the following: a) frying chicken; b) baking a meatloaf; c) making a cheesecake; d) cooking beans very quickly?

18. **CRITICAL THINKING** Why do you think separate tools are needed to measure liquid and dry ingredients?

19. What tool or equipment would you use for the following: a) chopping vegetables for a stir-fry; b) snipping fresh herbs; c) whipping egg whites; d) serving soup; e) checking the temperature of thin meat; f) cleaning spots on a pan?

20. Why should tools and equipment used in the kitchen and for grilling be cleaned after every use?

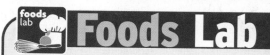

Apply Your Learning

1. **Kitchen Floor Plans.** Make a photo display of kitchen floor plans from magazines. Label work centers, indicate work triangles, and evaluate for convenience.

2. **MATH** **Financial Arrangements.** Research the financial arrangements for purchasing a major appliance. Compare with paying cash.

3. **Appliance Comparison.** Comparison shop for one of these appliances: refrigerator-freezer, gas or electric range, convection or microwave oven, or dishwasher. What would you recommend buying and why?

4. **Equipping a Kitchen.** Assume you're equipping your first kitchen (in a small apartment). What items from the chapter do you need? What do you need now, soon, and in the future?

5. **Use-and-Care Demonstration.** Demonstrate how to use and clean the following safely: a small appliance; cookware item; knife, including how to sharpen; mixing, cooking, or baking tool.

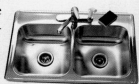

Foods Lab

Work Centers in the Foods Lab

Procedure: Prepare a simple recipe that requires the use of all three basic work centers. Pay special attention to how well the lab layout and design of each station accommodate more than one person at a time.

Analyzing Results

❶ Is the lab convenient for one person to use? For more than one person? Why or why not?

❷ Are items arranged conveniently in each work center? What would you improve?

❸ Are the lab, cookware, and supplies accessible to people of varying abilities? In what ways? How might any problems be corrected?

Food Science Experiment

Heating Properties of Metals

Objective: To compare how well various metals transfer heat.

Procedure:

1. Lightly grease and flour the bottom of a skillet. Tap out any excess flour.

2. Using medium heat, preheat the largest heating unit on the cooktop for two minutes. Place the skillet on the unit. Record the time needed for the flour coating to turn golden brown. Also note any unevenly browned spots.

3. Repeat Steps 1 and 2 to test skillets of different metals. Use the same heating unit for

each test. Compare your findings with those of other lab teams.

Analyzing Results

❶ Which skillet heated most quickly? Least quickly?

❷ Which skillet heated most and least evenly? Were these also the two you named in answering question 1?

❸ What might have caused any differences in team results?

❹ Which skillet do you think is more likely to retain heat longer: the one that heated most quickly or most evenly? Explain.

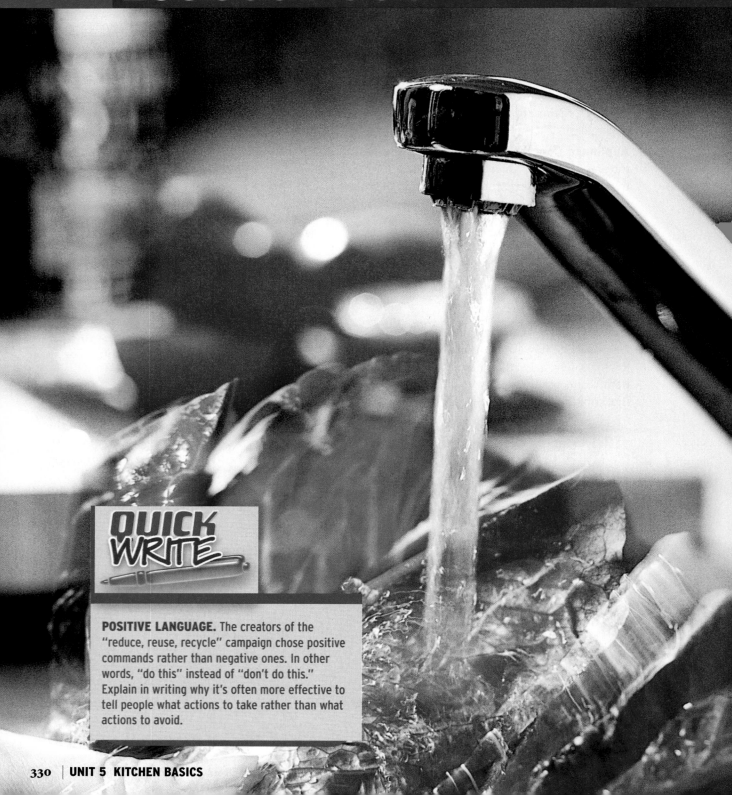

Conserving Resources

QUICK WRITE

POSITIVE LANGUAGE. The creators of the "reduce, reuse, recycle" campaign chose positive commands rather than negative ones. In other words, "do this" instead of "don't do this." Explain in writing why it's often more effective to tell people what actions to take rather than what actions to avoid.

To Guide Your Reading:

Objectives

▶ Explain conservation and its importance.
▶ Describe efficient ways to use kitchen appliances.
▶ Explain water-saving techniques in the kitchen.
▶ Summarize ways to reduce trash, reuse items, and recycle materials.

Terms

biodegradable
conservation
food waste
nonrenewable resources
recycle
renewable resources
sanitary landfill

THE STORY IS TOLD OF A MAN WHO FOUND A young child on the beach throwing starfish that had been stranded by the tide back into the ocean.

"But there are hundreds," the man said. "You can save just a few. Do you really think it makes a difference?"

The child held up one starfish and replied, "It makes a difference to this starfish," and flung it into the surf.

That child illustrates the spirit of **conservation**—concern for the environment and its future, shown by managing its resources wisely. What's more, the child understood that one person's actions can make a difference—for better and for worse.

WHY CONSERVE?

Where does the electricity that runs your appliances come from? Chances are it's generated by burning coal, natural gas, or oil—fossil fuels formed in the earth by plant and animal remains. These **nonrenewable resources** are continually produced in nature, but at a rate too slow to keep up with demand. The gas that heats an oven today—and then is gone—was millions of years in the making. With use of these fuels almost doubling every 20 years, supplies are rapidly dwindling. What's more, burning fossil fuels releases pollutants into the environment. Using these resources sensibly benefits present as well as future generations.

Conservation is equally important for renewable resources, including water, timber, and solar energy. See **Fig. 23-1** on page 332. **Renewable resources** replace themselves rather quickly, sometimes immediately, yet they also need careful management. For example, in 2002 beaches across the United States were closed thousands of times due to pollution. Only a drought in some states kept the problem from being worse. The rains that often cause sewage systems to overflow and contaminate rivers and lakes never fell. Unfortunately, the same drought contributed to the worst wildfires in the western part of the United States in 50 years.

Finally, consider one more resource. The average U.S. family spends over $1,400 a year on energy bills. Conserving natural resources conserves a family's financial resources. The kitchen, with its energy-hungry appliances, is a good place to start.

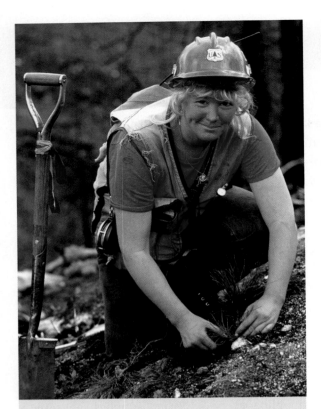

Fig. 23-1 Caring for timberland and managing the use of trees help ensure that this resource will be available in the future. As trees are used, they need to be replaced.

USING ENERGY EFFICIENTLY

The next time you open the refrigerator, try this test. Hold a dollar bill against the frame and close the door on it. If the door doesn't hold the dollar securely, it isn't holding cold air inside the refrigerator or keeping warm air out. The refrigerator has to work harder to chill the incoming air. Repairing or replacing the rubber gasket around the door might improve efficiency by creating a tighter seal. Another simple energy-saving step is to vacuum the condenser coils at least twice a year. Removing dust helps the condenser release heat removed from the interior.

If a little warm air uses a little extra energy, imagine the effect when the door is wide open. To avoid this waste, decide what you want from the refrigerator before opening the door. Keep the refrigerator and freezer well organized so you can find food quickly.

The same thing happens in reverse to the oven. Each time you open the door, heat escapes, the oven temperature drops, and more energy is needed to raise it again. Use the oven light to check on foods, at least during the early stages of cooking.

Also, try to plan meals to cook several foods at the same time. Use glass cookware if possible. Glass absorbs heat better than metal, so oven temperatures in recipes can be lowered by 25°F. Except for baked goods, most recipes do not need a preheated oven. They may not need an oven at all if they can be made in an electric skillet, slow cooker, or microwave oven. Microwave ovens use about half the energy of conventional ovens.

When you use a cooktop, you can save energy with a few simple habits. Liquid in a covered pot boils more quickly than in an uncovered one, so put on the cover. The cover holds the heat inside, allowing the temperature to rise faster. Lower the heat after liquids come to a boil, using just enough to keep them bubbling. On an electric cooktop, match the pan to the same-size heating element. You can turn off the element a few minutes before the food is done. Enough heat will remain in the coils to finish the job.

When it's time to replace an appliance, compare EnergyGuide labels to find the most efficient model. Also look for the ENERGY STAR® label shown in **Fig. 23-2**. This mark, found on refrigerators, dishwashers, and lighting fixtures, indicates that the item exceeds the federal government's minimum standard for energy efficiency. When choosing a refrigerator-freezer, consider that models with a top-mount freezer use the least energy.

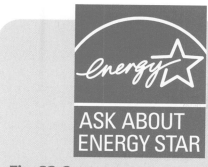

Fig. 23-2 When buying a refrigerator, dishwasher, or lighting fixture, look for this label. What does it mean?

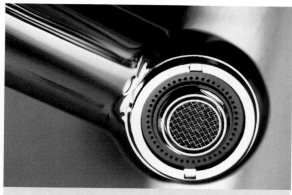

Fig. 23-3 A low-flow aerator can help decrease water use. How does it work?

Lighting too holds energy-saving possibilities. For some jobs, task lighting is more efficient than general lighting. You can cut up to 75 percent from energy bills by replacing incandescent bulbs with compact fluorescent bulbs, which also last much longer. To avoid using electricity, when possible, take advantage of sunlight.

USING WATER WISELY

Does your kitchen faucet drip? Water dripping at the rate of one drop per second can waste about 700 gallons a year. Fixing that faucet could save enough water to cook 5,600 servings of spaghetti or make 11,200 glasses of lemonade. You could save about 3 gallons more each day by installing a low-flow aerator if a faucet doesn't have one. This simple attachment mixes air with water to maintain water pressure but reduce water flow. See **Fig. 23-3**.

Other conservation measures help when preparing and serving meals. Wash vegetables under just enough running water to get them clean. Choose cooking methods that use less water—for example, steaming or microwaving instead of boiling. Ask whether people want water to drink with their meal before pouring.

Kitchen cleanup does take a lot of water, but maybe less than some people use. Hand washing dishes doesn't take constantly running water. Wash all the dishes first. Then rinse them all as quickly as possible. If you use a dishwasher, scrape dishes instead of rinsing them before loading. This removes more food and saves water.

Run the appliance with full loads only. Turn it off after the final rinse to let dishes air-dry.

Don't dump hazardous household chemicals into the water system. Call your local sanitation department to learn how to dispose of them safely.

TAKING OUT THE TRASH

The Environmental Protection Agency (EPA) estimates that the United States produces about 4.5 pounds of trash per person each day. Where does it all go?

Some trash is burned, which reduces the volume but adds to air pollution. Much of it ends up in dumps, where it attracts pests, breeds harmful bacteria, and pollutes the land and water. About half of the trash is buried in sanitary landfills. A **sanitary landfill** is an area insulated with clay and plastic liner, where trash is thinly spread, compacted, and covered with a layer of soil. The process is repeated until the area is full.

Landfills avoid the drawbacks of other options, but they are not a long-term solution. Despite the many precautions taken, landfills can leak or overflow and pollute soil and water. Once full, in fact, they are monitored for 30 years for leakage or release of harmful gas.

A more common problem, however, is how quickly they fill up. Some materials are **biodegradable**, meaning they break down, but others are not. While nature is very efficient at

What's in the Trash?

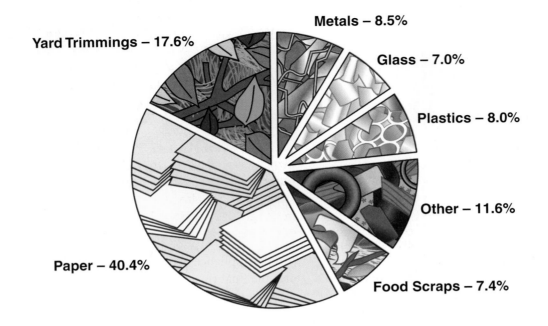

Metals – 8.5%

Glass – 7.0%

Plastics – 8.0%

Other – 11.6%

Food Scraps – 7.4%

Paper – 40.4%

Yard Trimmings – 17.6%

Source: U.S. Environmental Protection Agency

Fig. 23-4 According to the EPA, Americans generate different kinds of trash and in different amounts. Are you surprised by these percentages? How do you think your trash disposal compares to these figures?

recycling its own products—a banana peel will degrade in about six weeks—several conditions greatly slow this process in a landfill.

First, manufactured items take longer to decay—up to 30 years for a petroleum-based plastic bag and up to 60 years for some paper. A disposable diaper may still be there 500 years from now, and a glass jar can last a million years. Some plastics and synthetic textiles, in theory, last forever. Also, covering and compacting trash interferes with degrading elements that would speed decay, especially bacteria.

Fig. 23-4 shows the types of trash Americans generate. Scientists are exploring more sustainable ways to manage the trash output. Meanwhile, you can do your part with a threefold plan of action: reduce, reuse, recycle.

Reduce

Did you know that the typical supermarket goes through the equivalent of two young trees each day in paper shopping bags? By carrying your groceries in your own canvas bags or used paper bags, you can save a sapling. Your neighborhood could save a small forest.

That's one example of precycling, or "source reduction." It's a way to reduce trash by making earth-friendly, "green" shopping choices. This not only helps the environment but can also save money.

Packaging is a leading source of trash in the grocery aisle and accounts for 10 cents of every dollar you spend on food. Avoid products wrapped in unneeded layers of paper or plastic. Fresh foods and bulk items, for instance, are almost package-free. Save juice boxes and other single-serving sizes for lunches, road trips, and similar situations.

In addition, limit your use of paper goods, which make up 40 percent of all trash generated. Use paper cups, plates, and napkins only if washing "real" tableware would take too much time and energy. Instead of paper towels, use a mop for spills on floors and a dishcloth for those on countertops.

Food Waste

Food waste is any edible food that is discarded, such as servings left uneaten on a plate. Food waste represents the loss not only of food, itself a valuable resource, but of all the resources used to produce it as well.

People in the United States, accustomed to abundance, waste large amounts of food. Perhaps as much as 20 percent of all edible food is thrown out, equaling about half a pound of garbage per person each day.

Good meal planning is one tool to reduce food waste. Know what you want to serve and shop accordingly. Store all foods properly, and make plans for leftovers while they're still usable. Cut dried-out bread into cubes for croutons or grate it for breadcrumbs. Use mashed potatoes to top meat pies, thicken soups, and make yeast rolls. Be creative. How many different ways can you combine hard-cooked eggs, cooked vegetables, and pasta in casseroles, salads, soups, stews, meat pies, stir-fries, and omelets?

Reuse

Reusing gives second life to inedible items in the kitchen. Clean plastic tubs from margarine, yogurt, and cottage cheese are useful for refrigerating leftovers, although not heavy enough for freezing. Glass jars and bottles with tight-fitting lids make good storage containers for rice, pasta, and dry beans. Wash the jars and lids carefully. Let open containers dry for at least 24 hours to remove odors.

TRENDS in TECHNOLOGY

"GREEN" PLASTICS

Someday every shopper may take home a bag of cornstarch—a bag made with cornstarch, that is—and other packages made from starch-based, "green" plastics.

Conventional, petroleum-based plastics are not biodegradable. They often wind up in landfills or waterways, posing a choking risk to wildlife. Increasingly, ocean-going plastics carry bacteria and other organisms to new environments, where they could upset a delicate ecological balance.

The new plastics are called bioplastics because they're made from living things. Corn is most popular, but potatoes and grains are being tried. Since they're starch-based, they dissolve when exposed to heat and water. They can be composted. In fact, one use so far is as ground sheeting around crops; they dissolve into the soil after harvest. Corn is a renewable, and more reliable, resource than oil.

These plastics are not ideal. While some require less energy to produce than oil-based plastics, production may be no cleaner. They cost packagers about three times as much as conventional plastics.

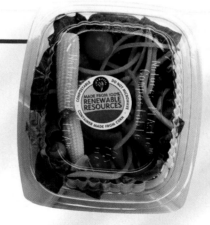

Since they dissolve in water, they also have limited use. You wouldn't package milk in a starch-based container.

Improved technology may solve the problems. Meanwhile "green" plastics are used selectively. One large manufacturer uses them for candy and cookie trays. Food vendors at the 2000 Olympics used only bioplastics and other biodegradable wrappers. Much of this waste was kept from landfills.

__**Think Beyond>>**__ Do you think food makers should be required to use bioplastics when possible? Why or why not?

Food containers can hold more than food. Egg cartons can store items ranging from jewelry to golf balls. Cereal boxes, with one corner and side cut diagonally, can organize manila folders. Cut lengthwise, they make trays for letters, greeting cards, or school papers. Convert smaller boxes into coupon organizers. Boxes of all sizes are good for wrapping gifts.

If you use grocery bags, give them a second career as trash bags or wastebasket liners. Paper bags can be used for lawn clippings, if kept dry.

Recycle

Some materials can be recycled. See **Fig. 23-5**. To **recycle** is to reprocess discarded products so they can be used again. Products are collected and sent to processing plants where the raw materials are recovered to make something new.

Recycling cuts down on trash and pollution. It conserves energy and other resources. For example, it takes 90 percent less energy to manufacture a product from recycled aluminum than from the raw material.

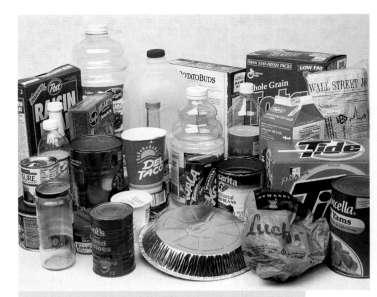

Fig. 23-5 Many materials can be recycled for additional use. How does your community support recycling?

Career Prep

Preparing a Resumé

LIKE A FULL-PAGE ADVERTISEMENT, your resumé must "hook" potential employers and invite a closer look. It must be clear and concise, fitting on one sheet of white, quality, bond paper. It must be error-free and typed in an easy-to-read font. Special software is helpful, but any word-processing program can give excellent results.

A resumé summarizes information about you. It starts with your name, address, and other contact information. You might briefly state your job objective, but the "meat" is your work history, educational background, and other experiences that show your strengths and qualifications, including awards and volunteer activities. Avoid giving personal information.

Employers in the United States cannot legally base hiring decisions on ethnicity, marital status, religion, or gender.

When sending your resumé, include a short cover letter to introduce yourself and explain why you're contacting the business—in response to a want ad, for example, or at the suggestion of your school counselor. Like the resumé, the letter should be professional but positive. Mention that you look forward to a response. Resumés can be prepared in several different formats.

● **Chronological.** Traditional resumés are organized chronologically, or by date. List work experiences first, starting with the most recent. For each entry, give the date of employment,

Learn which packaging materials are recyclable in your area and how they should be sorted or prepared. In most communities, public or private facilities accept newspapers, tin cans, aluminum cans and foil, glass bottles, and some plastics. Many supermarkets accept plastic shopping bags.

Some communities have curbside pickup for recycled materials. In others, residents bring items to collection centers. Some communities pick up items for recycling for free but charge for every container of trash. Families save money by recycling more and throwing out less.

When you shop, it's important to choose items made from recycled materials as well. Look for the word "post-consumer" on cardboard or plastic containers. This supports the recycling industry and lets manufacturers know that protecting the environment matters to you.

A WORLD PERSPECTIVE

A few years ago, the World Wildlife Fund, a conservation group, figured that the earth has the equivalent of about 28 billion acres worth of natural resources. With a global population of 6 billion, that comes to 4.7 resource-acres for each person.

The problem is that humans now use about 5.6 acres per person—and some use far more. Industrialized nations' high standard of living comes at a high cost in natural resources. Each European uses about 12.4 acres per person, and Americans average 23.7 acres, five times "their share." In comparison, Africans and Asians use less than 3.5 acres. That figure will rise, however, as developing countries industrialize and improve their standard of living. As the world's population grows, so too will the strain on the world's resources.

People around the world are practicing solutions and looking for new ones. Composting, home gardens, wetland restoration, and even refillable beverage containers are some. A compost pile, for example, holds decaying organic material that becomes fertilizer for gardens and shrubs. What role can you take in the effort?

position or job title, and employer's name. Then briefly describe your duties. Education and achievements go under separate headings. This arrangement lets you highlight promotions and career advances.

- **Functional.** Functional resumés may outline your work history but focus on skills, which you can organize to stress the most important ones. If you were applying for a nutrition writer's job, you could lead with previous communications experience.

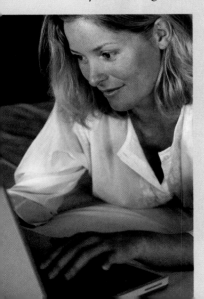

  - **Key word.** This format is designed for employers or resumé banks that scan resumés into databanks. It lets them store and search resumés by certain key words you've used.

Common key words include job titles, skills, and industry terms.

- **ASCII.** American Standard Code for Information Interchange (ASCII) is the "universal language" of text formatting. This is preferred for sending resumés by e-mail. When using ASCII, limit lines to 80 characters. Use the "enter" key or other hard return to start a new line. Indent and center text with spaces, rather than tabs or other command keys. Save the copy as plain text. To see how your resumé will look, send a copy to yourself and to someone who has a different e-mail program.

Career Connection

Comparing formats. Find models of two different resumé formats. Try writing your own resumé using each one. Which would you submit to an employer and why?

Summarize Your Reading

▶ Everyone can take part in the conservation effort.

▶ One way to conserve resources is to use appliances efficiently.

▶ Purchasing energy-efficient appliances with the ENERGY STAR label conserves energy and energy costs.

▶ Using less water when preparing foods also saves energy and energy costs.

▶ Sustainable ways to manage trash include reducing, reusing, and recycling.

▶ People who practice recycling save and put out recyclable materials for pick-up. They also choose items made from recycled materials when purchasing products.

Check Your Knowledge

1. What is **conservation**?

2. What are **nonrenewable resources**?

3. What problems are caused by using fossil fuels?

4. What are **renewable resources**, and why do they need management?

5. How can you conserve energy when using a refrigerator?

6. Why should you use the oven light to check on foods?

7. Why is it more efficient to cover the pot when boiling water?

8. How can you save energy costs when purchasing lightbulbs?

9. How can you use less water when cooking?

10. Describe a **sanitary landfill**.

11. What are ways to reduce your use of paper?

12. Why are plastic bags an environmental problem?

13. Describe bioplastics and list their positive and negative qualities.

14. How can you avoid **food waste**?

15. Describe kitchen uses for reusable food containers.

16. List common household items that can be **recycled**.

17. If resource-acres are divided by the number of people on earth, what is each person's fair share, and how many acres does the average American use?

18. **CRITICAL THINKING** Do you think one person can make a difference when it comes to saving earth's resources? Explain.

19. **CRITICAL THINKING** Which areas of resource conservation do you think are the most critical? Why?

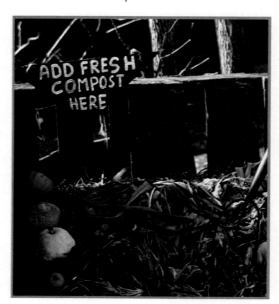

Apply Your Learning

1. **Condenser Coils.** Demonstrate how to clean the condenser coils on the lab refrigerator. Use the instruction booklet to locate the coils. What is their function?

2. **Package Reduction.** In supermarkets and other stores, find products with excess packaging. Make recommendations about ways to reduce their purchase and use.

3. **SCIENCE** **Composting.** Prepare a display on how to compost kitchen and table scraps. Why is composting useful?

4. **Self-Challenge.** For three days, monitor your own use of resources. How can you improve? Set two goals and evaluate your progress at specific intervals.

5. **SOCIAL STUDIES** **EPA Exploration.** Learn more about the U.S. Environmental Protection Agency (EPA). How is the agency organized? What does it do?

6. **Disposal of Chemicals.** Contact the sanitation department or a local or state department of environmental services to find information on household hazardous waste collections in your area.

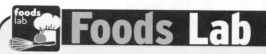

Foods Lab

Resource-Saving Recipes

Procedure: Find a recipe that uses—or can be adapted to use—as few natural resources as possible. Determine what resources were used to process, package, and store the ingredients; how much water is needed for preparation; and what food waste occurs. Prepare the recipe that you think is the most resource friendly. Modify it if needed. Share and compare finished products with other lab teams.

Analyzing Results

1. What types of food seemed best suited for this lab? Why?
2. How did you modify cooking techniques to use less energy?
3. Evaluate your team's success in conserving resources.

Food Science Experiment

Household Cleaners

Objective: To compare commercial and homemade cleaning products.

Procedure:

1. Perform a cleaning trial, as assigned: a) Streak the outside of two glass containers lightly with vegetable oil. Wipe one streak with a commercial glass cleaner. Wipe the other with a mixture of 1 Tbsp. vinegar and 1 cup water. Compare results. b) Polish three stainless steel utensils with a commercial, nonabrasive cleanser. Polish three identical utensils with a mixture of 1 Tbsp. baking soda and 2 tsp. water. Compare results.

2. Share results with other teams.

Analyzing Results

1. How did commercial and homemade cleaning products compare in effectiveness?
2. Compare the cost per use for commercial and homemade products. Which is more economical?
3. Vinegar and baking soda are used in many homemade cleaning products. What makes them effective?

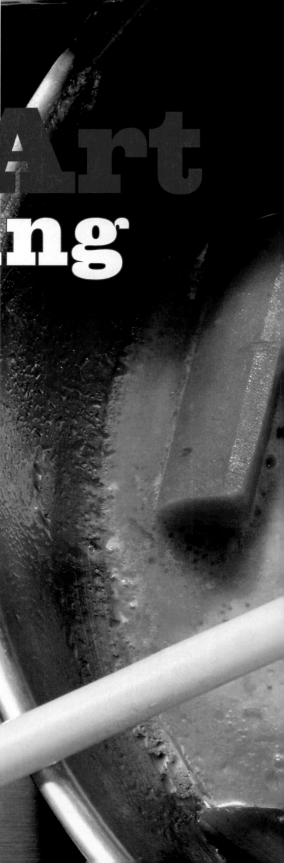

UNIT 6

The Art of Cooking

CHAPTER 24 **Using Recipes**

CHAPTER 25 **Preparation Techniques**

CHAPTER 26 **Cooking Methods**

CHAPTER 27 **Developing a Work Plan**

CHAPTER 28 **Creative Additions**

CHAPTER 29 **Preserving Food at Home**

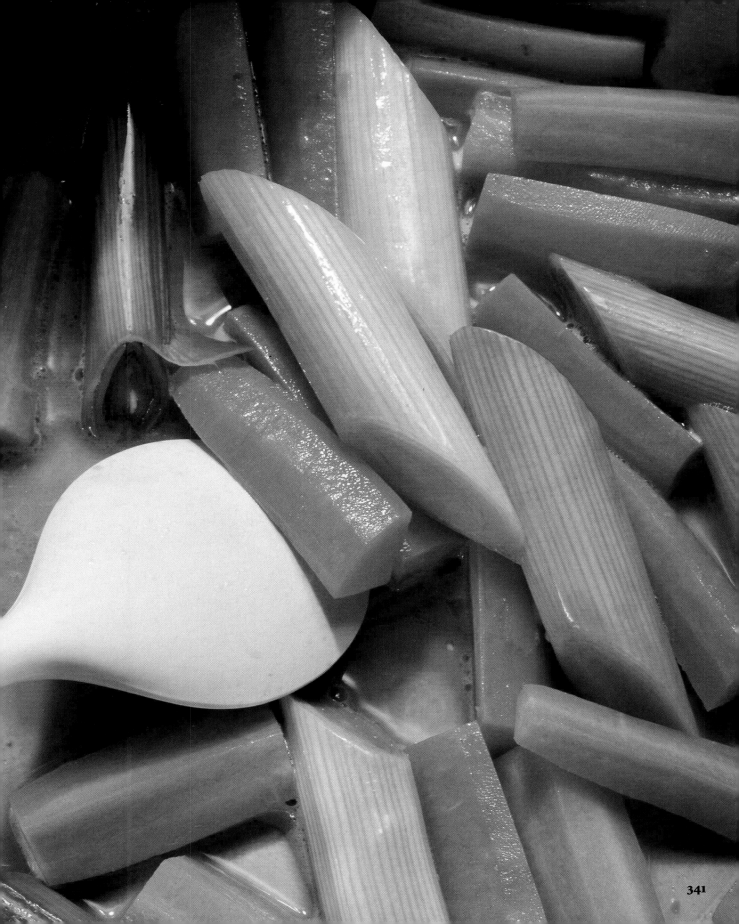

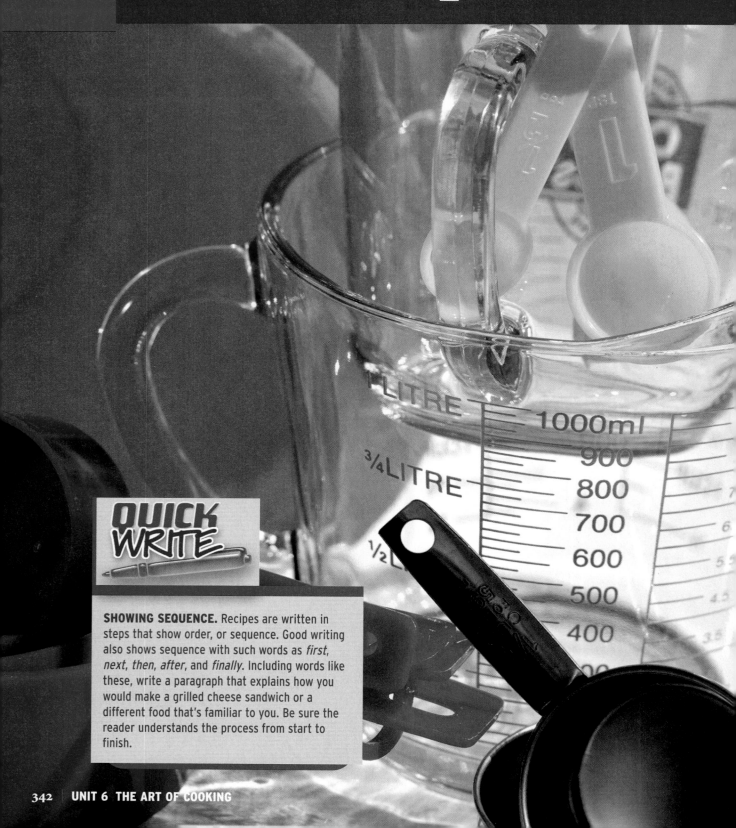

QUICK WRITE

SHOWING SEQUENCE. Recipes are written in steps that show order, or sequence. Good writing also shows sequence with such words as *first*, *next*, *then*, *after*, and *finally*. Including words like these, write a paragraph that explains how you would make a grilled cheese sandwich or a different food that's familiar to you. Be sure the reader understands the process from start to finish.

Objectives

▶ Evaluate the clarity and completeness of a recipe.

▶ Compare different units and systems of measurement used in recipes.

▶ Explain how and why a recipe might be modified.

▶ Describe how to find and organize recipes.

Terms

customary system

equivalents

high-altitude cooking

metric system

recipe

volume

weight

yield

I MAGINE THESE DIRECTIONS FOR MAKING A cake: "Beat a good lump of butter with a teacup of sugar. Mix in 2 scoops of flour, a pinch each of salt and soda, 2 eggs, and enough milk to make a thin batter. Add a handful of nuts. Pour in the pan and bake in a quick oven until done."

If you lived 150 years ago, following that recipe (or receipt, as it was called then) might have worked. You would have known which teacup and pan to use. Of course, relatives might not agree on exactly what a "thin batter" is, so the cake might have looked and tasted different depending on the preparer. Most home cooks didn't see the need for precise measurements and proportions of ingredients until the publication of Fannie Farmer's *Boston Cooking School Cookbook* in 1896.

Today's cooks can have more confidence that a **recipe**, a set of directions for making a food or beverage, will produce successful results. A good recipe complements the skills of a good cook.

THE WELL-WRITTEN RECIPE

Reading the cake recipe above, did you sense something was missing? Besides a title that names the dish, the essential parts of a recipe are described here. Which of these does the cake recipe lack?

- **List of ingredients.** Ingredients are given in exact amounts and in the order of use. This makes it easier to follow the recipe without leaving anything out.
- **Yield.** The **yield** is the number of servings or amount the recipe makes.

Consumer FYI

Recipe trends. Busy and beginning cooks might start a recipe collection in the supermarket. Recipes on food labels are getting simpler and shorter, with an average of six ingredients and four steps. Unusual herbs and spices are avoided, since some busy cooks may not have them. Single-pan recipes are preferred. Recipes often feature such food trends as low-fat or ethnic cuisine.

To help ensure success, test-kitchen chefs try to duplicate home cooking conditions. Recipes are tested with readily available, store-bought ingredients and prepared with typical kitchen utensils. They're evaluated on cost, preparation time—under 30 minutes—and ease of cleanup. Taste and appearance are still important, especially since recipes designed for busy families have to appeal to children as well as cooks.

- **Temperature and time.** Oven temperatures and times are usually for conventional ovens, unless stated otherwise. Recipes for baked goods may remind you to preheat the oven. Temperature and time may be indicated in such techniques as these: "fry until golden" or "chill until set."
- **Container size and type.** Containers are described in as much detail as needed. A brownie recipe may specify "a large bowl" for mixing and "an 8-inch square pan" for baking.
- **Step-by-step directions.** Directions should be in logical order, clear, and easy to follow. Steps may be numbered to help you keep your place and carry out each one in order. Directions for both conventional and microwave ovens are common.
- **Nutrition analysis.** Although not needed for preparation, this information can help you choose recipes that fit your eating plan. You might see the number of calories and grams of fat, sodium, and fiber per serving. Some recipes include values for carbohydrates, protein, cholesterol, vitamins, and minerals.

The most common format for a recipe lists the ingredients first, followed by the step-by-step directions. Recipes in your text use this format. See **Fig. 24-1.** You may also see recipes written with the ingredients incorporated into the directions. This space-saving design is often used on food labels.

WEIGHTS AND MEASURES

"This is delicious! How did you make it?" What cook doesn't want to hear these words? Recipe success hinges greatly on putting ingredients together in the right proportions.

When recipes are written, ingredient amounts are listed using one of two measurement systems. The **customary system**, also called U.S. standard or English, was brought to the United States long ago by colonists from England. It has been used in the United States ever since. Most other countries of the world use the **metric system**, which is based on multiples of ten. For instance, just as one dollar contains 100 pennies, one meter contains 100 centimeters.

Fig. 24-1

Try This! **Recipe**

Granola

Yield	Nutrition Analysis
8 cups granola (16, ½-cup servings)	***Per Serving:*** 260 calories, 5 g protein, 36 g total carbohydrate, 3 g dietary fiber, 20 g sugars, 12 g total fat, 2 g saturated fat, 0 g trans fat, 15 mg sodium ***Percent Daily Value:*** vitamin A 4%, vitamin C 6 %, calcium 2%, iron 8%

Ingredients
3 cups rolled oats
1 cup mixed seeds or grains
   (sunflower or sesame seeds, wheat germ, shredded wheat)
1 cup crisp rice cereal

½ cup vegetable oil
½ cup honey
1 cup raisins
1 cup diced, dried fruits
   (apricots, dates)

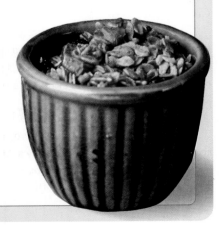

Directions
1. Preheat oven to 300°F.
2. Mix all ingredients except raisins and dried fruit in large bowl.
3. Spread in single layer on baking sheet.
4. Bake for 30 minutes, stirring often, or until golden brown.
5. Remove from oven and stir in raisins and dried fruit. Cool.

Since the United States has been gradually converting to metric, examples of metric are all around you. Scientists routinely work in metric. Food service operations often measure in metric. Beverages are sold by the liter, and food labels indicate weight in grams.

When cooking, you can use recipes that are written in customary or metric. **Fig. 24-2** is an example of a metric recipe. For either system, you need measuring tools that are sized or marked for the particular system. You need a kitchen scale to weigh ingredients.

Units of Measure

In the two systems of measurement, different units express volume, weight, dimensions, and temperature in recipes. See **Fig. 24-3** on page 346. **Volume** is the amount of space an ingredient takes up. For example, a salad recipe might list "½ cup chopped celery" or "250 mL milk." **Weight** measures the heaviness of an ingredient, as in "1 lb. ground beef" or "50 g chopped walnuts." Dimensions commonly describe bakeware lengths and widths. Temperatures, of course, indicate range settings and food temperatures.

Fig. 24-2

Try This! **Recipe**

Griddled Potato Scones

Yield	Nutrition Analysis
8 scones	**Per Serving:** 90 calories, 4 g total fat, 3 g saturated fat, 0 g trans fat, 10 mg cholesterol, 180 mg sodium, 11 g total carbohydrate, 1 g dietary fiber, 0 g sugars, 2 g protein
	Percent Daily Value: vitamin A 2%, vitamin C 4%, calcium 4%, iron 2%

Ingredients

1 large potato (about 250 g), peeled and cubed
25 g unsalted butter
50 g all-purpose flour
2.5 mL salt
1 mL baking powder
25 g shredded cheddar cheese
2.5 mL chopped fresh rosemary
4.7 g butter for greasing griddle or skillet

Directions

1. In a medium saucepan, cover potato cubes with cold water and cook over medium heat until fork tender.
2. Drain potato cubes and place in a bowl with the butter. Mash until the consistency of mashed potatoes.
3. In a bowl, sift flour, salt, and baking powder. While the mashed potatoes are still warm, incorporate the flour mixture, cheese, and rosemary, making a soft dough.
4. With floured hands, form the dough into two balls. On a lightly floured surface, roll out each ball with a rolling pin to a 5 mm disk.
5. Cut each disk into four quarters and pierce with a fork.
6. Heat griddle or skillet over medium-high heat. Coat surface with a little butter. When butter is hot and melted, add dough quarters and cook for 3 to 4 minutes on each side or until golden brown.
7. Transfer scones to a wire rack and cool slightly; eat warm and serve with butter.

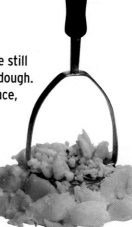

Units of Measurement

Fig. 24-3

Type of Measurement	Customary Units of Measurement	Metric Units of Measurement
Volume	teaspoon (tsp.); tablespoon (Tbsp.); cup (c.); pint (pt.); quart (qt.); gallon (gal.) fluid ounce (fl. oz.)	milliliter (mL); liter (L)
Weight	ounce (oz.); pound (lb.)	milligram (mg); gram (g); kilogram (kg)
Dimensions	inches (in.)	centimeter (cm)
Temperature	degrees Fahrenheit (°F)	degrees Celsius (°C)

Working with Units of Measurement

In the customary system, notice that "ounces" express weight but "fluid ounces" indicate volume. To understand the difference, suppose you measure a cup of popcorn and a cup of brown rice. Since 1 cup equals 8 fluid ounces, both of these ingredients have the same volume. What about their weights? Because popcorn is mostly air, it is much lighter in weight than rice. You can find out how many ounces each weighs with a kitchen scale.

When you work with a recipe, math skills help you determine quantities. What if you want to make a fruit salad recipe that calls for 1½ cups of blueberries, but the store only sells them by the pint? How many pints do you buy? Cooks use equivalents to get answers.

Equivalents are different units of equal measure. For example, look at **Fig. 24-4**, which shows volume and weight equivalents used in food preparation. Under the customary measurements, you'll see that 2 cups equal 1 pint. One pint of blueberries would be enough for the salad, with some left to sprinkle on your cereal.

Converting Between Systems

Some people have recipes they want to convert from one measuring system to the other. One person, for example, had an old family recipe that he wanted to send to a friend in England. First, he planned to convert the recipe into metric.

In conversions, results are likely to be close but not exact. For example, suppose you want to convert 8 fluid ounces to metric. This equals 236.5 mL, or 240 mL rounded. Since metric markings on a liquid measuring cup don't include this measurement, you would measure almost to the 250-mL mark, which works for many recipes. Conversion accuracy is more critical for some dishes you make than it is for others.

When converting recipes, good results also depend on the ingredients. Recipes from other countries may have ingredients that differ from those used in the United States. For example, crème fraîche (krehm fraysh), an ingredient in some English recipes, is similar to sour cream but not exactly the same.

To convert a recipe or to see how measurements in the two systems compare, conversion charts and formulas can help. You can use the equivalents in **Fig. 24-4**. **Fig. 24-5** on page 348 shows formulas to use when converting numbers yourself.

Here's how to convert temperatures:

- **To get degrees Fahrenheit.** Multiply the Celsius temperature by 9. Then divide by 5 and add 32.
- **To get degrees Celsius.** Subtract 32 from the Fahrenheit temperature. Then multiply by 5 and divide by 9. For example, to convert 350°F, subtract 32 from 350 to get 318. Multiplying

318 by 5 yields 1,590. Dividing that by 9 yields 176.66°C, or about 180°C.

CHANGING A RECIPE

From time to time, you may wish to change a recipe. Do you need to increase or decrease the yield? Maybe you need to substitute an ingredient for health reasons. On the other hand, you might just want to be creative.

Some recipes handle change better than others. In mixtures where ingredients act more or less independently of each other—fruits in a salad, for example, or vegetables in a stir-fry—changes have little effect. You can experiment with different flavors and textures and still have a successful outcome.

On the other hand, baking takes precise measurements. Recipes for baked items are like chemical formulas. Because each ingredient does a specific job in the recipe, ingredients must be used in exact amounts that are in the right proportion to each other. If one amount is changed or one ingredient omitted, you risk a ruined product. Unless a recipe for a baked product can be cut in half exactly, decreasing it isn't recommended. See **Fig. 24-6** on page 348.

Changing the Yield

Most recipes, including those for baked goods, can be doubled successfully by doubling the amount of each ingredient. Cooking times may need adjusting. Be sure you have larger equipment for mixing and cooking, if needed. For a double recipe of a baked product, use two baking pans of the original size rather than one large pan.

Recipes for casseroles, stews, and other mixtures can usually be decreased. The steps are fairly simple.

Fig. 24-4

Volume and Weight Equivalents			
Customary Measurements			**Approximate Metric Measurements***
Volume			
¼ tsp.			1 mL
½ tsp.			2 mL
1 tsp.			5 mL
1 Tbsp.	3 tsp.	½ fl. oz.	15 mL
⅛ cup	2 Tbsp.	1 fl. oz.	30 mL
¼ cup	4 Tbsp.	2 fl. oz.	50 mL
⅓ cup	5 Tbsp.	3 fl. oz.	75 mL
½ cup	8 Tbsp.	4 fl. oz.	125 mL
⅔ cup	11 Tbsp.	5 fl. oz.	150 mL
¾ cup	12 Tbsp.	6 fl. oz.	175 mL
1 cup	16 Tbsp.	8 fl. oz.	250 mL
1 pint	2 cups	16 fl. oz.	500 mL
1 quart	2 pints (4 cups)	32 fl. oz.	1 L
1 gallon	4 quarts (8 pints; 16 cups)	128 fl. oz.	4 L
Weights			
	1 oz.		28 g
1 lb.	16 oz.		448 g
2.2 lb.	35 oz.		1000 g or 1 kg

*Volumes have been rounded to correspond to metric measuring tools.

1. Divide the desired yield by the recipe's yield. Suppose a lasagne recipe yields 12 servings and you want only 6. Divide 6 by 12, which gives 0.5, or ½.

2. Multiply each ingredient amount by the result in Step 1. This keeps the ingredients in the same proportion as in the original recipe.

3. Convert the measurements into logical, manageable amounts. Suppose the lasagne recipe calls for ¼ cup of parsley. Half of ¼ cup is ⅛ cup. Since ⅛ cup equals 2 tablespoons, you can measure the parsley easily by using a tablespoon.

4. Make any needed adjustments in equipment, temperature, and time. Try to use a pan that maintains the depth and shape of the original recipe. If a 13 x 9 inch baking dish holds the larger lasagne, a 10 x 6 inch dish will hold your

Fig. 24-5

Conversion Chart

To Convert From	Multiply By	To Get
Volume		
fl. oz.	30	mL
mL	0.03	fl. oz.
c.	0.2368	L
L	4.22675	c.
pt.	0.47	L
L	2.1	pt.
qt.	0.95	L
L	1.06	qt.
gal.	3.8	L
L	0.26	gal.
Weight		
oz.	28.35	g
g	0.03527	oz.
lb.	0.45	kg
kg	2.2	lb.

6-serving version proportionally. Because the amount is smaller, however, you may still need to decrease the oven temperature or cooking time.

If decreasing a recipe is not workable, you may want to prepare the original amount. Freeze the leftovers for another meal or share them with friends.

Substituting Ingredients

Suppose you want to try a recipe for buttermilk dressing, but you don't normally use buttermilk and you don't want to buy a whole carton. In a situation like this, substituting ingredients may be the answer. **Fig. 24-7** gives some common substitutions that work.

As with other changes, recipes for baked goods are the most sensitive to substitutions. Replacing a nonessential ingredient with a similar one—exchanging walnuts for raisins in cookie dough, for instance—has little effect on the final product. Substituting basic ingredients, even ones as similar as butter and margarine, may change the recipe's appearance, taste, or texture. Experienced cooks often make these changes intentionally. Although many new dishes and baked items are created by altering basic recipes, the beginning cook needs to be careful about making revisions.

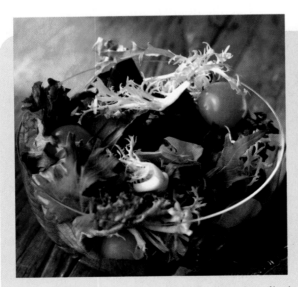
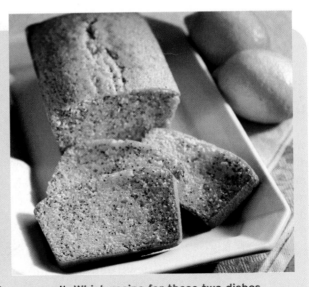

Fig. 24-6 Some recipes can be altered easily, but some can't. Which recipe for these two dishes could you easily change? Why would the other one be more difficult to alter?

High-Altitude Cooking

Imagine you move from a coastal town to a mountain village, and you invite your new neighbors to a dinner of homemade bean soup and corn bread. You've made both recipes dozens of times, yet this time the beans are tough and the corn bread is crumbly.

The unfortunate results are likely due to the difference in altitude. Like most recipes, yours were probably developed for altitudes of 3,000 feet or below. As the altitude gets higher, air pressure gets lower. This affects food preparation in two ways.

First, water boils at a lower temperature. Liquids come to a boil sooner, but foods simmered in them take longer to cook. The soup you simmered for 30 minutes may now need 10 more minutes. You may also have to increase the water to replace any that evaporated while simmering.

In addition, gas bubbles that form in liquids escape from mixtures more readily. This includes gases that raise baked goods. Baked products may rise before the batter is set, causing them to collapse in the center. For more success with future pans of corn bread, you might use less baking powder and sugar and increase the oven temperature. Adding a little extra liquid helps compensate for the dry air of high altitudes.

Making recipe corrections that allow you to prepare foods successfully where the altitude is high is called **high-altitude cooking**. Many packaged foods include special directions to use for high elevations. People who live in these areas can learn about adapting recipes from the nearest cooperative extension office, utility company, or newspaper.

COLLECTING RECIPES

If you haven't already begun a recipe collection, now is a good time to start. What you learn in this course will help you choose recipes that you can prepare successfully and "troubleshoot" problems that might arise. As you develop skills and understanding, a recipe that once seemed too challenging might become your specialty.

Fig. 24-7

Ingredient Substitutions	
When you don't have . . .	**Substitute . . .**
Baking chocolate, unsweetened, 1 oz.	3 Tbsp. cocoa + 1 Tbsp. butter, margarine, or vegetable oil
Bread crumbs, fine, dry	Equal amount cracker or cornflake crumbs
Buttermilk, 1 cup	1 Tbsp. lemon juice or vinegar + enough fat-free milk to equal 1 cup, or use 1 cup plain, nonfat yogurt
Cake flour, 1 cup	$^7/_8$ cup ($^3/_4$ cup + 2 Tbsp.) sifted all-purpose flour
Corn syrup, 1 cup	1 cup granulated sugar + $^1/_4$ cup water
Cornstarch (for thickening), 1 Tbsp.	2 Tbsp. flour
Garlic, 1 clove	$^1/_8$ tsp. garlic powder
Herbs, 1 Tbsp. fresh, chopped	1 tsp. dried, crushed herbs
Lemon juice	Equal amount vinegar
Milk, fat-free, 1 cup	$^1/_3$ cup nonfat dry milk powder + $^7/_8$ cup water
Mustard, dry, 1 tsp.	1 Tbsp. prepared mustard
Onion, 1 small	1 Tbsp. dried, minced onion or use 1 tsp. onion powder
Tomato sauce, 1 cup	6 T. tomato paste + $^1/_2$ cup water
Worcestershire sauce, 1 Tbsp.	1 Tbsp. soy sauce + dash red pepper sauce

Where can you find recipes? Cookbooks are one reliable source. Basic cookbooks give a broad range of foods and reinforce essential cooking skills. Your classroom or school library probably has at least a few. The public library is another source. If you don't find a cookbook you like, ask your teacher for recommendations. You can also try family and friends, magazines, newspapers, and package labels. An Internet search of your favorite food may turn up an amazing number of results.

Before you decide to try a recipe, study it carefully. Does it suit your cooking skills and budget? Does it give all the needed information? If ingredients are given without directions for using them or if directions refer to an ingredient not listed, look for another recipe.

If you plan to use a new recipe for a special occasion, try it ahead of time. Practice helps you work out any problems. You can make sure the recipe turns out as expected and decide whether to add it to your collection.

Organizing Recipes

Like an organized kitchen, an organized recipe collection makes cooking easier and more enjoyable. Many cooks write or paste recipes on index cards and store them in a card file box. Recipe cards are specially designed with lines for the recipe's name, yield, and source, but plain ones work just as well.

You can also write or type recipes on pages of a divided notebook or binder. Label each tab with a category based on food types or your interests, such as vegetarian, low-fat, or dessert recipes. An expanding file with tabbed, accordion-like pouches also holds clipped recipes. Expanding wallets fit smaller papers and cards. Photo albums not only store recipes but also display them conveniently under easy-to-clean plastic film.

You can also save recipes on a computer, using a word processing file, a data base, or special software. You'll be able to print out recipes as needed, which is handy for sharing with friends. You could even compile and print your own cookbook.

Career Prep

Applying for a Job

AFTER FINDING SOME PROMISING JOB openings, what steps do you take to land a job? The process is fairly simple. A little preparation can make it positive and successful as well.

MAKING CONTACT

First, write down the contact information from your job lead—whether you should call, stop in, or write a letter of application, for example. Remember that your evaluation as a potential employee starts with first impressions. Show confidence but be polite. Using correct grammar, explain your purpose and ask for the contact person by name if you know it. When applying in person, present a clean and well-groomed appearance.

THE APPLICATION FORM

Early in the hiring process, you'll probably need to fill out a job application. These forms vary, but all ask for some relevant personal information to assess your suitability. To create the best impression, read instructions first. Then fill out the form completely, printing neatly in black or blue ink. Be ready with your Social Security number, the address and phone number of past employers, and dates of employment. Answer items that don't apply with "N/A" or "not applicable." If possible, get two copies: one for practice, the other to return. You can also find sample job applications on the Internet.

RECIPE FILES

When many cooks talk about their recipe files, they mean a collection of index cards or binders, but that's changing. Files today may be electronic, and recipes may be a small part of what they contain. Recipe software and CD-ROMs give modern cooks access to more information more conveniently than ever. These are some popular software functions:

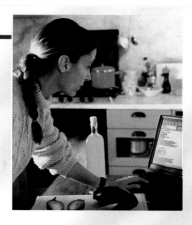

- Search recipes by cuisine, food group, or occasion.
- Avoid recipes that use certain ingredients, as for restricted diets.
- Save a photo with a recipe.
- Convert between metric and customary.
- Increase or decrease recipe yield.
- Estimate the cost of a recipe.
- Do a nutrition analysis.
- Suggest recipes from ingredients you enter.

- Learn cooking history, tips, and definitions of terms.
- Organize shopping lists by supermarket aisle.
- Access on-line databases to swap recipes with people across the world.
- Format electronic recipes for index cards, complete with dotted lines for cutting.

__Think Beyond>> Do you think using recipe software takes the creativity from cooking?

The application may ask for names, addresses, and phone numbers of references, people who know you and can recommend your character and abilities. Teachers, former employers, and supervisors in volunteer and school activities are good choices. Friends and family members are not considered to be objective. Ask permission before listing anyone as a reference.

THE LETTER OF APPLICATION

In a letter of application, you provide some of the same information as on an application form, but in your own words. You can expand and highlight points you think are important. If

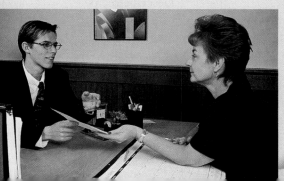

working as a camp counselor helped you relate to families of diverse backgrounds, that's a point that might be included. Keep the letter under one page in length.

Applying for a job may involve "working papers" as well. Workers under age sixteen need a work permit. Some states require those under eighteen to get an Employment/Age Certificate. A health certificate is required for some jobs in the foods industry. Check with your school counselor or state department of employment to learn what documents you need.

Career Connection

Troubleshooting. Bring a job application from a Web site or a local business to class. Compare with those found by classmates. Do any items seem unclear, irrelevant, or too personal? Discuss how to handle these and other problems people might have in filling out an application.

Summarize Your Reading

▶ Recipes today provide precise measurements and proportions of ingredients to produce exacting and successful results.

▶ Two systems of measurement are used to express ingredient amounts in recipes: the customary system (also called U.S. Standard or English) and the metric system, used in most other countries.

▶ Cooks use math skills to determine quantities, using their knowledge of equivalents, or different units of equal measure.

▶ Most recipes can be modified to increase or decrease the yield, and some recipes, but not all, allow for substituting ingredients.

▶ Recipes can be obtained from many sources. Organizing a recipe collection makes recipes easier to find and use.

Check Your Knowledge

1. What might cause a **recipe** to look and taste different each time it's prepared?

2. Describe the essential parts of a well-written recipe.

3. **CRITICAL THINKING** Evaluate the granola recipe on page 344 for completeness and clarity.

4. Compare the **customary system** with the **metric system** of measurement.

5. What tools does a cook need for measuring in each system?

6. Explain the difference between **volume** and **weight** measurements.

7. How would the volume and weight of a cup of oatmeal and a cup of almonds compare?

8. **CRITICAL THINKING** If you need 6 cups of milk for a recipe and you have ⅔ of a cup in the refrigerator, what size milk container or containers would you need to buy?

9. Why are conversion formulas and charts with measurement **equivalents** useful?

10. How can you convert oven temperature from Celsius to Fahrenheit?

11. What is the Celsius temperature of 375°F?

12. In what kinds of recipes is it easy to change ingredient amounts? Why?

13. Why isn't it a good idea to change ingredient amounts when baking?

14. What adjustments should you keep in mind when doubling a recipe?

15. What steps should be followed to decrease the size of a recipe?

16. Should a beginning cook substitute basic ingredients in a bread recipe? Explain.

17. How does **high altitude** affect the preparation of soup?

18. Why might a corn bread recipe need to be altered when prepared at high altitude? What should be done?

19. Why is it a good idea to try out a recipe before making it for a special occasion?

20. What are some sources for recipes?

21. **CRITICAL THINKING** Describe recipe organization methods and evaluate them to determine what type would work the best for you.

Apply Your Learning

1. **LANGUAGE ARTS** **Writing Recipes Right.** Choose a snack that you usually prepare without a recipe, such as s'mores. Write a recipe for the snack in correct form. Include ingredient measures and directions.

2. **MATH** **Conversion.** Change a recipe from customary to metric. If possible, prepare the recipe with metric measuring tools. Evaluate the results.

3. **MATH** **Changing Yield.** Choose several recipes from home or class. Double the recipes, indicating the ingredient amounts needed. Then cut the recipes in half. How will pan sizes change with the new amounts?

4. **SOCIAL STUDIES** **Elevation.** Use a map to find the elevation where you live. Are you higher or lower than 3000 feet? Locate places where the elevation is high enough to require changes in recipes. What changes would be needed?

Foods Lab

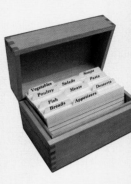

Altering Recipes

Procedure: Choose a recipe (not a baked item) and change it in some way to improve its nutrient profile. Depending on the recipe, you might reduce or replace some ingredients or increase others. Prepare and evaluate your modified recipe, including before and after nutrition analyses.

Analyzing Results

❶ How and how much did your change improve the recipe nutritionally?

❷ Did the modified recipe need any changes in preparation? Why or why not?

❸ Was this recipe a good choice for the change you made? Why or why not?

Food Science Experiment

Measuring Methods

Objective: To compare the accuracy of different measuring methods.

Procedure:

1. Make sure all lab team members are using the same measuring utensils and the same measuring system. Working alone, measure the volume specified for each of the following ingredients: ¼ cup (50 mL) flour; ⅓ cup (75 mL) brown sugar; and 1 cup (250 mL) water. Then weigh each result and record the weights.

2. Measure the weight specified for each of the following ingredients: 8 oz. (250 g) flour; 4 oz. (125 g) brown sugar; and 12 oz. (750 g) water. Then measure the volume of each ingredient. Record the volumes.

3. Compare your numbers with those obtained by lab team members.

Analyzing Results

❶ For which measurements are team members' numbers more in agreement: for volumes that were weighed or for weights that were then measured in volume? What might explain this result?

❷ Which ingredient was measured most consistently by all team members? Why do you think that happened?

❸ How can lab members help ensure consistency of measurement when working together on recipes?

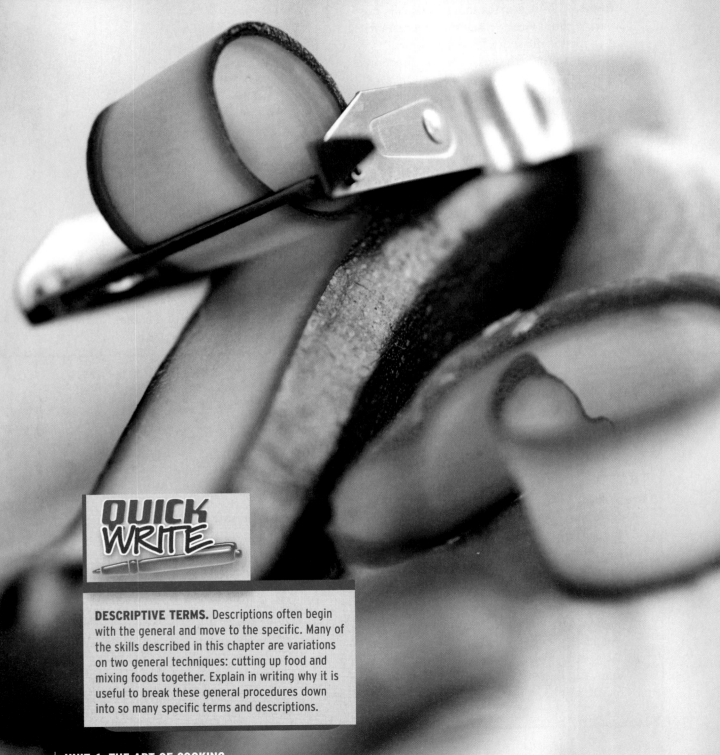

Preparation Techniques

QUICK WRITE

DESCRIPTIVE TERMS. Descriptions often begin with the general and move to the specific. Many of the skills described in this chapter are variations on two general techniques: cutting up food and mixing foods together. Explain in writing why it is useful to break these general procedures down into so many specific terms and descriptions.

W HAT DO YOU DO WITH A RECIPE THAT TELLS you to "bread" one food and to "cream" another, yet neither bread nor cream is listed in the ingredients? If you're familiar with a chef's vocabulary, you'll recognize these terms as two basic techniques that are used in food preparation. Mastering such skills is essential for success in the kitchen, whether you're making a three-step recipe or a gourmet meal.

MEASURING INGREDIENTS

Although a teacup, a soup spoon, and a little judgment might have enabled a cook to measure ingredients many years ago, cooks today rely more on standard measuring tools. To get the best results from most recipes, you need precise amounts and ratios.

Most recipes are developed with standard measuring cups and spoons. Since coffee mugs, soup spoons, and juice glasses vary in size, they can't give needed accuracy. See **Fig. 25-1**.

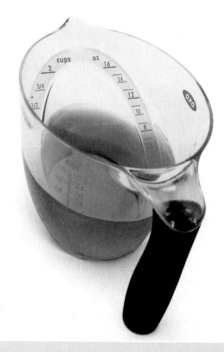

Fig. 25-1 Although some measuring tools are standard, today's marketers offer many variations. This liquid measuring cup allows you to see how much liquid is in the cup by looking into the cup from above rather than the side. What other modern measuring tools have you seen?

Other tools also help ensure accuracy in measuring. A straightedge spatula works well for leveling off dry ingredients, and a rubber scraper is handy for removing all ingredients from measuring cups.

Liquids, dry ingredients, and fats each take slightly different measuring methods. A few pointers apply to them all, however. First, don't measure ingredients over the bowl in which you are mixing. Anything you spill will land in the bowl, and you may not be able to remove it.

Another common question is how to measure amounts that are not marked on any measuring tool. For these in-between fractions, you need a combination of different standard-size measures. Suppose you cut a recipe in half and come up with a measurement of ⅝ cup. The standard measure closest to ⅝ cup is ½ cup ($½ = ⁴⁄₈$). This leaves you needing ⅛ cup more. For an amount this small, you can use measuring spoons. Look again at the equivalents on page 347. You'll see that ⅛ cup equals 2 tablespoons. Just add 2 tablespoons to ½ cup to get ⅝ cup.

Some amounts can be accurately measured by subtracting a smaller quantity from a larger one. To get ⅞ cup of milk, for instance, first measure one cup and then remove 2 tablespoons.

Measuring Liquids

Liquid measuring cups are used for larger amounts of flowing ingredients, including oils and syrups. To measure liquids accurately, follow these steps:

1. Set the cup on a level surface. A cup in the hand can be tilted, resulting in an incorrect reading, or jostled, resulting in a spill.
2. Pour the liquid into the measuring cup.
3. Bend down to check the measurement at eye level. Looking down at an angle can distort the reading. See **Fig. 25-2**.
4. Add more liquid or pour off the excess, if needed, until the top of the unmoving liquid is at the desired measurement mark.
5. Pour the ingredient into the mixing container. If needed, use a rubber scraper to empty the cup completely.

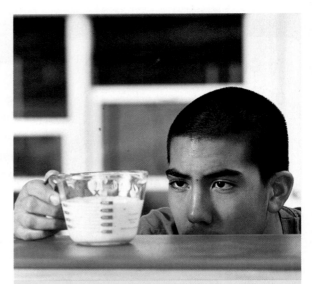

Fig. 25-2 When measuring a liquid, you need to wait until the liquid remains still. Why is this teen viewing the liquid at eye level?

For small amounts of liquids, use measuring spoons. To measure ⅛ teaspoon, dribble the ingredient into the ¼-teaspoon measure until it looks half full. Some spoon sets have a ⅛-teaspoon measure.

Measuring Dry Ingredients

Before measuring dry ingredients, check whether you need to sift it first. Flour, granulated sugar, and confectioners' sugar are often sifted to add air or remove small lumps. Whole-grain flours, however, are too coarse to go through the sifter. Instead, stir them with a spoon before measuring.

As a general rule, such ingredients as flour, granulated sugar, and confectioners' sugar should be spooned lightly into measuring cups. You will probably get too much of an ingredient if you shake the cup or pack the ingredient down. See **Fig. 25-3**.

To measure dry ingredients, follow these steps:

1. Place a piece of wax paper under the proper-size measuring cup to catch any extra ingredient. If you need ¾ cup, use the ½-cup and ¼-cup measures. For ⅔ cup, measure ⅓ cup twice.
2. Fill the cup with the ingredient.

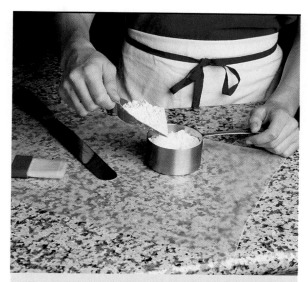

Fig. 25-3 When placing flour in a measuring cup, you should spoon it in lightly. Why is this technique recommended?

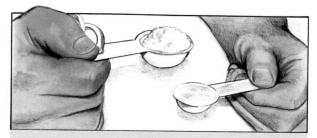

Fig. 25-5 When a recipe calls for a teaspoon of an ingredient, assume that you are to level off the ingredient. Only when the recipe says "heaping" should you leave the ingredient mounded in the spoon.

3. Level off the top of the cup, using the straight edge of a spatula. Let the excess fall on the wax paper and return it to its original container. See **Fig. 25-4**.

4. Pour the ingredient into the mixture, using a rubber scraper if needed.

Despite the name, not all ingredients measured in dry measuring cups are dry. Jam and yogurt are two examples. Depending on their consistency, such foods can be spooned or scraped into and out of the cup. Since brown sugar contains moisture and tends to be fluffy, it should be packed down firmly into a measuring cup with the back of a spoon. When you empty the cup, the sugar should hold its shape.

For amounts smaller than $\frac{1}{4}$ cup, you need measuring spoons—and a bit more judgment. Dry ingredients are usually measured by leveling them off evenly at the rim of the spoon. Sometimes, however, a recipe calls for a "heaping" teaspoon. In that case, leave the ingredient piled in the spoon. It should equal almost twice the amount you would get if you leveled it off. See **Fig. 25-5**. If you need $\frac{1}{8}$ teaspoon of a dry ingredient, fill the $\frac{1}{4}$-teaspoon measure and level it off. Then remove half the ingredient with the tip of a straightedge spatula or table knife.

Some recipes ask for a dash or a pinch of an ingredient, typically an herb, spice, or other seasoning. This is an even smaller quantity, measured as the amount that can be held between the thumb and finger.

Measuring Solid Fats

Depending on their type, solid fats can be measured in several ways.

- **Stick method.** This convenient method is used for fat that comes in $\frac{1}{4}$-pound sticks, usually butter and margarine. The wrapper is marked in tablespoons and in fractions of a cup. You simply cut off the amount you need, cutting through the paper with a serrated knife.

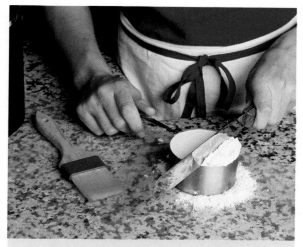

Fig. 25-4 A tool with a straight edge is needed for measuring dry ingredients. Is there any way that a table knife could be used?

- **Dry-measure method.** This is a common method for measuring shortening. Pack the fat into a dry measuring cup, pressing firmly to eliminate pockets of space and to remove air bubbles. Level off the top. Use a rubber scraper to remove as much of the fat as possible. Follow the same steps when using a measuring spoon.
- **Water-displacement method.** Some cooks prefer this technique, which takes a liquid measuring cup. First, subtract the amount of fat you want to measure from one cup. Pour that resulting amount of water into the measuring cup. If you need $\frac{1}{4}$ cup of shortening, for example, use $\frac{3}{4}$ cup of cold water. Cold water keeps the fat from melting. Add fat until the water reaches the 1-cup mark. Hold the fat down to keep it completely below the surface of the water. Don't push the utensil below the water surface or it could affect the measured amount. Lift the fat from the water with a slotted spoon. See **Fig. 25-6**.

Measuring by Weight

Amounts of ingredients may be given by weight. Sometimes the weight is the package size in which the food is sold, such as a 10-ounce bag of frozen vegetables. Weight is a more exact measurement than volume. For example, four ounces of shredded cheese may fill between 1 and $1\frac{1}{2}$

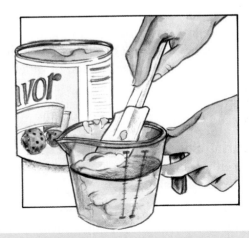

Fig. 25-6 With the water-displacement method, you can measure shortening and keep the cup fairly clean. When measuring, why must the utensil stay above the water?

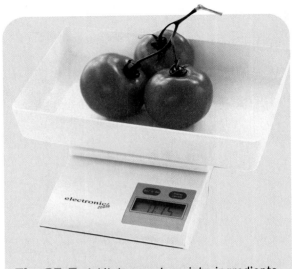

Fig. 25-7 A kitchen scale weighs ingredients. If you are going to put an ingredient in a container, first place the empty container on the scale. Press the tare button to set the scale back to zero. Then add the ingredient. The scale will register that weight only.

cups, depending on how firmly it packs. Professional chefs typically weigh ingredients to get accurate results.

Weighing ingredients takes a kitchen scale. Procedures vary, depending on whether you use a spring scale or an electronic model. Follow the manufacturer's directions for the type of scale you use.

You also need a container to weigh small pieces of food, such as rice or chopped vegetables. Remember to adjust the scale by **taring**, or subtracting the weight of the container to find the weight of the food alone. See **Fig. 25-7**.

CUTTING FOODS

Cutting means dividing a food into smaller parts, using a tool with a sharp blade. That tool is usually a knife. Safety plays a large role in cutting techniques. Remember to start with a sharpened knife to help prevent accidents and make the work easier.

A cutting board is also essential for safe and efficient cutting. It protects the countertop and the cook. Place a wet paper towel or dishcloth under it to prevent slipping. For most cutting

SAFETY ALERT

Review the guidelines. As you practice the preparation techniques in this chapter, remember the safety guidelines you learned in Chapter 21. This is a good time to review them, particularly those related to sharp edges and steam.

tasks, hold the food firmly on the board *with* your hand, not *in* your hand, curling your fingertips away from the blade. Grasp the knife by its handle with the other hand, avoiding the sharp edge of the blade. For a potato or other rounded food, cut a thin slice from the bottom so it sits flat on the board. Grip the knife securely. Face the blade away from your body. See **Fig. 25-8**.

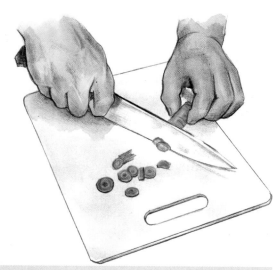

Fig. 25-8 To protect yourself from injury, hold the knife correctly when cutting foods. What guidelines are demonstrated here?

Now that you have the proper stance, you need certain techniques to cut food in different ways.

- **Chop and mince.** Chopping means to cut food into small, irregular pieces. To mince is to chop finely. Use a chef's knife for both tasks. Hold the knife handle with one hand, pressing the tip against the cutting board. Guide the blade by resting the other hand lightly on the back of the blade near the tip. Rock or pump the knife handle up and down carefully, keeping the tip of the blade on the board as the blade chops the food. See **Fig. 25-9**.

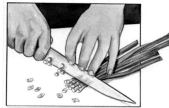

Fig. 25-9 Chopping and Mincing Food

- **Cube and dice.** Both of these terms refer to cutting food into small, square pieces. Cubed pieces are about $\frac{1}{2}$ inch square. To dice, make them $\frac{1}{8}$ to $\frac{1}{4}$ inch square. See **Fig. 25-10**.

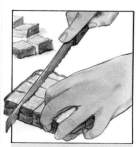

Fig. 25-10 Cubing and Dicing Food

- **Pare.** To cut off a very thin layer of peel with a paring knife. A peeler can also be used. See **Fig. 25-11**.
- **Score.** To make straight, shallow cuts with a slicing knife in the surface of a food. Scoring is often done to tenderize a meat like ham and let sauces sink in.

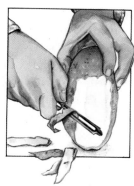

Fig. 25-11 Paring Food

- **Slice.** To cut a food into large, thin pieces with a slicing knife. Use a sawing motion while pressing the knife down gently. See **Fig. 25-12**.
- **Sliver.** To cut a food, such as almonds, into very thin strips.

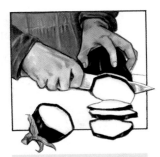

Fig. 25-12
Slicing Food

The cutting techniques just described are only a few ways to change the size and shape of food. Other techniques and tools produce different effects.

- **Crush.** To pulverize food into crumbs, powder, or paste with a rolling pin, blender, or food processor.
- **Flake.** To break or tear off small layers of food, often cooked fish, with a fork.
- **Grate and shred.** To cut food, such as cheese or carrots, into smaller pieces or shreds by pressing and rubbing the food against the rough surface of a grater. See **Fig. 25-13**. To shred cooked meat, pull it apart with a fork.

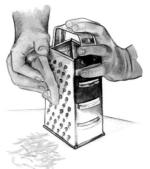

Fig. 25-13
Grating Food

- **Grind.** To use a grinder to break up a food into coarse, medium, or fine particles. Meat and coffee beans are often ground.
- **Mash.** To crush food into a smooth mixture with a masher or beater.
- **Purée.** To grind or mash cooked fruits or vegetables until they are smooth. Tools for this task include a blender, a food processor, a food mill, and a sieve.
- **Quarter.** To divide a food into four equal pieces.
- **Snip.** To cut food into small pieces with kitchen shears. This technique is usually used with fresh herbs or dried fruit.

MIXING INGREDIENTS

Most recipes require some form of **mixing**, combining two or more ingredients thoroughly so they blend. Useful tools for these tasks range from a spoon to a food processor. The terms "mix," "combine," and "blend" all refer to the basic process. Other terms describe more specific techniques that produce a particular effect. Sifting, as you have read, adds air and lightness. Other techniques include the following:

- **Beat.** To mix thoroughly and add air to foods. Use a spoon and a vigorous over-and-over motion or a mixer or food processor. See **Fig. 25-14**.
- **Cream.** To beat ingredients, such as shortening and sugar, combining until soft and creamy.
- **Fold.** Used to gently mix a light, fluffy mixture into a heavier one. Egg whites are often folded into a cake batter, for instance.

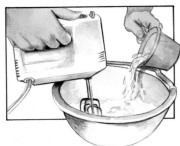

Fig. 25-14
Beating Ingredients

Place the light mixture on top of the heavier one in a bowl. With a rubber scraper or spoon, cut down through the mixture and move the tool across the bottom of the bowl to the side. Bring it back up to the surface, along with some of the mixture from the bottom. See **Fig. 25-15**. Don't lift the tool out of the mixture.

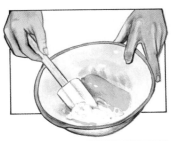

Fig. 25-15
Folding Ingredients

Give the bowl a quarter-turn and repeat until well blended.

- **Stir.** Often applies to food that is cooking. Mix with a spoon or wire whisk in a circular motion. This distributes heat and keeps foods from sticking to a pan. See Fig. **25-16**.

- **Toss.** To mix ingredients, such as salad greens and dressing, by tumbling them with tongs or a large spoon and fork.

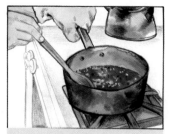

Fig. 25-16
Stirring Ingredients

- **Whip.** To beat quickly and vigorously to incorporate air into a mixture, making it light and fluffy.

COATING TECHNIQUES

Another common preparation technique is to **coat** food with a thin layer of another food. Coating adds flavor and texture. It also helps food brown better and retain moisture.

A coating may be a dry ingredient, such as flour or cornmeal. These are especially popular for meat, poultry, and seafood. A convenient way to apply a dry coating is to place it in a large plastic bag and add the food to be coated. Shake the bag until the food is completely covered. Remove the food from the bag and shake off the excess coating.

Coatings can be liquid as well. Foods may be brushed with a sauce or dipped in a batter, which is a dry coating mixture with liquid added.

The technique used to coat food varies, depending on the ingredients and the desired results.

- **Baste.** To pour liquid over a food as it cooks, using a baster or spoon. Foods are often basted in sauces or pan juices.
- **Bread.** To coat a food with three different layers. The food is first coated with flour. This provides a dry surface for the next layer, which is a liquid such as milk or beaten egg. Finally, the food is usually coated with seasoned crumbs or cornmeal. See **Fig. 25-17**.
- **Brush.** To use a pastry brush to coat a food with a liquid, such as melted butter or a sauce.
- **Dot.** To put small pieces of food, such as butter, on the surface of another food.

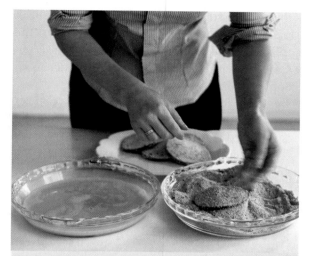

Fig. 25-17 To bread a food, both liquid and dry coatings are used. In what order are they applied to the food? Why?

- **Dredge.** To coat food heavily with flour, breadcrumbs, or cornmeal.
- **Dust.** To lightly sprinkle a food with flour or confectioners' sugar.
- **Flour.** To coat a food, such as chicken or fish, with flour.
- **Glaze.** To coat a food with a liquid that forms a glossy finish.

OTHER TECHNIQUES

As you do more cooking, you'll come across many techniques that are used in particular situations. While some terms may be unfamiliar, the procedures are fairly simple to learn.

- **Blanch.** To dip a food briefly in boiling water and then in cold water to stop the cooking process. Blanching is one step in canning and freezing fruits and vegetables. Blanched peppers and almonds are more easily peeled for roasting.
- **Candy.** To cook a food in a sugar syrup. Some root vegetables, fruits, and fruit peels are prepared in this way.
- **Caramelize.** To heat sugar until it liquefies and darkens in color. Other foods may be caramelized to release their sugar content.
- **Clarify.** To make a liquid clear by removing solid particles. A broth is clarified by removing

the fat and straining. Clarified butter has been melted and the butterfat poured off from the milk solids.

- **Core.** To remove the center of a fruit, such as an apple or pineapple.
- **Deglaze.** To loosen the flavorful food particles in a pan after food has been browned. The food is removed from the pan and excess fat poured off. A small amount of liquid is added, stirred, and simmered. The resulting sauce is served with the cooked food.
- **Drain.** To separate water from solid food, such as vegetables or cooked pasta, by putting the food in a colander or strainer. See **Fig. 25-18**.
- **Marinate.** To add flavor to a food by soaking it in a cold, seasoned liquid. The liquid is usually discarded.
- **Mold.** To shape a food by hand or by placing it in a decorative mold.
- **Pit.** To remove a stone or seed from fruit using a sharp knife.

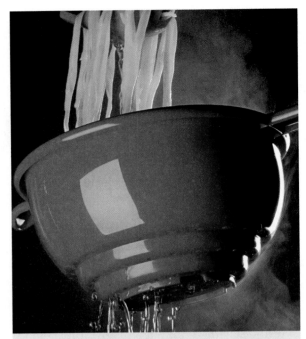

Fig. 25-18 A colander is used to separate solid foods from water. Since it has smaller holes, a strainer can be used for the same purpose as well as for straining solid particles from liquids. When might you use each tool?

Job Interviews

PREPARATION IS YOUR BEST DEFENSE against the job-interview jitters. Most people feel at least a little nervous about talking with a potential employer. Knowing what to expect and preparing for it, however, can ease your mind. Use the suggestions here for the job interviews in your future.

- **Locate information.** Using the library, newspaper, or Internet, find information on the business. You'll be able to respond better if the interviewer asks, "Why do you want to work here?"
- **Dress appropriately.** Since appearance counts, wear an outfit that is clean, pressed, and fits well. Jeans, T-shirts, athletic shoes, and unconventional garments are not acceptable.

- **Be on time.** Before you go to the interview, check the location and the route.
- **Arrive alone.** Anyone who accompanies you should wait outside.
- **Greet the interviewer.** If a handshake is offered, respond with a firm grasp. Smile and make eye contact. When invited, sit down and place any items you're carrying on the floor rather than on the interviewer's desk.
- **Try to relax.** Avoid slumping in the chair. Instead of fidgeting with your hands, place them in your lap.
- **Respond appropriately.** Speak clearly, without using slang. Give a little more than just yes and no answers. If you talk about belonging to a club, add details about skills you've gained.

- **Reduce.** To boil a mixture in order to evaporate the liquid and intensify the flavor. Also called "cooking down."
- **Scald.** To heat liquid to just below the boiling point. Also, to blanch food.
- **Season.** To add such flavorings as herbs and spices to a food.
- **Shell.** To remove the tough outer coating of a food, such as eggs or nuts.
- **Steep.** To soak dry ingredients, such as tea or herbs, in hot liquid to extract flavor or soften the texture. The mixture is strained and the particles are discarded. See **Fig. 25-19**.
- **Strain.** To separate solid particles from a liquid, such as broth, by pouring the mixture through a strainer or sieve.
- **Vent.** To leave an opening in a container so steam can escape during cooking.

By practicing all of these preparation techniques, you will expand your store of cooking skills. You'll be better equipped to add new recipes to your list of favorites.

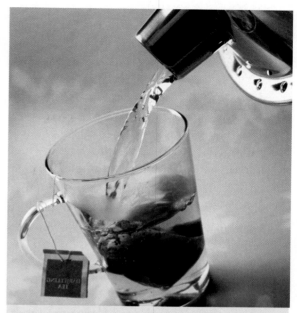

Fig. 25-19 To steep is to soak dry ingredients in a hot liquid to extract flavor or soften the texture. Timing is significant. Some teas, for example, become bitter if steeped too long.

- **Answer honestly.** If negative information must be mentioned, briefly explain how you've learned from mistakes and negative experiences. Avoid blaming and criticizing.
- **Show interest.** You might ask about duties and advancement opportunities.
- **Show enthusiasm.** Be positive about the work opportunity.
- **Thank the interviewer.** As the interview ends, express appreciation for the time spent

with you. You may wish to follow up later with a letter of thanks.

Missing out on a job that you wanted can be disappointing, but it isn't unusual in a job search. Multiple interviews may be needed to find the right position. Each interview is an opportunity to analyze what went well and what didn't. By making improvements—speaking up more, speaking up less, polishing a resumé—you may be the candidate who is chosen the next time.

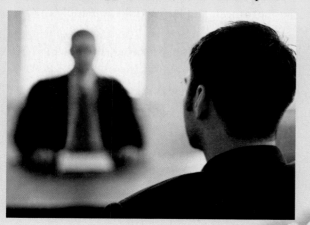

Career Connection

Interview practice. Interviewers often ask similar questions. Look on the Internet or in other resources for lists of typical interview questions. Then with a partner, plan an imaginary interview for a job related to food or nutrition. Take turns playing the roles of interviewer and applicant as you ask and answer interview questions.

Summarize Your Reading

▶ Cooking requires knowledge of a chef's specialized vocabulary, terms that describe tools and methods of food preparation.

▶ Liquids, dry ingredients, and fats each take slightly different measuring methods.

▶ Safety plays a large role in using knives for cutting techniques.

▶ Tools for mixing range from a spoon to a food processor.

▶ Coating foods with either dry or liquid ingredients adds flavor and texture. This process helps food brown better and retain moisture.

▶ Many specialized cooking techniques are used to make candy, add flavor, and prepare foods.

Check Your Knowledge

1. How can a straightedge spatula and rubber scraper help when measuring foods?

2. Should you measure ingredients over the bowl you're using for **mixing**? Explain.

3. How could you measure 1⅞ cups of a dry ingredient?

4. What is the correct method for measuring liquids?

5. Why might some ingredients, such as flour and confectioners' sugar, need to be sifted before measuring?

6. What is the proper method for measuring dry ingredients?

7. Compare the methods for measuring confectioners' sugar and brown sugar.

8. How are dry ingredients in amounts less than ¼ cup typically measured?

9. Describe two ways to measure a fat that doesn't come in a stick.

10. What is **taring** and why is it done when measuring foods by weight?

11. What general guidelines should be followed when **cutting** foods?

12. Describe how chopping, mincing, cubing, and dicing differ.

13. How do you pare, score, slice, and sliver foods?

14. Explain how flaking, grating, shredding, and quartering foods differ.

15. Describe the cutting techniques that require use of a grinder, blender, or food processor.

16. **CRITICAL THINKING** Predict outcomes that might result if a cook doesn't know what different cutting terms mean and how to do them.

17. **CRITICAL THINKING** Why should you fold egg whites into a cake batter instead of beating or creaming?

18. How would you mix ingredients when making a salad?

19. What foods might you **coat** with flour or cornmeal, and how would you apply the coating?

20. What do basting, brushing, and glazing have in common?

21. How does a glaze differ from other coatings?

22. Why would you blanch, reduce, and steep foods?

23. Why might a cook want to core, shell, or pit food before serving?

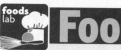
Apply Your Learning

1. **MATH** **Measurement Comparison.** Conduct an experiment to compare the volume of standard measuring cups and spoons to tableware teaspoons and tablespoons and beverage cups. What differences do you find?

2. **Measurement Alternatives.** What does it mean to eyeball ingredients? When close measurements will do in a recipe, this technique can work. A fist, for example, is about the size of a cup. If measuring tools aren't available, what items in the kitchen could you use to get approximate measurements?

3. **LANGUAGE ARTS** **Methods Demonstration.** Demonstrate the following: a) cutting safely with knives; b) measuring liquid and dry ingredients; c) measuring solid fats; d) measuring by weight; e) methods for cutting foods; f) mixing methods; and g) coating techniques.

4. **Recipe Techniques.** Find a recipe that uses various preparation techniques from the chapter. Share the recipe with classmates and quiz them on the definitions.

Foods Lab

Making a Streusel

Procedure: A streusel is a crumb topping for baked goods. Prepare two recipes for streusel, using different techniques. For both recipes, use 2 Tbsp. flour, 2 Tbsp. sugar, and 2 Tbsp. margarine. For the first recipe, sift together the flour and sugar; then cut in the margarine. For the second recipe, cream the margarine and the sugar; then cut in the flour. Compare the results.

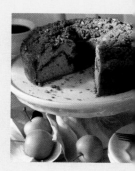

Analyzing Results

❶ Which technique produced the more crumbly mixture? Why?

❷ What could you do to "rescue" the other mixture and create a crumbly consistency?

❸ How else might you use the less crumbly mixture?

Food Science Experiment

Measuring Techniques

Objective: To compare measuring techniques.

Procedure:

1. Measure 1 cup of flour by scooping the flour out of the container, using the measuring cup itself as the scoop. Don't tap the cup. Weigh the flour and record the result.

2. Measure 1 cup of flour by spooning flour lightly into the cup, using a tablespoon. Don't tap the cup. Weigh the flour and record the result.

3. Measure 1 cup of flour by spooning the flour into the cup with a tablespoon and tapping the cup on the countertop after each flour addition. Weigh the flour and record the result.

Analyzing Results

❶ How do your results compare?

❷ Are your results similar to those of other students?

❸ What do you conclude? What impacts could different measuring techniques have on cooking and baking?

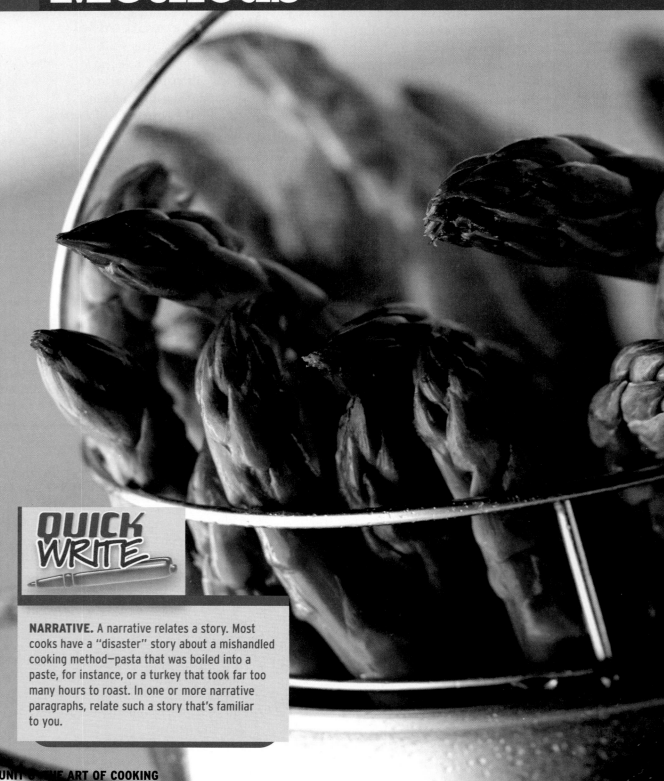

Cooking Methods

QUICK WRITE

NARRATIVE. A narrative relates a story. Most cooks have a "disaster" story about a mishandled cooking method—pasta that was boiled into a paste, for instance, or a turkey that took far too many hours to roast. In one or more narrative paragraphs, relate such a story that's familiar to you.

S KIM THE PAGES OF MOST COOKBOOKS AND you're bound to find recipes that use a variety of cooking methods. The section on chicken alone might include baked chicken, grilled chicken, and chicken stir-fry. Why are foods cooked in so many different ways? What happens to food in the process? Knowing the answers to these questions can help you choose methods and learn skills that add nutrition and appeal to meals.

HOW FOOD COOKS

The simplest method for cooking might be: "Get food. Add heat." Adding heat means transferring it from a source—a cooktop or campfire, for example—to the food, often passing through metal or glass cookware. If you add enough heat to a substance, the molecules within vibrate. The greater the heat, the more intense the vibration is. Although you can't see the process, you can see, feel, and eventually taste the results.

Transfer of heat occurs in three main ways: conduction, convection, and radiation.

Conduction

Conduction is a method of transferring heat by direct contact. Heated molecules pass their heat to neighboring molecules. In this way, heat is conducted within an object and to other objects. See **Fig. 26-1**.

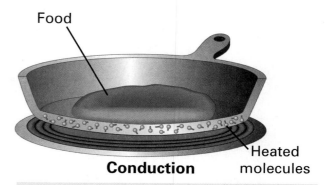

Food

Conduction

Heated molecules

Fig. 26-1 Through conduction, heat moves from one object to another when the two are in contact. Here, the heating element heats the pan, which in turn, heats the food in the pan.

As an example, think of a pancake cooking in a skillet. Heat from the heating unit is conducted into the skillet, which, in turn, passes the heat to the bottom of the pancake. The heat from the bottom of the pancake is conducted to the rest of the batter. To cook the pancake evenly, you flip it over so the top comes in contact with the hot pan.

Convection

Convection is the movement of molecules through air or liquid. Warm air is less dense than cool air because the molecules vibrate more quickly, driving them farther apart. As air is heated, it rises. Cooler and denser air immediately sinks to replace it. The cycle continues, forming a convection current. The process continues until all of the air is evenly heated. See **Fig. 26-2**.

Convection also occurs in heated liquids. Suppose you're heating a pan of water. The water nearest the bottom of the pan warms and rises through cooler water to the surface. This cooler water is forced downward, where it absorbs heat and rises.

Radiation

In **radiation**, heat is transferred as waves of energy. Unlike convection, which relies on rising heat, radiant heat flows evenly from the source in every direction. This is how the sun warms the earth and how flames from a broiler cook food on the pan below it. See **Fig. 26-3**.

Most cooking methods use a combination of heat-transfer processes. In baking, for example, the surface of a food is heated by convection. The heat then travels through the food by conduction.

Effects on Food and Nutrients

Applying heat with care and understanding creates delightful changes in food's sensory qualities. Heat releases flavor and aroma, which mingle pleasingly when different foods are cooked together. The combination of raw meat, vegetables, seasonings, and water that goes into a pot emerges from the oven as a savory stew.

Heat also changes the texture of foods. Some foods get firm or crisp; others turn soft or tender. The effect on color is equally varied. Heat lightens some foods and darkens others. Many vegetables grow brighter; some become duller.

Conventional oven

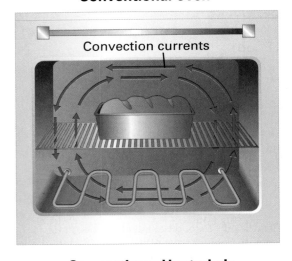

Convection—Heated air

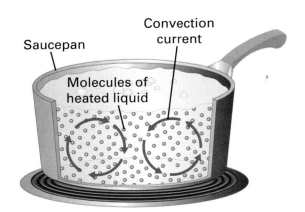

Convection—Liquid

Fig. 26-2 Heat transfer occurs through convection as molecules move through air or water. Convection currents flow through the air in a conventional oven and through the liquid in a saucepan. What keeps the currents moving?

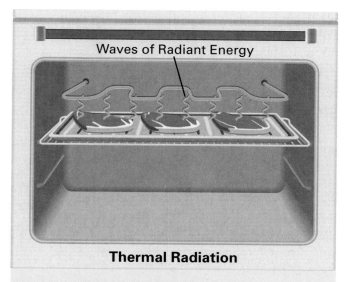

Waves of Radiant Energy

Thermal Radiation

Fig. 26-3 Another method of heat transfer is radiation. Waves of radiant energy, which are emitted from the heat source, strike the food.

The brown exterior that you see on cooked roasts and baked and fried foods adds flavor as well as color. Browning occurs when heat provokes a series of chemical reactions between certain sugars and proteins in the food. Known as the **Maillard reaction**, this browning effect was named for the person who described it, Dr. L.C. Maillard.

Nutritionally speaking, heat produces both positive and negative effects. Cooking breaks down some forms of fiber, making them easier to eat and digest and thus more useful to the body.

At the same time, heat destroys some nutrients, especially vitamin C and the B vitamins. Minerals are generally more resistant, so cooked foods usually retain their mineral values. Very little protein is lost during cooking, but animal proteins are sensitive to high temperatures. Have you had scrambled eggs that were rubbery instead of fluffy or steak that was so chewy it was almost inedible? Those are signs of overcooking.

COOKING RATES

As you'll see, each process transfers heat at a different rate, which affects the time foods need to cook. Other food-related factors also influence cooking rates.

- **Density.** Density measures a food's weight compared to its size. A 3-inch cube of meat is denser than a 3-inch cube of potato, for example. Since added density slows heat transfer, the meat takes longer to cook.
- **Shape and size.** The more surface area a food has, the greater its exposure to heat. Thus two, 1-inch carrot slices cook more quickly than a single 2-inch chunk. Their uniform size also helps them cook evenly. Suppose you leave the carrot whole. Which end will finish cooking first, the narrow or the thick one?
- **Amount.** The more food in the cooking area, the longer it takes heat to reach each item. Foods closer to the heat source cook more quickly. The impact varies with food size, shape, density, and other factors. The smallest potato still takes less time than the largest one, but four potatoes don't necessarily take four times longer to cook than one.

How heat is applied—that is, the cooking method—also affects food's appeal and nutritional value. Food can be cooked by three basic methods: in moist heat, in fat, and in dry heat.

MOIST-HEAT COOKING

In **moist-heat cooking**, food is cooked in hot liquid, steam, or a combination of the two. Moisture allows heat transfer by both conduction and convection. Moist-heat cooking helps tenderize food and blend flavors. It's the only way to prepare rice, dry beans, and other foods that must absorb liquid to be edible.

Food can be cooked using moist heat in a pan, with or without a tight-fitting lid. A lid prevents liquid from evaporating, so foods don't burn. Evaporation may be useful at times, however, to concentrate flavors or thicken a sauce. A slow cooker and microwave oven also use moist heat.

Moist heat can be produced through a variety of techniques. Their differences make some methods better choices for certain foods.

Boiling

A liquid at a boil has reached its highest temperature possible under normal conditions. The temperature varies depending on the liquid. Water, for example, boils at 212°F. In boiling, air bubbles in a liquid continuously rise, break the surface, and escape as steam. This is a vigorous, rolling action that propels pieces of food against each other. These tiny collisions can break up foods and break down texture, color, and flavor.

Boiling is suitable for the relatively few foods that need this high degree of energy, such as corn on the cob and pasta. It toughens animal proteins, as seen in the texture of hard-cooked eggs. It also results in the greatest loss of nutrients of all cooking methods, particularly if food is overcooked. Water-soluble vitamins dissolve in the liquid.

When you boil foods, use a pot or saucepan large enough to hold the liquid and the food, with space left to allow for bubbling. Bring the liquid to a boil and add the food. Be sure the liquid continues to boil as the food cooks. To save any water-soluble vitamins, save the liquid to make a sauce or to cook rice.

Simmering

To simmer means to cook food in a liquid at temperatures just below boiling. Water, for instance, simmers at about 185°F to 210°F. When a liquid simmers, air bubbles rise slowly and just barely break the surface. Since this method is gentler on foods than boiling, it is less destructive to shape, flavor, color, and texture. Water-soluble vitamins are still diminished, so save the liquid for another recipe.

Simmering is useful for cooking many types of foods: fish, rice, firm or dried fruits, and less tender cuts of poultry. Some foods, such as meat and dry beans, can be simmered in a slow cooker.

Poaching

In poaching, whole or large pieces of food are cooked in a small amount of liquid at temperatures just below simmering. The pan may or may not be covered. This gentle cooking method helps retain the shape and tenderness of delicate foods, including fish, fruit, and eggs without the shell. For added flavor, the liquid is often seasoned or sweetened.

Steaming

Steaming is a method of cooking food over, but not in, boiling water. See **Fig. 26-4.** The food is placed in a perforated steamer basket that fits inside a pan. Water is placed in the pan below the level of the basket. The pan is covered with a tight-fitting lid to trap the steam, which is created as the water boils. Foods don't make contact with the water. Thus, while they take longer to cook, they retain their appearance and flavor better than in boiling or simmering. You may need to add water to keep the pan from boiling dry. Using an electric steamer eliminates this concern.

Most types of food can be successfully steamed, including vegetables, seafood, poultry, and meat. Steamed breads and puddings are holiday traditions in some cuisines.

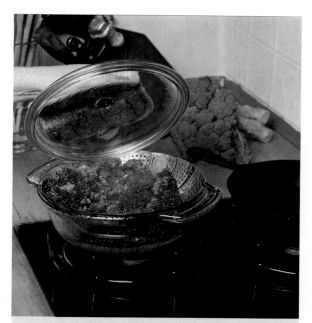

Fig. 26-4 Different pans and devices are available for steaming foods. Why is this a nutritious way to prepare vegetables?

Pressure-Cooking

A pressure cooker, you might recall, creates a high-pressure atmosphere by trapping steam in an airtight chamber. This added pressure raises the boiling point. Water can reach temperatures of around 250°F, so foods cook in one-third or less the time usually needed. Thus fewer nutrients are lost.

Pressure-cooking is convenient for foods that normally have long cooking times, including potatoes, dry beans, and less tender cuts of meat. Those that cook quickly, however, soon turn to mush. Follow the manufacturer's directions carefully when using a pressure cooker.

Braising

Braising takes advantage of both simmering and steaming. A large piece of food, usually a less tender cut of meat or poultry, is placed in a small amount of liquid in a Dutch oven or a pan with a tight-fitting lid. The food cooks in the liquid and trapped steam. See **Fig. 26-5**.

Meats are usually browned before braising. Carrots and other vegetables can be added near the end of the cooking time. Braising is also a way to flavor tender foods, such as fish or pork chops, by using a seasoned sauce as the liquid.

Food may be braised on top of the range or in the oven, or a slow cooker or pressure cooker may be used. On a cooktop, the liquid should simmer just enough to create steam. Oven braising uses similarly low temperatures, around 325°F. Check the pan occasionally. Add a little hot liquid if more is needed; cold liquid slows the cooking process.

Stewing

To stew means to cover small pieces of food completely with a liquid and simmer slowly in a covered pan. This method is often used for less tender cuts of meat and for poultry, fish, and fruit.

COOKING IN FAT

As with moist-heat methods, cooking food in oil or melted fat applies heat through convection and conduction. Fats, however, can be heated to

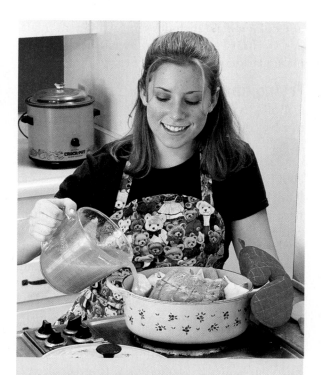

Fig. 26-5 With braising, food is cooked slowly. Sometimes the flavorful liquid is made into gravy to go with the meal.

much higher temperatures than liquids. As a result, foods brown, develop a crisp crust, and acquire the characteristic fried flavor.

Fats can flavor foods in less desirable ways too. Every type of fat has a **smoking point**—the temperature at which it begins to break down. Heated above this temperature, fats not only smoke but also discolor and develop an unpleasant odor and flavor, which they impart to food.

Animal fats have low smoking points. Butter starts to break down at around 300°F, lard at 375°F. Vegetable oils have relatively high smoking points—450°F for corn oil, 495°F for soybean oil. Adding a little oil to butter raises the butter's smoking point, making it useful for more frying tasks. The smoking point drops about 10°F each time an oil is re-used, as exposure to food, heat, and air degrades its quality. Therefore the fresher the oil is, the better the results.

Remember that moisture in food can make fats spatter, burning anyone in range. Also, fats ignite easily at temperatures over 600°F. For frying safely, dry food and a fire extinguisher nearby are essential.

Cooking in fat includes several different methods. Contrary to what many people believe, some methods add little fat to recipes.

Frying and Sautéing

Both frying and sautéing (saw-TAY-ing) involve cooking food in a small amount of hot fat in a skillet over moderate heat. Of the two methods, frying uses more fat and is designed for larger pieces of food, including seafood, eggs, and tender cuts of meat and poultry. The food may need to be turned a few times while frying to cook completely and evenly, but generally it's allowed to brown and cook undisturbed. If the pieces are thick, the pan may be covered to retain heat. Frying is also called pan-frying.

Sauté comes from the French word for "jump." Sautéed foods "jump" as the pan is occasionally shaken, a traditional technique that lets them cook quickly in small amounts of fat without burning. Sautéing is often used to precook vegetables for use in a recipe, such as chopped onions and celery for a poultry stuffing. Small pieces of fish and tender meats may also be sautéed.

Pan-Broiling

In pan-broiling, food cooks in an uncovered skillet in its own natural fat, with no fat added. It's most often used for thin cuts of tender meat that cook quickly, including hamburgers, steak, and some cuts of pork. The food retains a minimal amount of fat. The excess is drained off. See **Fig. 26-6**.

Pan-broiling is often used to **sear** meat, or brown it quickly over high heat, before it's cooked in moist heat. The high heat and a hot skillet give an attractive, flavorful brown crust that moist-heat cooking does not provide. A broiler may also be used for searing.

Deep-Fat Frying

Deep-fat frying is often called "french frying." Both terms describe a process in which foods cook by immersion in hot fat, without making contact with the cooking vessel. Seafood and vegetables are breaded or coated with a batter first. Sweet doughs are deep-fat fried to produce a variety of breads and pastries.

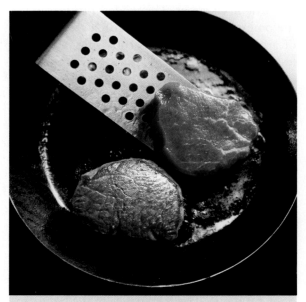

Fig. 26-6 This food is being pan-broiled. How is the technique different from frying?

To deep-fat fry, fill a deep kettle no more than half full of oil. Bring the oil to the temperature specified in the recipe, usually around 350°F. Monitor the temperature with a deep-fat frying thermometer. If the temperature is too low, the food soaks up the fat. If too high, the food burns on the outside yet remains undercooked inside.

Add food carefully to the hot oil. Place small pieces of solid food in a wire frying basket, which can be gently lowered and easily removed. Turn large pieces of food with tongs or a slotted spoon, not a fork. A fork will pierce the food, releasing its juices. This lowers the temperature of the fat and allows fat to enter the food. The juices that are released may also cause the fat to bubble over or ignite. Overcrowding the kettle also lowers the oil temperature.

After the food is fully cooked, carefully remove it from the kettle and drain it on a baking sheet lined with paper towels. Some people use a cooling rack so food doesn't sit in its own fat. Let the fat return to the proper temperature before adding another batch of food. When done cooking, allow the oil to cool and discard it.

Stir-Frying

In stir-frying, small pieces of food are stirred constantly and cooked quickly over high heat in a small amount of oil until just tender. Foods are usually sliced into thin, uniform pieces to ensure fast, even cooking. Those that take the longest to cook are started first, and others are added accordingly. You might begin with chicken strips and stir in sliced green pepper a few minutes later. Vegetables in a stir-fry remain crisp.

When cooking is almost complete, a small amount of seasoned liquid is added, which thick-ens when cooked. Flavors blend and the liquid glazes the ingredients as they finish cooking. Some recipes call for covering the pan toward the end.

A special bowl-shaped pan called a **wok** is the traditional cookware for stir-frying. A skillet with a tight-fitting lid makes a serviceable substitute.

DRY-HEAT COOKING

Dry-heat cooking is cooking food uncovered without added liquid or fat. The idea of cooking with dry heat might make you think the results will be dry food, yet this is the method that produces soft, chewy brownies in the oven and juicy hamburgers on the grill. Dry, radiant heat gives food a crisp brown crust with a distinctive flavor, while the inside remains moist and tender. It also helps retain water-soluble vitamins.

Dry-heat methods include roasting or baking, broiling, and grilling. The placement of the heat source distinguishes one method from the others.

Roasting and Baking

Roasting and baking both refer to cooking foods surrounded by heat in an oven. Meat and poultry are said to be roasted. The food, usually a large, tender cut, is held in a shallow roasting pan, uncovered. See **Fig. 26-7**. Placing the food on a rack inside the pan allows fat to drain away.

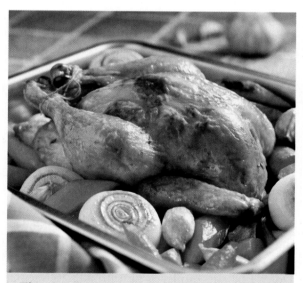

Fig. 26-7 Roasted foods cook in dry heat, without liquid or fat. Vegetables, poultry, and meats can all be roasted.

Baking is a way to cook vegetables, fruits, casseroles, fish, and of course, baked goods. Moisture loss is more likely, and sometimes desirable, in baking. A baked cake is drier than the uncooked batter, and steam escaping from a potato creates a fluffy interior.

All ovens use convection as well as radiation to cook foods; however, a convection oven has a fan to circulate the heated air. The moving air delivers more heat energy, which promotes browning and crispness. Depending on the food, you can reduce oven temperatures in recipes by 25°F to 50°F when using a convection oven.

Broiling

Cooking food under direct heat is called broiling. The food is placed on a pan below the heating unit, which may be in a special compartment or in the oven. The broiler pan has two pieces: a slotted grid that holds the food and a shallow pan below that catches the fat drippings, usually called the drip pan. The heat radiates down from the heating unit, cooking the food rapidly. Large pieces of food are turned to brown both sides. Tender cuts of meat and poultry are good candidates for broiling, as are seafood, fruits, and some vegetables.

While some ranges have more than one broil setting, most have just one, which turns on the broiling unit. Cooking is controlled by adjusting the distance of the pan from the heat. Tomato slices might be placed 4 inches below the heat source and chicken pieces 6 inches. To position specific foods for broiling, follow directions in the appliance owner's manual.

When broiling, be sure food is dry. Moisture can keep food from browning and getting crisp. If needed, salt foods after broiling. Salt draws moisture to the surface, which interferes with browning and dries the interior.

To help keep foods from sticking, start with a cold broiler pan. Remove the pan before preheating the broiler. Make sure the pans are clean in case you want to use the drippings to make gravy. Don't line the broiler grid with foil to keep it clean. Any liquid that drips from the food will turn to steam, which defeats the purpose of broiling. Also, the fat that doesn't drain away may start to smoke, spoiling the food's taste. Worse yet, it could ignite.

Broiling takes relatively little time but a lot of attention. Food that is just inches from an open flame can go from nearly done to completely burned in several seconds.

Grilling

The broiling position of food and flame is reversed when grilling. Food is placed on a grate over an open flame, and heat radiates upward. See **Fig. 26-8**. As with broiling, cooking time depends on the kind and thickness of food and its distance from the heat. The methods are suited to the same types of food. In addition, corn on the cob and potatoes grill nicely in a skillet or wrapped in heavy-duty, aluminum foil, a method that also works for warming breads and rolls.

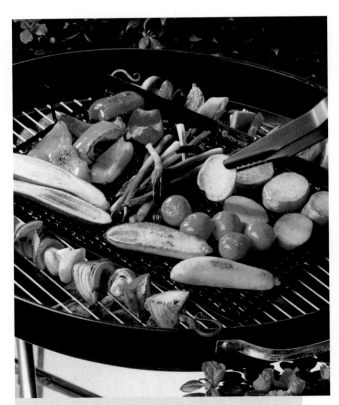

Fig. 26-8 Grilling gives foods special flavor. What other foods besides meats and poultry can be grilled?

Besides the safe grilling habits you've already learned, you might want to consider the safety of the food itself. Some health experts have voiced concern that chemical compounds produced in meats by rapid cooking over high heat may cause cancer. Other possibly hazardous compounds are sometimes formed when fat drips on hot coals. While the exact risk is yet unclear, the following precautions will keep the formation of these substances to a minimum:

- Marinate food, even briefly, before grilling. It can reduce—and in some cases, all but eliminate—the amount of cancer-causing agents.
- Raise the grate a few inches to cook food farther from the flame at a lower temperature.
- Precook meat and poultry in the microwave oven to cut down on grilling time. Finish the cooking immediately to prevent bacterial growth.
- Cut food into small pieces to speed cooking.
- Turn food frequently while grilling so it doesn't char. Remove any charred parts before serving.

MICROWAVE COOKING

In **microwaving**, foods cook from energy in the form of electrical waves. Microwaves cook quickly, with little or no added water. Therefore foods retain more nutrients, especially water-soluble vitamins, than in other methods. In fact, microwaving has been shown to be the best method for preserving nutrients in vegetables.

How Microwaves Cook

While microwaves are a form of radiant energy, they are not a form of heat energy. Microwaves flow in an electric current that causes food molecules to vibrate. Vibration creates friction, which produces the heat that cooks the food. Thus microwaved foods are sometimes said to cook themselves. Also, because microwaves do not generate heat, the chemical reactions that brown foods and develop crisp crusts don't occur.

Microwaves are fast moving but relatively weak, penetrating food to a depth of $1\frac{1}{2}$ inches at most. Conduction, a slower process, moves the heat deeper into thick foods to complete the cooking. Such foods as pasta and rice, which need to absorb liquid as they cook, take the same amount of time in a microwave oven as on a cooktop.

Microwaves penetrate foods unevenly. They affect water molecules most, so foods with high water content cook more quickly. This makes microwaving well suited for foods that can be cooked in moist heat. It also poses problems for cooking potatoes, hot dogs, or butternut squash. These foods have a skin thick enough to prevent moisture inside from evaporating. Steam can build and the food could split and even explode. Slit or pierce firm-skinned foods before microwaving. Don't microwave eggs in the shell.

Fat, sugar, and salt also absorb microwaves efficiently. Concentrations of these ingredients can become "hot spots." If you microwave a jelly doughnut, you might burn your mouth on scorching hot jelly, while the doughnut itself feels only warm. Salting foods before microwaving can lead to uneven cooking.

Power Settings

Microwaves generate power but not heat, so oven controls are not marked with temperature settings. Instead, you choose a **cooking power**,

---

SAFETY ALERT

Heating water. Use caution when heating water in the microwave oven. Because microwaves heat water so quickly and uniformly, the water can become superheated, rising above the boiling point before forming bubbles. The risk is greater with a new container, which lacks tiny scratches where air bubbles begin to form as the temperature rises. Superheated water is very unstable. It can erupt violently at the slightest agitation, causing serious burns. To avoid this hazard, follow recommended microwave times. Use oven mitts to remove the container, holding it away from your face. To be doubly safe, microwave the water with a wooden skewer in the container. Bubbles will begin forming on the surface, allowing normal boiling.

the amount of energy the oven uses to generate microwaves. The energy is measured as watts of electricity rather than degrees Fahrenheit. The higher the cooking power is, the more quickly foods cook.

On some microwave ovens, the power setting is expressed as a percentage, such as 50 or 100 percent power. On others, it is a description, such as "low" or "medium." **Fig. 26-9** gives typical equivalents for the two kinds of settings. Microwave ovens differ in energy capabilities. At 30 percent power, a 900-watt oven cooks with more energy than a 700-watt oven does at the same setting. To avoid overcooking or undercooking, check the owner's manual regarding power settings.

When set at less than full power, the microwave oven cycles on and off during cooking. For instance, at half power, or 50 percent, microwaves are created during only half the time.

Microwave Cookware

Special cookware for microwave ovens is available, but many types of tableware and conventional cookware are just as suitable. You can use glass, china, pottery, and paper. Microwaves pass through these materials to heat only the food. Be sure paper containers are strong enough to hold the food. Avoid products containing recycled paper, which may contain metal fragments or chemicals that could catch fire. All containers should be heat-resistant to withstand the heat transferred from the food.

Use only plastic items marked "microwave-safe." Plastic and Styrofoam™ containers from store-bought or take-out foods may blister, warp, or melt. Chemicals from the plastic may contaminate the food. Even containers from microwavable foods, such as cups from shelf-stable soups, shouldn't be reused. See **Fig. 26-10**.

Generally, metal is a microwaving hazard. Metals, even trims on dishes and screws in handles, reflect microwaves. This can cause **arcing**, electrical sparks that can damage the oven or start a fire. Never leave a metal tool or utensil in any food while microwaving. Use aluminum foil only as the owner's manual or recipe specifies. Small pieces of foil are sometimes used to shield the bony end of chicken legs, for instance.

If you're not sure whether a container is microwave-safe, use this simple test. Put a cup of cold water in a glass measuring cup and place it in the microwave oven next to the empty container you're testing. Heat for 2 minutes on high (100 percent power). If the water has heated and the empty container is still cool, it's microwave-safe. If the container is warm or hot, it isn't safe. Can you explain why?

The size and shape of microwave cookware also affect the way food cooks and the cooking time. Pans should be shallow, with straight sides. Round pans promote even cooking. Food in square or rectangular pans may overcook in the corners.

Fig. 26-9

Microwave Power Levels	
Description	Percentage of Power
High	100
Medium-High	70
Medium	50
Medium-Low	30
Low	10

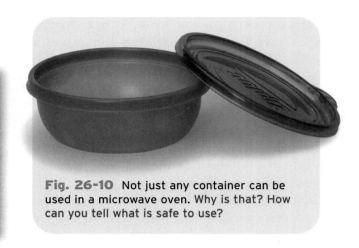

Fig. 26-10 Not just any container can be used in a microwave oven. Why is that? How can you tell what is safe to use?

Techniques for Microwaving

Due to the way microwaves favor some food molecules over others, certain techniques are particularly important for thorough, even cooking. Some general principles are described here. A good microwave recipe gives specific instructions on how to use the oven to prepare a particular food.

Food Placement

Food should be arranged to let microwaves enter from as many sides as possible. A ring is the most effective shape. You can mold meatloaf into a ring or make a circle of whole potatoes, end to end. Leave space between them to allow better microwave penetration.

As a rule, food in the center of the oven cooks more slowly. Arrange food like the spokes of a wheel, with the thickest or toughest parts toward the outside and the thinnest or most tender parts toward the center. See **Fig. 26-11.** Asparagus spears, for example, would be placed in a dish with stalks pointing outward and the tips in the center. Some recipes call for rearranging the food partway through cooking.

Covering Food

Covering helps foods retain moisture as well as cook more evenly. It also keeps them from spattering in the oven. The kind of cover you use depends on the results you want.

- **Paper towels.** Paper towels absorb excess moisture. When you heat breads and sandwiches, keep them from getting soggy by wrapping them in paper towels. Choose paper towels labeled "microwave-safe." Other towels may contain synthetic fibers that could melt.
- **Wax paper and cooking parchment.** Wax paper and silicone-coated parchment paper retain heat while allowing some moisture to escape. They are sometimes specified for microwaving commercially frozen entrées.
- **Plastic wrap.** Plastic wrap is best for holding in moisture. It is used for foods that may dry out, such as casseroles, or to keep liquids from evaporating. Use only microwave-safe plastic wrap, never plastic storage bags or other wrappers.

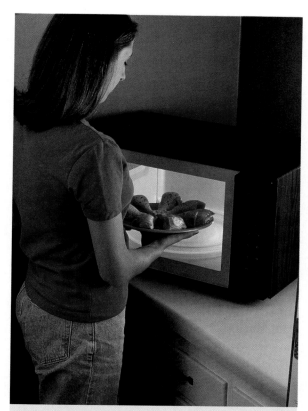

Fig. 26-11 This food was arranged in a particular pattern for a reason. Can you explain what it is?

Cover the container loosely or slit the wrap so steam can escape. Keep the plastic from touching the food to prevent chemical contamination. Some plastic wrap calls for at least 1 inch of space between food and plastic.

Foods may also be covered with an inverted plate or a loose-fitting glass or plastic lid. Tight-fitting lids, however, may cause the contents to erupt. Remember too that heat and steam build under any type of cover. Remove a cover with a potholder or an oven mitt, tilting the cover away from you to shield against escaping steam.

Stirring, Rotating, and Turning

Microwaves may not be distributed evenly throughout the oven. To compensate, most ovens have turntables that rotate food as it cooks. Even so, it's often helpful to stir or turn foods, usually halfway through cooking. Turn dense foods over with tongs. To rotate a pan by hand, grasp it with a potholder and turn it half way.

Cooking Times

In microwave recipes you'll probably see two kinds of time: microwave time and standing time. Each is important.

Microwave time is the actual time the food cooks with microwave energy. Most recipes give a range of time, such as 2 to 2½ minutes. Check the food after the shorter time. Continue microwaving if necessary, but beware: food overcooks quickly in a microwave oven, turning hard or tough.

Don't be surprised if food is slightly undercooked even after the maximum time. Cooking is completed by the built-up heat in a food during **standing time**, as molecules continue to vibrate until they lose energy and the food starts to cool. To retain heat and continue cooking, let food stand on a potholder on a countertop or other solid surface. It should be covered, even if uncovered during microwave time.

To be sure that meat, poultry, fish, and casseroles are thoroughly cooked, use an instant-read food thermometer after the standing time. Insert the thermometer in several different areas to check for cold spots, which may result from uneven cooking.

Getting the Most from a Microwave Oven

As in conventional ovens, built-up dried food absorbs energy in microwave ovens, reducing cooking power. Clean the microwave oven regularly, wiping the interior with a clean, wet dishcloth and drying thoroughly. Use a mild detergent if needed, never an abrasive cleanser. Keep the door seal clean so the door shuts tightly. Check the owner's manual for other care directions to follow.

These ovens also have some particular maintenance needs. Never turn on an empty oven. The accumulated microwaves could cause damage. Don't attach kitchen magnets, which can affect the oven's electronic controls.

Microwave leakage from a properly used and cared for oven is very rare. If this is a concern, however, the manufacturer or the state health department can explain how to have the oven tested by a qualified service. Leakage meters for home use are available but generally not reliable.

Although microwave ovens are standard equipment in many kitchens, adjusting to their speed and method of cooking may involve some trial and error. A good, general microwave cookbook can teach basic techniques and help you know what results to expect. As you grow familiar with microwave recipes, you can try adapting some conventional ones, making your oven and your recipe files more useful. See **Fig. 26-12**.

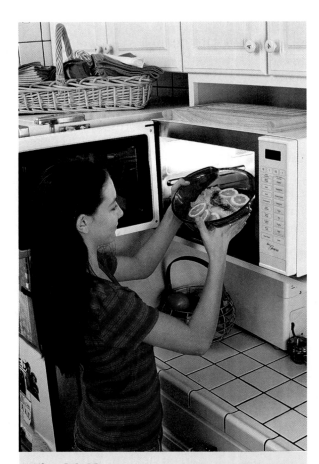

Fig. 26-12 In many homes, the microwave oven comes in handy for reheating foods, but it can be used in other ways too. What are some ideas?

Radio Show Host

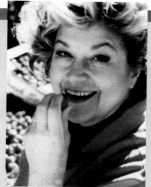

LYNNE ROSSETTO KASPER: What does food mean to you? For Lynne Rossetto Kasper, food has too many meanings to be explored in a lifetime. She has tried—as author, educator, historian, and talk show host—only to discover, "You will never know it all."

Feasting on Food Lore. Growing up in an Italian family, Lynne was fascinated by food early on. Even then, she found traditional food careers lacking. "No one I knew worked in food as I envisioned working in food. Everything intrigued me, from hands-on work, to theory, to history, to anthropology." She satisfied this wide-ranging interest with an equally varied education. She studied language, theatre, and chemistry in college; practiced culinary techniques in cooking school; and learned to cut beef from her butcher.

By the late 1960s, Lynne had braided such diverse strands of schooling into a career as a cooking instructor and writer in New York City. In 1976, she moved to Denver, Colorado. There she opened a cooking school that became the largest in the state.

In 1981, her husband's job took them to Europe. "The experience changed my work dramatically," she recalls. "At last I had time to explore the connection between food and cultures, why food changes from valley to valley, and what shapes its future." Ten years of research and talking to farmers, artisan bakers, scientists, and artists produced her first book, *The Splendid Table: Recipes from Emilia Romagna, the Heartland of Northern Italian Food.* The book is the only one to earn Cookbook of the Year awards from both the James Beard Foundation and the International Association of Culinary Professionals.

Spreading the Table. In 1995, Lynne's career path took another tailor-made turn: her show, "The Splendid Table," produced and distributed by American Public Media, debuted on National Public Radio. The program examines food in all its facets. A food writer's discovery of a humble, back-roads pie shop might be followed by a physicist explaining the structural similarities between the universe and milk foam on Italian coffee. Listeners' calls on far-ranging food topics are a favorite feature. In between are consumer tips, humorous commentaries—and even recipes.

Some people might think that a subject as visual as food and cooking would be limited by radio. Lynne finds the medium ideal. On radio, "we can take you to places, create a picture and flavor sensation in ways a visual medium rarely does. We are about imagination. As for communicating taste, just ask our listeners. Their main complaint is not being able to concentrate on driving because we make them so hungry."

In a way, "The Splendid Table" is one more vehicle to carry Lynne's advice on appreciating food and life, the message she continues to promote: "Get the broadest education possible. Chemistry, the arts, languages, and history are all going to feed you for the rest of your life."

On-line Connections

1. To learn more about topics in this article, search the Internet for these key words: The Splendid Table; artisan baking; Emilia Romagna.

2. To learn about related careers, search the Internet for these key words: culinary historian; restaurant reviewer.

Summarize Your Reading

▶ Food is cooked through the transfer of heat in three main ways: conduction, convection, and radiation.

▶ Such food factors as density, shape and size, and amount of food all affect cooking rates.

▶ Foods can be cooked by many different methods. These different methods affect food's appearance, taste, texture, and nutritional value.

▶ In microwaving, foods cook from energy in the form of electrical waves, so foods retain more nutrients.

Check Your Knowledge

1. What happens when heat is added to food for cooking?

2. Compare heat transfer by **conduction**, **convection**, and **radiation**.

3. Describe the combination of heat transfer that bakes a cake.

4. How do density, shape and size, and amount affect cooking rates?

5. What is **moist-heat cooking**, and how is it used in cooking?

6. What is the difference between boiling and simmering water?

7. **CRITICAL THINKING** After boiling rice for a dish, a beginning cook wondered why it didn't turn out right. What could go wrong and why?

8. What advantages does steaming vegetables have over boiling or simmering them?

9. What are the benefits of pressure cooking?

10. List the steps to follow when braising meat in the oven.

11. What are the effects of cooking food in oil or melted fat?

12. What is **smoking point**? Why shouldn't foods be cooked above the smoking point?

13. Compare frying and sautéing.

14. Why is pan-broiling hamburgers considered to be cooking with fat even though no oil is added to the pan?

15. Compare deep-fat frying and stir-frying.

16. What is **dry-heat cooking**? Give examples of the methods.

17. What are tips to follow when broiling foods?

18. What are possible health risks of eating grilled foods? What precautions can be taken?

19. How does a microwave oven cook food?

20. What problem can occur when baking a potato in a microwave oven? How can the problem be avoided?

21. Why should you only use microwave-safe cookware in a microwave oven?

22. How should you arrange food in a microwave oven?

23. What is the difference between **microwave time** and **standing time**?

24. What can you do to take care of a microwave oven? Why is this necessary?

Apply Your Learning

1. **Heat Transfer Graphic.** Draw a graphic or make a model that shows the three methods of heat transfer. Explain how they differ.

2. **SCIENCE Effects on Color.** Conduct a cooking experiment with fresh broccoli to test color change, using different cooking methods and times. Chart the results. Which methods preserve color best?

3. **Cooking Methods.** Find eight recipes that use different cooking methods. Choose two to describe to the class.

4. **SCIENCE Microwave-Safe.** Conduct careful experiments with available kitchen equipment to see which are safe for use in a microwave oven. Explain your conclusions to the class.

5. **Microwave Cooking.** Change a recipe so it can be partly or fully prepared in a microwave oven. Predict results. Prepare the recipe and compare your predictions to actual results.

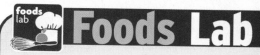

Foods Lab

Microwave Recipes

Procedure: Find a recipe that gives directions for both microwave cooking and another cooking method. Prepare the recipe twice, using both cooking methods. Evaluate the finished products for taste, appearance, and texture.

Analyzing Results

❶ How was using the microwave recipe more convenient than the alternate method? How was it less convenient, if at all?

❷ Compare the finished products for appearance, taste, and texture. Which was more appealing? What would you do differently for either method?

❸ Do you think the recipe is a good choice for microwave cooking? Why or why not?

Food Science Experiment

Browning Foods

Objective: To compare methods for browning foods (the Maillard reaction).

Procedure:

1. Weigh a 4-ounce portion of ground beef. Shape the beef into a patty ½ inch thick.

2. Prepare a skillet, using the method assigned to you.
   Method 1: Do not preheat skillet. Cook with low heat.
   Method 2: Do not preheat skillet. Cook with medium heat.
   Method 3: Preheat skillet over low heat for one minute. Cook with low heat.

Method 4: Preheat skillet over medium heat for one minute. Cook with medium heat.

3. Cook the patty as follows: Place the patty in the skillet. Cook for 3 minutes. Turn the patty and cook until the internal temperature reaches 160°F.

Analyzing Results

❶ Compare patties on appearance, texture, and taste. Which method browned the beef best? What factors seemed to affect this outcome?

❷ How did browning, or lack of it, affect the texture and taste of each patty?

❸ Do you think the results would be the same when cooking potatoes? Pancakes? Why or why not?

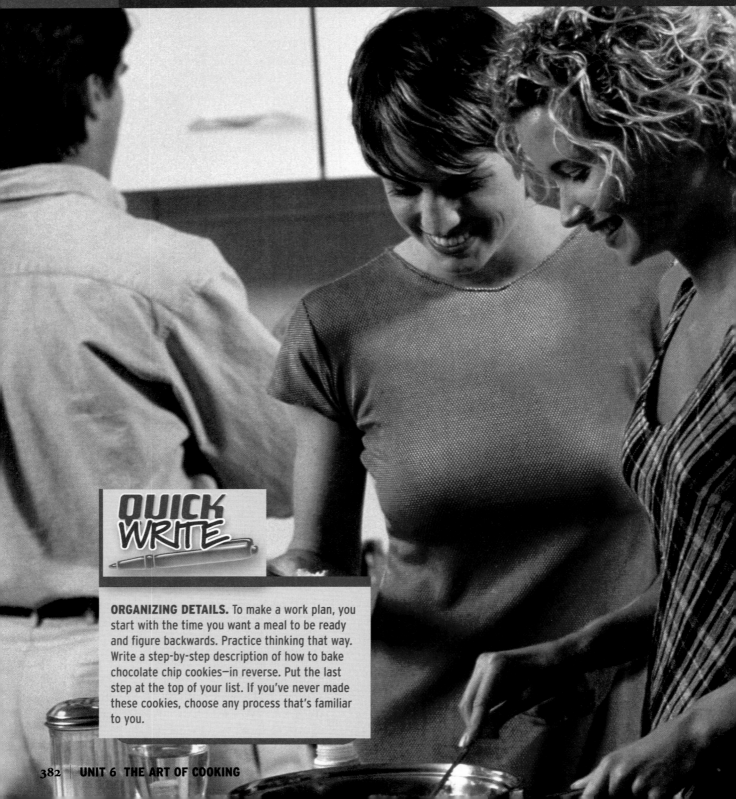

QUICK WRITE

ORGANIZING DETAILS. To make a work plan, you start with the time you want a meal to be ready and figure backwards. Practice thinking that way. Write a step-by-step description of how to bake chocolate chip cookies—in reverse. Put the last step at the top of your list. If you've never made these cookies, choose any process that's familiar to you.

Objectives

▶ Explain how to create a timetable and a work plan.

▶ Develop a work plan for preparing a meal.

▶ Point out ways to improve efficiency when carrying out food preparation tasks.

▶ Explain how teamwork skills can help people work more effectively in the foods lab and the home kitchen.

Terms

dovetail

pre-preparation

teamwork

timetable

work plan

W HETHER YOU'RE PREPARING A FAMILY dinner or working in the foods lab, timing is usually a concern—as in getting preparation tasks accomplished and all foods ready to eat at the same time. What's the secret to this management feat? It all starts with a plan—a work plan.

THE WORK PLAN

A **work plan** is a list of all the tasks it takes to prepare a meal. The tasks are listed in chronological order based on their starting time. A work plan fits into a larger process that includes reading recipes beforehand, listing the tasks, developing a timetable, making and carrying out the work plan, and evaluation.

Like a meal, a useful work plan starts with a detailed menu. Write down every food you plan to serve. With this, you'll be less likely to leave something out and have to rework the plan. A menu for a Sunday brunch, for example, might look like the one shown in **Fig. 27-1**. With the menu set, you can start on the work plan.

Read Recipes Beforehand

Read the recipes carefully, including instructions on any packaged food you plan to use. Make note of the following:

Fig. 27-1

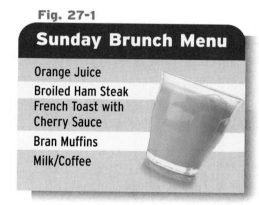

Sunday Brunch Menu

Orange Juice
Broiled Ham Steak
French Toast with Cherry Sauce
Bran Muffins
Milk/Coffee

• The food and equipment you need. Check your supply of ingredients.
• The oven temperature and whether preheating is required.
• The cooking time for each food.
• The food preparation techniques to use. Consider your skill at each one.

List the Tasks

Begin by listing the tasks involved in preparing each recipe. Then write down other jobs, such as setting the table and gathering food and equipment. As you identify each task, look for ways to speed and simplify the work. Ask the following:

- Could any food products or equipment save some effort? Would a different cooking method be more efficient?
- Can any foods be prepared safely ahead of time? A dessert might be baked a day in advance, for instance.
- Can any steps be done as pre-preparation? **Pre-preparation** includes tasks that can be done before you begin to put the recipes together. You might open packages, chop and measure ingredients, and grease baking pans. Having ingredients and equipment ready when you need them saves time. List all pre-preparation tasks together.
- How many tasks can be dovetailed? To **dovetail** means to fit different tasks together to make good use of time. Not every preparation step needs your undivided attention. For example, clean-up tasks can often be dovetailed with others. Fill the sink or dishpan with hot, sudsy water before you start to work. Whenever you have a few free minutes, wash the equipment

you have finished using. Keep a clean, wet dish-cloth handy to wipe up spills as they happen. Put away leftover ingredients after using them.

Develop a Timetable

With all the tasks listed, you can make a timetable. A **timetable** shows the total time needed to complete preparation tasks and the time to start each one. It serves as the basis for your work plan.

To make a timetable, work backwards from the time you want to have everything ready to serve the meal. To serve brunch at 11 a.m., you might plan to have all preparations finished at 10:55 a.m. To prepare a timetable, follow these steps:

1. Divide a sheet of paper into five columns with these headings: Task; Preparation Time; Cooking Time; Total Time; and Starting Time. See **Fig. 27-2**.
2. List tasks in the first column. Group any tasks with optional start times.

Fig. 27-2

Sunday Brunch Timetable

Task	Preparation Time	Cooking Time	Total Time	Starting Time
Tasks with Optional Start Times				
Set table.	10 min.	--	10 min.	To be decided
Gather food and equipment.	10 min.	--	10 min.	To be decided
Pre-preparation: Open packages; measure ingredients; wrap muffins in paper towels and put in microwave; fill coffeemaker; arrange cleanup area.	20 min.	--	20 min.	To be decided
Food Preparation and Serving Tasks				
Broil ham steak: Put ham steak on broiler pan and into broiler; set timer to remind.	2 min.	13 min.	15 min.	10:40 a.m.
Prepare French toast: Mix batter; heat skillet; dip bread; fry.	5 min.	15 min.	20 min.	10:35 a.m.
Prepare orange juice: Mix frozen concentrate in pitcher; refrigerate.	5 min.	60 min. (to chill)	65 min.	9:50 a.m.
Prepare cherry sauce: Pour cherries into pan; mix cornstarch and water; stir in and cook.	2 min.	3 min.	5 min.	10:50 a.m.
Warm bran muffins: Start microwave.	--	2 min.	2 min.	10:50 a.m.
Prepare coffee: Turn on coffeemaker.	--	10 min.	10 min.	10:45 a.m.
Serve food on plates in kitchen; pour beverages.	5 min.	--	5 min.	10:55 a.m.

3. Estimate preparation times and write them in the second column. It's better to allow too much time than not enough. Record cooking times in the third column.

4. For each food task, add preparation and cooking times to find the total time needed. Write this in the fourth column. Carry over the times for other jobs from the second column.

5. Determine when you need to start preparing each food by deducting the total time from the time the meal should be ready. Enter this starting time in the last column. As you can see in **Fig. 27-2**, preparing the ham steak for the brunch takes a total of 15 minutes. To be ready at 10:55, it should go on the broiler pan at 10:40 (10:55 − 15 = 10:40). Tasks that can be done ahead or dovetailed need no start time at this point. Instead, choose these times when you make the work plan. For example, table setting might be done while a food bakes.

Make and Carry Out the Work Plan

A work plan organizes information in the "Starting Time" column of the timetable. It's a start-to-finish road map for getting your meal to the table, as shown in **Fig. 27-3**.

To make a work plan, list the tasks in chronological order according to start times. For tasks with optional start times, choose times that fit with other tasks. You might take care of some jobs before getting involved with the cooking or during a lull in the activity. Dovetail tasks when you can. Allow the time needed for each task as you plan, but make logical changes. For instance, in **Fig. 27-3** note when the orange juice will be mixed. Why was this time chosen?

In a more elaborate meal than the brunch, the work plan can be tailored to stagger the timing of different courses. To serve a dessert warm from the oven, your serving time might be 30 minutes later than that of the main course. In fact, the more complicated the meal, the more important a work plan becomes.

With a work plan made, you're ready to carry it out. Before you start to work, gather all the needed equipment, tools, and ingredients. A tray or cart may be helpful for this. Place them near your work area so everything is at hand. While

Fig. 27-3

Work Plan for Sunday Brunch

Time	Task
9:50 a.m.	Mix frozen juice in pitcher; refrigerate.
9:55 a.m.	Set table.
10:05 a.m.	Gather equipment and ingredients.
10:15 a.m.	Do pre-preparation: Open packages; measure ingredients; wrap muffins in paper towels; fill coffeemaker; get cleanup area ready.
10:35 a.m.	Start French toast: Mix batter; heat skillet; dip bread in batter; fry.
10:40 a.m.	Put ham in broiler; set timer.
10:45 a.m.	Start coffee.
10:50 a.m.	Prepare cherry sauce. Finish French toast.
10:50 a.m.	Warm bran muffins in microwave oven.
10:55 a.m.	Put food on plates in kitchen. Pour beverages.
11:00 a.m.	Start brunch.

you work, check off each task as you complete it so no step is left out.

Evaluate the Work Plan

After the meal is over, review your work plan. Ask yourself these questions:

- Did I complete the meal on time?
- Did I feel hurried or pressured at any point? If so, when?
- Was the work plan flexible enough to handle problems?
- Could I have worked more efficiently? How?
- What changes, if any, would I make in the work plan to prepare the same meal again?

TEAMWORK IN THE SCHOOL FOODS LAB

As any coach will tell you, a good team whose members work together can beat a more gifted team whose members do not. Why? It takes organization, cooperation, and communication to bring together each player's individual talents and efforts, especially in a game situation.

Working in the foods lab at school is also a game situation. You and other members of your lab team combine individual efforts to reach one shared goal. You work under the pressure of needing to complete all tasks within a limited period of time. Only with teamwork is success possible. **Teamwork** includes the following:

- **Organizing jobs.** In a foods lab, several people work on different tasks at the same time. An expanded version of the basic work plan is essential to organize their efforts. Team members need to decide not only when each task should start but also who will do it. They need to consider work space and equipment. It may be helpful to use a schedule that has five-minute blocks of time down the left-hand column, with each person's name across the top. This lets all team members know what they and every other person should be doing throughout the lab period.
- **Cooperating.** Team members should be resources for each other. Ask for help if you have a question or problem. In return, be will-

ing to help someone who falls behind or makes a mistake. In either case, keep a sense of humor. Showing respect and using tact also promote a cooperative spirit.
- **Communicating.** Think of the many things you need to communicate in the kitchen. You talk about recipes, warn of potential safety hazards, and update others on progress. Equally important is the communication that occurs later, when you evaluate the preparation process and the finished product. Learning from the experience takes honest and thoughtful discussion. This is especially true if the lab was less than successful. What do you say if the food didn't turn out as expected, if preparations bogged down, or if your team didn't work well together? Do you lay blame, or do you suggest ways to improve your performance next time?
- **Taking responsibility.** Even in a team effort, the outcome ultimately rests on each person doing his or her part. Taking responsibility means learning your job and doing it carefully and efficiently. It means accuracy when preparing a recipe and safety at all times. Carelessness,

Dressing for Work

YOU'VE BEEN LEARNING TO CHOOSE "appropriate" clothing since you were old enough to dress yourself. You base your choice on personal tastes, fashion trends, practicality, and the opinions of others.

Similar standards apply in the work world, although the priorities may be different. Coworkers are team members, and your dress should reflect that.

Like schools, most workplaces have a written or unwritten dress code, rules that describe appropriate clothing. Some work dress codes include a uniform, or clothes of a certain style or color. The more choices you have in dress, the more you need to consider the following:

- **Comfort and safety.** As in the foods lab, many jobs in foods and nutrition, from fast-food fry cook to chemical lab technician, involve physical work and potential hazards. Choose clothes that reduce the risk to you and others.
- **Fitting in.** Dressing in the accepted style shows team spirit. While still at the interview, note what other employees are wearing and plan to dress similarly. In a larger company, consult the human resources department if you're not sure. Otherwise, play it safe until you get a better idea of what's acceptable. Choose something too conservative rather than too showy.

whether measuring flour or mopping a spill, can be costly to the whole team.

Extend the spirit of teamwork to the lab group that follows your own. Leave the lab as you like to find it yourself. Be sure all equipment, appliances, and work surfaces are clean and dry. Return everything to its proper place. Dispose of waste properly. Otherwise, you will slow down the next team. Remember that cleaning as you go makes end-of-class cleanup easier and faster.

TEAMWORK AT HOME

Your home kitchen may not be as busy as your school lab, but the same skills help the work run smoothly. See **Fig. 27-4**. What's more, these qualities can foster a relaxed, enjoyable atmosphere. Teaching a younger brother or sister how to thicken a sauce can build confidence as well as cooking skills. Trying a new recipe may be the start of a family tradition—and the makings of good family memories. Will helping prepare family meals be a chore or a chance to build togetherness? The choice is up to you.

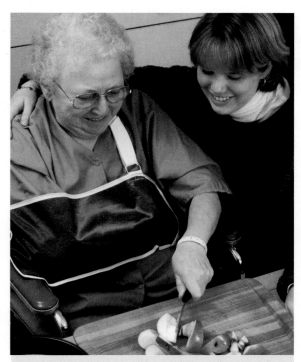

Fig. 27-4 The same teamwork skills you learn in the foods lab can work well for you at home. How do cooperation, communication, and responsibility affect family relationships?

- **Public image.** A business's reputation and relationship with clients is central to its success. When you're on the job, you're expected to promote the company's image. Whether you're selling ice cream cones to families or selling a new brand of ice cream to store owners, dress to meet expectations.

- **Business casual.** Many people have trouble defining this style. Although it has become common in the workplace, some businesses have moved away from it. Career consultants suggest thinking of the style as "casual for business." Whereas a suit is business formal, business casual might be a collared shirt or

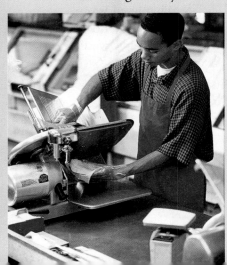

good sweater and a nice pair of slacks or a skirt for women.

Regardless of what you wear, some basic rules of dress apply to any workplace. These include the following:

- Keep all clothing and shoes clean and in good repair.

- Nails and hair should be clean. Neither should interfere with your ability to do a good job.

- To help advance your career, dress "up." Wear the styles of those who are one position above your own.

Career Connection

Wardrobe watch. Learn the expectations for dress in a foods and nutrition job that interests you. Make sketches or gather photos of this attire, noting how it relates to issues in this article. Share the results in class.

Summarize Your Reading

▶ Developing a work plan helps a cook accomplish tasks so that all foods are ready at the same time when preparing a meal.

▶ A work plan for cooking a meal includes a list of tasks in the order in which they need to be done.

▶ Writing down a work plan provides a start-to-finish road map for getting a meal on the table.

▶ Dovetailing tasks and looking for shortcuts when cooking can be useful as long as food safety isn't compromised.

▶ Teamwork is important when sharing the kitchen with other cooks to prepare a meal.

Check Your Knowledge

1. What is a **work plan**?

2. List the five steps included in a work plan.

3. **CRITICAL THINKING** Why is it important to read recipes before you start to prepare dishes?

4. Why might you want to make a dessert the day before it will be served with a meal?

5. What tasks would be examples of **pre-preparation**?

6. What does **dovetailing** tasks mean?

7. How could you save time when measuring flour, sugar, and shortening for a cake?

8. What is the basic way to make a **timetable** for preparation tasks?

9. What are the five basic components in a timetable for cooking a meal?

10. **CRITICAL THINKING** Why doesn't setting the table have a specific start time in a timetable for meal preparation?

11. When could the table be set as part of a work plan?

12. **CRITICAL THINKING** Why do you suppose one of the last tasks on the work plan for the Sunday brunch menu is to warm the bran muffins?

13. **CRITICAL THINKING** Why is a work plan especially useful when preparing an elaborate meal with several courses?

14. How can evaluating your meal plan after the meal is over be helpful?

15. When evaluating a work plan, what questions should you ask yourself?

16. Why is **teamwork** important in the school foods lab?

17. List the four skills that are part of teamwork.

18. Why is it important to organize jobs in the school foods lab?

19. What are signs of a cooperative spirit?

20. Why does much of the learning in a school foods lab take place during the evaluation?

21. **CRITICAL THINKING** What would your feelings be about a team member who does not take responsibility seriously? How would you react?

22. What are the benefits of using teamwork to prepare foods at home?

Apply Your Learning

1. **Pre-Preparation Tasks.** Plan menus and locate recipes for the three meals in one day. Study these and list specific pre-preparation tasks for each meal and when the tasks could be done.

2. **LANGUAGE ARTS** **Skits.** Create and perform a short skit for the class on one of these topics: a) team members in the foods lab disagree on who should do what tasks; b) a team member wastes time instead of doing assigned tasks; c) team members disagree on how a cooking task should be done; d) one team member works much more slowly than the others; e) in a busy family, one member feels overburdened with all meal preparation. Include a resolution to the problem.

3. **Evaluation Form.** Develop an evaluation form to use after classroom cooking labs. Focus on work plan effectiveness and teamwork skills.

Foods Lab

Implementing a Work Plan
Procedure: With a team of students, plan a lunch menu to prepare and eat together. Gather appropriate recipes. Create a timetable and work plan for the meal. Then prepare, serve, and eat the meal.

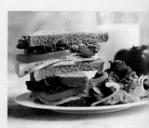

Analyzing Results
❶ How were tasks dovetailed, if at all?
❷ What meal preparation problems did you have? How were they resolved?
❸ Evaluate the effectiveness of the work plan.
❹ Evaluate teamwork skills, including an analysis of task organization, cooperation, communication, and responsibility.
❺ What improvements would you suggest for next time?

Food Science Experiment

Surface Area and Cooking Rate

Objective: To observe how a food's surface area affects its cooking rate.

Procedure:
1. Cube a potato and then weigh it. Divide the potato cubes into two samples of equal weight.
2. Dice one sample of potato.
3. Bring 1 cup of water to a boil in each of two equal-sized saucepans. Add one sample to each pan.
4. Test pieces of each sample for doneness at one-minute intervals by inserting a toothpick through the center. Record the degree of doneness at each interval. For example, record: uncooked, slightly tender, or partly cooked. Use the same wording for each sample.
5. When the toothpick easily pierces the pieces, remove that sample from the heat. Record the total time needed to cook the potato in each sample.

Analyzing Results
❶ Which sample cooked more quickly? What explains this result?
❷ Suppose that your work plan for a meal is on a very tight schedule. How can the knowledge from this experiment be useful?

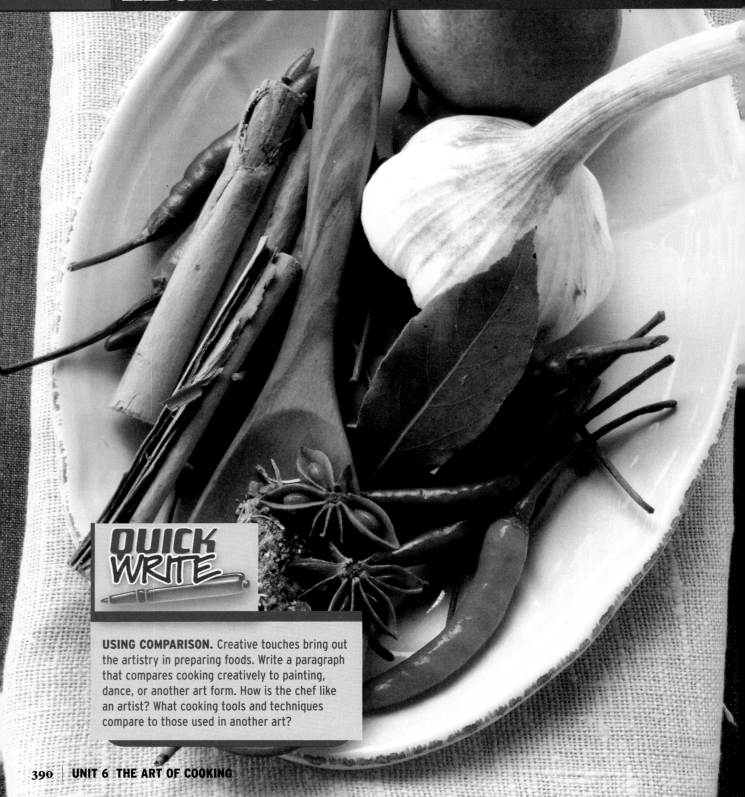

CHAPTER
28 Creative Additions

QUICK WRITE

USING COMPARISON. Creative touches bring out the artistry in preparing foods. Write a paragraph that compares cooking creatively to painting, dance, or another art form. How is the chef like an artist? What cooking tools and techniques compare to those used in another art?

Objectives

▶ Compare characteristics of different herbs and spices.

▶ Explain how to use, buy, and store herbs and spices.

▶ Choose seasonings that will add desired flavors to foods.

▶ Use garnishes and other techniques to make dishes appealing.

▶ Suggest creative ways to present foods as gifts.

Terms

bouquet garni
condiments
garnish
herbs
seasoning blends
spices

CHILDREN ARE OFTEN TOLD "DON'T PLAY with your food," yet the same creative spirit is an asset to someone with growing kitchen skills, knowledge, and food appreciation. With creativity, you can add appeal to the most ordinary meal—without making faces in the mashed potatoes.

SEASONINGS

Seasonings are ingredients that are used in small amounts to flavor food. In recipes, they're typically the smallest items in quantity, yet they make a big difference. Salt has been the most popular seasoning worldwide since ancient times. Exploring the incredible variety of other choices not only opens doors to creative cooking but also avoids problems associated with high-sodium diets.

Herbs and Spices

The words *herbs* and *spices* are often used interchangeably, but there is a difference. **Herbs** are the flavorful leaves and stems of soft, succulent (fleshy and moisture-rich) plants that grow in a temperate climate. Both fresh and dried herbs are available. See **Fig. 28-1** on pages 392 and 393.

Spices are the dried buds, bark, fruits, seeds, stems, and roots of aromatic plants and trees that grow in tropical or subtropical regions. Most are sold whole or ground. A few, such as ginger root, are also sold fresh. See **Fig. 28-2** on page 394.

Seasoning blends are convenient combinations of herbs and spices. A **bouquet garni** is a bundled or bagged blend that flavors foods while cooking and is later removed. Popular seasoning blends include the following:

- **Curry powders.** Blends of as many as 20 herbs and spices in different combinations. Cinnamon, ginger, and various peppers are commonly featured. Curries are essential in Indian cooking.
- **Five-spice powder.** A staple in Chinese and Japanese cuisine. It contains equal parts of ground cinnamon, cloves, fennel seed, star anise, and Szechuan peppercorns.
- **Chili powder.** A mix of ground, dried chiles, garlic, oregano, cumin, coriander, and cloves. It's the hallmark of Tex-Mex dishes and, of course, chili.

Using Herbs and Spices

Although certain herbs and spices are often used with specific foods, no combination is right or wrong. Creativity, after all, includes seasoning foods to your liking. Some guidelines, however, are worth remembering:

- Unless otherwise noted, recipes use dried herbs.
- Begin with a few of the basic herbs and spices. Once you learn how to use them, you can add others.
- Herbs and spices vary in strength and so are used in different amounts. As a rule, start with ¼ teaspoon of dried herbs and spices for every four servings. You can always add more if desired.

- Herbs are more potent dried than fresh. Generally, 1 tablespoon of fresh herbs equals 1 teaspoon of dried, crushed herbs or ¼ teaspoon of ground herbs.
- Wash fresh herbs before using them. Shake off the excess water. Snip them with scissors or chop them by hand. If the stems are tough, use only the leaves.
- To release flavors, crush dried leaf herbs, such as oregano and rosemary, before adding them to foods.
- In hot foods, add herbs and spices at least 10 minutes before the end of the cooking time to

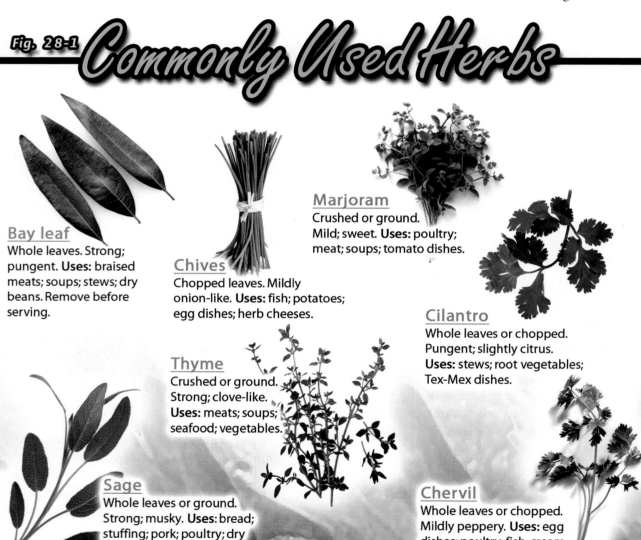

Fig. 28-1 *Commonly Used Herbs*

Bay leaf
Whole leaves. Strong; pungent. **Uses:** braised meats; soups; stews; dry beans. Remove before serving.

Chives
Chopped leaves. Mildly onion-like. **Uses:** fish; potatoes; egg dishes; herb cheeses.

Marjoram
Crushed or ground. Mild; sweet. **Uses:** poultry; meat; soups; tomato dishes.

Cilantro
Whole leaves or chopped. Pungent; slightly citrus. **Uses:** stews; root vegetables; Tex-Mex dishes.

Thyme
Crushed or ground. Strong; clove-like. **Uses:** meats; soups; seafood; vegetables.

Sage
Whole leaves or ground. Strong; musky. **Uses:** bread; stuffing; pork; poultry; dry beans.

Chervil
Whole leaves or chopped. Mildly peppery. **Uses:** egg dishes; poultry; fish; cream soups; spring vegetables.

let the heat activate their oils. Add herbs no more than 30 minutes before serving. They lose flavor if overcooked.

- In cold mixtures, such as a salad dressing, add herbs and spices 30 minutes to several hours before serving so that flavors can be released.

Buying and Storing Dried Herbs and Spices

Because dried herbs and spices are used sparingly, consider buying them in bulk. That way you can buy only as much as you can use in a short time.

Light, air, and heat degrade the oils that carry flavor in herbs and spices. Store the dried forms in a cool, dark place in tightly closed, opaque containers. Mark containers with the purchase date. Dried, crushed herbs keep their flavor for about six months if properly stored. To test for freshness, rub a bit of the herb in the palm of your hand with your thumb for five to ten seconds. If the aroma is weak, the herb is probably too old to use. It might impart a bitter flavor.

Ground spices hold their flavor for about a year. Whole spices last much longer, some for several years.

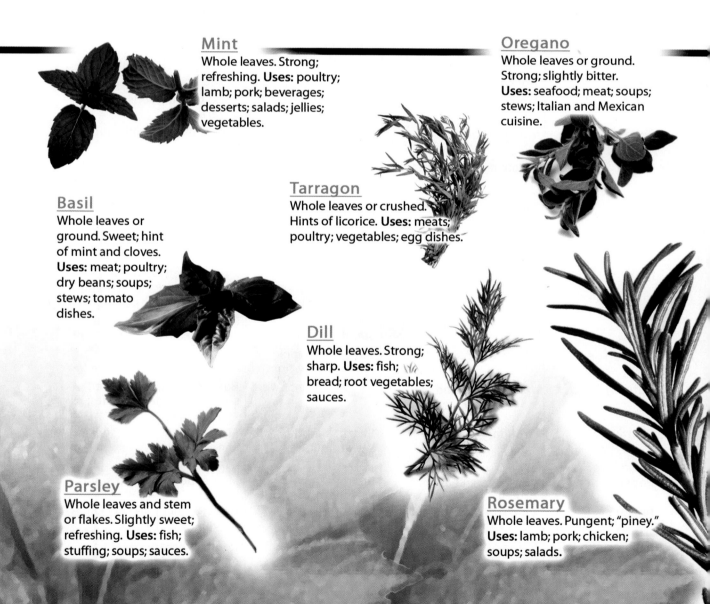

Mint
Whole leaves. Strong; refreshing. **Uses:** poultry; lamb; pork; beverages; desserts; salads; jellies; vegetables.

Oregano
Whole leaves or ground. Strong; slightly bitter. **Uses:** seafood; meat; soups; stews; Italian and Mexican cuisine.

Basil
Whole leaves or ground. Sweet; hint of mint and cloves. **Uses:** meat; poultry; dry beans; soups; stews; tomato dishes.

Tarragon
Whole leaves or crushed. Hints of licorice. **Uses:** meats; poultry; vegetables; egg dishes.

Dill
Whole leaves. Strong; sharp. **Uses:** fish; bread; root vegetables; sauces.

Parsley
Whole leaves and stem or flakes. Slightly sweet; refreshing. **Uses:** fish; stuffing; soups; sauces.

Rosemary
Whole leaves. Pungent; "piney." **Uses:** lamb; pork; chicken; soups; salads.

Fig. 28-2

Commonly Used Spices			
Spice	**Forms**	**Flavor**	**Uses**
Allspice	Whole berries or ground	Sweet; slightly peppery	Meats; baked goods; Caribbean cuisines
Anise seed	Whole or ground	Similar to licorice	Baked goods; fish; Middle Eastern and Indian cuisines
Caraway seed	Whole or ground	Slightly sweet; tangy	Breads; soups; German cuisine
Cardamom	Whole seed or ground	Slightly sweet; lemony	Baked goods; cheese dishes; British cuisine
Cayenne	Ground	Pungent; very hot	Meats; poultry; egg dishes; Cajun cuisine
Celery seed	Whole or ground	Slightly bitter; similar to celery	Fish; soups; salads
Chili powder	Ground	Hot; peppery	Meats; stews; salsas
Chiles	Whole or ground	Mildly to very hot	Meats; stews; salsas
Cinnamon	Stick or ground	Warm; sweet	Baked goods; beverages
Cloves	Whole or ground	Pungent; slightly hot	Pork; baked goods; beverages
Coriander seed	Whole or ground	Musky; slightly citrus	Meats; baked goods; Indian cuisine
Cumin	Whole seed or ground	Musky; slightly bitter	Legumes; soups; rice; vegetables; Middle Eastern, Asian, and Tex-Mex cuisines
Dill seed	Whole	Sharp; slightly bitter	Seafood; bread; salad and slaw dressings
Fennel seed	Whole, cracked, or ground	Similar to licorice	Seafood; breads; pasta sauces
Garlic	Whole cloves, minced, ground, or flakes	Sharp, pungent when raw; sweet, nutty when cooked	Meats; poultry; soup; tomato dishes; Italian and Mediterranean cuisines
Ginger	Whole root or ground	Sweet; hot; pungent	Baked goods; vegetables; Asian cuisines
Mustard seed	Whole or ground	Pungent; moderately to very hot	Egg dishes; salad dressings; sauces
Nutmeg	Whole or ground	Mellow; nutty; sweet	Baked goods; milk-based soups and sauces; fruits; vegetables
Paprika	Ground	Sharp; slightly sweet; moderately hot	Fish; poultry; egg dishes; cheese dishes
Pepper	Whole, cracked, or ground	Sharp; tangy; moderately to very hot	Meats; poultry; fish; soups; sauces
Poppy seed	Whole	Mild; nutty	Breads; pasta dishes; salad dressings
Sesame seed	Whole	Mild; nutty	Poultry; breads; pasta dishes; stir-fries

Buying and Storing Fresh Herbs

Fresh herbs are often sold packaged. Look for bright color with no wilting, browning, or damage. They keep for about five days in the refrigerator, wrapped in a slightly damp paper towel and sealed in a plastic bag with the air pressed out. For longer storage, dry or freeze them.

- **To dry fresh herbs.** First, tie them in bunches. Label and hang them in a dry, shaded, well-ventilated area. They should dry within two weeks. To dry herbs in the microwave oven, place them between several layers of paper towels. Microwave on high (100 percent power) for 15 to 30 seconds at a time until they are crumbly.
- **To freeze fresh herbs.** Spread them on a baking sheet in a single layer and freeze overnight. Store in a freezer container for up to a year.

Condiments

Condiments are liquid or semi-liquid accompaniments to food. They also make imaginative seasonings. A tomato-based ketchup can add spicy sweetness to a recipe. Salsa, popular in Tex-Mex cuisine, is made with tomatoes, chili peppers, and seasonings chosen to give the desired degree of heat. Other condiments offer a range of flavor possibilities. How would you use the following condiments to liven up a dish?

- **Mustard.** Ground or powdered mustard seeds are combined with vinegar and various seasonings in this tangy blend. Relatively mild American mustards are bright yellow from the spice turmeric. Darker French and Chinese varieties, plus many variations, range from spicy hot to honey sweetened.
- **Sauces.** Sauces are zesty, sometimes intensely flavored, liquids. Hot pepper sauce is made from chili peppers and is so fiery that it's doled out in drops. Worcestershire (WUS-tuhr-shir) sauce combines vinegar, soy sauce, garlic, molasses, and a tropical fruit called the tamarind. Soy and tamari (tuh-MAHR-ee) sauces are made from fermented soybeans. Soy sauce has a sharp, pungent flavor; tamari is thicker and mellower.
- **Vinegar.** Souring or fermenting cider or wine creates mildly acidic liquids called vinegars. Colors and flavors vary, depending on the base. Distilled white vinegar, a product of white grapes, has a sour, pungent taste. Rice vinegar, used in Asian cooking, adds a slight sweetness and golden color to recipes. Balsamic (bawl-SA-mik) vinegar is aged in wood barrels for years, giving it a sweet, pungent flavor and dark color. Herb vinegars are flavored by soaking various herbs in the vinegar.

GARNISHES

What seasonings are to the taste buds, a garnish is to the eye. A **garnish** is a small, decorative piece of food used to enhance the appearance of a dish. Color, shape, or texture is creatively used as a finishing touch. See **Fig. 28-3.**

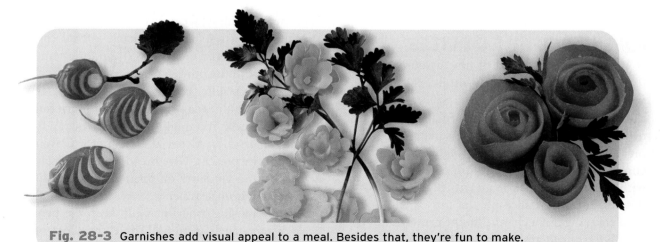

Fig. 28-3 Garnishes add visual appeal to a meal. Besides that, they're fun to make.

Making Garnishes

Fruits and vegetables are the most common garnishes. With some practice, you might create some eye-catching effects.

- **Carrot curls.** Peel carrots. With a vegetable peeler, cut carrots into paper-thin strips lengthwise. Roll up and fasten with a wooden pick. Chill in ice water. Remove picks before using.
- **Radish roses.** Remove the stem. Cut thin petals around the edges. Chill in ice water to open and make crisp.
- **Citrus twists.** Slice unpeeled orange or lemon crosswise. Cut the slice just to the center, separate, and twist.
- **Celery twirls.** Cut celery stalks into 3-inch lengths. Slit both ends into narrow strips, but do not cut through the center. Chill in ice water.

Spur-of-the-moment garnishes can be equally appealing. It takes only a second to hook a candy cane over the rim of a mug of hot cocoa. You can frame a sandwich on a bed of lettuce with cheese strips at the corners. Try floating croutons, chopped fresh herbs, a spoonful of yogurt, or a sprinkling of cheese in a bowl of soup. Any ingredient in a salad can also serve as a garnish: olives, grapes, chopped nuts, cherry tomatoes, croutons, wheat germ, tomato wedges, or rings of green bell pepper or red onion.

Simple or elaborate, a garnish should complement—not compete with—a dish. It should be small in comparison to the food and serving container. Food and garnish should be compatible in color and flavor.

FRESHENING UP FAVORITES

When people get tired of how a room looks, they often rearrange the furniture. The same approach might work when a favorite recipe starts to seem stale. Vary the presentation. Instead of serving a bowl of chili and a square of cornbread, spread the cornbread batter in muffin cups, top with the cooked chili, and bake. Garnish with shredded cheese or green bell pepper. For dessert, cut a thin slice off the top of an angel food cake, dig out a channel in the center, and fill it with fresh fruit and chunks of cake.

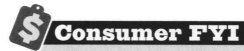

Consumer FYI

Cookie cutter art. Cookie cutters do more than cut cookie dough. They can double as an inexpensive decorator kit.

- **Baked goods.** Cut shapes from the top crust of two-crust pies to suit the season. Scatter autumn leaf shapes over a pumpkin pie. You can even custom-cut store-bought, refrigerated, biscuit dough.
- **Side dishes.** Stamp shapes from pieces of fruits, vegetables, and other ingredients. A thick slice of tomato becomes a red heart in a heart-healthy salad. Cheddar cheese diamonds dress up a mound of mashed potatoes.
- **Sandwiches.** Sandwiches don't have to be square. Crescent moon sandwiches are more appealing than rectangles. For a sunburst effect, cut sandwich meat into stars.

Do you have a pastry bag to decorate cakes? Use it to swirl mashed potatoes into a fluffy basket filled with colorful cooked broccoli. Ring a roast with a decorative border of mashed sweet potato. For snacks or appetizers, pipe a creamy tuna salad or seasoned cheese spread into celery sticks or atop crackers or bread rounds.

FOOD AS GIFTS

For many people, homemade food is the perfect example of a gift from the heart. Cakes, cookies, and pies are often given at holidays and birthdays. Homemade breads and jams help make new neighbors feel welcome.

Making a casserole or preparing a meal can ease the physical and emotional strain for a family dealing with the burden of illness.

As with any gift, the wrapping can show as much thoughtfulness as the food. Aluminum foil has a festive look. You might find cookie or candy tins at garage sales. A special container can even be part of the present. Give bread baked in a clay flowerpot to a gardener or small cakes made in jelly jars to a home canner.

When choosing food for a gift, keep the person's dietary needs in mind. The extra effort of finding a diabetic or low-fat recipe makes the gift even more meaningful.

Career Pathways

Graphic Designer

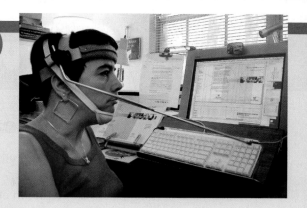

LEIGH-ANNE TOMPKINS: Leigh-Anne Tompkins knows what it takes to be a successful graphic designer: first, a college education; second, patience; but also creativity, networking, meeting deadlines, and energetic self-promotion. What it doesn't take is a fully functioning body. One working foot and a head for visuals do fine.

Toehold on Technology. Leigh-Anne has cerebral palsy. The disorder, which affects muscle coordination, has impaired her hearing and speech and left her limbs mostly unresponsive. At age nine, however, she discovered a flair for drawing—with her good right foot. Later, her brother Eric, a computer engineer, helped her learn her way around computers. Vocational rehabilitation engineers helped her acquire and use assistive technology, including a head stylus, which is a headband with an attached pointer that serves as Leigh-Anne's typing hand. Leigh-Anne herself thought of some adaptations. She turned a trackball shaped like a billiard ball into a mouse alternative by placing it on the floor beneath her reliable right foot.

Career plans started to fall into place when Leigh-Anne entered the University of North Florida. "I didn't know what graphic design was until my counselor in college suggested it," she recalls. "My professor, Fred Elliott, was my mentor, and he actually taught me the real world of graphic design." She graduated in 1992 with a bachelor's degree in the field, bolstered by certification courses in various graphic design programs. A former schoolmate, who is senior graphics designer for a large international corporation, helped Leigh-Anne land her first big job: a multimedia promotional campaign for the firm, designing brochures, videos, Web sites, and more. Equally important, Leigh-Anne says, her friend

"gave me a chance to teach her co-workers that my disability doesn't stop me."

Visualizing Goals. Eventually, Leigh-Anne set up shop as Graphics Afoot Studio Design, in Jacksonville, Florida. Today, clients include communications giant AT&T and health insurer Blue Cross and Blue Shield of Florida. She also designs menus for local, chef-owned restaurants. The goal here, as Leigh-Anne describes it, is to capture the restaurant's atmosphere in words and images. "One must be concerned with the ambience the owner wishes to portray: whether to be formal or informal; and whether to be serious about the restaurant and menu theme or be light and charming. The menu should reflect the chef, his or her style and panache."

Between projects, Leigh-Anne plans to return to college for her master's degree in computer graphics. The advanced education could open more doors professionally, with the result, she hopes, that "people will think more positively about my work and less negatively about my disability." "Besides," she adds, a master's degree "looks good on your resumé."

On-line Connections

1. To learn more about topics in this article, search the Internet for these key words: graphic designer; cerebral palsy; assistive technology.

2. To learn about related careers, search the Internet for these key words: Web designer; restaurant design.

Summarize Your Reading

▶ Creative use of seasonings adds flavor and appeal to ordinary meals.

▶ Different seasoning blends are staples in ethnic cooking.

▶ Herbs can be purchased fresh, or they can be dried or frozen.

▶ Varying the presentation of foods by using aromatic fruits and vegetables, adding garnishes, and by varying the shape and size of foods can add freshness and appeal.

▶ Foods can be given as gifts by using festive wrappings and unusual containers.

Check Your Knowledge

1. How are **herbs** and **spices** different?

2. What herbs could you use when cooking chicken?

3. What spices are commonly used in Asian dishes?

4. Define and give examples of **seasoning blends**.

5. What herbs and spices might you expect to find in chili powder?

6. As a rule, what amount of dried herbs and spices should a cook add to a dish that serves four people?

7. How do fresh herbs compare to dried herbs in potency?

8. Why should you add herbs no more than 30 minutes before serving?

9. How should you store dried herbs and for how long?

10. How do you test dried herbs for freshness?

11. For how long can ground and whole spices be stored?

12. How should fresh herbs be stored and for how long?

13. Define and give examples of **condiments**.

14. Compare Worcestershire sauce, soy sauce, and tamari sauce.

15. What is the difference between distilled white vinegar, rice vinegar, balsamic vinegar, and herb vinegars?

16. What is a **garnish**?

17. Describe several common garnishes.

18. What guidelines should you follow when choosing a garnish?

19. **CRITICAL THINKING** Think of five of your favorite dishes. Suggest how the foods might be garnished for added visual appeal.

20. What are some homemade food gifts that are suitable for specific occasions?

21. How might you wrap or present food as a gift?

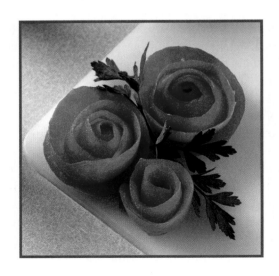

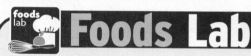
Apply Your Learning

1. **SOCIAL STUDIES** **Salt Research.** Research the history of salt. Make a timeline showing its history and uses.

2. **Demo Area.** Help set up a demonstration area where classmates can see and smell various herbs, spices, and seasoning blends. Choose an herb or spice that is new to you and then find and try a recipe that uses it.

3. **SCIENCE** **Herb Gardening.** Interview an herb gardener. Find out what is needed to grow herbs successfully. Then grow one or more herbs in the classroom. Try freezing and drying them for preservation.

4. **Garnishes.** Find a garnish idea, and demonstrate how to make it.

5. **Fund-Raiser.** Plan a food gift that your class could make and sell as a fund-raiser. For example, you could make and package a valentine cookie for students to buy and give to someone special. Determine all costs to price the item correctly. Project sales carefully so you make a profit.

Foods Lab

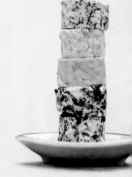

Herb Butters
Procedure: With your lab team, use a variety of herbs and other seasonings, if you wish, to develop a recipe for an herb butter. Work with the recipe in very small quantities, using softened butter or margarine, until the recipe is approved by the team. Keep track of amounts and proportions as you work. Sample the flavors on plain crackers or on pita bread. Then make a batch of the final product to share in a taste test with other lab teams.

Analyzing Results
1. How did your team reach consensus on the recipe? Was compromise needed?
2. Evaluate your final recipe. What improvements, if any, might still be needed?
3. Which herbs do you think made the best herb butters? Why?

Food Science Experiment

Packaging Foods

Objective: To analyze the effects of packaging different foods together.

Procedure:
1. Place half an apple and a graham cracker together in a plastic storage bag. Seal the bag securely.
2. Repeat Step 1 twice, packaging half an apple with a potato chip, and a graham cracker with a potato chip.
3. Leave all three bags on the same counter or table overnight. Then remove the foods and evaluate the results.

Analyzing Results
1. Describe any changes in the foods' appearance, taste, and texture.
2. What components in the foods may have played a role in the changes you noted?
3. Do you think refrigerating the foods would have affected the results? Why or why not?
4. Based on your findings, what advice would you give for packaging different foods for gift giving?

Preserving Food at Home

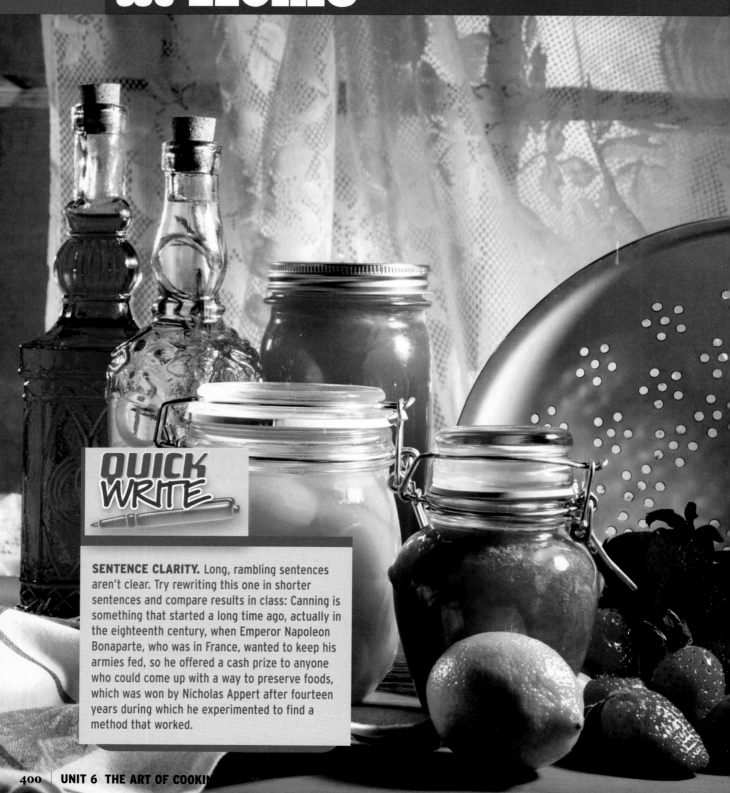

QUICK WRITE

SENTENCE CLARITY. Long, rambling sentences aren't clear. Try rewriting this one in shorter sentences and compare results in class: Canning is something that started a long time ago, actually in the eighteenth century, when Emperor Napoleon Bonaparte, who was in France, wanted to keep his armies fed, so he offered a cash prize to anyone who could come up with a way to preserve foods, which was won by Nicholas Appert after fourteen years during which he experimented to find a method that worked.

AT ONE TIME, IF YOU WANTED CORN OR peaches in the winter, you didn't go to the supermarket. You went to your kitchen pantry. There you found jars or canisters of foods you had "put up," or preserved, during the growing season. To **preserve** is to prepare food in a way that allows it to be safely stored for later use. For most of history, preserving food by canning, freezing, or drying was a do-it-yourself project. For some people, it still is.

PRAISE OF PRESERVING

Today, with grocery store aisles lined with cans, jars, and pouches of foods, why do the work yourself? For many people, preserving offers both fun and savings. Fresh foods in season are often a good value. If you can buy produce at bargain prices from local farmers, an investment in the containers and equipment needed for home preserving may save money over time.

Some people preserve foods they raise themselves. They literally enjoy the fruits (or vegetables) of their labor long after the harvest, along with the satisfaction of knowing that none of the crop was wasted. See **Fig. 29-1**.

Preserving food can be a family affair. A family may work together tending a garden all summer or spend a day picking produce at a local orchard or farm. Like cooking meals, freezing or canning

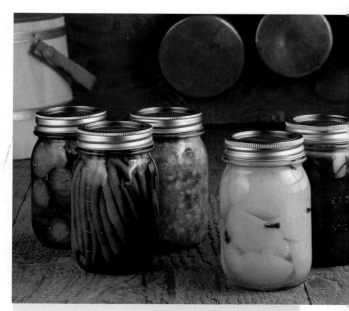

Fig. 29-1 What advantages are there to preserving foods you've grown or purchased at the farmers market?

the food is a chance to grow closer and create memories. Preserving food can also preserve traditions. A recipe for an unusual family favorite like red pepper jam might be handed down for generations.

Preserving food at home can give you more "quality control" over what you eat. You can choose high-quality food and decide whether it will contain salt, sugar, or other additives. Also, if you've created the perfect salsa recipe, you can put up a year's supply in one afternoon.

PREPARING TO PRESERVE

For any preserving project, these guidelines can lead to safe and successful results:

- Decide what foods to preserve, how much, and by what method. Buy only as much as you can prepare in the time available.
- Be sure that any supplies on hand are in usable condition.
- Always use high-quality food: ripe, firm fruit and young, tender vegetables. Look for varieties that are noted for preserving well.
- Choose tested, up-to-date recipes and follow them exactly. See **Fig. 29-2**. Don't take short-cuts or experiment. Get reliable information from a cooperative extension office or Web site.
- Wash food carefully and prepare it according to recipe directions. Keep both cleanliness and food safety in mind.

Fig. 29-2

Try This! **Recipe**

Kiwifruit Leather

Yield	Nutrition Analysis
About 50 servings	*Per Serving:* 100 calories, 0 g total fat, 0 g saturated fat, 0 g trans fat, 0 mg cholesterol, 0 mg sodium, 24 g total carbohydrate, 2 g dietary fiber, 22 g sugars, 0 g protein *Percent Daily Value:* vitamin A 2%, vitamin C 450%, calcium 2%, iron 2%

Ingredients
1 bag of kiwifruit (5 lbs.)
Strained juice of 1½ lemons
3⅔ cups sugar

¾ cup Sure•Jell® Fruit Pectin
 (1 box = about ⅓ cup)
nonstick vegetable spray

Directions
1. Halve each kiwifruit. Scoop out fruit and purée in blender or food processor.
2. On a long table, lay out 3 sheets parchment paper (16 x 24 inches) and lightly spray with nonstick spray.
3. Place kiwifruit and lemon juice in large, heavy, nonreactive pot. Set over medium-high heat.
4. In another bowl, combine sugar and Sure•Jell®. Add to purée and whisk ingredients to combine. Bring mixture to boil while whisking constantly. Continue to boil for 3 minutes.
5. Remove from heat source, and ladle out on prepared parchment paper. Spread with large offset spatula until thin, even, and opaque. Allow to cool and dry overnight. Make sure table is undisturbed and free of insects.
6. Cut into strips of desired size (will feel a little sticky). Roll up, leaving parchment attached for separation and easy peel. Store in heavy, plastic freezer bags.

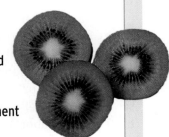

Variation: Cut leather into ravioli shapes and fill with sweetened ricotta cheese.

- Have all equipment and supplies ready before you begin to work with the food.

FREEZING FRUITS AND VEGETABLES

Freezing preserves food at a temperature of 0°F or below. It's the most convenient method and useful for most produce. Exceptions are those foods with high water content, including salad greens and celery. As the water freezes, it expands and explodes the food's cell structure, leaving it soft and soggy when thawed. Frozen tomatoes would be fine for a sauce but less appealing in a salad. The same is true of citrus fruits, although their juices freeze well alone.

Foods must be frozen quickly for the same reason. Slow freezing allows large ice crystals to form, damaging food texture. To promote quick and even chilling, freeze foods in small containers and small batches. Overloading the freezer slows the process.

Fruits and vegetables can be frozen individually on a tray or baking sheet and then packed in containers. This helps retain quality in small, whole foods, such as berries and peas. It makes it easier to remove just the amount needed. Foods can also be frozen directly in containers. Because they freeze as a solid block, this method is convenient when the entire amount will be used at the same time.

Before certain fruits and vegetables can be frozen, enzyme activity must be stopped. Otherwise, color, flavor, and texture suffer. Nutrients are lost. The method used to deactivate enzymes depends on the food.

Freezing Fruits

Prepare the fruit the way you plan to use it—sliced or peeled, for example. Look for information on freezing specific fruits.

To disable enzymes, some fruits need to be treated with a commercial ascorbic acid (vitamin C) mixture. In general, ascorbic acid is either sprinkled on the fruit or added to a syrup. The package gives directions. Apples, apricots, peaches, and nectarines, in particular, need this treatment.

Freeze the fruit with one of these methods:

- For the **sugar-pack method**, toss the fruit in sugar until well coated. Pack into freezer containers. The sugar helps retain the fruit's color and texture and combines with the juice to form a syrup when defrosted.
- To use the **syrup-pack method**, make a syrup by dissolving sugar in water. Pack fruit in freezer containers and cover it with the chilled syrup. Keep the fruit under the syrup with a small piece of crumpled wax paper on top of the fruit.
- The **tray-pack method** works well with blueberries, cranberries, and other fruits that freeze well whole without sugar. Place the prepared fruit on a tray or baking sheet, leaving space between pieces. Cover tightly with aluminum foil and freeze just until frozen. Then pack pieces into freezer containers.
- The **dry-pack method** is for unsweetened fruit. Pack the fruit directly into freezer containers. Small whole fruits work best.

Freezing Vegetables

Except for tomatoes, vegetables require **blanching**, or brief cooking in boiling water, to neutralize enzymes. To blanch vegetables, use 1 gallon of boiling water in a large pot for 1 pound of vegetables. Place the prepared vegetables in a large strainer and immerse them in the water for the time recommended in blanching charts.

When the time is up, remove the strainer of vegetables and plunge it into a large pot of ice water until cool. Add ice cubes as needed to keep the water ice-cold. Drain the vegetables on clean, dry towels. Pat them dry to prevent ice crystals from forming as they freeze. Pack them into freezer containers.

Don't use a microwave oven for blanching. Microwaves do not cook evenly, so they cannot blanch evenly.

Packing and Freezing

When you pack foods, leave a 1-inch space between the food and the lid of the container. Called **headspace**, this area allows for expansion as water in and around the food freezes. If using plastic bags, squeeze out as much air as possible before sealing. Wipe containers clean. Label them with the date, contents, and amount.

Freeze foods as soon as they are packed. Arrange containers in a single layer with plenty of space between them. This promotes air circulation and rapid, even freezing. Don't place food in the freezer door, which tends to be warmer than the rest of the compartment.

In about 24 hours, when the food has frozen, stack the containers close together to save space. So you can find them easily, stack the same kinds of food together.

CANNING FRUITS AND VEGETABLES

Canning is the most demanding preservation method. You need special equipment to pack and process foods at a specific temperature for a specific length of time. These features all aim to destroy microorganisms and enzymes, saving food from spoilage and saving you and your family from foodborne illness. The time, effort, and expense are well invested.

Jars and Lids

Despite the name, foods are canned in jars. Canning jars are strong, with a flat rim and threaded neck that promote an airtight seal with the lid. Jars from mayonnaise, peanut butter, and other commercial products lack these features. Furthermore, only canning jars in perfect condition can be used. Inspect the rim for chips or nicks. Discard any jars with tiny cracks that could fracture when heated.

Canning lids have two metal pieces. The flat top is rimmed with a rubber compound that molds to the jar when processed. The screw band holds it in place. See **Fig. 29-3**. Bands can be reused as long as they remain in good condition, but tops are used only once. Older, porcelain-lined lids and one-piece lids with separate rubber rings should not be used at all.

Just before canning, wash the jars and lids in hot, sudsy water. A dishwasher is convenient for large canning projects. Rinse the jars well. Keep them immersed in clean, hot water until needed.

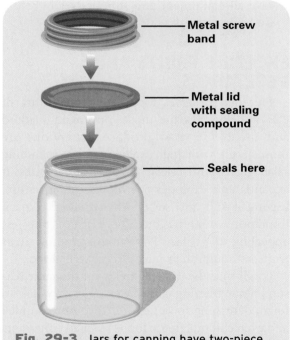

Metal screw band

Metal lid with sealing compound

Seals here

Fig. 29-3 Jars for canning have two-piece lids. Why do you think the metal lid can only be used once?

Packing Methods

You can use one of two methods to pack food into jars.

- For the **raw-pack method**, put the prepared raw food into the jars. Pour in a hot liquid, such as syrup, water, or juice. Raw packing helps delicate foods retain their shape and texture.
- To use the **hot-pack method**, simmer the food briefly. Place the food and some of the liquid into the jars. The light cooking "preshrinks" foods. They fit together more closely, leaving less air in the jar. This increases the vacuum effect, which improves the food's quality.

When you pack jars, leave about $\frac{1}{2}$ to 1 inch of headspace for the food to expand. Run a spatula between the food and the jar to remove any air bubbles. Wipe the jar top clean. Apply the lid and screw on the band until just tight. A lid that's too tight might not allow air to escape during processing.

Some microorganisms may survive the heat of blanching and packing. To finish them off, food must be processed at boiling temperatures or higher.

Processing Methods

For home canning, foods are divided into two classes—high acid and low acid. Each type is processed differently.

Most fruits are high-acid foods. Their natural acidity prevents the growth of microorganisms after canning. They can be processed in a **boiling-water bath**.

All other foods, including tomatoes, are low-acid foods. Low acid and a tightly sealed jar create a prime breeding ground for the deadly *botulinum* bacteria, which can withstand the heat of boiling. Processing these foods requires **pressure canning**, where temperatures above 212°F are possible.

- **Boiling-water bath.** A water-bath canner is a large, deep kettle with a tight-fitting lid. The jars are covered with boiling water and processed for a specified length of time. A removable, divided rack separates and holds the jars off the bottom of the kettle, increasing water circulation.
- **Pressure canning.** A pressure canner is similar to a large pressure cooker. Jars of food are processed in steam under pressure. The dial gauge should be checked annually to ensure an accurate reading. This can be done at the cooperative extension office. Read the manufacturer's directions carefully before using the canner. See **Fig. 29-4**.

After processing, place the jars on a rack or clean dish towel away from drafts until completely cool, usually 12 hours or longer. During this time, the lids "pop"—music to the ears of home canners. This sound indicates that the jar and lid have formed the perfect seal needed to prevent spoilage. To make sure, press the center of the lid. It should stay down when released, due to the vacuum created inside. Tap it with a spoon. It should give a clear ring.

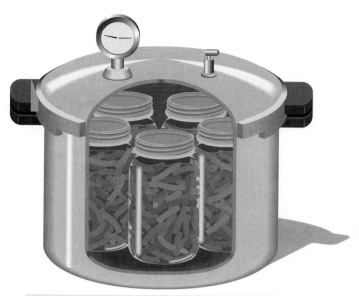

Fig. 29-4 If you're preserving low-acid foods, you need a pressure canner like this one. Why can't you use a water-bath canner?

Any jars that didn't seal can be safely reprocessed within 24 hours, using a new lid; however, food quality will suffer. You may want to remove the food and refrigerate or freeze it.

To allow flavors to develop, you should store home-canned foods in a clean, cool, dry area for at least two weeks before using. Remove or loosen the screw bands to prevent them from rusting. This is not only unsightly but can also mask a faulty seal.

SAFETY ALERT

Unsafe methods. The open kettle method was once a standard way to preserve foods. Cooked foods were sealed in jars with no further treatment. This technique is now recognized as unsafe because the food never gets hot enough to kill all microorganisms. Likewise, food processed in a conventional or microwave oven cannot reach temperatures higher than the boiling point of water. Moreover, as heat causes food and air to expand, the internal pressure could overwhelm the external pressure and the jars could explode.

Fruit and Vegetable Spreads

Homemade fruit and vegetable spreads are also preserved by canning. Jellies are made from juice and sugar, firmed with a gelling agent. Preserves are whole fruits or large pieces cooked with sugar. Jams use chopped fruits or vegetables. Butters are puréed fruit pulp cooked with sugar and spices until smooth and creamy.

Cook these recipes in a large, wide pot with a flat bottom so the mixture has room to boil and foam without bubbling over. Prepare small batches so the food cooks quickly. Process the mixture in a boiling-water bath. To use less sugar, follow a specifically designed, low-sugar recipe.

Pickled Foods

Pickled foods are packed in a mixture of pickling salt, vinegar, water, and spices. This is how cabbage becomes sauerkraut and cucumbers become pickles. You can also pickle mixed vegetables in bean salads. Relishes are often pickled, as are sweetened combinations of chopped fruits, vegetables, or both. Hard-cooked, pickled eggs are a regional favorite. Pickled fruits are simmered in a spicy, sweet-sour syrup that complements naturally tart foods, including crabapples and watermelon rind.

Due to the acidity of the liquid, all pickled recipes can be processed in a boiling-water bath.

DRYING FOOD

Drying, or dehydration, preserves food by depriving microorganisms of the moisture they need for survival. This method is the oldest type of preservation yet requires special equipment. Food must dry slowly and evenly, retaining enough water to be edible but not enough to breed microorganisms.

The most convenient, reliable way to achieve this result is by using a food dehydrator. Unlike the sun, oven, or microwave oven, this appliance provides a balance of moderate temperatures, low humidity, and adequate circulation to dry foods safely. Most dehydrators have a 24-hour timer and an adjustable thermostat to dry each food with the proper time and temperature.

Career Prep

Wages and Benefits

JOB SATISFACTION IS IMPORTANT when choosing a career, and earning good wages and benefits contributes to job satisfaction. Each company sets its policy, which employees can learn by reading the company manual.

WAGES

Entry-level workers usually earn an hourly wage, often starting at the legal minimum wage. Food servers may earn less; they usually increase their earnings through tips. Wages increase with experience and the demands of the job.

Higher positions often bring a yearly salary, a set amount regardless of hours worked. Salaried positions usually involve broader responsibilities and may have less regular hours.

Many employers have a schedule of pay raises. For example, a first raise might come after the first 60 days or perhaps six months. Also, workers may get regular performance reviews or evaluations. Positive reviews can bring a higher wage. Much depends on the business and the economy in general. The best strategy for getting a raise is to earn it by working conscientiously.

BENEFITS

Most employers provide full-time employees with added compensations called benefits. A typical benefits package might include health insurance, paid vacation and sick days, and savings or investment plans. The popular 401(k), for example, allows workers to invest a percent-

Almost any kind of food can be dried. Apples, berries, peaches, and pears are some of the most successfully dried fruits. Peppers, peas, corn, onions, and green beans are most suitable among vegetables. As with freezing, fruits are treated with ascorbic acid and vegetables are blanched. The dehydrator owner's manual gives recommendations for drying different foods.

Store home-dried produce as you would the store-bought variety, in glass jars or sturdy plastic containers or bags. Containers should close securely to keep out moisture.

USING HOME-PRESERVED FOOD

Dried foods make nutritious snacks and interesting "chips" for dipping. When added to soups, they **rehydrate** as the liquid simmers and water reenters and softens the food. After an hour or two of soaking in water or juice, they're ready for use in recipes.

Properly frozen fruits and vegetables keep their quality for 12 to 18 months. They lose texture on thawing, however. The effect is less noticeable in foods cooked in recipes. To use fruits uncooked, serve them while still slightly frozen. Except for corn on the cob, which should be partially thawed, vegetables can be cooked frozen.

Before using canned foods, take prudent precautions. Examine jars carefully before opening. Bulging lids and liquids trickling from under the lid are signs of spoilage. Discard the food without tasting it.

Examine jars when you open them too. Check for mold, unusually soft food, or cloudy, bubbling, or spurting liquid. If any of these signs are present, destroy the food immediately, so that no person or animal can even taste it.

No matter how carefully low-acid foods have been processed, *never taste them cold*. Canned foods containing *botulinum* bacteria often look and smell normal and edible, yet even a teaspoon can be fatal. Boil low-acid foods for 10 to 15 minutes before tasting them. Use a conventional cooktop only. A microwave oven heats too unevenly to kill all the microorganisms.

age of their wages in investment plans. Some firms will match all or part of an employee's investment.

An employer may also provide a severance package to workers who are fired through no fault of their own, as due to a lay-off. These workers may receive extra pay, sometimes equal in value to unused holidays or sick days; services to help them find a new job; and the use of fax machines to send resumés.

More companies are offering a growing variety of perquisites (PUR-kwuh-zuts), or perks, bonuses in addition to traditional benefits. Among the perks most in demand by workers are flexible hours, casual dress, and the option to telecommute, or work from home. On-site child care, health clubs, and paid leave to care for family members are also valued.

Some workers give benefits little weight when considering a job, reasoning that they don't need health insurance or severance pay. Unexpected situations can happen to anyone, however. Benefits are a valuable part of working, and they grow more important as you plan for your own or your family's future security.

Career Connection

Comparing benefits. Use local or Internet sources to learn what wages and benefits are offered for an entry-level, technical-level, or professional job in foods and nutrition. Compare findings in class. How do you explain any differences?

Summarize Your Reading

▶ Foods can be preserved at home, much as people used to preserve foods before the advent of supermarkets and cans, jars, and pouches of food.

▶ Preserving food at home can be a satisfying family affair that preserves such traditions as making an unusual family recipe.

▶ Canning foods takes special equipment to pack and process foods at a specific temperature for a specific length of time.

▶ Preserved foods can be used in many ways, from adding canned tomatoes to a stew to enjoying dried vegetables with a dip.

Check Your Knowledge

1. What does it mean to **preserve** foods?

2. How does preserving foods offer people money savings?

3. Why do people who preserve their own food have more quality control over what they eat?

4. **CRITICAL THINKING** How do you think these factors affect whether a family or individual decides to preserve foods: income; time schedule; size of family? Explain your reasoning.

5. Why can't some produce be preserved by freezing?

6. How would you freeze peas that you will use in small amounts?

7. Compare the **sugar-pack** and **syrup-pack methods** of freezing fruit.

8. What is **blanching**?

9. How are vegetables blanched?

10. Why must you allow **headspace** when packing foods to be frozen?

11. When arranging containers in a freezer, why should you place them in a single layer with plenty of space around them?

12. How can you tell that jars and lids are safe for canning?

13. In canning, what's the difference between **raw pack** and **hot pack**?

14. Describe the basic process for packing food into jars.

15. Why must low-acid foods be processed at a higher temperature than high-acid foods when canning?

16. When is **pressure canning** used?

17. What is a **boiling-water bath**? Which foods can be processed with it when canning?

18. How can you tell whether canned foods have sealed safely?

19. Compare these fruit spreads: jellies, preserves, and butters.

20. What are pickled foods? Give two examples.

21. Why is a food dehydrator a better way to dry foods than the sun, oven, or microwave oven?

22. What are external and internal signs that canned food should be discarded?

23. Why should low-acid, canned foods not be tasted cold?

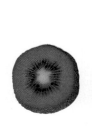
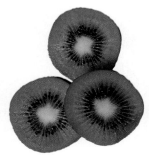

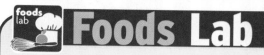
Apply Your Learning

1. **SOCIAL STUDIES** **Preservation History.** Research the history of canning and freezing foods. How did they begin? What challenges did the pioneers of these processes encounter? Report your findings.

2. **SCIENCE** **Pectin Research.** Find information about pectin. What role does pectin play in food preservation? Compare products made with different kinds of pectin.

3. **MATH** **Cost Comparison.** Calculate the cost of homemade jam or jelly and compare it to the cost of a similar purchased product. Show results in a chart. Why might someone make jam or jelly?

4. **Recipe Preparation.** Find recipes for fruit jams and jellies. Prepare one in class.

5. **SCIENCE** **Botulism.** Research botulism. What is it and why is it important in food preservation?

Foods Lab

Dehydrating Foods

Procedure: Use a dehydrator to dry two different fruits. Consult a reliable resource for instructions and advice. Compare the methods used for each fruit and evaluate the results.

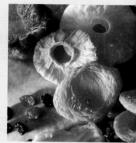

Analyzing Results

1. How did you prepare the two fruits for dehydration? Why was each preparation needed?
2. How were the drying methods similar and different?
3. Which of the foods gave better results? What do you think affected the outcome?
4. Would a dehydrator be a worthwhile investment for you? Why or why not?

Food Science Experiment

Blanching Vegetables

Objective: To analyze the effects of blanching on vegetables.

Procedure:

1. Prepare assigned vegetable as instructed. Rinse the vegetable pieces thoroughly under cold water. Divide them into two equal portions.
2. Dry one portion, pack it in a plastic freezer bag, and label the bag.
3. Blanch the second portion. Add water to a large saucepan half way to the top and bring to a rolling boil. Add vegetables and boil for 3 minutes.
4. Remove the vegetables and immediately submerge them in a bowl of ice water for 5 minutes.
5. Dry and pack the vegetables as in Step 2.
6. Remove the two portions after two weeks. Defrost and cook them in separate saucepans in a small amount of boiling water until tender. Evaluate the results.

Analyzing Results

1. How did the portions compare on appearance, texture, and taste? What do you think caused these results?
2. How might the results have been different if you stored the vegetables for only two days? For a month? Why?

UNIT 7

Food Preparation

CHAPTER 30 **Fruits**

CHAPTER 31 **Vegetables**

CHAPTER 32 **Grain Products**

CHAPTER 33 **Legumes, Nuts & Seeds**

CHAPTER 34 **Dairy Foods**

CHAPTER 35 **Eggs**

CHAPTER 36 **Meat**

CHAPTER 37 **Poultry**

CHAPTER 38 **Fish & Shellfish**

CHAPTER 39 **Beverages**

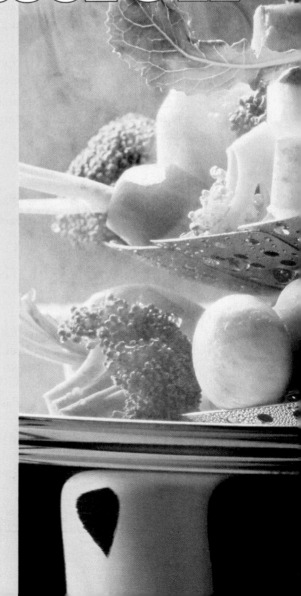

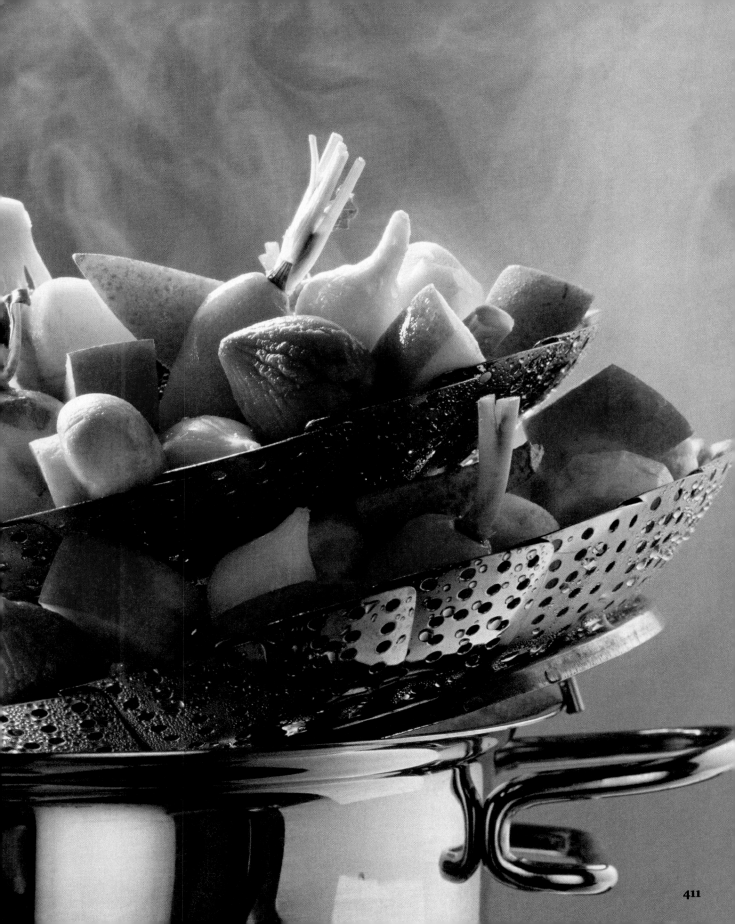

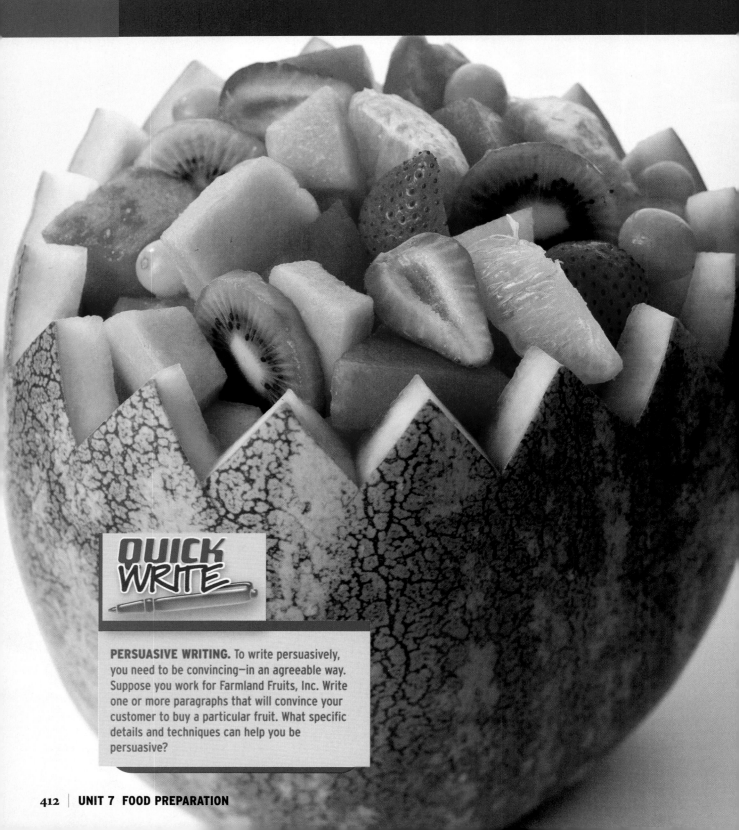

30 Fruits

QUICK WRITE

PERSUASIVE WRITING. To write persuasively, you need to be convincing—in an agreeable way. Suppose you work for Farmland Fruits, Inc. Write one or more paragraphs that will convince your customer to buy a particular fruit. What specific details and techniques can help you be persuasive?

412 | **UNIT 7 FOOD PREPARATION**

FRUITS ARE NATURE'S OWN CONVENIENCE FOOD, ready to eat and enjoy. Think about it. To savor a luscious orange, all you have to do is wash it, peel it, and eat. Many fruits don't even have to be peeled.

Fruits are colorful, flavorful, and easy to prepare, making them ideal for snacks as well as meals. Fruits also supply a wide variety of nutrients.

NUTRIENTS IN FRUITS

Fruits are an important source of dietary fiber and carbohydrates. They are fat-free, low in calories, and low in sodium.

Fruits are an excellent source of vitamin C, potassium, and such phytochemicals as beta carotene. Some fruits are good sources of other nutrients. For instance, oranges provide folic acid. Bananas are a source of magnesium. Raisins and other dried fruits provide iron.

IDENTIFYING FRUITS

A **fruit** is the part of a plant that holds the seeds. Fruits are categorized by certain characteristics that set them apart from each other.

● **Berries.** These small fruits are juicy and have a thin skin. Examples are strawberries, cranberries, grapes, and blackberries.

Nutrition Connection

How much do you need? On a diet of 2,000 to 2,600 calories, a person needs 2 cups of fruit each day. This equals four ½ cup servings. For example, you could eat one small banana, one large orange, and ¼ cup of dried apricots.

? Why might eating a fresh orange be better for you than drinking a glass of orange juice?

● **Melons.** A thick rind, or outer skin, characterizes melons. They are juicy and usually have many seeds. Watermelons, cantaloupes, and casaba (kuh-SAH-buh) are examples.
● **Citrus fruits.** Besides a thick rind, citrus fruits have a thin membrane separating inner flesh segments. Citrus fruits include oranges, tangerines, grapefruits, lemons, and limes.
● **Drupes.** A single hard seed, also called a pit or stone, identifies fruits known as **drupes.** The inner flesh is soft and covered by a tender, edible skin. Drupes include cherries, apricots, peaches, nectarines, and plums.

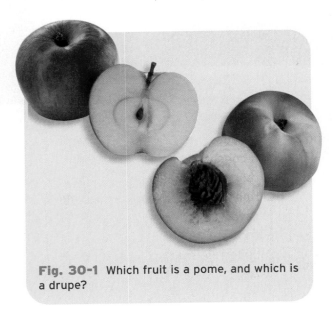

Fig. 30-1 Which fruit is a pome, and which is a drupe?

- **Tropical fruits.** Tropical fruits are grown in tropical and subtropical climates. They include bananas, guavas, papayas, and mangos.

Fig. 30-2 on pages 415 to 418 describes many fruits. Can you place them in the categories just described? Note the typical uses of these fruits. They are used in many sweet dishes, but also in **savory** dishes that are not sweet.

Unusual Fruits

Identifying an apple and a banana is easy, but would you recognize a carambola (kar-uhm-BOH-luh) or a cherimoya (cher-uh-MAWY-uh)? Many less familiar fruits like these are native to countries around the world. Modern transportation ships these fruits quickly from any part of the globe to U.S. markets. As interest grows in these fruits, some are being grown commercially in the United States. See **Fig. 30-3**.

- **Carambola.** Also called star fruit, this fruit has an oval shape with four to six prominent ribs and edible skin. When sliced horizontally, it

- **Pomes.** A **pome** has thick, firm flesh with a tender, edible skin. The central core contains several small seeds. Apples and pears are pomes. See **Fig. 30-1**.

Fig. 30-3

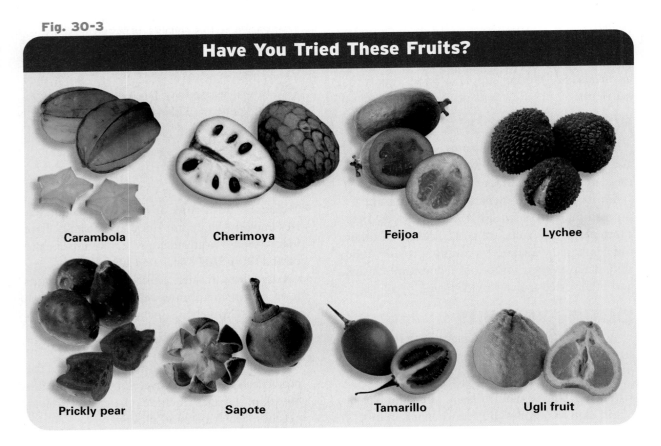

Have You Tried These Fruits?

Carambola

Cherimoya

Feijoa

Lychee

Prickly pear

Sapote

Tamarillo

Ugli fruit

Fig. 30-2

Fruit Descriptions and Uses

Apples

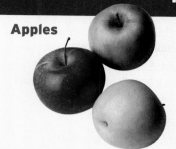

Red, green, and yellow varieties. Variety determines best use since some hold shape better, partly due to cell structure. Vibrant color, firm, no bruises.

Uses: Braeburn—raw and cooked; Gala—raw; Golden Delicious—raw; Granny Smith—cooked; McIntosh—raw; Red Delicious—raw; Rome—cooked. Many desserts; sautéed; salads; cider; sauce; dried; some savory dishes.

Apricots

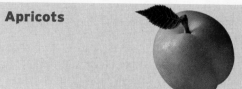

Smaller than peach and dryer flesh. Oval. Even, golden color. Slightly fuzzy skin. Pit removes easily. Peeling not usually necessary.

Uses: Raw; jam; dried; baked with other stone fruits in crisp or tart.

Avocados

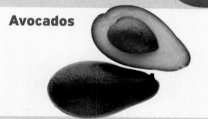
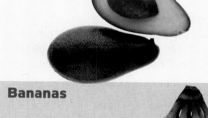

Green to black. Very dark when ripe and only ripens after harvesting. Gives to slight pressure, but shouldn't be too soft or sunken. Light green flesh darkens with oxygen exposure. Large seed in center. High in fat, but mostly monounsaturated.

Uses: Raw; guacamole dips; salads.

Bananas

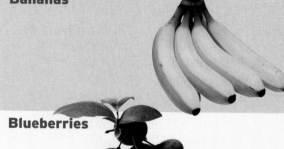

Yellow, red (very sweet with creamy texture), baby, and plantains (look like overripe yellow bananas). Picked green. Ripe when fully yellow, with only a few black spots. Spots indicate starch is turning to sugar, for sweet taste.

Uses: Raw; fruit salads; smoothies; pancakes; quick bread; pies.

Blueberries

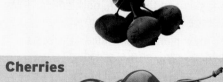

Dark bluish purple, often with silvery surface. No aroma. Choose plump and unwrinkled.

Uses: Raw; cereal topping; muffins; jam; desserts; pancakes; pie; tarts; syrup; dessert sauce; dried.

Cherries

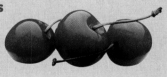

Varieties include dark red Bing cherries and light red Queen Anne. Sweet to tart. Darker is typically sweeter. Bright, plump, and firm. Won't ripen after harvesting.

Uses: Raw; pie; cobbler.

Clementines

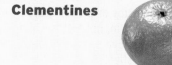

Smaller than tangerine and orange, with loose, easy-peel rind. Very sweet. Nearly seedless.

Uses: Raw; savory and sweet dishes, especially sauces. Often substituted for orange sections in recipes to save peeling time.

Fig. 30-2 (continued)

Fruit Descriptions and Uses

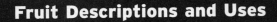

Cranberries

Tart, hard berries. Light to dark red. Dry and sour. Should be shiny and plump, not shriveled.

Uses: Usually cooked. Sauces; jelly; relishes (some raw); juice; quick bread; many desserts and savory dishes; dried like raisins.

Gooseberries

Green, red, purple, golden, and milky-white varieties. Tart, similar to green grapes. Should be firm, not hard.

Uses: Jam; jelly; crisp; pie; with sugar added.

Grapefruits

Yellow rind. Rosy blush where hit by sun. Tart to sweet, and juicy. Flesh white/yellow or pink, with pink being sweeter.

Uses: Raw; juice; salads.

Grapes

Varieties include green seedless; deep purple, red, or white Concord; and red seedless. Plump, bright, and firm when ripe. Raisins are dried grapes.

Uses: Raw; juice; jam; jelly; salads.

Kiwifruits

Small and egg-shaped with thin, fuzzy brown skin and soft green flesh. Tiny, black edible seeds. Sweet. Peel to eat. Slightly soft is ripe.

Uses: Raw; smoothies; fruit salad.

Kumquats (KUHM-kwahts)

Small and round or oblong. Orange color. Citrus family. Sweet skin and tart flesh, both edible. Juicy, with sour-orange flavor.

Uses: Raw; jelly; marmalade; salads; desserts. Often candied, pickled, or preserved.

Lemons and Limes

Lemons are yellow and limes, green. Heavy for size indicates less skin, more juice. Both very tart. Plump, with glossy skin. Key limes are very small and light green.

Uses: Make **zest** (small strips or pieces grated or shaved with peeler) from skin, not bitter white underneath. Squeeze and remove seeds for juice. Use zest or juice to flavor dishes. Soups; stews; rice and bean dishes; on fish, vegetables, fruit and vegetable salads; desserts.

Fig. 30-2 (continued)

Fruit Descriptions and Uses

Mangos

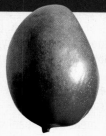

Large, oval fruit. Red, yellow, green, orange, or a combination. Usually tinged yellow when ripe. Golden orange flesh that is juicy and sweet. Fruity aroma from stem end. Peel and remove seed to eat.

Uses: Raw; fruit salads; marinades; desserts; some main dishes.

Melons

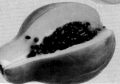

Varieties include: cantaloupe with sweet, juicy, orange flesh and rough rind; honeydew, with green juicy flesh; muskmelon with bright orange flesh; watermelon with sweet, juicy, red flesh. Watermelon may be seedless.

Uses: Raw; fruit salads.

Oranges

Thin or thick rind. Orange color. Most sweet but some bitter. Navel orange is large, seedless, and easy to peel, good for eating. Blood orange is red inside.

Uses: Raw; juice; salads; marmalade.

Papayas

Resemble pears. Yellow skin when ripe. Small, black, edible seeds. Juicy and sweet.

Uses: Raw; salads; main dishes; enzyme used in meat tenderizers.

Peaches and Nectarines

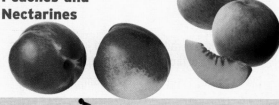

Peaches yellow with reddish blush. Fuzzy skin. Sweet and juicy. Many varieties. "Freestone" and "clingstone" refer to whether flesh is attached to pit. Pleasing aroma. Nectarines similar to peaches, but smooth skin.

Uses: Raw; pies; cobbler; desserts.

Pears

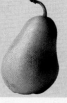

Varieties include: Bartlett—yellow or red; Bosc—brown with long neck; and D'Anjou—yellow. Won't ripen after picking. They get softer, but flavor doesn't increase.

Uses: Raw; poached; baked.

Persimmons

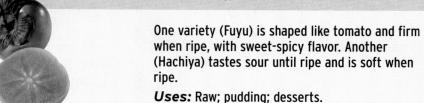

One variety (Fuyu) is shaped like tomato and firm when ripe, with sweet-spicy flavor. Another (Hachiya) tastes sour until ripe and is soft when ripe.

Uses: Raw; pudding; desserts.

Fig. 30-2 (continued)

Fruit Descriptions and Uses

Pineapples

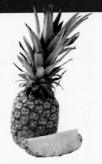

Large, with spiky leaf crown. Tough, prickly skin. Golden cast indicates ripeness. Juicy flesh is white to yellow. Gold variety very sweet, with deep yellow flesh. Won't ripen or sweeten after picking. Fresh pineapple has enzyme that prevents gelatin from setting.

Uses: Raw; juice; meat accompaniment; salads; upside-down cake; desserts. Use canned in gelatin dishes.

Plums

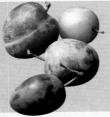

Many varieties in green, red, and purple shades and different sizes. Smooth skin. Common variety has yellowish flesh. Slightly soft when ripe. Very juicy, which affects use. Prunes are dried plums.

Uses: Raw; jam; cobbler.

Pomegranates (PAH-muh-GRA-nuhts)

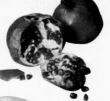

Round. Yellow with reddish overlay when ripe. Red flesh and many seeds, with sweet-tart flavor. Remove inedible membrane around flesh.

Uses: Raw; juice; sauces. Seeds can be sprinkled on salads, roasts, ice cream, pie.

Quinces

Round to pear shape. Can be size of grapefruit. Usually yellow, fuzzy skin. Dry white flesh with pineapple taste. Eaten cooked.

Uses: Peel and core for poaching, stewing, baking, braising.

Raspberries

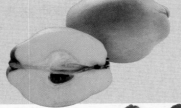

Red, black, or white. Sweet and juicy. May have "hairs" on surface. Bright, plump, and firm.

Uses: Raw; syrup; desserts; jam; jelly.

Strawberries

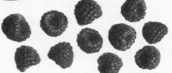

Bright red berries with exterior seeds and green stem cap attached. Some markets offer pick-your-own.

Uses: Raw; jam; jelly; shortcake; cobbler; pie; desserts.

Tangerines

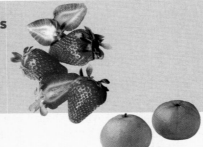

Deep orange color. Citrus. Skin loosely attached. Sweet to tart flavor. Juicy. Typically many seeds.

Uses: Raw; juice.

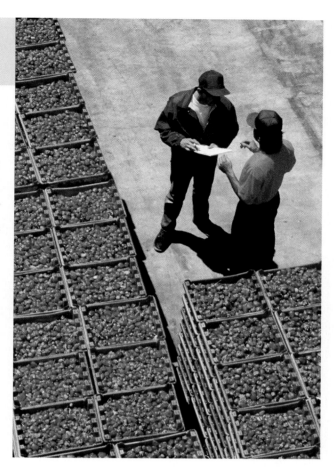

Fig. 30-4 Strawberries must be harvested when they are fully ripe. What impact does this have on getting the berries to market?

forms a star shape. Ripe fruits are yellow-gold, with a slight browning on the ribs. Flavor is similar to a combination of plums, apples, and citrus. The fruit doesn't darken when cut.

- **Cherimoya.** Called a "custard apple," this fruit has a custard-like texture when chilled. It is heart-shaped, with green skin that's imprinted with petal shapes. The flavor is like a blend of strawberries, pineapples, and bananas. To eat, spoon the flesh from the shell.
- **Feijoa (fay-YOH-uh).** This small, egg-shaped fruit has thin, bright green skin and fragrant, cream-colored flesh. Flavor resembles a combination of pineapple and mint. Peel the fruit before eating.
- **Lychee (LEE-chee).** Also spelled litchi, this small fruit has a rough red shell and a single seed. The flesh is creamy white, juicy, and sweet. To eat, remove the shell and seed. When the fruits are dried, they are called "lychee nuts" because the shell turns dark brown and the flesh turns crisp and brown.
- **Prickly pear.** This is the delicious fruit of several varieties of cactus; thus it's also called cactus pear. The fruits are like a pear in size and shape and range in color from yellow to red. Flesh is soft and yellow, with a melon-like aroma and sweet flavor. Peel, section, and remove the seeds and serve the fruits cold.
- **Sapote (sah-POH-tay).** This medium-size, plum-shaped fruit has a thin, olive-green skin. The creamy, custard-like flesh has a sweet flavor that resembles a combination of peach and vanilla. Peel and remove the seeds before eating.
- **Tamarillo (ta-muh-RIH-loh).** Small and egg-shaped, this fruit has a tough, bitter, varicolored skin and a flavorful, tart, pink flesh. Peel, remove seeds, and add sugar before eating.
- **Ugli fruit.** This fruit is about the size of a grapefruit. It has a rough, thick, yellow-green skin and juicy, yellow-orange flesh that is divided into sections. It can be eaten like grapefruit.

SELECTING FRESH FRUITS

Some fresh fruits are available all year. Apples, oranges, and bananas are among these. Others, including peaches and berries, are seasonal and can typically be purchased only during certain months. Together, fresh fruits and vegetables are agricultural products known as **produce.**

Fruits must be picked when mature. **Mature fruits** have reached their full size and color. When a mature fruit reaches its peak of flavor and is ready to eat, it becomes a **ripe fruit.** At this point, fruits are tender and have a pleasant aroma. See **Fig. 30-4.**

When a mature fruit is picked, it may be ripe or underripe. **Underripe fruits** are very firm, lack flavor, and have not yet reached top eating quality. Most fruits are picked when underripe to prevent them from spoilage during shipping. They ripen while en route to the consumer and after purchase. Grapes, berries, cherries, citrus fruits, pineapples, and melons, however, won't ripen after harvest and must be picked when fully ripe.

If a fruit is picked before it's mature, it never ripens. Fruits that are picked too soon are called **immature fruits**. They are usually small for their size and have a poor color and texture.

To test fruits for ripeness, press very gently. Ripe fruit gives slightly under the pressure. Don't press so hard that you damage the fruit since damaged fruit spoils faster.

Some fruits have natural blemishes that don't affect their quality. Grapefruits and oranges may have brownish surface areas. Some oranges experience **regreening**. In warm weather, chlorophyll, the greening substance in plants, returns to the skins of ripe oranges. Bright lights in the produce department can also cause regreening. Green oranges are fully ripe and have the same sweet flavor as those with an orange color.

Buy only good-quality fruits. Immature, overripe, and damaged fruits are no bargain at any price. Nutrients have been lost. Flavor and texture are poor, and the fruit won't keep well. As you choose fruits, inspect them carefully. To avoid buying poor-quality fruit, look for the following:

- **Condition.** Avoid fruits with bruised or damaged spots or decay.
- **Denseness.** Fruit should be plump and firm. Avoid those that are dry, withered, very soft, or very hard.
- **Color.** Color should be typical for the particular fruit.
- **Aroma.** Ripe fruit usually has a pleasant, characteristic aroma. If it has been refrigerated and is still cold, however, it may not have an aroma.
- **Size.** Fruit should be heavy for its size. Heaviness usually means the fruit is juicy.
- **Shape.** Each type of fruit has its own characteristic shape. If misshapen, it probably has poor flavor and texture.

Since most fruits are highly perishable and lose quality quickly, buy only what you can use and store for about a week. Buy fruits that are at the stage of ripeness you want. For example, choose ripe ones if you want to use them right away and less ripe if you plan to use them a few days later.

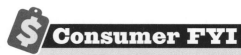

For cooking, choose fruits that are ripe but firm so they will hold their shape.

Storing Fresh Fruit

Never wash fruits before storing them. Instead, wait until you're ready to use them. If you wash fruits before storing, any remaining moisture encourages bacteria to grow. The fruits spoil faster and get moldy.

To store fruit correctly, use the right method for the fruit. Follow these guidelines:

- **Underripe fruits.** Keep at room temperature to ripen. To speed ripening, put the fruit in a brown paper bag. You can add an apple, which produces harmless ethylene, a fruit-ripening gas. If you use a plastic bag for storage, make holes in the bag to allow moisture to evaporate.
- **Bananas.** Store bananas uncovered at room temperature. They can be refrigerated after ripening. The skin turns dark, but the bananas keep their eating quality. See **Fig. 30-5**.
- **Berries, cherries, and grapes.** Sort these fruits to remove any that are damaged or decayed. Refrigerate in a perforated, plastic bag or container, in a covered, shallow container, or uncovered in the refrigerator crisper. Use the fruits as soon as possible.

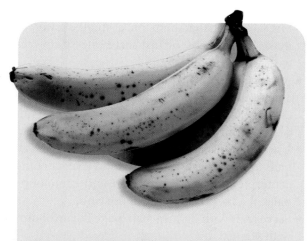

Fig. 30-5 As bananas ripen, green areas on the skin turn yellow and dark spots form on the skin. More ripening increases the dark areas as well as the sweet taste.

- **Citrus fruits.** Store citrus fruits at room temperature. Refrigerate them uncovered for longer storage.
- **All other ripe fruits.** Refrigerate other fruits uncovered in the crisper or in a perforated plastic bag. To keep melon's aroma from flavoring other foods, store them in a closed container or plastic bag.
- **Cut fruits.** Refrigerate in an airtight container or plastic bag.

The keeping quality of fruits depends on how fresh they were when you bought them, how they were handled, and the temperature in your refrigerator. Except for citrus, most fresh fruits should be used within a few days. Citrus fruits can last longer.

PREPARING FRESH FRUITS

Fruits can be prepared with minimal effort. Whether you peel fruits or not, always wash them first under cool, running water. The running water provides a scrubbing action that loosens and washes away dirt and microorganisms that can cause illness. Thick-skinned fruits can be brushed. Avoid soaking fruits in water since flavor and nutrients can be lost.

Have you ever wondered why some fruits are shiny, particularly apples and oranges? Some fruits are waxed to make them look more attractive and to prevent moisture loss so they last longer. The waxes, which are on the FDA list of GRAS chemicals, are not water-soluble and therefore cannot be washed off. Many fruits also have pesticide residues. To remove the wax and pesticides, pare a thin layer of skin from the fruit.

Never use detergents to wash fruits. Detergents may react chemically with any pesticides and waxes on the fruit to create harmful compounds.

As you prepare fruits, remove any stems or damaged spots. Then pare the fruit if needed. Pare thinly in order to retain nutrients that are right under the skin. Since such fruits as apples, peaches, and pears have a tender, edible skin, paring is optional. Some fruits, such as oranges and bananas, must be peeled before using. Others, such as melons, must be cut and have the seeds removed.

Suppose you're freezing a large quantity of peaches and you want to remove the skin as quickly as possible. The skin slides off easily with this method: lower the fruit gently into simmering water for about 15 seconds; then use a slotted spoon to switch the fruit to ice water for two minutes.

Fresh fruits are easier to eat when cut into pieces. To retain nutrients, keep the chunks fairly large and serve them as soon as possible. If you don't plan to serve cut fruit immediately, cover it tightly with plastic wrap and squeeze out as much air as possible. Refrigerate until serving time.

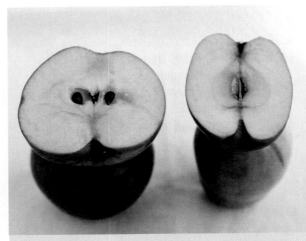

Fig. 30-6 Some fruits have enzymes that react chemically with oxygen in the air, turning the fruit brown. How can you prevent this reaction?

Preventing Fruits from Darkening

When you see the flesh of an apple, banana, or peach turn brown, you're seeing science in action. This darkening occurs after exposure to oxygen in the air. The oxygen reacts with an **enzyme**, a special protein, making the fruit turn brown. This chemical reaction is called **enzymatic browning** (en-zuh-MA-tik). See **Fig. 30-6**.

How can you stop this reaction? Ascorbic acid, which is vitamin C, destroys the enzyme so that it can't react with oxygen. Since lemon, grapefruit, and orange juices all contain vitamin C, you can dip the fruit into one of these juices to prevent browning. Another option is to buy ascorbic acid powder to mix with water and sprinkle on the cut fruit.

SERVING FRESH FRUIT

Because it's nutritious and delicious, fresh fruit ranks high as a meal accompaniment and also as a snack or party fare. Why not try these ideas for serving fresh fruit?

- Experiment with shapes for different uses. Bananas and kiwifruit can be sliced. Peaches can be cut into wedges. Citrus fruits can be sectioned. See **Fig. 30-7**. Cut fruits into bite-size pieces and string them on a small skewer to make fruit kebabs, or just serve bite-size pieces with wooden picks.
- Arrange different fruits in circles or wedges on a large platter. Color contrast makes a pleasing display. Cover the arrangement tightly with plastic wrap and refrigerate until serving time.
- Use a melon-ball tool or small scoop to make balls of soft-flesh fruits. For an eye-catching centerpiece, place watermelon and cantaloupe balls in a basket made from the rind.
- Serve fruit with dip. You can make flavorful dips with yogurt.
- Make frozen fruit bites. Freeze whole berries or grapes on trays to make frozen candy-like snacks.
- Make a **trifle** (TRI-fuhl), a refrigerated dessert with layers that may include cake, jam or jelly, fruit, custard, and whipped cream. You might try alternating layers of fruit, sponge cake, and sweetened whipped cream or yogurt. You can experiment with other layers, such as nuts or oatmeal.

COMMERCIALLY PROCESSED FRUITS

Do you need a quick meal accompaniment or a convenient snack to pack for a trip? Canned, frozen, or dried fruit may be the answer. Each of these commercially processed fruits has its own advantages. As a general rule, fresh and frozen fruits are more nutritious than canned. Canned fruits are convenient and easy to store. Dried fruits are nutritious, although they have a high concentration of natural sugar.

When you buy fruits in these varied forms, follow the guidelines you learned in Chapter 17. Review Chapter 20 for storage guidelines.

Canned Fruits

Canned fruits come in many forms—whole, halved, sliced, and in pieces. Some are packed in light or heavy syrup, which sweetens them. Heavy is sweeter and higher in calories. For fewer calories, look for fruits packed in water or their own juices. They have no added sugar and about the same number of calories as fresh fruit.

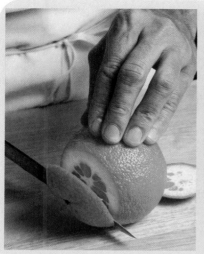
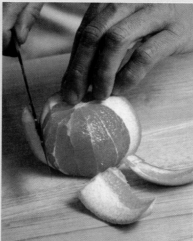
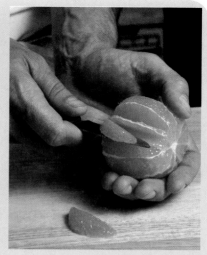

Fig. 30-7 Here's an easy way to section citrus fruits. First, slice off both ends (left photo). Then cut off the skin (center photo). Finally, cut along both sides of each dividing membrane to loosen the sections (right photo). Then lift the sections out. You can work over a bowl to save juice.

As you scan supermarket shelves, you'll notice options besides just plain fruit. Pears might be flavored with vanilla. Cinnamon might be added to apples. When buying canned fruits, read the labels to be sure you're getting the kind you want. Buy the form best suited for your needs.

Canned fruits can often be served in place of fresh. For a quick dessert, purée canned fruits in a blender and serve over angel food cake.

Frozen Fruits

Since frozen fruits come with or without sugar, check the label to get what you want. Frozen fruits taste similar to fresh fruits, but the frozen version has a softer texture when defrosted. Freezing damages the cell walls, allowing water to run out as fruits thaw.

If you have enough freezer space, consider buying fruit in large plastic bags. You can remove only the amount you need and leave the remainder in the freezer.

When serving frozen fruit plain, thaw it only partially so that ice crystals remain and help keep the fruit firm. If thawed completely, the fruit gets mushy and loses its shape. For a dish like a gelatin dessert with fruit as an ingredient, however, complete thawing may be needed.

Dried Fruits

Although many fruits are dried, the most common ones include raisins, prunes, dates, peaches, apples, apricots, and cranberries. Typically, they are packaged in boxes or plastic bags, but some stores sell them loose by the pound.

When you buy dried fruits, look for good color. Choose fruit that is fairly soft and pliable. Hard fruits have become too dry.

Store unopened packages in a cool, dry place. After opening, store dried fruits in an airtight container in the refrigerator.

Dried fruits make nutritious snacks. Often they're mixed with other foods like nuts and seeds to make tasty combinations. Dried fruits are also used for cooking and baking. Some recipes call for **reconstituting** dried fruit so it cooks faster. This process restores a dried food to its former condition by adding water.

COOKING FRUITS

When you think about cooking foods, do fruits come to mind first? Perhaps not, yet fruits are as versatile as many other foods when it comes to cooking. They are featured in many desserts—the classic apple pie, for example—but they can also be part of a main course. See **Fig. 30-8** on page 424 for a recipe idea.

Fig. 30-8

Try This! Recipe

Peach-Blueberry Crisp

Yield	Nutrition Analysis
2 servings	*Per Serving:* 290 calories, 7 g total fat, 1 g saturated fat, 0 g trans fat, 0 mg cholesterol, 100 mg sodium, 55 g total carbohydrate, 4 g dietary fiber, 27 g sugars, 5 g protein
	Percent Daily Value: vitamin A 15%, vitamin C 25%, calcium 4%, iron 10%

Ingredients

¼ cup crispy rice cereal
¼ cup regular or quick-cooking oats (not instant)
¼ tsp. cinnamon
3 Tbsp. brown sugar, packed

1 Tbsp. melted margarine or butter
1 cup peaches, peeled and sliced
1 cup blueberries
1½ Tbsp. water
1½ tsp. lemon juice

Directions

1. Preheat oven to 375°F.
2. Combine cereal, oats, cinnamon, and brown sugar in a bowl.
3. Stir in melted margarine or butter; set aside.
4. Arrange fruit in a small baking dish or loaf pan.
5. Combine water and lemon juice; pour over fruit.
6. Top with cereal-oat mixture.
7. Bake at 375°F for about 35 minutes or until peaches are tender but not mushy and top is lightly browned.
8. Serve warm or cold.

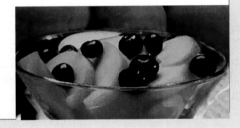

What if fruits have become too ripe to eat out of hand? Instead of throwing the fruits away, cooking them is an economical option.

To cook successfully with fruits, you need to know what happens to fruits during cooking. Several changes occur.

- **Nutrients.** Cooking results in a loss of heat-sensitive nutrients, especially vitamin C.
- **Color.** Colors change, depending on the fruit. Some become lighter, while others develop a deeper color.
- **Flavor.** Fruit flavors usually change slightly during cooking. They become mellow and less sharp and acidic. If overcooked, fruits tend to lose their flavor or may develop an unpleasant flavor.
- **Texture and shape.** When heat is applied to fruits, the cells in the fruits lose water and soften. As the structure breaks down, the fruits fall apart, becoming more tender and easier to digest. At the same time, shape is lost. To keep the shape, add sugar to the cooking water. Sugar draws some water back into a fruit's cells, which strengthens them. Understanding this effect helps you cook fruits successfully in moist heat.

Cooking Fruits in Moist Heat

Fruits can be cooked in moist heat in two ways: to hold their shape or to make a thick sauce. The result you want determines when you add sugar to the mixture. Use a saucepan with a tight-fitting lid.

If you want cooked fruits to retain their shape, poach them. See **Fig. 30-9.** Use firm fruits, such as apples, peaches, plums, or pears. Leave them whole or cut them into fairly large pieces. Quarters and eighths work well. After placing the fruits in a saucepan, add sugar and enough water to cover them. Cover the pan and simmer gently just until tender. Rapid boiling breaks the fruit apart.

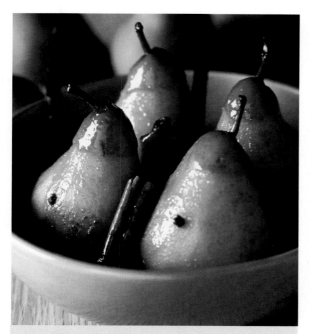

Fig. 30-9 Poached pears make an elegant dessert. How can you cook them so they keep their shape?

To make a sauce, cut fruits into small pieces. Leave small berries whole. Add a small amount of water, just enough to cover the bottom of the pan. Fruit has a high water content. As it cooks and the cell walls break down, the juices are released. Do not add sugar at this point. Simmer in a tightly covered pan, stirring occasionally to break the fruit apart. At the end of the cooking time, add sugar, honey, or another sweetener if you wish.

You can add extra flavor to the fruits with lemon juice, lemon or orange rind, vanilla, a cinnamon stick, or other spices.

Frying Fruits

Some fruits may be fried, usually as a side dish. Fried apple slices, for instance, are often served with pancakes or roast pork. Pineapple slices and banana halves are other options for frying.

Fruits for frying should be firm enough to hold their shape. If you use canned fruits, drain them well.

Fruits may be sautéed in a small amount of butter or margarine until lightly browned. Another way to fry fruit is to make **fritters**. Dip cut-up fruits in a batter and deep-fry until golden brown. See **Fig. 30-10**.

Baking Fruits

Fruits can be baked alone or as part of a recipe. For example, pineapples or dried prunes are often baked with pork. Fruits can be baked whole, peeled, or cut into pieces. Use apples, pears, bananas, or other firm fruits that hold their shape well. As you'll read in a later chapter, fruits are also used in many baked goods, including pies, cakes, cobblers, and muffins.

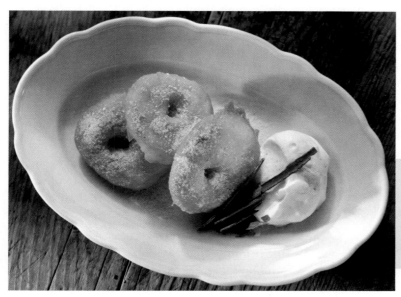

Fig. 30-10 When dipped in batter and deep-fried, apple slices make fritters. A light sprinkling of powdered sugar can be added. Why are fritters best eaten occasionally rather than often?

Apples are probably baked whole more often than other fruits. They are easy to prepare and make a delicious ending to a meal. See **Fig. 30-11**. Before cooking, core the apples and cut a thin strip of skin from around the middle. This allows the apples to expand as they cook so they won't burst. You can fill the cavity with raisins, nuts, and a spicy sugar mixture. Place the apples in a baking dish and pour hot water around them to a depth of ¼ inch. Bake at 350°F until tender, about 45 to 60 minutes, depending on the size of the apples.

Broiling Fruits

Broiling cooks fruits slightly and browns them. Any tender fruits that hold their shape may be broiled. You might try bananas, peaches, grapefruit halves, or pineapple slices. You can also broil canned fruits.

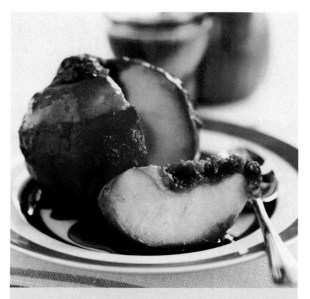

Fig. 30-11 Firm apples are best for baking. These are a few varieties that bake well: Rome, Granny Smith, Gala, Braeburn, Jonagold, Cortland, and Winesap.

Career Prep

Verbal Communication

IT ALMOST GOES WITHOUT SAYING: good verbal skills can help you in any job, starting with the interview and continuing through your career. Even if you work mostly alone or with machines or equipment, at some point you'll need to share information personally. Good verbal communication can contribute to your success and to a pleasant working environment.

Verbal communication includes two important elements: speaking and listening.

SPEAKING

"It isn't what you say; it's how you say it." Keep that in mind the next time you speak. Pay attention to:

● **Word choice.** Be specific. "Set the box on the counter" is more helpful than "Put that there."

Be tactful; avoid blame and hurt feelings when possible. Also, while slang may be fine for friends and family, standard English is clearer to the varied clients, co-workers, and supervisors you may encounter.

● **Enunciation.** Speak clearly, especially when talking on the telephone.

● **Tone.** The same message can encourage or criticize, depending on the tone used in delivering the message. A positive, sympathetic tone helps build cooperation.

● **Organization.** Relate ideas in a more or less logical order, such as time sequence or order of importance.

● **Posture.** Words sound clearer if spoken with the head raised. People are more attentive if you look them in the eye.

Because fruits have no fat, they must be protected to keep them from drying out. Brush the surface with melted butter or margarine or use a topping, such as brown sugar or seasoned crumbs.

Grilling Fruits

Grilling fruits gives them a delicious flavor and a caramelized color. Choose firm, ripe fruits. Fruits that are overripe fall apart too easily. Cantaloupes, apples, pears, or peaches can be cut into slices for grilling. Banana halves also grill well. Another idea is to cut the fruits into pieces and thread them on a small skewer.

Before grilling, brush a little oil on the grate. Place the fruits on the grate and grill until grill marks form. Turn to cook the other side. The fruit should soften but not be mushy.

Microwave Cooking

Fruits are easy to prepare in the microwave oven. They cook quickly, keep their flavor and shape, and retain the most nutrients. Because they are so tender, however, they can easily overcook. Watch the timing carefully.

Cover fruits when you microwave them, but leave a small opening for steam to escape. If you are cooking whole fruits, such as plums, pierce them with a fork in several places to keep them from bursting. Refer to the owner's manual or a microwave cookbook for power levels and cooking times.

- **Timing.** Pick a time when your message will be best received. Make an appointment, if needed.

- **"I" messages.** This technique focuses on your feelings or viewpoint. It is more persuasive and more honest than criticizing. "I get angry" is a factual statement. "You make me mad" judges another person. "I" messages suggest solutions. Compare "I find this method easier" to "You're doing that wrong."

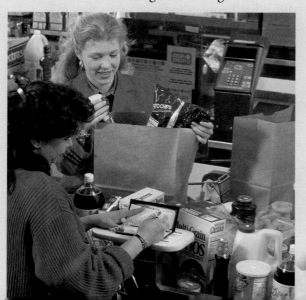

LISTENING

Verbal communication is a two-way street. Speaking alternates with listening. In fact, some studies show that the average worker spends twice as much time listening as speaking.

Strive to listen as carefully as you speak. If you let your mind wander, you may miss the message. Focus on the speaker. Listen actively, using thinking skills to process what is being said. Reflect on the entire message before reacting. Repeating the message in your own words gives the other person the chance to clear up any misunderstandings or fill in any blanks.

Career Connection

Communication skills. With other students, write a short skit showing weak and strong verbal communication skills in the workplace. Possible situations are: a) someone interviewing for a job; b) a job trainee making several mistakes; and c) an employee giving a supervisor verbal notice of quitting. Perform your skit for class analysis.

Summarize Your Reading

▶ Fruits can be categorized according to their different characteristics.

▶ Fruits provide vital nutrients for good health.

▶ Fruits can be purchased fresh, canned, frozen, and dried. Each form has particular qualities that affect selection and storage. Each form also affects how you use the fruits.

▶ Fruits can be prepared and enjoyed in many different ways. Careful cooking can help preserve the nutrients in fruits.

Check Your Knowledge

1. What six categories distinguish different fruits?

2. Why are fruits nutritious? Give examples.

3. Compare **drupes** with **pomes**.

4. In **Fig. 30-2** on pages 415 to 418, identify a fruit that fits each of these descriptions: a) very dark when ripe; b) plantain is one type; c) has a fuzzy, brown skin; d) makes prunes when dried.

5. Describe three unusual fruits.

6. **CRITICAL THINKING** Why do you think the length of time that many fresh fruits are available in supermarkets has increased?

7. Compare the following terms as they relate to fruit: **mature**; **ripe**; **underripe**; and **immature**.

8. **CRITICAL THINKING** The owner of an apple orchard places a metal ring around an apple on the tree and tests a drop of juice. Why do you think the owner does this?

9. Can oranges that experience **regreening** be eaten? Explain.

10. What would you look for when evaluating fresh fruits for purchase?

11. Why shouldn't fruits be washed before you store them?

12. How would you store each of the following: a) an underripe banana; b) fresh grapes; c) oranges to be eaten soon?

13. Why must fruits be washed before use?

14. Why is it best to pare only a thin layer of skin from fruit?

15. **CRITICAL THINKING** Predict what will eventually happen if you pare an apple and let it sit. Why does this happen? How could you prevent this occurrence?

16. What is a **trifle**?

17. What advantage is there to buying fruit packed in its own juice?

18. How should dried fruits be stored?

19. What happens to fruits when they're cooked?

20. How does added sugar affect fruit as it cooks?

21. Describe a method for cooking each of the following: a) apples; b) bananas; c) peaches; d) pineapple.

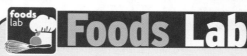

Apply Your Learning

1. **Tropical Fruit Tasting.** Bring in samples of tropical fruits for a taste test. Share information about the fruit you brought. Which fruits do students like the most and the least? Why?

2. **Nutrition Check.** Keep a list of the fruit servings you eat for three days. Compare results to nutrition guidelines.

3. **SCIENCE Ripening Rates.** Compare ripening rates with four green bananas, equally unripe. Leave one uncovered on a counter under dim light, one in a sunny windowsill, one in a paper bag with an apple, and one in a bag without an apple. Record changes twice a day until all are ripe. How do ripening rates compare?

4. **MATH Cost Comparison.** Compare the cost per ounce of fresh, frozen, canned, and dried versions of three fruits. Chart the results. What do you conclude?

5. **Demonstration.** Demonstrate the following procedures: a) peeling and coring a pineapple; b) creating lemon zest; c) peeling a peach; d) sectioning an orange.

Foods Lab

Baking Apples

Procedure. With your lab team, create an original recipe for stuffing a baked apple. What kind of apple and ingredients will you use? Write your recipe, and then bake the apples in the oven or microwave oven. Conduct a taste test of teams' recipes.

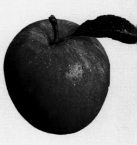

Analyzing Results

❶ How did the ingredients and ovens used by different teams affect taste?

❷ How would you revise your team's recipe?

❸ How well did your team work together in creating the recipe and product? What would you do differently the next time?

6. **Cooking with Fruit.** Choose a fruit and a method for preparing it. Try out the recipe at home or in the foods lab. Evaluate the results.

Food Science Experiment

Enzymatic Browning

Objective. To identify fruits subject to enzymatic browning and determine reaction rates.

Procedure:

1. Cut a pear, banana, orange, peach, cantaloupe, and any other fruits into small cubes and place them on a glass plate.

2. At two-minute intervals, inspect the fruits for discoloration. Keep track of total minutes during the experiment. List the fruits on paper and record when enzymatic browning starts to occur for each fruit.

3. Repeat the experiment with fresh cubes of fruit, but use only the kinds of fruit that previously turned brown. This time drizzle lemon juice over the cubes.

Analyzing Results

❶ Which fruits underwent enzymatic browning? How long did the process take for each fruit?

❷ What was the effect of the lemon juice?

❸ How can this information help you when preparing fruits for a dish?

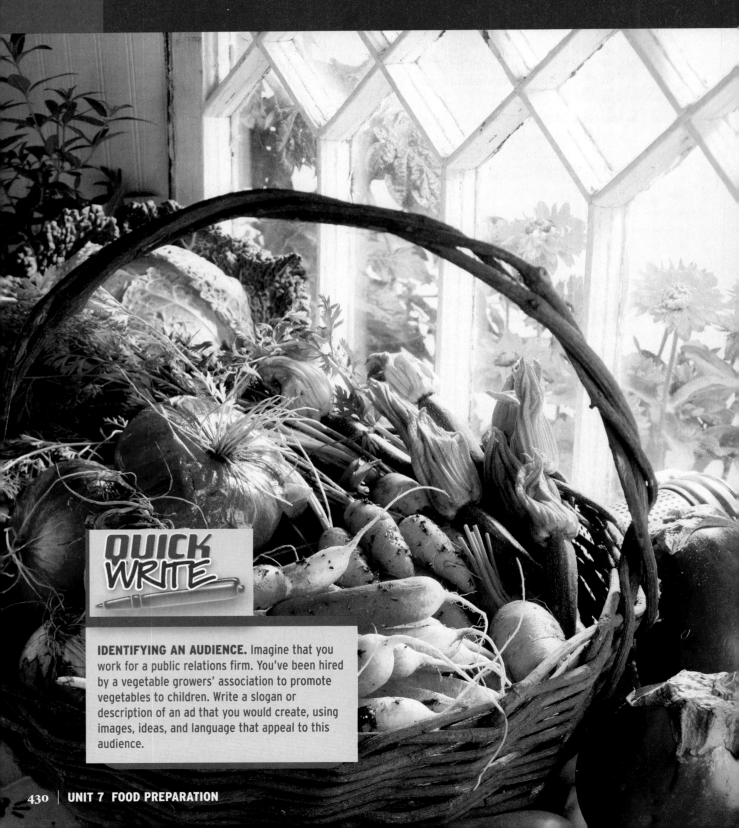

31 Vegetables

QUICK WRITE

IDENTIFYING AN AUDIENCE. Imagine that you work for a public relations firm. You've been hired by a vegetable growers' association to promote vegetables to children. Write a slogan or description of an ad that you would create, using images, ideas, and language that appeal to this audience.

Objectives
▶ Identify vegetables and their uses.
▶ Explain the value of vegetables in the diet.
▶ Explain how to select and store vegetables.
▶ Describe and demonstrate methods for preparing, cooking, and serving vegetables.

Terms
aromatic vegetables
carrageen
cooking greens
salad greens
sea vegetables
solanine
tuber

ONG BEFORE PEOPLE LEARNED TO GROW vegetables, they found food in the edible plants that grew naturally around them. Today people raise many different vegetables—on farms and in gardens. Through experimentation and creativity, they have found endless ways to prepare and serve vegetables. People enjoy these versatile foods both raw and cooked. They use them in appetizers, side dishes, soups, salads, breads, and main dishes. Vegetables add flavor, color, and texture to meals. Not only that, they contribute significantly to health.

NUTRIENTS IN VEGETABLES

Because vegetables are rich in many vitamins and minerals, they are among the most nutritious foods around. For instance, bell peppers, tomatoes, and raw cabbage are good sources of vitamin C. Leafy green vegetables provide folic acid, vitamin K, calcium, and magnesium.

Vegetables are also an important source of fiber, carbohydrates, and phytochemicals. They contain no cholesterol, and most are low in calories, fat, and sodium. Since many vegetables contain antioxidants, including vitamins A and C and lycopene, eating them may lower your risk of some cancers and heart disease.

Nutrition Connection

Colorful servings. On a diet of 1,800 to 2,000 calories, a person needs 2½ cups of vegetables each day. This equals five ½ cup servings. For 2,200 to 2,400 calories, 3 cups are recommended. Choose a colorful variety of vegetables, especially dark green and orange. Different colors have different nutrients.

 What are some easy ways to increase vegetable servings in an eating plan?

TYPES OF VEGETABLES

Carrots may be easy to identify, but would you know a jicama (HEE-kuh-muh) from a rutabaga? **Fig. 31-1** on pages 432 to 436 describes vegetables, some more familiar than others. Which ones do you eat regularly?

As you look at all the different vegetables, you'll notice many variations in structure. That's because vegetables come from different plant parts. What's edible on one plant might not be on another. Sometimes the entire plant can be eaten, as with lettuce. Plants that provide beans and broccoli, however, have only certain edible parts.

Fig. 31-1

Vegetable Descriptions and Uses

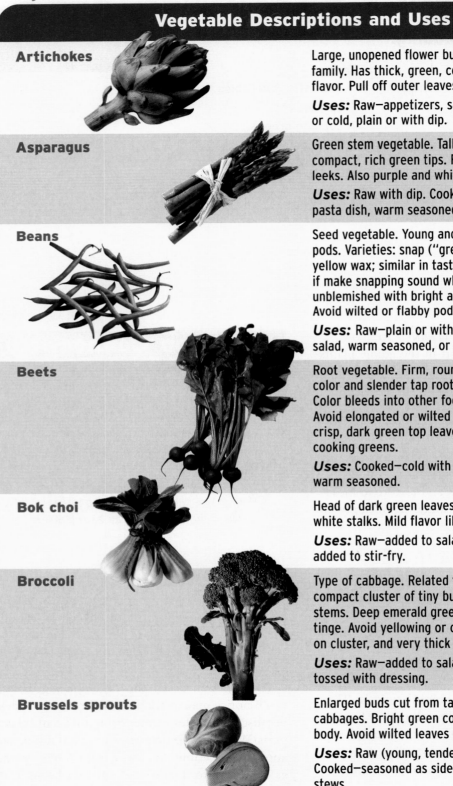

Artichokes

Large, unopened flower bud of plant in thistle family. Has thick, green, compact scales. Nutty flavor. Pull off outer leaves.

Uses: Raw—appetizers, salad, entrée. Cooked—hot or cold, plain or with dip.

Asparagus

Green stem vegetable. Tall stalks with closed, compact, rich green tips. Related to onions, garlic, leeks. Also purple and white varieties.

Uses: Raw with dip. Cooked—cold in salad or pasta dish, warm seasoned.

Beans

Seed vegetable. Young and tender, with firm, crisp pods. Varieties: snap ("green" or "string") or yellow wax; similar in taste and texture. Fresh if make snapping sound when bent. Choose unblemished with bright appearance, good color. Avoid wilted or flabby pods or thick, tough pods.

Uses: Raw—plain or with dip. Cooked—cold in salad, warm seasoned, or added to stir-fry.

Beets

Root vegetable. Firm, round, smooth, with deep red color and slender tap root. Crisp with sweet flavor. Color bleeds into other foods, even when cooked. Avoid elongated or wilted beets. Beet greens are crisp, dark green top leaves of beets, used as cooking greens.

Uses: Cooked—cold with dressing or in salad; warm seasoned.

Bok choi

Head of dark green leaves on thick, crisp, edible white stalks. Mild flavor like cabbage.

Uses: Raw—added to salads. Cooked—side dish, added to stir-fry.

Broccoli

Type of cabbage. Related to cauliflower. Firm, compact cluster of tiny buds on stout, edible stems. Deep emerald green, with possible purple tinge. Avoid yellowing or open buds, watery spots on cluster, and very thick stems.

Uses: Raw—added to salads. Cooked—seasoned, tossed with dressing.

Brussels sprouts

Enlarged buds cut from tall stem. Look like small cabbages. Bright green color, compact leaves, firm body. Avoid wilted leaves or yellow or black spots.

Uses: Raw (young, tender buds)—with dip. Cooked—seasoned as side dish, added to soups and stews.

Fig. 31-1 (continued)

Vegetable Descriptions and Uses

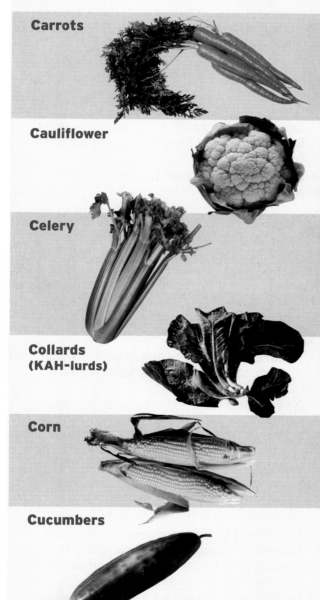

Cabbage

Short, broad stem; compact, heavy head of leaves or flowers. Strong flavor. Varieties include green, red, savoy (milder flavor), kale. Napa cabbage has elongated head and thick-veined, crinkly leaves; cream-colored with green tips, mild flavor.

Uses: Raw—shredded for salads or slaws. Cooked—side dish, stir-fries; leaves used to wrap meat fillings.

Carrots

Root vegetable. Lacy greens and long, slender, orange root. Crunchy. Avoid wilted, flabby carrots. Baby variety available.

Uses: Raw—out of hand, shredded or sliced for salads. Cooked—side dish or added to breads, soups, stews, roasts.

Cauliflower

Type of cabbage. Compact, tiny white or creamy white florets in clusters on stalks surrounded by green leaves. Avoid brown spots.

Uses: Raw—with dip or in pasta salad. Cooked—seasoned, stir-fried, added to soups.

Celery

Glossy, light- to medium-green stalk containing individual ribs with green leaflets. Crisp; bland to slightly sweet flavor. "Hearts" are innermost tender ribs. High water content.

Uses: Raw—with dip; added to meat, potato, or pasta salads. Cooked—added to soups, stews, stir-fries, stuffing.

Collards (KAH-lurds)

Cruciferous vegetable. Large, dark green leaves on tall stems. Flavor is cross between cabbage and kale.

Uses: Same as cabbage.

Corn

Ears of plump kernels enclosed in green husks with moist, golden silk. Seed kernels may be yellow, white, or both. Sweet and juicy. Silk ends should not be decayed or have worm injury.

Uses: Cooked—on ear or removed.

Cucumbers

Related to pumpkins, watermelon, and squash. Deep green skin covering cool, moist, whitish flesh with edible seeds. Often waxed to keep in moisture. Avoid overly large diameter and shriveled ends.

Uses: Raw—plain or with dip, slices added to tossed or creamy salads, shredded.

Fig. 31-1 (continued)

Vegetable Descriptions and Uses

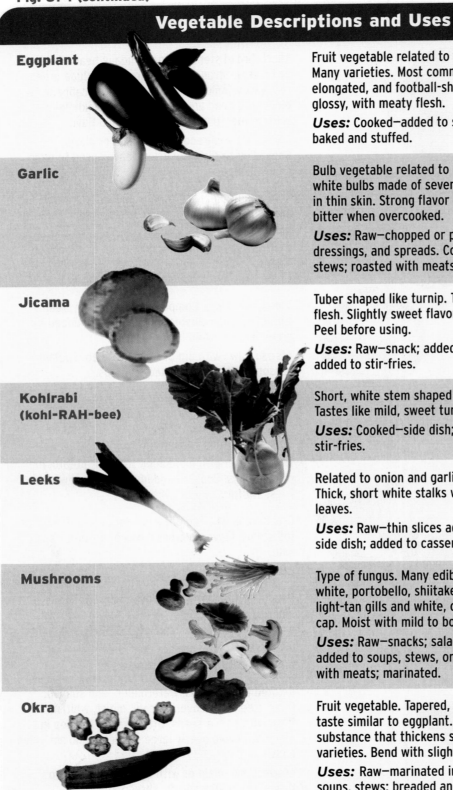

Eggplant

Fruit vegetable related to tomatoes and potatoes. Many varieties. Most common is dark purple, elongated, and football-shaped. Firm, smooth, and glossy, with meaty flesh.

Uses: Cooked—added to stir-fries and stews; baked and stuffed.

Garlic

Bulb vegetable related to onions and leeks. Plump white bulbs made of several small cloves encased in thin skin. Strong flavor mellows with cooking but bitter when overcooked.

Uses: Raw—chopped or pressed and added to oils, dressings, and spreads. Cooked—added to soups, stews; roasted with meats; baked whole.

Jicama

Tuber shaped like turnip. Tough brown skin. White flesh. Slightly sweet flavor, crunchy texture, juicy. Peel before using.

Uses: Raw—snack; added to salads. Cooked—added to stir-fries.

Kohlrabi
(kohl-RAH-bee)

Short, white stem shaped like globe; green leaves. Tastes like mild, sweet turnip.

Uses: Cooked—side dish; added to soups, stews, stir-fries.

Leeks

Related to onion and garlic; milder, sweet flavor. Thick, short white stalks with crisp, blue-green leaves.

Uses: Raw—thin slices added to salad. Cooked—side dish; added to casseroles, soups, stews.

Mushrooms

Type of fungus. Many edible varieties, including white, portobello, shiitake. Short stem with pink or light-tan gills and white, creamy, or light brown cap. Moist with mild to bold flavor.

Uses: Raw—snacks; salads; stuffed. Cooked—added to soups, stews, omelets, stir-fries; served with meats; marinated.

Okra

Fruit vegetable. Tapered, oblong fuzzy pods with taste similar to eggplant. When cut, gives off sticky substance that thickens soups. Dark green and red varieties. Bend with slight pressure.

Uses: Raw—marinated in salad. Cooked—added to soups, stews; breaded and fried.

Fig. 31-1 (continued)

Vegetable Descriptions and Uses

Onions

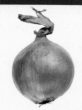

Bulb vegetable. Green (scallions)—very young onion; long, straight green leaves with small white bulb, mild flavor. Yellow, white, and red—firm, round, and dry with small necks. Juicy flesh surrounded by papery skin. Mild to strong flavor. Vidalia—crisp, juicy, sweet.

Uses: Raw—chopped in salads, fillings, stir-fries, soups. Cooked—added to soups, stews, roasts.

Parsnips

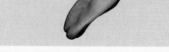

Root vegetable. Whitish color, similar in shape to carrots. Firm with sweet, nutty flavor.

Uses: Cooked—seasoned; mashed; added to stews.

Peas

Crisp, bright green pods filled with small, sweet peas. Snow pea pods are flat. Sugar snap pea pods are plump.

Uses: Raw—snack; added to salads. Cooked—side dish; added to dishes.

Peppers

Fruit vegetable. Sweet (bell, banana, pimiento) or hot (chile). Bell peppers bright and glossy; may be green, red, yellow, orange, or purple. Bell-shaped, firm, hollow, with short, thick stem and three to four lobes. Have seeds. Crunchy. Green less sweet. Hot chile peppers include jalapeño, cayenne, habanero. Range of spiciness.

Uses: Raw—sliced; chopped; whole as snack; added to salsa, salads. Cooked—added to stir-fries, soups, stews, chili; bell peppers stuffed with cooked rice, meats.

Potatoes

Tubers. Varieties include: Idaho or russet (dark brown), new (freshly harvested), white, Round Red, and blue or purple. Firm, heavy, round to oval, with thin skin. White, starchy flesh. Purple has purple flesh. Texture varies with type. New, whites, and Round Reds keep shape, so good for boiling, frying, and salads. Russets loosen up easily and bake well.

Uses: Cooked—side dish; added to soups, stews, cold salads.

Pumpkins

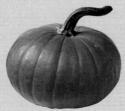

Large, round, orange gourd, related to squash. Thick rind, orange flesh with seeds. Sweet, mild flavor. Seeds can be husked and roasted. Nutty taste. Small pumpkins best for cooking.

Uses: Cooked—side dish; added to soups, casseroles, pies.

Fig. 31-1 (continued)

Vegetable Descriptions and Uses

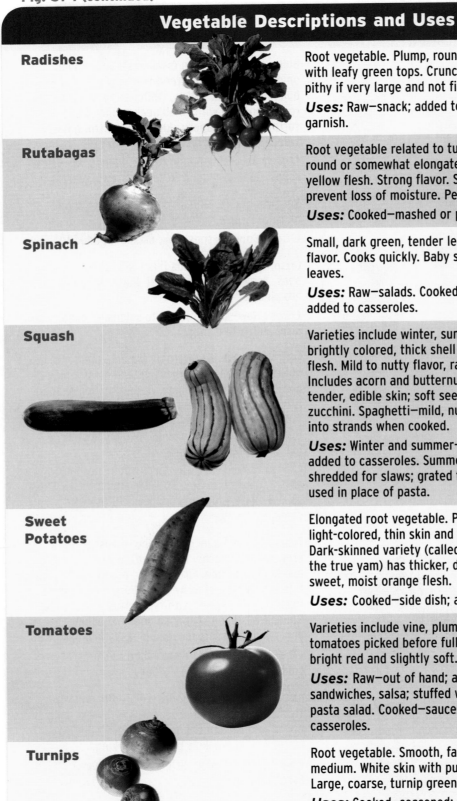

Radishes

Root vegetable. Plump, round, firm, often bright red with leafy green tops. Crunchy and flavorful. May be pithy if very large and not firm.

Uses: Raw—snack; added to salads, sandwiches; garnish.

Rutabagas

Root vegetable related to turnips. Large, smooth, round or somewhat elongated; firm, dense. Sweet, yellow flesh. Strong flavor. Skin may be waxed to prevent loss of moisture. Peel before cooking.

Uses: Cooked—mashed or puréed, seasoned.

Spinach

Small, dark green, tender leaves with slightly bitter flavor. Cooks quickly. Baby spinach has very small leaves.

Uses: Raw—salads. Cooked—seasoned side dish; added to casseroles.

Squash

Varieties include winter, summer, spaghetti. Winter—brightly colored, thick shell with yellow or orange flesh. Mild to nutty flavor, range of sweetness. Includes acorn and butternut. Summer—glossy, tender, edible skin; soft seeds; mild flavor. Includes zucchini. Spaghetti—mild, nutty flesh that separates into strands when cooked.

Uses: Winter and summer—cooked for side dish; added to casseroles. Summer—raw as snack; shredded for slaws; grated for breads. Spaghetti—used in place of pasta.

Sweet Potatoes

Elongated root vegetable. Pale-skinned variety has light-colored, thin skin and pale yellow, dry flesh. Dark-skinned variety (called "yam" but not related to the true yam) has thicker, dark orange skin with sweet, moist orange flesh.

Uses: Cooked—side dish; added to soups and stews.

Tomatoes

Varieties include vine, plum, cherry, beefsteak. Some tomatoes picked before fully ripe. Fully ripe tomatoes bright red and slightly soft. Juicy flesh with seeds.

Uses: Raw—out of hand; added to salads, sandwiches, salsa; stuffed with chicken, seafood, pasta salad. Cooked—sauces; canning; added to casseroles.

Turnips

Root vegetable. Smooth, fairly round, firm, small to medium. White skin with purple tinge, white flesh. Large, coarse, turnip greens can be cooked.

Uses: Cooked—seasoned; mashed; puréed.

The plant parts shown in **Fig. 31-2** are described here.

- **Flowers.** Broccoli and cauliflower are the flowers of a plant. They are tender and can be eaten raw or cooked.
- **Fruits.** Most vegetables from the fruit part of a plant, such as tomatoes, cucumbers, and peppers can be eaten raw. Others, such as eggplant and squash, are usually cooked.
- **Seeds.** Seeds are the plant part that grows new plants. Seeds are high in nutrients and require minimal cooking. Beans, corn, and peas are seeds. Although corn is a grain, people eat a sweet variety of the grain as a vegetable.
- **Stems.** Edible stems are tender, needing minimal cooking. Some, like celery, can be eaten raw. Certain vegetables that are classified as stems include both the stem and the flower. Asparagus is an example.
- **Leaves.** Familiar leaf vegetables include cabbage, lettuce, Brussels sprouts, and spinach. They are tender and many can be eaten raw. Others need minimal cooking.
- **Roots.** Roots store a plant's food supply. Many can be eaten raw, but others must be cooked. Roots include carrots, turnips, and radishes.
- **Tubers.** The potato is a familiar **tuber**—a large, underground stem that stores nutrients. This part of the plant must be cooked.

- **Bulbs.** Bulbs have layers of fleshy leaves surrounding the underground part of the stem. They can be eaten raw or cooked and used in many recipes. Onions and garlic are bulbs.

Some vegetables that come from leaves are called leafy greens. When eaten raw, they are known as **salad greens**. Many lettuce varieties are in this category. They are described in Chapter 41, where salads are discussed. **Cooking greens**, as the name indicates, are typically cooked before being seasoned and eaten. They may also be added to soups, sauces, and other recipes. Cooking greens include collards, dandelion greens, kale, mustard greens, chard, and spinach.

Sea Vegetables

Sea vegetables have been used as food for centuries in coastal regions around the globe. Also known as seaweeds, these vegetables grow in waters with filtered sunlight. Many are grown in Japan. Sea vegetables are classified as algae, not plants. They are low in fat and a rich source of vitamins and minerals; however, they contain more sodium than other vegetables. See **Figs. 31-3** and **31-4** on page 438.

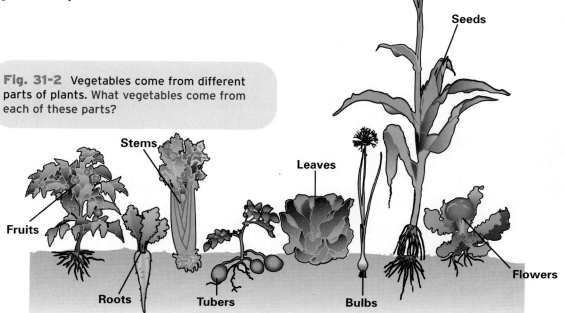

Fig. 31-2 Vegetables come from different parts of plants. What vegetables come from each of these parts?

Seeds

Stems

Leaves

Fruits

Flowers

Roots

Tubers

Bulbs

Fig. 31-3

Common Sea Vegetables

Name	Description	Uses
Arame (ah-rah-meh)	Dark brown with mild, slightly sweet flavor.	Used without cooking in salads; sautéed.
Kombu (KOHM-boo), or kelp	Dark brown or black. Delicate flavor. Sold in sheets or strips. White powder covering the surface adds flavor.	Used in soups, stews, stir-fries, and salads or cooked as vegetable.
Laver (LAY-vuhr)	Dark purple with strong, tangy, slightly sweet flavor. Sold in sheets.	Used in soups or deep-fried as appetizer.
Wakame (WAH-kah-meh)	Deep green. Treated as vegetable.	Adds richness to soups and salads.
Nori (NOH-ree)	Dark green, dark purple, or black with sweet flavor. Comes in sheets.	Used to wrap seafood and rice rolls, sushi (SOO-shee).
Dulse (duhls)	Dark pink to brick red color. Pungent, salty flavor.	Used in soups or as condiment. Also eaten like beef jerky.
Hijiki (hee-GEE-kee)	Black with mild, salty, sea-like flavor. Highest mineral content of all sea vegetables.	Used as a vegetable in soups, stews, and stir-fries.
Agar (AH-gur)	Tasteless. Acts as a vegetarian gelatin. Sold in blocks, flakes, or powder.	Can be used as a substitute for gelatin. Will set at room temperature.

If you've eaten ice cream, you may have eaten sea vegetables without knowing. **Carrageen** (KAR-uh-geen) is a sea vegetable that helps produce the consistency of such products as ice cream, salad dressings, soups, and pudding mixes.

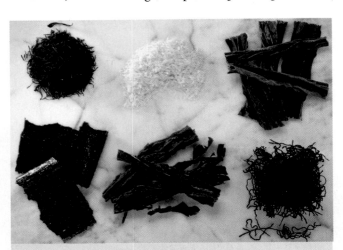

Fig. 31-4 Sea vegetables, sometimes called seaweeds, are often used in Asian dishes. Pictured here are assorted seaweeds. Seaweeds are used both fresh and dried.

FRESH VEGETABLES

Fresh vegetables are appealing for their taste, appearance, versatility, and nutritional value. As with fruit, the summer months bring a bounty of vegetables to the marketplace. Quality generally peaks during this time, and prices are typically lower. Through modern processing, transportation, and storage methods, however, you can enjoy fresh vegetables year round.

When you grow your own vegetables, you have fewer to buy. Gardening is a popular hobby in the United States today. For information on starting a vegetable garden, visit a Cooperative Extension office. Garden shops and books also offer help.

Buying Fresh Vegetables

Depending on where you shop, fresh vegetables may be available loose, in a plastic-covered tray, or in a pre-packaged bag. Some, like broccoli and parsley, usually come in bunches held together with a rubber band or plastic tie. When you buy vegetables, look for these signs of quality:

- **Ripeness.** Since vegetables are harvested when ripe, buy only what you can use during the storage life of the vegetable. Most fresh vegetables should be used within two to five days, although root vegetables last from one to several weeks. Underripe vegetables have poor texture and flavor.
- **Color and texture.** Vegetables should have a bright, characteristic color and crisp texture. Avoid green potatoes. The green color, usually caused by exposure to light, may indicate the presence of a bitter, toxic compound called **solanine** (SOH-luh-neen). If green parts develop during storage, cut them away before cooking.
- **Shape.** The shape should be typical for the vegetable. Misshapen ones usually have inferior texture and flavor.
- **Size.** A vegetable should feel heavy in relation to its size. Extra-large vegetables may be overripe, tough, and have poor flavor. Extremely small ones, which are immature, also lack flavor.
- **Condition.** Avoid choosing wilted, decayed, or damaged vegetables. They have lost nutrients and won't last long. Unless you plan to use the tops of root vegetables, such as carrots and beets, buy them without the tops. The tops draw moisture from root vegetables, making them wilt. Root vegetables, bulbs, and tubers should not be sprouting. Sprouts, or new growth as offshoots, indicate that the vegetables have been stored too long.

Storing Fresh Vegetables

Except for roots, tubers, and bulbs, most vegetables are highly perishable and should be refrigerated as soon as you bring them home. Wash before refrigerating only if dirt is visible, since moisture speeds up bacterial action and causes mold to grow. If you do wash vegetables before storing them, dry them thoroughly.

To maintain the freshness of vegetables, follow these storage tips:

- **Potatoes.** Store potatoes, including sweet potatoes, in a cool, dark, dry place. If you must store them at room temperature, buy only what you can use in a short time. Don't refrigerate them since refrigerator humidity can cause mold and spoilage. In addition, the cold temperature

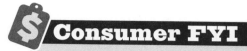

Consumer FYI

Baby vegetables. Two-inch ears of corn and egg-size eggplant aren't agricultural accidents; they're just two examples of baby vegetables. Some are regular vegetables picked while immature. Most are full-grown miniatures.

Baby vegetables, first introduced in restaurants, have found their way into supermarkets. Produce growers and nutritionists hope consumers are won over by the novel appearance and appealing names, like teardrop tomatoes and turnip pearls. Studies show that relatively few Americans eat enough vegetable servings, and baby vegetables are as nutritious as "grown-up" varieties.

Because they're so delicate, baby vegetables cook more quickly; however, they must be used sooner. Given their small size, that's not difficult. You might eat half a dozen ears of baby corn, cob and all, in one serving.

turns the starch in potatoes into sugar, making them slightly sweet. Storing potatoes in a dark place prevents them from turning green. If you don't have a dark storage area, put potatoes in a paper bag.
- **Onions.** Store onions in a cool, dry area. Place them in a basket or loosely woven bag so air can circulate around them. If onions are refrigerated or stored in plastic bags, they get moldy. Avoid storing them in the same bag or bin with potatoes. Onions will absorb moisture from the potatoes and become moldy, and the potatoes will sprout faster.
- **Other vegetables.** Most vegetables should be stored in the refrigerator in plastic bags, airtight containers, or the refrigerator crisper. Use perforated plastic bags to allow moisture to escape. Let tomatoes ripen before refrigerating them.

Washing and Serving Fresh Vegetables

Fresh raw vegetables make an attractive presentation because of their different colors and textures. You can serve many vegetables raw, including celery, cucumbers, radishes, tomatoes, peppers, turnips, carrots, cabbage, cauliflower, and broccoli.

Whether you plan to eat them raw or cook them, wash all fresh vegetables thoroughly. Remember that edible parts of most vegetables grow close to the ground, so they may carry dirt and harmful bacteria. Even vegetables that you will peel need to be washed first to prevent transferring dirt and bacteria to edible parts.

Wash tender vegetables under cool, running water. Scrub potatoes, root vegetables, and thick-skinned vegetables, such as winter squash, with a stiff brush to remove dirt. Don't wash vegetables by soaking them in water or using detergents. Soaking causes nutrient loss, and detergents can react with waxes or pesticide residues on vegetables to form harmful compounds.

After washing, some vegetables—like potatoes—may need to be peeled with a vegetable peeler. You also need to remove any inedible parts, including seeds, stems, and soft spots. To retain more nutrients, eat edible skins instead of peeling them away. For instance, you don't have to peel cucumbers.

Raw vegetables can be served on a relish tray, in salads, or as a snack. To prepare a relish tray as an appetizer, cut vegetables into small pieces that can be picked up easily. Experiment with a variety of shapes for extra appeal. On a serving plate, you might arrange rings, wedges, and sticks in a design that shows off colors and shapes.

To keep a supply of nutritious vegetable snacks on hand, simply cut up raw vegetables and refrigerate them in a covered container or sealed plastic bag. Add a few ice cubes or a tablespoon or two of cold water to the container to keep the vegetables crisp. You can restore crispness to a vegetable like celery by placing it in ice water for a short time.

Cooking Fresh Vegetables

Many vegetables must be cooked to make them edible and easy to digest. Fresh vegetables can be cooked by several different methods. The method you choose and the length of cooking time depends on the vegetable, its tenderness, the size of pieces, and your own taste preferences.

How Cooking Affects Vegetables

Cooking affects not only the look of a vegetable but also its flavor, texture, and nutritional value. In order to avoid unpleasant changes, cook most vegetables for a short time in a small amount of water. Cooking causes these changes in vegetables:

- **Nutrients.** Some nutrients in vegetables dissolve in cooking water or are destroyed by heat. Vitamin C, for instance, is both water soluble and heat sensitive. Vitamin B is lost in water.
- **Texture.** Heat softens the cellulose, or fiber, in cell walls of vegetables, making them tender. If overcooked, vegetables become mushy. Cooked vegetables are most appealing and nutritious when they are still somewhat firm.
- **Color.** When properly cooked, vegetables remain colorful. Green vegetables get their color from chlorophyll, the chemical compound that plants use to turn the sun's energy into food. These vegetables can turn an unpleasant olive color if overcooked. Heat doesn't destroy the carotene that gives some vegetables a yellow or orange color.
- **Flavor.** Cooking releases flavors, making vegetables taste more mellow and delicious. When overcooked, vegetables lose their flavor or may even develop an unpleasant flavor.

Simmering Vegetables

To simmer most vegetables, put a small amount of water in a medium-size saucepan, cover, and bring to a boil. Add the vegetables, re-cover, and bring to a boil again. Then lower the heat until the water simmers. Cook covered, just until the vegetables are tender yet somewhat firm. Drain the vegetables before serving.

For tender vegetables like green beans, broccoli, corn, and peas, allow about ½ cup of water for four servings. Nutrient loss is less with small amounts of water. Spinach, chard, and other greens should be cooked only in the water that clings to their leaves after washing. Tomatoes, too, do not need water added for cooking—just cut them into pieces and cook in the juices that flow out. When water or juice is minimal, keep the heat low enough to prevent scorching.

TALENTED 'TATERS

Have you eaten a potato today? The answer may be yes if you've eaten soup from a can or muffins from a mix. Potatoes are as versatile in food processing as they are on the dinner plate. In fact, about two-thirds of all potatoes sold are used in packaged foods.

Potatoes adapted for processed foods undergo a rigorous ordeal. First they are steam-peeled, then machine-scrubbed. (The peels are used in cattle feed.) Under carefully controlled conditions, the potatoes are partially cooked, cooled, and then cooked again. The resulting mash is thinly spread onto a hot drum and dried. This sheet of pulverized potato is crumbled into fine flakes. Dehydrated potato flakes are not only found in such starchy foods as breads and noodles, but their bland taste and binding quality also make them good filler for meat and fish products.

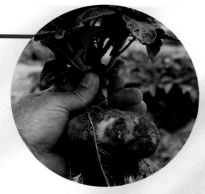

If you like baked or fried snacks, you may have eaten potatoes in another form. To make crunchy, cheese-coated balls and curls, bits of processed potato are forced from a high-pressure machine called an extruder. As each piece shoots out, it rapidly expands into a light, airy snack. The process is called "explosion puffing." Commercially prepared french fries are made this way. To improve the nutrient profile of these snacks, a new method adds dietary fiber using dairy proteins.

__**Think Beyond>>**__ Why are potatoes well suited for the uses described?

Potatoes and beets take longer to cook than many other vegetables. Cover them with water, put on the lid, and simmer until the vegetables are tender. To help retain nutrients, cook both potatoes and beets with skins on. If you prefer to eat them without the skins, peel them after the vegetables have been cooked.

Mashed is one favorite way to prepare potatoes. After the potatoes are cooked, drain the water, add seasonings, and mash with an electric mixer or by hand. A little butter adds rich flavor. Gradually adding a little milk as you beat produces a fluffy texture. Control the amount of milk so that the potatoes don't get too soggy.

In hard-water areas, minerals in cooking water can change the color of red vegetables, such as red cabbage, to purple or purplish-green. To prevent this undesirable color change, add a small amount of acid—vinegar or lemon juice—to the cooking water. Tomatoes retain their color when cooked because nature has provided them with acid.

To allow the true flavor of vegetables to come through, don't add salt during or after cooking. Instead, experiment with flavor by adding herbs or spices or use the cooking water to make a seasoned sauce. Because the cooking liquid contains nutrients, serving it with the vegetables or saving it to use in sauces, soups, or stews is better than discarding it.

Steaming Vegetables

Steaming is a nutritious way to cook vegetables. Because the vegetables are not cooked in water, fewer water-soluble nutrients are lost.

To steam, place a steamer basket in a saucepan with a tight-fitting lid. Add water to a depth just below the bottom of the basket. Cover the pan and bring the water to a boil. Then add the vegetables to the steamer basket and re-cover. Steam until the vegetables are tender. Green beans and other tender vegetables will cook more quickly than such firm vegetables as potatoes and carrots. Thicker pieces also take longer.

Pressure-Cooking Vegetables

A pressure cooker is a handy way to prepare vegetables that need a long cooking time, such as beets, turnips, whole carrots, and potatoes. These foods cook quickly under the high temperature in a pressure cooker. As with steaming, nutrient loss is minimal. Follow the manufacturer's directions carefully when using the cooker.

Braising Vegetables

Onions, carrots, parsnips, and potatoes are often added to braised dishes, a pot roast, for example. You can also braise vegetables for a side dish. Carrots, potatoes, and eggplant work well. Cut them into large pieces and place in a heavy pan with a small amount of water or other liquid. Season them as you like. Cover tightly and bake in the oven at 375°F until the vegetables are tender and browned and the liquid is reduced to a sauce.

Frying Vegetables

Vegetables may be sautéed, fried, stir-fried, or deep-fried. Some **aromatic vegetables**, including onions, garlic, celery, and bell peppers, are sautéed to add flavor and aroma to dishes. Sautéing brings out flavor. See **Fig. 31-5**.

Potatoes and other cooked vegetables may be fried in a small amount of butter or margarine to make them crusty. Hash browns are made this way from shredded cooked potatoes. You can also fry raw vegetables, like potatoes and carrots; however, they take longer to cook when raw.

To speed cooking time for raw vegetables, add a small amount of water to the pan and then cover it so the vegetables also cook in moist heat. Add the water carefully to prevent spatters.

French-fried potatoes are among the deep-fried favorites. Eggplant, onion rings, zucchini, and mushrooms can be dipped in a batter and then deep-fried.

Baking Vegetables

Baking is a simple way to cook many vegetables, including onions, tomatoes, winter squash, potatoes, and eggplant. For instance, you can cut winter squash in half, remove the seeds, and place the halves on a baking sheet. Bake at 350°F for 30 min-

Fig. 31-5

Try This! Recipe

Sautéed Greens

Yield	Nutrition Analysis
4 servings	***Per Serving:*** 70 calories, 1.5 g total fat, 0.5 g saturated fat, 0 g trans fat, 5 mg cholesterol, 570 mg sodium, 9 g total carbohydrate, 6 g dietary fiber, 1 g sugars, 8 g protein ***Percent Daily Value:*** vitamin A 220%, vitamin C 90%, calcium 20%, iron 25%

Ingredients

1½ lb. cooking greens (beet greens, collards, kale, mustard greens, Swiss chard, or turnip greens)

½ cup diced lean ham

¼ cup chopped onion

2 tsp. vinegar

⅛ tsp. pepper

Directions

1. Wash and drain greens. Trim off tough stems. Chop or tear leaves into pieces.
2. Sauté ham in skillet until browned. Remove ham and set aside.
3. Sauté onion in ham drippings until soft.
4. Add greens, vinegar, and pepper. Cover. Cook over medium heat, stirring occasionally, until greens are tender, about 10 to 15 minutes.
5. Return ham to skillet. Mix well and heat through. Serve hot.

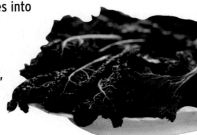

utes or longer, until tender. The exact amount of time depends on the variety and size of the squash.

When you bake whole potatoes in the skin, be sure to poke holes in them first to allow steam to escape. Otherwise, the potatoes may explode. Place the potatoes directly on the oven rack. If you like crispy skin, rub them with oil before placing in the oven. Since potatoes can bake at any temperature between 300°F and 450°F, you can bake them with other foods that need more exact temperatures. For instance, you can bake muffins at 375°F and bake potatoes at the same time. The baking time for the potatoes, of course, will vary with the temperature. They are done when a fork easily pierces the potato.

Roasting Vegetables

Any vegetable can be roasted. See **Fig. 31-6**. Brussels sprouts, carrots, onions, turnips, and asparagus are particularly good prepared this way. Cut the vegetables into pieces of similar size. Drizzle with oil, sprinkle with seasonings, and toss lightly to coat. Then place them on a baking sheet in a single layer. Roast at 425°F until browned, tender, and caramelized. To assure even roasting, turn the vegetables over about halfway through the cooking time.

Potatoes, onions, and carrots can be roasted in the same pan with a roast. Pare the vegetables. Then place them in the pan around the roast. Cut large pieces into halves or quarters. Turn occasionally to moisten them with the drippings. Although this method adds fat to vegetables, it also browns them and produces a tasty crust.

Grilling Vegetables

Grilling is a nutritious, flavorful way to cook vegetables. Keep in mind that vegetables cook at different rates. Since the center of the grill is usually the hottest, use this space for potatoes and other long-cooking vegetables. Large pieces can be wrapped in heavy-duty foil and placed on the grate; small pieces can be grilled in a vegetable basket or on skewers.

Here are some additional guidelines:

- Brush the grate with oil to keep vegetables from sticking.

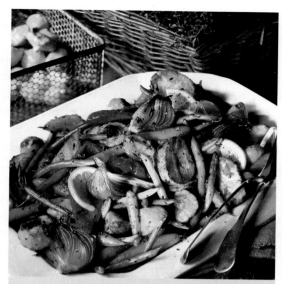

Fig. 31-6 Roasted vegetables take on a delicious flavor when the outside forms a brown, caramelized crust.

- To shorten grilling time, blanch less tender vegetables, such as carrots, before grilling.
- Marinate vegetables for added flavor.
- To keep vegetables from drying out, brush them with an oil and herb mixture.
- When grilling vegetables on skewers, arrange those with similar cooking times together.

Microwaving Vegetables

A microwave oven cooks vegetables quickly, using only a small amount of water. As a result, vegetables lose few nutrients and retain color, texture, and flavor.

Large vegetable pieces take longer to cook than small ones. If parts of a vegetable are less tender, such as broccoli stems, arrange tender parts toward the center and less tender ones toward the edge of the baking dish. Cover the container to retain moisture, and stir the vegetables during cooking to allow for better heat distribution. When cooking potatoes, squash, and other whole vegetables that have a skin, first pierce the skin with a fork to keep the vegetables from bursting.

Follow directions in the owner's manual for cooking times, power settings, and any special instructions.

CONVENIENCE FORMS OF VEGETABLES

Busy cooks appreciate the convenience forms of vegetables: canned, frozen, and dried. As the name implies, convenience vegetables are handy and generally fuss-free. They can be stored longer than fresh vegetables, can be prepared quickly, and are often used in recipes. No matter what the season, convenience vegetables are always available and often at a lower cost than fresh vegetables.

Although canned and frozen vegetables may have a different texture and taste than fresh vegetables, they generally contain similar amounts of vitamins and minerals. This is because processing techniques preserve much of their nutritional value, while fresh vegetables can lose nutrients during handling, storage, and cooking.

When buying convenience vegetables, use the guidelines you learned in Chapter 17. To prepare them, use the tips that follow.

Canned Vegetables

Vegetables are canned whole, sliced, or in pieces. Although most are packed in water, some, such as Harvard beets and creamed corn, are packed in sauces. Salt is generally added to canned vegetables as a preservative, but you can usually find no-salt versions.

Canned vegetables can be used the same way you use cooked fresh vegetables—for instance, as a side dish or in a salad. Since canned vegetables have already been cooked during the canning process, just heat the vegetables in their liquid in a saucepan on the stove until heated through. You can also heat them in the microwave oven. Take care not to overcook them, as they will soften and lose nutrients and color.

Frozen Vegetables

Frozen vegetables are closest in nutrients, color, and flavor to fresh varieties, although texture may be different. They are packaged whole or in pieces. You can also buy combination vegetables, often used in stews or stir-fry dishes, and vegetables packed in cheese or butter sauces. Frozen vegetables usually come in cartons or plastic bags of various sizes. Just pour out what you need and store what's left in the freezer. Some come in a plastic pouch for heating.

Frozen vegetables take less time to cook than fresh vegetables because they are preheated prior to freezing. To cook frozen vegetables, follow the directions on the package. As with canned vegetables, frozen varieties retain flavor, color, and nutrients best if they are heated for the least amount of time necessary.

Dried Vegetables

Dried vegetables come in different forms. Mushrooms, tomatoes, and potatoes are among the vegetables that can be dehydrated and later reconstituted, mainly for use in recipes. Dried vegetables are reconstituted, or restored to their former condition, by adding water.

Many vegetables, including onions, parsley, chives, and garlic, are dried for use as flavorings in entrées, side dishes, and soups. Follow package directions for use.

USING LEFTOVER VEGETABLES

Leftovers don't have to be boring. Try marinating cold, cooked vegetables in a tangy salad dressing and serve on a bed of lettuce. You can add cooked vegetables to a stir-fry dish or mix them into a casserole. With a little creativity, you can come up with many ideas. See **Fig. 31-7**.

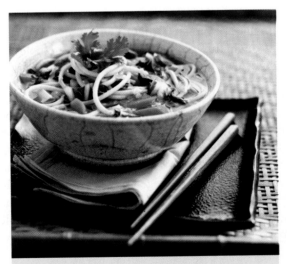

Fig. 31-7 You can make good use of leftover vegetables by adding them to soup.

Television Chef

CURTIS AIKENS: For Curtis Aikens, it all started in a garden—his grandfather's vegetable garden in Georgia. There, as a child, his love of fresh foods sprouted along with the collards and beans. Working at a supermarket in high school, he was drawn to the produce department, "where all the action was." Equally inspiring was his mother's cooking. He even took pictures of her making biscuits in the morning—"it was such a beautiful, loving sight." With warm associations like these, a career in foods was calling.

Uprooted. A vacation in California convinced Curtis to relocate to the San Francisco Bay area in the early 1980s. Within a year, he opened his own produce company, aptly named Peaches, yet his rising success was threatened by a painful secret. At age twenty-six, Curtis couldn't read. In school, his gift for talking plus an outgoing personality had carried him through. Those skills could get him only so far in business, so overcoming his deep embarrassment and aided by literacy volunteers, he began making up for lost time. Today, reading is a favorite pastime.

In 1986, Curtis headed for New York. As head of the produce departments of several large wholesalers, he fed diplomats at the United Nations and tennis fans at the U.S. Open Tournament. He styled hamburgers in ads for McDonald's. A few years later he was back in Georgia, running Aikens Family Produce. One of his clients, ironically, was his old school.

A Star Is Born. Curtis began his road to celebrity with a local weekly foods column focused on fresh produce. This led to spots on the news. Curtis's obvious enthusiasm for food and greater delight in people shined on television. By the early 1990s he was a regular on *Good Morning America*, with appearances on *The Oprah Winfrey Show* and CNN. He has hosted a series of shows on the Food Network since its beginning.

In 1991, Curtis released his first cookbook. *Guide to the Harvest* shares a wealth of wisdom in choosing and using fruits, vegetables, nuts, and herbs. "Down home" recipes like stewed okra share space with California-inspired creations like eggplant enchiladas. Later books, written after Curtis was diagnosed with diabetes, emphasize heart-healthy eating. By donating part of his royalties, his books help fund literacy projects.

Yielding Good Fruit. What drives Curtis more than foods and cooking is the love he shares while showing people how to enjoy food and nourish their families. The desire to touch others energizes his crusade for literacy, with appearances at the White House and on the PBS series *Reading Rainbow*, and spurs his promotion of diabetes awareness in the African-American community. Lately, it has inspired him to return to school for a degree and teaching certificate. He wants to be a high school teacher by the time his own two sons are teens. "When you do what you love," he says, "everything will follow that."

On-line Connections

1. To learn more about topics in this article, search the Internet for these key words: literacy programs; heart-healthy recipes.

2. To learn about related careers, search the Internet for these key words: produce buyer; organic farming.

Summarize Your Reading

▶ Edible plants, from artichokes to zucchini, come from different plant parts. They are a nutritious part of a healthy diet.

▶ Fresh vegetables must be selected carefully and stored correctly for quality and safety. Most vegetables need to be refrigerated to ensure freshness.

▶ Cooking affects not only the look of a vegetable but also its flavor, texture, and nutritional value. Vegetables can be cooked in many different ways, including simmering, steaming, pressure-cooking, braising, frying, baking, roasting, grilling, or microwaving.

▶ Convenience forms of vegetables include canned, frozen, and dried.

Check Your Knowledge

1. What makes vegetables a healthful part of an eating plan?

2. Compare broccoli, cabbage, and cauliflower.

3. How would you use garlic?

4. For each plant part, name an edible vegetable that comes from that part.

5. How are **tubers** and bulbs different?

6. What are examples of **cooking greens**?

7. Describe **sea vegetables** and their nutritional value.

8. Why should you avoid purchasing potatoes that are green or sprouting?

9. Should you buy carrots and beets with the tops? Explain.

10. **CRITICAL THINKING** You're headed to the farmers market to buy vegetables to use in the next few days. What will you look for to get the best produce?

11. How should potatoes and onions be stored, and why?

12. How and why should vegetables be washed?

13. **CRITICAL THINKING** A teen plans to bake acorn squash halves. Since the skin won't be eaten, he doesn't wash the squash. Evaluate this decision.

14. What changes occur in vegetables when cooked and overcooked?

15. When simmering vegetables, why should you use only a small amount of water?

16. Why is steaming a nutritious way to cook vegetables?

17. Which vegetables might you cook in a pressure cooker, and why?

18. Explain the difference between braising and frying vegetables.

19. How would you prepare potatoes for baking whole and for roasting?

20. What are some guidelines to follow for grilling vegetables?

21. What precaution should be taken when baking a potato in the microwave oven? Why?

22. What advantages do convenience vegetables have?

23. How are dried foods reconstituted?

24. How can leftover vegetables be served creatively?

Apply Your Learning

1. **LANGUAGE ARTS** **Puppet Play.** Develop a puppet play for young children about the benefits of eating vegetables. Perform it for young children.

2. **Nutrition Comparison.** Make a chart that compares the nutritional value of three of your favorite vegetables and three of your least favorite. Summarize your conclusions in writing.

3. **Vegetable Exploration.** Research one topic and report to the class: a) squash identification; b) mushroom identification; c) potato identification; d) baby vegetables; e) starting a vegetable garden; f) less familiar vegetables (for example, fiddlehead ferns, celeriac, broccoflower, fennel).

4. **MATH** **Cost Comparison.** Conduct a cost comparison of fresh, canned, frozen, and dried vegetables. Include both store brands and national brands. Which is the least expensive?

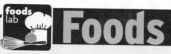

Foods Lab

Vegetable Recipes

Procedure: With your team, find recipes that use vegetables from the plant part assigned to you (for example, stem or root vegetables). Choose one recipe to prepare and offer for a class taste test. The recipe you choose should use one or more of the vegetables as primary ingredients.

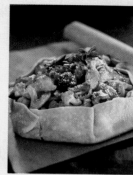

Analyzing Results

❶ How would you rate your dish on appearance, taste, and ease of preparation? Why?

❷ Of all the dishes prepared, which ones score highest on nutrition? Why?

❸ Were any of the vegetables or dishes new to you? Would you eat them again? Explain.

Food Science Experiment

Water Absorption in Vegetables

Objective: To compare water absorption in different vegetables.

Procedure:

1. Pour ½ cup of water into each of two glasses. Tint each with one drop of blue food coloring. Cover both glasses tightly with aluminum foil.

2. Cut the bottom off a stalk of celery. Poke a hole in the foil on one glass and place the cut end of the celery in the water.

3. Slice the top off a carrot. Repeat Step 2, using the other glass.

4. Leave the glasses together in the same place overnight. The next day, slice each vegetable lengthwise and observe the interior. Measure the water in each glass.

Analyzing Results

❶ Which vegetable absorbed more water? How was the water absorbed?

❷ Explain the reason for the results you noted in the previous question, based on the part of the plant each vegetable comes from.

❸ How might these findings help you decide how to prepare different vegetables?

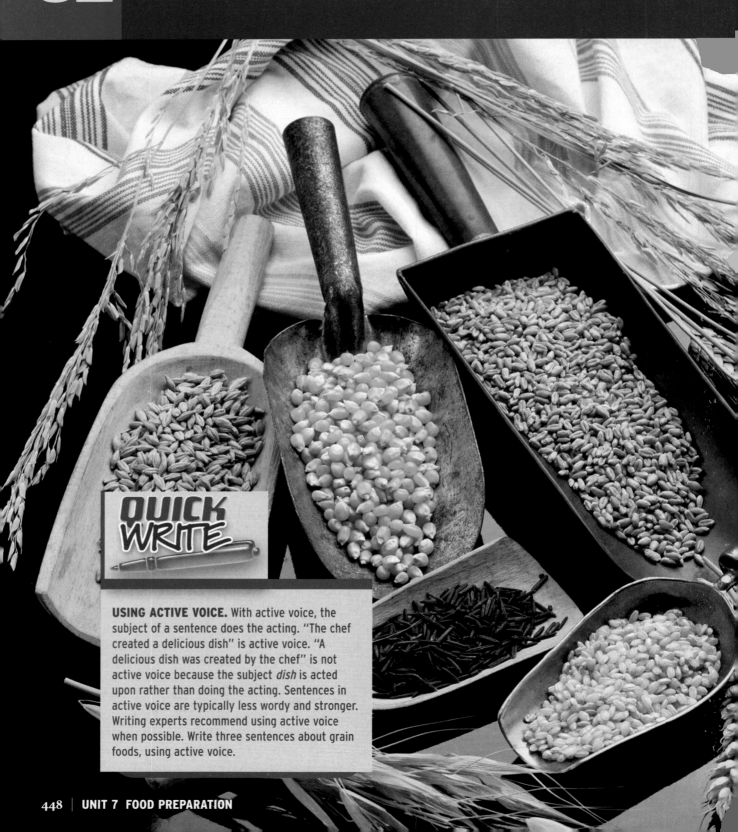

QUICK WRITE

USING ACTIVE VOICE. With active voice, the subject of a sentence does the acting. "The chef created a delicious dish" is active voice. "A delicious dish was created by the chef" is not active voice because the subject *dish* is acted upon rather than doing the acting. Sentences in active voice are typically less wordy and stronger. Writing experts recommend using active voice when possible. Write three sentences about grain foods, using active voice.

Objectives

▶ Identify grain products and their uses.

▶ Explain the value of grains in the diet.

▶ Explain how to select and store grains.

▶ Describe and demonstrate methods for preparing, cooking, and serving grains.

Terms

- al dente
- bran
- endosperm
- flatbread
- germ
- grains
- hull
- kernels
- leavened bread
- macaroni
- noodles
- pasta
- rice
- wheat
- whole grain
- whole wheat

BEFORE YOU START TO READ THIS CHAPTER, list the grains that are familiar to you. Are you stumped after just a few? Many people are, yet the list of grains is surprisingly long. Perhaps no other foods are as universal and versatile as grains. Properly prepared, they are not only a nutritious, flavorful addition to meals but also an economical way to stretch a food budget.

WHAT ARE GRAINS?

All plants in the grass family are **grains**, sometimes called cereals. Common grains in North America include wheat, corn, rice, oats, rye, barley, buckwheat, and millet. Grains produce many small, separate dry fruits called **kernels**, which are harvested and processed for food. Because grain kernels are fruits, grains are sometimes called berries, as in wheat berries.

Every grain kernel has three main parts. The **bran** is the edible, outer layer of the kernel. The **endosperm**, the largest part of the kernel, is made of proteins and starches and contains the plant's food supply. The **germ** is the seed that grows into a new plant. Some grains are covered with an inedible outer coat called the **hull**, which is removed after harvesting. See **Fig. 32-1**.

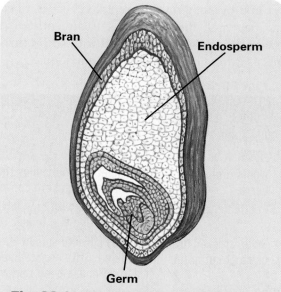

Fig. 32-1 A grain kernel has three main parts. All three parts are used to make whole-grain products. The parts are separated and used individually to make other grain products.

Grains are processed into several forms for different uses. For instance, oats can be rolled and flaked for use in hot cereals and cookies, or they can be ground into flour. **Fig. 32-2** on page 450 shows several common grain forms.

NUTRIENTS IN GRAINS

Whole grains are rich in nutrients. The endosperm consists mostly of complex carbohydrates and proteins, and the bran contains dietary fiber, B vitamins, and minerals. The germ provides protein, unsaturated fats, B vitamins, vitamin E, iron, and zinc, as well as other minerals and phytochemicals.

Before consumers can use them, all grains must be processed. The type of processing affects a grain's nutrient value. **Whole-grain** products, including whole-wheat flour and whole-grain breakfast cereals, are made of the entire kernel and so contain most of the original nutrients.

Very often during processing, the bran and germ are removed, leaving only the endosperm. As a result, most of the vitamins, minerals, phytochemicals, and dietary fiber are also removed. White flour and many breakfast cereals are made this way. According to federal law, some nutrients lost in processing must be replaced. As described in Chapter 4, this is called enrichment. Some grain products may be fortified with such nutrients as iron to make them more nutritious.

GRAINS AND GRAIN PRODUCTS

Grains have been a food staple in the world for thousands of years. Because grains are abundant, they offer many dining options. Grains can be eaten plain or topped with vegetables, seasonings, and sauces. They are used in side dishes, casseroles, soups, and baked goods. Sometimes they thicken soups and stews. Cooked grains can be eaten as hot breakfast cereals. **Fig. 32-3** shows a recipe idea. You might eat hot oatmeal for breakfast, a whole-wheat sandwich for lunch, and

Fig. 32-2

Grain Forms		
Form	**Description**	**Typical Uses**
Whole grains or berries	Complete kernel minus the hull. They cook slowly and are chewy.	Processed into other forms or used in side dishes, cereals, soups, and stews.
Pearled grains	Whole grain with bran layer removed. Fast cooking and tender texture.	Processed into other forms or used in side dishes, cereals, soups, and stews.
Grits, cracked grains, or steel-cut grains	Grains cut into small pieces to speed cooking. Grits are steamed and soaked, and germ has been removed.	Cereals, side dishes, and baking.
Flakes or rolled grains	Grains that have been steamed, flattened between rollers, and flaked.	Hot cereals, cookies, breads, soups, and casseroles.
Meal	Gritty, ground, whole grains. Stone-ground meal has been ground between stones.	Hot cereals and breads.
Bran	Outer layer of grain. Rich in fiber.	Cereals; baked goods; topping for fruits and desserts.
Germ	The seed of the kernel. Rich in nutrients.	Breads; cereals.
Flour	Grain ground to a fine powder.	Baked goods; thickener.

Pearl barley

pasta for dinner. Grains even become desserts by adding sweeteners or fruits. Not many meals go by that don't include at least one of the grains described here.

Wheat

Wheat is one of the oldest food plants. Thousands of wheat varieties exist. These are some of the grain products made from wheat:

- **Wheat berries.** The entire wheat kernel, including bran and germ. This very chewy form of wheat can be cooked as a cereal or used in grain-based dishes.
- **Bulgur.** Wheat kernels that have been steamed, dried, and crushed. Bulgur is tender, with a chewy texture, and is used in main dishes, in salads, and as a side dish. One common dish is *tabbouleh* (tuh-BOO-lee), a Middle Eastern salad with chopped tomatoes, onions, parsley, mint, lemon juice, and olive oil.
- **Cracked wheat.** Made from crushed wheat berries. Cracked wheat has a tough, chewy texture and is often added to bread.

Rice

Rice is the starchy seed of plants grown in flooded fields in warm climates. Much of the rice produced grows in Asian paddies, or wetlands, but some is grown in a few parts of the United States.

A common way to categorize rice is by grain length. Each type has a different purpose.

- **Long grain.** This is the most-used rice in the United States. When cooked, the grains are fluffy and they stay separated. Long-grain rice

---

Fig. 32-3

Try This! **Recipe**

Apple and Spice Oatmeal

Yield	Nutrition Analysis
2 servings	**Per Serving:** 270 calories, 4.5 g total fat, 0.5 g saturated fat, 0 g trans fat, 0 mg cholesterol, 40 mg sodium, 50 g total carbohydrates, 5 g dietary fiber, 21 g sugars, 8 g protein **Percent Daily Value:** vitamin A 4%, vitamin C 4%, calcium 10%, iron 15%

Ingredients

²/₃ cup fat-free milk
²/₃ cup unsweetened apple juice
½ cup chopped, tart, cooking apple
⅛ tsp. grated orange peel
dash cinnamon
dash allspice

²/₃ cup quick-cooking oatmeal (not instant)
2 Tbsp. chopped dates
½ tsp. honey
1 Tbsp. chopped walnuts

Directions

1. Combine milk, apple juice, chopped apple, orange peel, cinnamon, and allspice in a 1-qt. saucepan. Bring to a boil.
2. Add oatmeal and dates.
3. Cook for 1 minute, stirring frequently.
4. Remove from heat and stir in honey.
5. Cover and let stand 2 minutes.
6. Spoon into serving bowls. Sprinkle each serving with some of the chopped walnuts and serve.

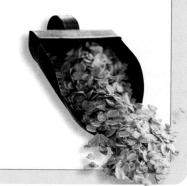

hardens when it cools, so it isn't recommended for puddings and cold salads. It is often used as a side dish. Basmati (bahz-MAH-tee) rice is a long-grain rice with a fine texture and fragrant, nutlike aroma and flavor.

- **Medium grain.** Shorter than long-grain rice, these grains are plump, tender, and moist. They stick together, but not as much as short grain. They can be used for puddings and cold salads.
- **Short grain.** These grains are almost round, and they have the highest starch content of the three types. When cooked, the grains are moist and stick together. Short-grain rice is usually used for creamy dishes and molded rice rings. Asian cuisine uses short grain because it's easy to eat with chopsticks. Italian arborio (ar-BOH-ree-oh) rice is a short-grain rice traditionally used to make risotto (rih-SAH-toh), a creamy rice dish.

Rice also varies in the way it's processed. Enriched, or white, rice is a favorite. The bran and germ are removed, leaving only the endosperm. Although enriched, white rice lacks some nutrients, phytochemicals, and dietary fiber.

Brown rice is the whole-grain form of rice. Only the hull has been removed. The bran, endosperm, and germ remain, along with all the nutrients and dietary fiber. Brown rice takes longer to cook than white rice and has a nutlike flavor and chewy texture.

Converted rice is steamed under pressure to save nutrients before the hull is removed. It is enriched and takes longer to cook than white rice.

Instant rice is precooked and dehydrated before packaging. Although it takes only a few minutes to prepare, it is the least nutritious. See **Fig. 32-4**.

Wild rice isn't actually rice; it's the seed of a water grass. With a crisp texture and nutlike flavor, wild rice is high in protein and dietary fiber. Because the supply is limited, it's very expensive and is often sold combined with long-grain rice.

Corn

As far back as 3500 B.C., people were raising corn in Central America. Corn has long been a

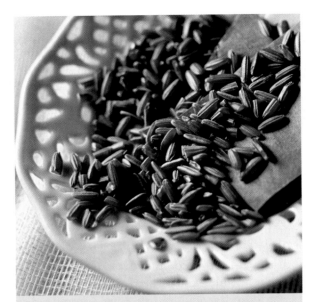
Fig. 32-4 Regular brown rice has a long cooking time. You can also buy instant brown rice, which cooks quickly.

fundamental food plant. Today the corn plant is used for many purposes other than food, including uses in making plastics and dyes.

Some familiar grain products are made from corn. Hominy is the dried kernel with the hull and germ removed, leaving only the endosperm. When hominy is coarsely ground, it becomes grits, which can be served as a side dish or used in casseroles. Cornmeal, used in recipes, comes from ground, dried, corn kernels. The endosperm of corn is also ground into a fine flour called cornstarch, used as a thickening agent in sauces and fillings.

Oats

If you've eaten oatmeal cookies, you've savored the pleasant, slightly sweet flavor of oats. Although most of the oat grain produced in the world feeds animals, a small portion is used by humans. This grain is usually eaten as a hot breakfast cereal or used in baked goods. Even though oats are processed, they contain considerable nutrients and dietary fiber. Quick-cooking types are available.

Other Grains

Although wheat, corn, rice, and oats are deeply rooted in the American past and used in countless ways today, many other grains are enjoyed as well.

- **Amaranth** (A-muh-ranth). Tiny round seeds, once the staple crop of the ancient Aztecs. When cooked, gets thick and sticky and has a sweet, nutty flavor. Can be used as a hot cereal or side dish or in puddings.
- **Barley.** Thought to be one of the most ancient grains. A staple in Asia, the Middle East, and parts of Europe. Unlike other grains, the entire kernel contains dietary fiber. Mild-flavored, chewy grain, usually used in soups and stews. Hulled barley has the outer hull removed but retains the bran, so it has more dietary fiber than other types of barley. Pearl barley, the most common form sold in supermarkets, has the outer hull and bran removed, but it still contains 50 percent of the original fiber. Scotch (or pot) barley is less processed than pearl barley and is used in salads, soups, and casseroles.
- **Buckwheat.** Has a nutlike, earthy flavor. High in protein and other nutrients. Commonly ground into flour or crushed and used as breakfast cereal.

- **Couscous** (KOOS-koos). Steamed, cracked endosperm of durum wheat, with a flavor similar to pasta. Used as a cereal, in salads and main dishes, or sweetened for dessert. A staple in North African cuisines.
- **Kasha** (KAH-shuh). Roasted buckwheat that is hulled and crushed. Has a pleasant, nutty flavor. Used extensively in Eastern European, Middle Eastern, and Asian cuisines. Used in the United States as a breakfast cereal or side dish.
- **Millet.** Small, yellow grains with a mild flavor. A staple in Europe, Asia, and North Africa. Used in breads and as a breakfast cereal or side dish.
- **Quinoa** (KEEN-wah). Small, ivory-colored, rice-like grain that was a staple of the Incas. Popular in South American cuisines. Cooks quickly and has a unique, mild flavor. Contains more protein than any other grain. Used as a side dish and in soups, puddings, and salads.
- **Rye.** Dark with hearty flavor. Common in northern Europe. Used in breads and crackers. Less nutritious than other grains but high in minerals. See **Fig. 32-5**.

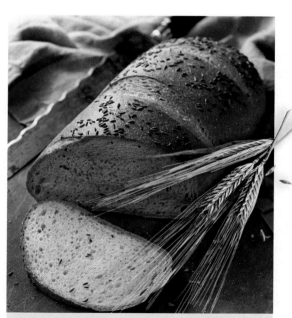

Fig. 32-5 Rye is a cereal grain that is similar to wheat. The seeds are ground to make rye flour.

- **Spelt.** Mellow, nutty flavor. Used for thousands of years in southern Europe. Tolerated by people with wheat allergies. Spelt flour can be substituted for wheat flour in baking. Available in natural foods stores.
- **Teff.** Tiny grain with mild, nutty flavor; brown and white varieties. Native to North Africa and a staple in Ethiopian cuisine for thousands of years. Used as a cooked cereal and in puddings.
- **Triticale (trih-tuh-KAY-lee).** A cross between wheat and rye, with more protein than wheat. Can be used in cereals and main dishes and combined with other cooked grains.

Pasta

Counting the ways that pasta can be served would surely be impossible. This food comforts and delights people in many parts of the world. **Pasta** is an Italian word meaning "paste," or dough made from flour and water. Pasta includes **macaroni** products, which are made from durum (DUR-uhm) wheat flour and water, and **noodles**, which have egg solids added for tenderness.

Durum wheat is grown especially for pasta. It is processed into semolina (seh-muh-LEE-nuh) flour, which gives pasta its characteristic yellow color and nutlike flavor. Durum wheat products hold their shape and firm texture when cooked.

After pasta dough is rolled thin, machines form it into hundreds of different shapes. **Fig. 32-6** shows some common pasta shapes. Certain sauces go best with specific shapes. For instance, smooth tomato and cream sauces and sauces with small pieces of food complement long, flat pasta. Large, hollow shapes are usually stuffed with a meat, vegetable, fish, or cheese mixture and baked in a sauce.

Pasta is sold in both dried and fresh forms. Dried pasta, the more common, is preserved by a drying process. Packages of dried pasta are found with other shelf-stable foods. Fresh pasta, which is perishable, is in the refrigerated section.

You can choose enriched or whole-wheat pastas. Whole-wheat pasta has more dietary fiber than the enriched kind. Some pastas are flavored and colored with carrots, spinach, tomatoes, and other foods.

In addition to traditional pasta, Asian noodles are sold in the ethnic section of many supermarkets. These noodles are made from many different flours, such as rice, potato, cornstarch, bean, and soy. Chinese cellophane noodles, for instance, are thin, translucent noodles made from mung-bean starch. Japanese ramen (RAH-mehn) are made from wheat flour and deep-fried, and Japanese soba (so-BAH) noodles are made from buckwheat flour.

CONVENIENCE FORMS OF GRAINS

With convenience forms of grain products, preparation is quick and easy.

Breakfast Cereals

Wheat, oats, and corn are some of the grains commonly made into breakfast cereals. These cereals may consist of whole grains; refined, enriched grains; or both. Dry breakfast cereals are ready to eat out of the container; other types need cooking.

Ready-to-eat cereals include puffed, rolled, flaked, granulated, and shredded types. Some are coated with sugar or other sweeteners, and they may have fruit, nuts, and other flavorings added.

Oats and other cereals that require cooking come in regular, quick-cooking, and instant forms. Often, sugar and other flavorings have been added. Instant cereal has usually been precooked and requires only mixing with boiling water.

Besides being flavorful, breakfast cereals can fit into a healthy eating plan. Be sure to read the Nutrition Facts panel on the box or bag and look for a product that is high in complex carbohydrates and dietary fiber. You don't need a cereal that provides 100 percent of the recommended daily requirement because other foods you eat also provide nutrients. You can often get a nutritious product at a lower cost by buying cereals that are not highly fortified.

Breads

When you walk into a bakery, you may notice the wonderful aromas first and then see the wide array of flavors, textures, shapes, and sizes. Breads and individual rolls are made from enriched white flour, whole wheat, and mixed whole

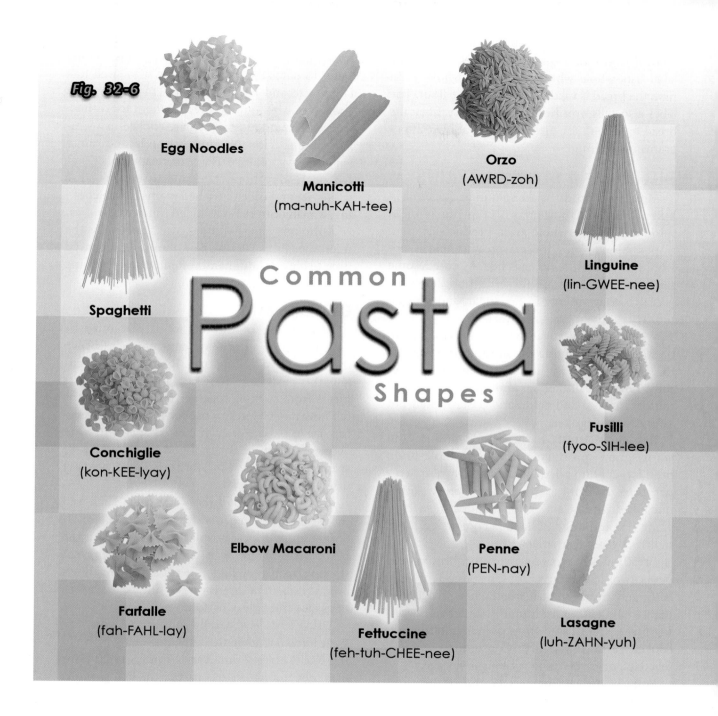

Fig. 32-6

Common Pasta Shapes

Egg Noodles

Manicotti
(ma-nuh-KAH-tee)

Orzo
(AWRD-zoh)

Linguine
(lin-GWEE-nee)

Spaghetti

Fusilli
(fyoo-SIH-lee)

Conchiglie
(kon-KEE-lyay)

Elbow Macaroni

Penne
(PEN-nay)

Farfalle
(fah-FAHL-lay)

Fettuccine
(feh-tuh-CHEE-nee)

Lasagne
(luh-ZAHN-yuh)

grains. **Leavened bread** (LE-vuhnd) is made with a leavening agent, such as yeast or baking powder, which makes the bread rise. **Flatbreads**, like tortillas, are unleavened, or made without leavenings. Pita bread is a flatbread that splits horizontally, forming a pocket to fill with foods.

When buying bread, read the label carefully. **Whole wheat** means that the product is made from the whole grain. **Wheat**, however, just means white flour. Some dark breads, such as pumpernickel, are made with white and rye flour and then colored with caramel or molasses.

Don't be misled by words like *multigrain*, *cracked wheat*, or *7-grain* on a label. Unless the label lists whole wheat or another whole grain first, the bread is made mostly of white flour. The label also tells you how much dietary fiber the bread has. Look for bread that has at least 2 to 3 grams per serving.

BUYING AND STORING GRAINS

Most grain products are sold in packages or in bulk. When you buy grains, keep nutrition in mind and choose whole-grain products as often as possible. If you choose a product that is not whole grain, be sure it's enriched. As noted, some ready-to-eat cereals are the exception. Look for products that are low in fat, sugar, and sodium too. Try different grains for variety.

When buying grains, read the label carefully to be sure you are getting the product you want. If the grain is visible in the package, inspect it carefully. Whole-grain kernels should be plump and uniform in size and color, and pasta should not be cracked or broken.

Refrigerate fresh pasta, whole grains, and whole-grain products. Because whole-grain products contain oil, they can spoil at room temperature if not used quickly. Store other uncooked grains and grain products, such as white rice and dried pasta, in a cool, dry place in tightly covered containers.

Breads may be stored short-term at room temperature or in the freezer for long periods of time. Although bread gets stale faster when refrigerated than when left out, in humid weather refrigerating bread keeps mold from growing. Refrigerate cooked grains if you plan to use them within a few days, or freeze them for longer storage.

You can review Chapters 17 and 20 for information on buying and storing packaged foods.

PREPARING GRAINS

Through photosynthesis, plants make simple sugars. As simple sugars link, they form complex carbohydrates, or starch. Grains are full of starch granules, which have many layers of tightly packed molecules. When you heat a grain in water, the molecules start moving, the chemical bonds break, and the tight layers loosen. This enables water to enter the starch, causing it to swell to a larger size and become softer. This is why you cook grains in liquid to prepare them for eating.

Even though most grains are cooked in a similar way, specific cooking methods and times vary. Always follow package or recipe directions. Unless the directions state otherwise, don't rinse white rice and other enriched grains before cooking. Rinsing can remove added nutrients.

Although many foods cook faster in the microwave, this isn't true of grains. Grains need time to absorb liquid and soften, so microwaving doesn't usually save time.

Cooking Pasta

Pasta is one of the few foods that must be boiled. Choose a pot that's large enough to keep the water from boiling over. Boiling helps circulate the pasta for even cooking and prevents pieces from sticking together. Package directions tell how much water to use for a particular serving size of pasta. For example, dry spaghetti takes about 1 quart of water for every 4 ounces of spaghetti. See **Fig. 32-7** for the cooked yields of dried pasta.

To cook pasta, boil the water first. Then add the pasta slowly so the water continues to boil. If boiling stops, the pasta will stick together. Stir the pasta occasionally as it cooks to help prevent sticking. Don't add oil to the cooking water, however, as it forms a slippery pasta surface that keeps the sauce from clinging to it.

Dried pasta is generally cooked to a doneness stage known as **al dente** (ahl DEN-tay), or firm to the bite. Cooking time varies from 5 to 20 minutes, depending on the pasta's thickness. If the pasta will be added to a dish for more cooking, as in lasagne, reduce the boiling time to keep the pasta slightly firmer. Unless directions state otherwise, fresh pasta cooks in a fraction of the time needed for dried pasta. Follow package directions to prepare pasta for the recipe in **Fig. 32-8**.

After cooking, drain the pasta in a colander or strainer. Never rinse cooked pasta. Doing so removes nutrients. To keep cooked pasta hot, set

Fig. 32-7

Dried Pasta Yields			
Type of Pasta	Dry Weight	Dry Volume	Cooked Yield (approximate)
Small pasta shapes: macaroni, shells, spirals, twists	4 ounces	1 cup	2½ cups
Long, slender, pasta strands: spaghetti, angel hair, vermicelli	4 ounces	1-inch-diameter bunch	2 cups

Fig. 32-8

Try This! **Recipe**

Molded Pasta Salad

Yield
8 servings

Nutrition Analysis
Per Serving: 370 calories, 16 g total fat, 4 g saturated fat, 0 g trans fat, 125 mg cholesterol, 700 mg sodium, 33 g total carbohydrate, 2 g dietary fiber, 4 g sugars, 23 g protein

Percent Daily Value: vitamin A 15%, vitamin C 40%, calcium 8%, iron 15%

Ingredients
2¾ cups elbow macaroni (6 cups cooked)
2½ cups smoked turkey, cut into ¼-inch cubes
2 cups chopped, frozen broccoli, defrosted
3 hard-cooked eggs, peeled and chopped into ¼-inch pieces
3 Tbsp. finely chopped green onions (green only)

1 Tbsp. unflavored gelatin
1 cup chicken stock (¼ cup cold and ¾ cup hot)
1 cup light mayonnaise
¾ cup light sour cream
⅛ tsp. cayenne pepper
1 tsp. salt
2 tsp. fresh sage (1 tsp. dried)

Directions
1. Cook macaroni according to package directions and cool slightly.
2. In large bowl, combine cubed turkey, chopped broccoli, chopped eggs, and chopped green onions with pasta. Gently mix with large rubber spatula.
3. In medium bowl, sprinkle gelatin over ¼ cup cold chicken stock. Let soften for 5 minutes. Add ¾ cup hot chicken stock and mix to dissolve. Cool for 15 minutes.
4. Whisk mayonnaise into gelatin mixture. Gently mix in sour cream with a rubber spatula. Add cayenne pepper, salt, and sage and adjust to taste.
5. Pour mayonnaise mixture over pasta mixture and gently mix with rubber spatula until well coated.
6. Spray 10- or 12-cup mold or tube pan with vegetable cooking spray. Pour mixture into mold and pack in evenly. Cover with plastic wrap. Chill until firm, at least 2 hours.
7. Unmold salad by holding it in sink with warm water for under a minute until it loosens. Turn onto a platter.

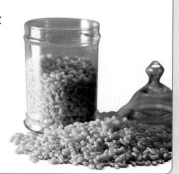

the colander or strainer over a pan of hot water and cover.

You can freeze leftover cooked pasta by itself, but it freezes best with a sauce. Freeze in serving-size portions.

Cooking Rice

White rice and brown rice are cooked in the same way, although brown rice needs more water and a longer cooking time. See **Fig. 32-9**. You can add extra flavor to rice by cooking it in milk, juice, or broth instead of water.

To cook rice, bring the liquid to a boil. Add the rice, cover, and bring to a boil again. Then reduce the heat so the rice simmers gently. Keep covered and stir the rice as little as possible, as stirring scrapes off the starch and makes the rice sticky.

Near the end of the cooking time, check the rice for doneness. It should be moist and tender but firm, with no liquid left in the pot. If any liquid remains, continue cooking without the lid until the excess liquid is absorbed or evaporates. If undercooked, rice is hard and gritty. Overcooked rice is soft and sticky. To cook converted and instant rice, follow package directions.

If you plan to use cooked rice in a recipe that needs further cooking, undercook the rice slightly. This prevents mushiness.

Keep rice warm by placing it in a colander and setting the colander over a pan of simmering water. Cover to allow the steam to warm the rice without making it sticky. You can also reheat rice by this method.

Refrigerate leftover rice immediately if you plan to use it within a few days, or freeze for longer storage. To reheat rice, add 2 tablespoons of water for each cup of cooked rice; then microwave or reheat on top of the range.

Cooking Other Grains

Barley, grits, kasha, and many other grains are cooked in much the same way as rice, although package directions may vary slightly. For most grains, boil the water, add the grain, cover, and bring to a boil again. Reduce the heat so the grain simmers gently. The cooking time can vary from 20 to 45 minutes, depending on the grain. **Fig. 32-9** gives the amounts of liquid needed to cook 1 cup of different types of grain, as well as the cooking time and approximate yield.

Career Prep

Unspoken Communication

ANYTIME YOU SEND A MESSAGE without speaking, you are still using some form of communication. In some work situations, silent communication is more effective than verbal. A press release, for example, must be written to be useful. A smile sends an immediate welcome to a client or co-worker.

Considering memos, reports, letters, proposals, and e-mail, you may read and write for a job as much as for school. Sharpening these skills now can help your future career.

READING AND WRITING SKILLS

The skills of previewing and skimming are time-savers when reading for information. To check an employer's policy on sick days in the company manual, you might find the section on benefits in the table of contents and then scan those pages for paragraphs dealing with sick days. Highlighting or taking notes might help you recall the information. Remember, too, that required reading for work often includes symbols, charts, and tables.

In the workplace, clear writing that uses correct grammar and spelling is easiest to understand. It also fosters a supervisor's and a client's confidence in your abilities. Avoiding bias and stereotypes in writing shows respect as well as your awareness of growing workplace diversity.

Stir grains occasionally to keep them from sticking, lumping, or scorching. If you over-stir them, they turn gummy and pasty. Grains are usually chewy if not cooked long enough and sticky if overcooked. Most grains have a delicate flavor, so don't add too much seasoning.

Bulgur requires a different preparation method. Pour boiling water on the dry grain and let it stand for 30 minutes.

Preparing Convenience Forms of Grains

Instant forms of grains take less time to cook than regular forms, and they can be served in the same ways. Instant may have more sodium than regular forms.

Both dry and hot breakfast cereals can be a tasty and nutritious way to start your day. Dry cereals are ready to eat; all you need to do is add milk and, if you wish, fresh or dried fruit—per-haps bananas, strawberries, raisins, or dried apricots. To prepare instant forms of hot breakfast cereals, follow the package directions. Usually, adding boiling water is all that's needed.

Fig. 32-9

Grain Cooking Times and Yields			
Grain (1 cup dry)	Liquid	Cooking Time	Yield (approximate)
Barley, pearl	3 cups	40 minutes	3 cups
Bulgur	2 cups	30 minutes of standing time	2½ cups
Cornmeal	4 cups	25 minutes	3 cups
Grits (regular)	4 cups	25 minutes	3 cups
Kasha	2 cups	20 minutes	2½ cups
Millet	2½ to 3 cups	35 to 40 minutes	3½ cups
Rice, brown (long grain)	2½ cups	45 minutes	3 cups
Rice, white (long or medium grain)	2 cups	15 minutes	3 cups

BODY LANGUAGE

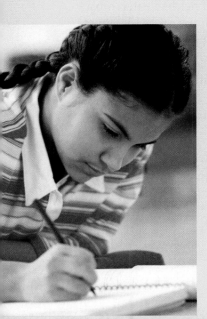

Gestures, facial expressions, and body posture can convey meaning swiftly and powerfully. This is their strength—and their weakness. Some types of body language are unmistakably positive. A smile, steady eye contact, and an open, relaxed posture project a friendly image. They invite further communication.

Negative body language is just as definite and effective. A tapping foot communicates impatience. Rolling eyes show disbelief or boredom. Folded arms express defiance. Use such gestures with care. They can sour the environment and discourage the respect that is needed among co-workers.

Also be careful how you interpret body language. Does a supervisor's frown show anger or concentration? Is a co-worker sighing from disgust or weariness? A negative message, sent or received, needs a follow-up with verbal communication—the sooner, the better. Problems between co-workers are resolved only when discussed openly and constructively.

Career Connection

Converting information. For two or three days, observe and record examples of body language. Include people in work settings. No names of individuals are needed. Write an analysis that explains one situation in which body language had impact. What was the outcome?

Summarize Your Reading

▶ Grains include all plants in the grass family and are also called cereals.

▶ Grains can be categorized according to their different forms.

▶ Nutrition is important to keep in mind when choosing grains. Some products are enriched to replace nutrients lost during processing. Some are fortified with nutrients to make them more nutritious.

▶ While most grains cook by simmering, pasta is boiled.

▶ Grains can be served as cereal and bread and also in many side dishes, main dishes, and even desserts.

Check Your Knowledge

1. Name and describe the three main parts of each grain **kernel**.

2. How is the **hull** used in **grain** products?

3. Name and describe eight grain forms.

4. Why are **whole-grain** products nutritious?

5. **CRITICAL THINKING** Why do you think grains have been a staple around the world for thousands of years?

6. What are some ways that grains can be combined with other foods to produce tasty dishes?

7. What do wheat berries, bulgur, and cracked wheat have in common? How are they different?

8. What qualities distinguish these forms of **rice**: long grain, medium grain, and short grain?

9. Compare white, brown, converted, and instant rice.

10. Compare these forms of corn: hominy, grits, cornmeal, and cornstarch.

11. Each of these grains is commonly used in what types of dishes: barley, buckwheat, couscous, kasha, quinoa, and teff?

12. How are **macaroni** and **noodles** different?

13. Why can dried **pasta** be stored in a cupboard while fresh pasta must be stored in the refrigerator?

14. Describe some different forms of breakfast cereals.

15. What is the difference between **leavened bread** and **flatbread**?

16. If you buy **wheat** bread with a brown color, is it **whole grain**? Explain.

17. Why should whole-grain products be stored in the refrigerator?

18. How do grains change when cooked in water?

19. **CRITICAL THINKING** While eating spaghetti with sauce, a diner had eaten most of the pasta but much of the sauce remained on the plate. How might cooking have caused this situation?

20. What does **al dente** mean and what is its purpose?

21. How do you cook rice? Why should rice not be stirred?

22. Are all grains cooked like rice? Explain.

23. What is the advantage of convenience forms of grains?

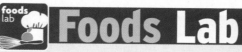
Apply Your Learning

1. **LANGUAGE ARTS** **Grains in the Diet.** Some fad diets suggest limiting grains. Write an article that counters this view. Review Chapter 6 and include specifics on the valuable role of grains in the diet. Make your article available for others to read.

2. **Grain Variety.** Survey supermarket shelves, health food stores, and ethnic food stores for different grain products. How many can you find? Purchase one unfamiliar grain to prepare and share with the class.

3. **SOCIAL STUDIES** **Grain Origins.** On a world map, locate where various grains originated and are grown today.

4. **SCIENCE** **Rice Experiment.** Design and conduct a cooking experiment that explores different kinds of rice. Compare taste, yield, uses, appearance, and cost.

5. **MATH** **Bread Crumbs.** Make your own bread crumbs. Compare the quality and cost to prepared crumbs from the supermarket. Chart the results.

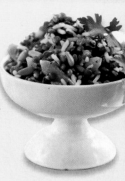

Foods Lab

Evaluating Grain Dishes

Procedure: Find three simple recipes that use rice, bulgur, and couscous. Follow package instructions to make the grains for the recipes. Make enough to sample plain and to use in the recipes. Then prepare the three recipes. Compare the grains on appearance, taste, and texture before and after the recipes are prepared.

Analyzing Results

❶ How did the grains compare on appearance, taste, and texture? How did the recipes affect the grains?

❷ Which grain was the easiest to prepare? Most time consuming? How might that affect menu planning?

Food Science Experiment

Preparing Pasta

Objective: To compare how the amount and temperature of water affect pasta when cooked.

Procedure:

1. Cook pasta, using the method below assigned by your teacher:

Method 1: In a large saucepan, bring 2 cups of water to a rolling boil. Gradually add 2 oz. of dried pasta. Stir gently. Return the water to a boil and cook at a boil.

Method 2: Use method 1, but lower the heat and cook the pasta at a simmer.

Method 3: Use method 1, but reduce the water to 1 cup.

2. Cook pasta for the amount of time listed on the package. Drain but reserve some of the water. Toss the pasta lightly with 1 tsp. of oil. Compare the pasta and water produced by the different cooking methods.

Analyzing Results

❶ Which cooking method gave the best results?

❷ What problems resulted from using the other two methods?

❸ Observe and feel the water left from each cooking method. What differences do you notice? How do they help explain the success or failure of each method?

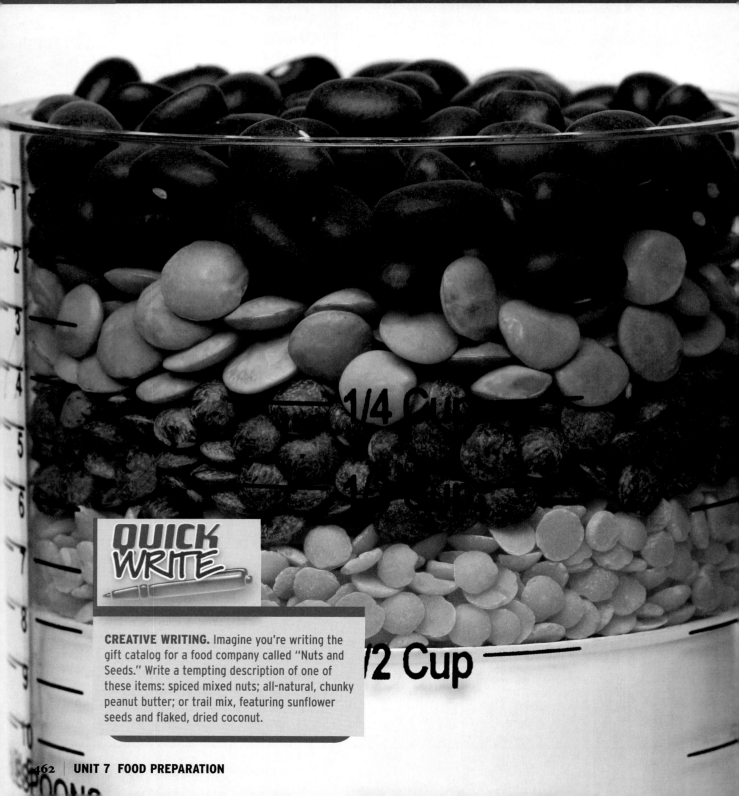

Legumes, Nuts & Seeds

QUICK WRITE

CREATIVE WRITING. Imagine you're writing the gift catalog for a food company called "Nuts and Seeds." Write a tempting description of one of these items: spiced mixed nuts; all-natural, chunky peanut butter; or trail mix, featuring sunflower seeds and flaked, dried coconut.

1/4 Cup

1/2 Cup

To Guide Your Reading:

Objectives

▶ Identify types of legumes, nuts, and seeds.

▶ Explain the value of legumes, nuts, and seeds in the diet.

▶ Explain how to select and store legumes, nuts, and seeds.

▶ Describe and demonstrate methods for preparing, cooking, and serving legumes, nuts, and seeds.

Terms

dry legumes

fresh legumes

hilum

legumes

nuts

seeds

tofu

P EOPLE ALL OVER THE WORLD HAVE EATEN legumes, nuts, and seeds for thousands of years. Their growing popularity in the United States is easy to understand. These foods are packed with nutrients and flavor, and a little recipe research will uncover many delicious uses for them.

LEGUMES

Legumes are plants with seed pods that split along both sides when ripe. Green beans, green lima beans, and green peas are examples of **fresh legumes** from young plants. As soon as fresh legumes are ripe, they are picked and sold as vegetables. Although fresh legumes are nutritious, they have fewer nutrients than dry legumes.

Dry legumes, including dry beans, peas, and lentils, are the seeds of mature plants left in the field to dry. In food preparation, the word *legumes* refers to the dry form rather than the fresh variety.

Nutrients in Legumes

Because seeds contain the food supply for a new plant, dry legumes are rich in nutrients. First, they are an excellent source of protein. Legumes work with grains to provide complete protein because each has amino acids the other lacks. By eating both, you can get all the essential amino acids needed for good health. They don't have to be eaten at the same meal. Combined grains and legumes make up about two-thirds of the proteins eaten by people all over the world.

Legumes are an economical source of protein. One-half cup of cooked legumes contains the same amount of protein as one ounce of cooked meat, yet legumes are less expensive than meat. Beans also double in volume when cooked, whereas meat, poultry, and other high-protein foods lose moisture and shrink during cooking. Therefore beans go further than a similar amount of meat.

Nutrition Connection

Daily Choices. Like meat, poultry, and fish, legumes are a protein source. On a 2,000-calorie diet, a person needs 5½ ounces of protein foods per day. One ounce equals ¼ cup of cooked dry beans or tofu or 1 tablespoon of peanut butter.

 Why are legumes a healthful alternative to meats?

Besides protein, legumes are rich in complex carbohydrates and dietary fiber. They're also high in iron, calcium, potassium, and some trace minerals. Since they are low in fat, calories, and sodium and contain no cholesterol, legumes are a healthful alternative to meats, which are often high in fat and cholesterol.

Types of Legumes

You might not think of beans as colorful, yet they are. White, pink, red, green, and black are among the choices. Whether small like black beans or large like lima beans, each kind has its own distinctive flavor and texture. Despite differences, some can be used interchangeably in recipes and side dishes. See **Fig. 33-1**. Split peas and lentils also come in several colors. If a supermarket doesn't carry the legumes you want, you might find them in ethnic markets. **Fig. 33-2** shows many types of legumes and their uses.

Some legumes are traditional in ethnic dishes. Pinto beans, for instance, are used in Tex-Mex cuisine, including burritos, enchiladas, nachos, and refried beans. Lentils are the main ingredient in *dal*, a traditional dish in India.

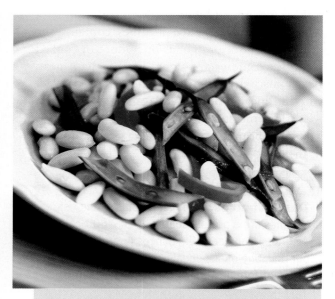

Fig. 33-1 Because legumes come from plants, they can be thought of as vegetables. As protein suppliers, they compare to meats and other protein foods. Either way, they offer delicious meal possibilities.

Selecting and Storing Legumes

Dry legumes are sold in packages or in bulk. When you purchase legumes, look for those that are firm and clean. Legumes with no visible damage and a uniform color and size have a better appearance, but nutritional quality and flavor are seldom affected by broken, wrinkled, or blistered legumes. Appearance won't matter in many dishes. Keep in mind that mixed sizes cause uneven cooking, since smaller legumes cook faster than larger ones.

To store dry legumes, put them in a cool, dry place. Once a package is open, transfer the remainder to a tightly covered container. Do not refrigerate dry legumes. Because legumes continue to dry out during storage, buy only the amount you will use within a reasonable length of time. With proper storage, legumes should keep for up to 12 months. The older and drier legumes become, the longer they take to cook.

Cooked legumes may be stored in the refrigerator if used within four days. For longer storage, freeze them in an airtight container.

Convenience Forms of Legumes

Most dry beans are available canned, although taste and texture are somewhat different. A 15-ounce can, when drained, yields about $1\frac{1}{2}$ cups of cooked beans. To remove excess sodium, rinse them well before cooking. Then use them as you would use cooked dry beans.

Are you in a hurry to eat? If so, legume dishes come in cans and packages that take little preparation. These include bean soups as well as baked beans and refried beans. Frozen legumes can be heated as a side dish or added to recipes. The frozen food section of supermarkets offers such entrées as burritos, soups, and curries.

Cooking Legumes

Legumes are dried in the field and then harvested and processed. Since moisture could make them sprout, they are not washed. For this reason, always inspect legumes for damage and foreign material. Remove any pebbles and stems. See **Fig. 33-3** on page 466. Then rinse the legumes well in cold water several times to wash off the field dust. Rinse until the water is clear.

Fig. 33-2

A Guide to Legumes

Black Beans (Turtle Beans) 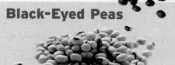 Small, black, oval beans with white dot at one end and cream-colored flesh. Sweet flavor and smooth texture. Used for soups and stews. Traditional in Mexican, Central and South American, and Caribbean cuisines. Used for Cuban rice and beans. Cooking time: 1 to 1½ hours.

Black-Eyed Peas 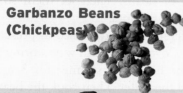 Medium-size oval beans. White with small black "eye" on one side. Light, smooth texture with distinct savory flavor. Used in curries and main dishes with ham or rice. Traditional in Southern cuisine. Mixed with rice and bacon to make Hoppin' John, traditionally served on New Year's Day to bring good luck. Cooking time: 30 minutes to 1 hour.

Garbanzo Beans (Chickpeas) 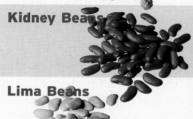 Medium-size, round, roughly shaped, beige beans with nutlike flavor and firm texture. Hold shape when cooked. Used in soups, stews, and salads and as snacks. Popular in European and Middle Eastern cuisines. Main ingredient in hummus (HUH-muhs), a Middle Eastern dip. Cooking time: 1 to 1½ hours.

Kidney Beans Large, deep-red, kidney-shaped beans with cream-colored flesh. Also come in light red. Hearty flavor and firm texture. Used in soups, stews, casseroles, and salads. Traditionally used in chili and in red beans and rice. Popular in Central American cuisines. Cooking time: 1½ to 2 hours.

Lima Beans Greenish-white, flat, oval beans with mild flavor and smooth, creamy texture. Used as a side dish and in soups and casseroles. Baby limas are small and cook in 1 hour. Large limas, also called butter beans, cook in 1 to 1½ hours.

Pinto Beans 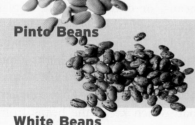 Medium-size, oval beans with mottled beige and brown skin. Turn brown when cooked. Flavorful, with creamy texture. Popular in most Spanish-speaking countries and in Tex-Mex cuisine. Served with rice or used in soups and stews. Used to make refried beans, which are mashed beans fried with fat. Cooking time: 1½ to 2 hours.

White Beans White beans with mild flavor. Used in soups, stews, casseroles, and salads. Several varieties. • Navy beans are small oval beans used in Boston baked beans and commercially prepared pork and beans. Also known as Yankee beans. Cooking time: 1½ to 2 hours. • Great Northern beans are about twice the size of navy beans. Cooking time: 45 minutes to 1 hour. • Cannellini beans (kan-eh-LEE-nee), also called white kidney beans, have smooth texture and nutlike flavor. Used in soups and bean salads. Cooking time: 1½ to 2 hours.

Split Peas 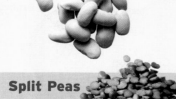 Whole dry peas, skinned and split. Green or yellow. Cook relatively fast and turn into thick, creamy purée. Common in soups. No presoaking necessary. Cooking time: 30 minutes to 1 hour.

Lentils Small, lens-shaped legume popular in Europe, the Middle East, and India. Mild flavor. Red, brown, and green varieties. Cook relatively fast, so do not presoak. Red lentils cook faster than others. Used in soups, stews, salads, and side dishes. Cooking time: 20 minutes to 1 hour.

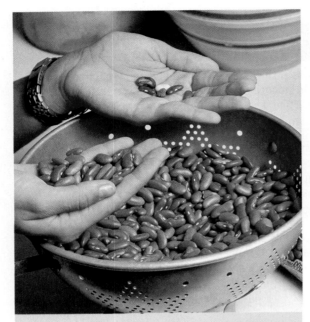

Fig. 33-3 Beans need to be sorted before cooking. Why is this done?

With legumes, if you don't think ahead, you may get more than you expect. On average, a 1-pound package of dry legumes contains about 2 to 3 cups. Because they expand during cooking, this amount yields about 5 to 6 cups of cooked legumes. The particular legume you're cooking determines the quantity.

Presoaking Beans

The thick skin, or coat, on beans affects their cooking time. Although they can be cooked in several ways, presoaking is usually a first step.

Beans must absorb water before they can begin to cook. If you presoak them, you lessen the cooking time. As beans soak, water enters first through the scar, called the **hilum** (HY-luhm), the place where the bean was attached to the stem in the pod. Once some water has been absorbed through this tiny opening, water starts to soak through the outer coat. See **Fig. 33-4**.

Soaking also dissolves some gas-causing substances, which makes beans easier to digest. According to researchers, no significant nutrient amounts are lost in presoaking.

Two methods work for presoaking beans. No matter which method you use, always discard the soaking water. For the first method, use 10 cups of water for each pound of beans. Since beans double in size, be sure the pot is large enough. Heat to boiling, reduce the heat, and let simmer for about 2 to 3 minutes. Remove from the heat and set aside. Let the beans soak for 1 to 4 hours. The longer the beans soak, the more water they absorb and the shorter the cooking time.

You can also presoak beans with the traditional overnight method. Use 10 cups of cold water for every 2 pounds of beans. Then let them soak overnight or at least 8 hours.

A slightly different method is used to presoak black-eyed peas. Cover them with water, bring to a boil, reduce the heat, and simmer for 3 to 4 minutes. Discard the water. Then cook the beans in fresh water for about 45 minutes.

Simmering Beans

Once beans have been soaked, you can drain them and cook them by simmering. Place the beans in a large pot and follow these steps:

1. Cover with 6 cups of fresh hot water for each pound of beans, or cover to about 1 inch above the beans.
2. Add seasonings if you like—perhaps chopped onions, garlic, or dried herbs—but don't add salt or acid ingredients like tomatoes until the beans are tender. They toughen the bean coat, which keeps the beans from absorbing water and softening.

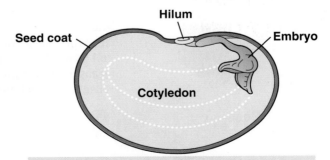

Fig. 33-4 On a legume, the cotyledon (kah-tuh-LEE-dun) stores energy and protein. It is attached to the embryo, consisting of a root, stem, and first pair of leaves. A hard seed coat covers the legume, with the only opening at the hilum.

3. Cover the pot. Bring to a boil, reduce the heat, and simmer until tender. If beans foam, tilt the lid slightly to keep the water from boiling over. Add hot water, if necessary, to keep beans covered with liquid.
4. Test beans frequently for doneness.

Cooking time depends on bean variety, bean age, water hardness, and the altitude of your area. Depending on intended use, cook beans until firm or soft. If you plan to freeze them or use them in a salad or a dish to be cooked, cook the beans to the firm stage. If you plan to mash or purée beans, cook them until soft. See **Fig. 33-5**.

Beans take longer to cook in hard water. To shorten the cooking time when you have hard water, use bottled, purified drinking water in place of tap water. Don't add baking soda to soften the water because it will give beans an off-flavor and destroy thiamin.

Although beans retain most of their nutrients when cooked, the cooking liquid is full of flavor. Serve it with the beans or save it for soups or sauces.

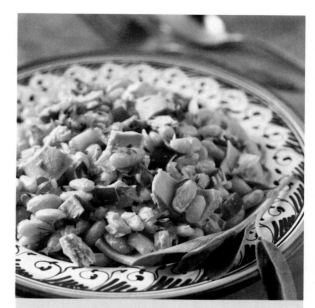

Fig. 33-5 When you cook beans, think about how they'll be used. How would you cook beans for this dish?

Pressure-Cooking Beans

To cook beans in a pressure cooker, cover them with water or broth first. Be careful not to fill the cooker more than halfway. Because foaming can clog the pressure cooker's vent, reduce the effect by adding 1 tablespoon of oil for every cup of beans. Cooking times vary, depending on the kind of bean and whether the beans were pre-soaked. Follow directions in the owner's manual for using the pressure cooker.

Slow-Cooking Beans

The slow cooker is ideal for cooking beans. Follow the directions in the owner's manual for using this appliance.

Beans usually don't need to be soaked first. After boiling the water separately, add it carefully to the beans in the slow cooker. Mix well and cover. The beans must simmer, so use the high setting. Slow-cooking generally takes 3 to 8 hours, depending on the bean.

Microwaving Beans

Presoak beans before microwaving them. If you wish to presoak them in the microwave, put 1 pound of beans in a 5-quart, microwavable container. Add 8 cups of water and cook on high (full power) for 8 to 15 minutes or until the water boils. Let stand for 1 hour or longer. Stir occasionally. Then drain.

To microwave presoaked beans, add 6 to 8 cups of fresh hot water to 1 pound of beans. Cover and cook on high (full power) for 8 to 10 minutes or until the liquid starts to boil. Reduce the power to 50 percent. Cook another 15 to 20 minutes or until the beans are tender. Cooking time depends on the bean used.

Cooking Split Peas and Lentils

Because of their thinner coat, split peas and lentils cook faster than dry beans and don't need to be soaked before cooking. To cook split peas, use 2 cups of water for 1 cup of peas. Boil for about 30 minutes or until the peas are tender. Cooked split peas break down into a creamy purée, so they work well for soups and stews.

To cook lentils, add 1 pound of lentils to 3 cups of water. Season the lentils as desired and simmer for about 45 minutes or until tender but not mushy. Lentils hold their shape.

Serving Cooked Legumes

Because of their mild flavor, legumes combine well with other foods. Once cooked, they can be served whole, mashed, or puréed. You can use them as a side dish or a main ingredient in casseroles, soups, stews, and salads. **Fig. 33-6** is a recipe for a favorite side dish—baked beans. Beans can also be eaten as snacks.

Tofu

Tofu is a custard-like product made from soybeans. A traditional food in Asian cuisines for centuries, tofu is used often in the United States today. Tofu is made by curdling soy milk, the liquid pressed from grinding soaked, cooked soybeans. The curd is poured into special pans, pressed, and cut into chunks.

Tofu has a creamy texture and bland flavor. Because it absorbs the flavors of other ingredients, it is very versatile. Tofu can be mashed, blended, sliced, cubed, or cut into any desired shape. As an excellent source of protein, it can be substituted for meat and poultry. You can use tofu in recipes that include casseroles, stews, soups, salad dressings, sauces, dips, stir-fries, and even desserts. Tofu can be sautéed, grilled, scrambled, fried, or marinated and barbecued.

Fig. 33-6

Try This! **Recipe**

Boston Baked Beans

Yield	Nutrition Analysis
4 servings (about ³⁄₄ cup each)	*Per Serving:* 280 calories, 1 g total fat, 0 g saturated fat, 0 g trans fat, 0 mg cholesterol, 310 mg sodium, 54 g total carbohydrate, 16 g dietary fiber, 15 g sugars, 15 g protein *Percent Daily Value:* vitamin A 0%, vitamin C 4%, calcium 15%, iron 35%

Ingredients

4 cups water
1¼ cups dry navy beans, sorted and rinsed
reserved cooking water
¼ cup onion, chopped
2 Tbsp. dark molasses

2 Tbsp. brown sugar
1 tsp. dry mustard
½ tsp. salt
½ tsp. vinegar
4 oz. salt pork

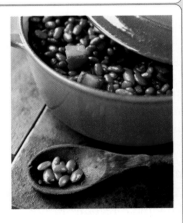

Directions

1. Combine 4 cups water and beans. Soak overnight.
2. Drain and discard soaking water.
3. Add fresh water to cover beans. Bring to boil in 2-qt. saucepan. Reduce heat and simmer, covered, for 30 minutes.
4. Drain beans and reserve cooking water.
5. In 2-qt. casserole dish, combine beans, ½ cup reserved cooking water, chopped onion, molasses, brown sugar, dry mustard, salt, and vinegar.
6. Cut salt pork into 4 pieces. Press into surface of beans.
7. Cover casserole dish. Bake at 250°F for 6 to 8 hours. If beans begin to dry out during cooking, add more reserved cooking water, heated to boiling; do not stir. (Beans should be moist but not soupy.) During the last 30 to 60 minutes of cooking, uncover the beans to let them brown. Discard salt pork before serving.

Tofu provides complete protein. It is low in sodium, contains no cholesterol, and is a good source of B vitamins and iron. Because tofu is made from soybeans, however, it contains more fat than other legumes.

Selecting Tofu

Fresh tofu is packaged in water-filled plastic tubs or in vacuum packs. Look for it in the refrigerated and produce sections of natural food stores and supermarkets. Tofu also comes in aseptic packages, found in the grocery section with other shelf-stable foods. Tofu is highly perishable, so check the date on the package label for freshness. To use freeze-dried tofu, reconstitute the product with boiling water.

Tofu comes in these three textures:

- **Firm tofu.** This dense solid holds its shape. It absorbs marinades well and is used in stir-fries and soups or for deep-frying or grilling. Squeeze out excess moisture before using.
- **Soft tofu.** With a softer texture, this tofu works in recipes that call for blending. You can also substitute soft tofu for eggs and cream cheese in many recipes.
- **Silken tofu.** This product is made by a slightly different process that creates a creamy texture. Sold only in aseptic packages, it is used in puréed or blended dishes, such as smoothies, sauces, dips, and desserts.

Storing Tofu

Keep fresh tofu refrigerated. If any is left after you open the package, rinse it with water, cover with fresh water, and refrigerate. Change the water daily to keep the tofu fresh, and use it within a week.

Aseptic packages can be stored in a cool, dry place. Once a package is opened, refrigerate it.

You can freeze firm tofu for up to five months. Over time, however, it turns light brown and the texture becomes spongy and chewy.

Cooking with Tofu

People who have never bought tofu before are often puzzled by how to use it. Here are some suggestions:

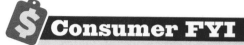

Consumer FYI

Soy for dessert? Soy can't turn brownies into health food, but it can improve nutrient profiles of many treats. In brownies and other baked goods, soy-and-wheat-flour blends boost protein content, while egg replacements made of powdered soy protein lower cholesterol content. "Soy nuts"—roasted, immature soybeans—replace high-fat nuts and seeds in some cereals, snacks, and spreads. Even fudge can be made more nutritiously with soy products.

Like many specialty foods, soy products may be costly. For people with allergies or diet restrictions, however, cost may not be an issue. Researchers are working to create soy ingredients with added appeal in taste and texture, increasing their usefulness in diets.

- Always cook tofu over low heat, as it will turn tough and dry if overcooked.
- Mix crumbled tofu into meatloaf or add it to soups, stews, casseroles, and stir-fries.
- Marinate tofu in barbecue sauce, grill until lightly browned, and serve on crusty bread.
- Make tacos by adding a package of taco seasoning mix to a pan of crumbled, fried tofu.
- For an onion dip, blend dried onion soup mix into soft or silken tofu.
- Mix tofu with reduced-fat sour cream and use as a topping on baked potatoes.
- Replace all or part of the cream in creamed soups with silken tofu.
- Substitute puréed silken tofu for part of the mayonnaise, sour cream, cream cheese, or ricotta cheese in recipes. Use in dips and creamy salad dressings.

NUTS

Early food gatherers in history were probably pleased to sit under a tree and have food fall in their lap. They may not have realized the nutritious contribution nuts made in their diet.

Nuts are edible kernels surrounded by a hard shell. You may be surprised to know that some foods you call nuts aren't technically nuts at all. Peanuts, for example, are actually legumes, and walnuts are seeds. Similarities to true nuts, including how they're used, commonly put peanuts and walnuts in the nut category. **Fig. 33-7** shows nuts that are enjoyed around the world today.

Nutrients in Nuts

Nuts are rich in nutrients. They are high in protein, dietary fiber, B vitamins, vitamin E, calcium, magnesium, potassium, and various trace minerals. They are also low in sodium and contain no cholesterol. Nuts are high in fat and therefore high in calories; however, most of the fat is unsaturated. When eaten in moderation, nuts can be a beneficial part of your eating plan.

Selecting and Storing Nuts

Generally, the more nuts are processed, the more they cost. They come in a variety of forms.

SAFETY ALERT

Peanut allergies. Although peanuts and peanut butter are favorite foods for many people, they are dangerous for those with peanut allergies. Serious reactions, even fatal, can occur. Many processed foods contain peanuts, often not clearly labeled. During manufacturing or preparation, foods without peanuts may pick up traces of peanut products. Be careful when serving foods to others and also when eating peanut products around those with this allergy.

- **In the shell.** Nuts in the shell store well and keep as long as a year. One pound of unshelled nuts makes about ½ pound of shelled nuts.
- **Shelled, unblanched.** These nuts have no shells but retain their skins, which add color, flavor, and texture.

Fig. 33-7

A Guide to Nuts

Almonds		Oval shape, with light brown, soft shell and delicate, slightly sweet flavor. Used in main dishes, desserts, and baked goods and as snacks and garnishes. Grown in California, the Mediterranean, South Africa, and Australia. Marzipan (MAHRT-suh-pahn) is mixture of almond paste and sugar, often tinted with food coloring, shaped into assorted forms.
Brazil Nuts		Large, triangular shape, with hard, dark brown shell and white kernel. Mild flavor and crisp, tender texture. High in selenium. Imported from Brazil.
Cashew Nuts	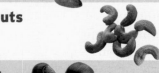	Medium-size, crescent shape, with sweet, buttery flavor and tender texture. Sold only shelled because shell is toxic. Imported from Brazil, India, and East Africa.
Hazelnuts	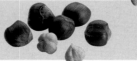	Also called filberts. Round, grape-size, with hard brown shell and white kernel. Mild, distinctive, slightly sweet flavor and tender, crisp texture. Grown in temperate climates.
Macadamia Nuts	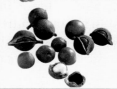	Grape-size, with slightly sweet, buttery flavor and tender texture. Shells are extremely hard, so nuts are sold shelled. Grown in Hawaii, California, and Florida.

- **Shelled, blanched.** Both the shells and skins have been removed from these nuts.
- **Shelled, blanched, and roasted.** Many varieties are roasted in oil, salted or unsalted. Dry-roasted nuts are roasted without oil and have fewer calories than regular roasted nuts.

Some nuts are ground into thick, spreadable pastes, such as almond butter and the ever-favorite peanut butter. These pastes can be used as spreads or ingredients in recipes.

Because of high fat content, nuts turn rancid quickly. If you plan to store them for a long time, buy nuts with shells. Shelled nuts won't last as long and are best purchased in small quantities to use quickly.

Nuts are sold in bulk, in boxes and plastic bags, and in vacuum-packed jars and cans. When buying nuts in the shell, look for unbroken ones and store them in a cool, dry place. Refrigerate or freeze shelled nuts in an airtight container to keep them from becoming rancid.

Using Nuts

If you like nuts, you probably appreciate their versatility. Nuts can be chopped, grated, ground, or slivered. You can buy slivered almonds or make your own—just peel off slivers carefully with a vegetable peeler. Slivered almonds can garnish cereals, salads, main dishes, and baked goods.

If you want to remove the skin on such shelled nuts as almonds, pistachios, and peanuts, you can blanch them yourself. Cover the shelled nuts with boiling water and let stand for 2 minutes. Drain and cool just until you can handle them easily; then slip off the skins.

Fig. 33-7 (continued)

A Guide to Nuts

Peanuts	Technically a legume but used the same as nuts. Long, rough, beige shell usually containing two kernels. Have a distinctive flavor and tender texture. Grown in southern United States. Half the peanut crop used for peanut butter. An important ingredient in Thai and some African cuisines.
Pecans	Large, oval shape, with smooth, thin, tan shell and light brown kernel. Have a distinctive, buttery flavor and tender texture. Native to America. A popular American dessert is pecan pie.
Pine Nuts	Small, oval shape, with thin shell and ivory-colored kernel. Have a light, delicate flavor and crisp texture. Grown inside pinecones of several varieties of pine trees in southwestern United States as well as China, Italy, Mexico, North Africa, Asia, and Mediterranean area.
Pistachio Nuts	Small, oval shape, with thin, tan, half-opened shell and pale green kernel. Mild flavor and tender texture. Popular in Middle Eastern, French, and Italian cuisines. Used as snack and in main dishes, sweets, and desserts. Unshelled nuts should be partially open. Closed shells indicate immaturity.
Walnuts	Large and round, with beige shell and light brown kernel. Distinctive, mild, sweet flavor and tender texture. Grown in temperate climates throughout the world. Used in main dishes, salads, baked goods, and as snacks.

Toasting nuts gives them added crunch and brings out flavor. To toast nuts, spread them on an ungreased baking sheet without covering. Roast at 350°F for 5 to 10 minutes or until light brown. The time varies with the type and size of nut. Watch so they don't burn.

Even a small amount of nuts can enhance a dish. They can be a garnish or an ingredient in salads, sandwiches, casseroles, stir-fries, desserts, and baked goods. When mixed with ready-to-eat cereals, dried fruits, or yogurt or when eaten alone, nuts make a delicious snack.

SEEDS

Seeds are the edible dried kernals of certain plants, such as the sunflower. Although seeds, like nuts, are high in fat and calories, they are rich in nutrients. They offer a needed source of protein in many areas of the world.

Also like nuts, seeds can be eaten plain or used in cooking. They add unique tastes to the same types of dishes listed for nuts, both sweet and savory. They are tasty as a garnish and add crunch to baked goods. Some seeds can be eaten as a snack. For extra flavor, toast seeds with the same method used for nuts. Through processing, some seeds are made into spreads and oils.

Selecting, Storing, and Using Seeds

You can buy seeds in bulk or in boxes and plastic bags. They are generally sold ready to use. As with nuts, buy seeds in small quantities to use right away. Since they can turn rancid quickly, store them in an airtight container in the refrigerator. Caraway and poppy seeds are two seeds used in recipes. Here are other common seeds:

- **Pumpkin seeds.** These are the small, flat, oval seeds inside pumpkins. The seeds have a white hull with a dull-green kernel inside. The kernels, called pepitas (puh-PEE-tuhs), are popular in Mexican cuisine. The hull, with the kernel

Career Prep

Electronic Communication

TECHNOLOGY HAS HAD GREAT IMPACT on workplace communications. New means of communicating call for new rules, yet they are based on traditional standards of politeness and professionalism. For example, e-mail and fax machines should be used only for work, just like business telephones and company stationery. Be aware of company policies about using electronic communications.

- **E-mail.** An electronic message deserves a prompt reply, even if only a note saying you received it and will respond fully as soon as possible. Formal greetings should include the recipient's name and title. Abbreviations, such as "U" and "thnx," and emoticons, punctuation that represents facial expressions, are fine with

friends, but a formal tone is more appropriate in business, especially with people you don't know well. When replying to an e-mail, address the sender the same way the message was signed. A few key words in the subject line identify your purpose. Ask before sending an attachment. Some e-mail programs automatically delete them to prevent the spread of viruses. Complicated and emotional issues should be handled in person, not in an e-mail. E-mails that accidentally go to the wrong person can cause embarrassment. If you say something you regret, apologize and offer to make amends. Be aware that some businesses monitor e-mails sent from company computers. Keeping a high standard in the way you handle e-mails is wise.

inside, can be roasted. Pumpkin seeds have a tender, crunchy texture and delicate flavor.

- **Sesame seeds.** These tiny, flat, beige seeds have a nutty flavor and crunchy texture. They are sold raw or roasted, shelled or unshelled, and are used in salads, sandwiches, casseroles, and baked goods. They are also ground to make *tahini* (tuh-HEE-nee), a thick paste common in Middle Eastern cuisine. Sesame paste is also used in Chinese cuisine. The paste can be used in spreads or as an ingredient in recipes. Sesame oil is used in margarine and as oil for cooking.
- **Sunflower seeds.** These are the medium-size, oval seeds of the sunflower plant. See **Fig. 33-8**. The beige kernel is removed from the hull. The kernel has a delicious flavor and crunchy texture. Sunflower seeds, which are high in many nutrients including vitamin E, are eaten as a snack or in cereals, salads, sandwiches, casseroles, stir-fries, vegetable dishes, and baked goods. Oil from the seeds is used in cooking.

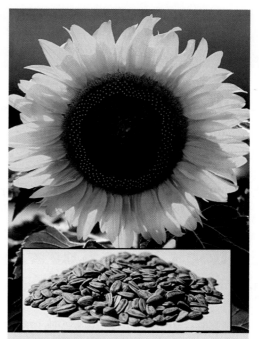

Fig. 33-8 Sunflower seeds are harvested from the center of the flower. The hull is removed to get the edible kernel.

- **Voice mail.** Voice mail acts as a sophisticated answering machine that can store or forward calls as well as record them. If you have a voice mailbox on the job someday, record a short greeting, updating it with your work hours or schedule. To leave a voice mail message, make it short and to the point, with just enough details to help the other party return the call.

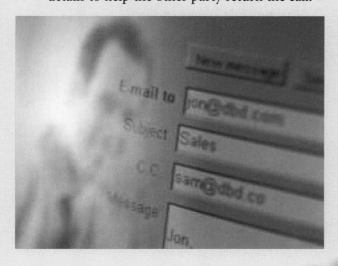

- **Conference calls.** These multiparty meetings can be held by phone or computer network. The rules of etiquette for personal meetings apply here. Introduce the speakers to each other. Write down their names, if needed, so no one is forgotten or left out. Be especially precise when you speak, since others can't pick up on nonverbal cues. Ask before using a speakerphone so people know their comments may be heard by others.
- **Faxes.** Send a fax only if requested. Include a cover letter with the recipient's name, the date, the number of pages, and any contact information.

Career Connection

Communications survey. Research and evaluate another electronic communication in the workplace, possibly Instant Messaging (IM), two-way radios, cell phones, or Webcams.

Summarize Your Reading

▶ Legumes, nuts, and seeds are high in nutrients and can be a beneficial part of a person's eating plan.

▶ Legumes are plants with seed pods that split along both sides when ripe and can be categorized as fresh legumes or dry legumes.

▶ Beans come in many different colors, sizes, flavors, and textures.

▶ Dry legumes take a long time to prepare.

▶ Nuts and seeds need to be purchased in small quantities and stored properly.

Check Your Knowledge

1. Define and give examples of **fresh legumes** and **dry legumes.**

2. How do **legumes** and grains work together nutritionally?

3. Compare legumes with meat as protein sources.

4. Describe types of white beans.

5. What are pinto beans and how are they used?

6. Suppose the beans you buy are broken and wrinkled. Should you throw them away? Explain.

7. How should dry legumes be stored? How do they change if stored for a long time?

8. How can convenience forms of legumes be used? Why are they handy?

9. Why should legumes be inspected before using them?

10. If you need 7 cups of cooked legumes for a recipe, will a 1-pound bag be enough? Explain.

11. Why are beans often presoaked?

12. Describe two methods for presoaking beans.

13. How do you cook beans?

14. How are beans cooked in a pressure cooker?

15. Why are lentils and split peas prepared differently from other dry legumes?

16. Suggest ways to serve legumes.

17. What is **tofu**?

18. **CRITICAL THINKING** "I don't like the taste of tofu," a person said. How would you respond?

19. Compare firm with soft tofu.

20. How should tofu be stored?

21. In what forms are **nuts** sold?

22. **CRITICAL THINKING** Why should shelled nuts be stored only for short periods of time?

23. What is the difference between nuts and **seeds**?

24. How are sesame seeds used in Middle Eastern and Chinese cuisines?

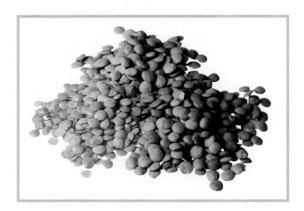

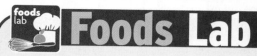
Apply Your Learning

1. **Sodium Check.** Read the Nutrition Facts panel for the amount of sodium in canned legumes. Which have the most and the least? Compare amounts with other processed foods. How can you reduce the sodium in canned legumes?

2. **Bean Comparison.** Prepare one type of bean, using dry beans. Compare this with the canned version of the same bean. How do you rate the appearance, taste, and texture of each? How would you use each type?

3. **SCIENCE Bean Experiments.** Develop and carry out one of these experiments to compare methods for cooking dry beans: a) simmering versus microwave cooking, pressure cooking, and/or slow cooking; b) cooking with and without presoaking; c) cooking with and without acid ingredients; and d) cooking with and without salt.

4. **MATH Cost Comparison.** Find several recipes for legume and meat main dishes. Calculate the cost per serving for each dish. What do you conclude?

Foods Lab

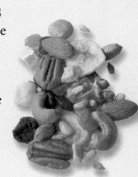

Trail Mix Recipes
Procedure: Develop a recipe for trail mix. Use nuts and seeds, as well as different cereals, dried fruits, and any other suitable foods. Prepare your recipe and share samples. Remember that some people have allergies to certain nuts and seeds.

Analyzing Results
❶ What was the ratio of nuts and seeds to other ingredients in your recipe? Why did you choose these proportions?
❷ What size serving would you suggest for your mix? Why?
❸ How does your recipe compare nutritionally to other typical snacks that you eat?

5. **Recipe Samples.** Using tofu or the legume assigned to you, find recipes that use this as an ingredient. Choose a recipe to make.

Food Science Experiment

Composition of Soybeans

Objective: To identify nutrients in soybeans.

Procedure:
1. Place ½ cup raw soybeans in a plastic freezer bag. Wrap the bag in a dishtowel and hit with a hammer until the beans are crushed.
2. Scrape the beans into a jar and cover with about 2 inches of hot water. Stir the mixture for 2 minutes. Cover the jar and let it sit overnight.
3. Observe the mixture the next day.

Analyzing Results
❶ Describe the appearance of the mixture. What do you think has occurred?
❷ What nutrient do you think the top layer is composed of? The middle layer? The bottom layer?
❸ Suppose you repeated this test using ground pork and again with a shredded apple. How do you think the results would compare?
❹ Review the discussion of cholesterol in Chapter 7. How does this experiment demonstrate a concept associated with cholesterol? (Recall that soybeans are cholesterol-free.)

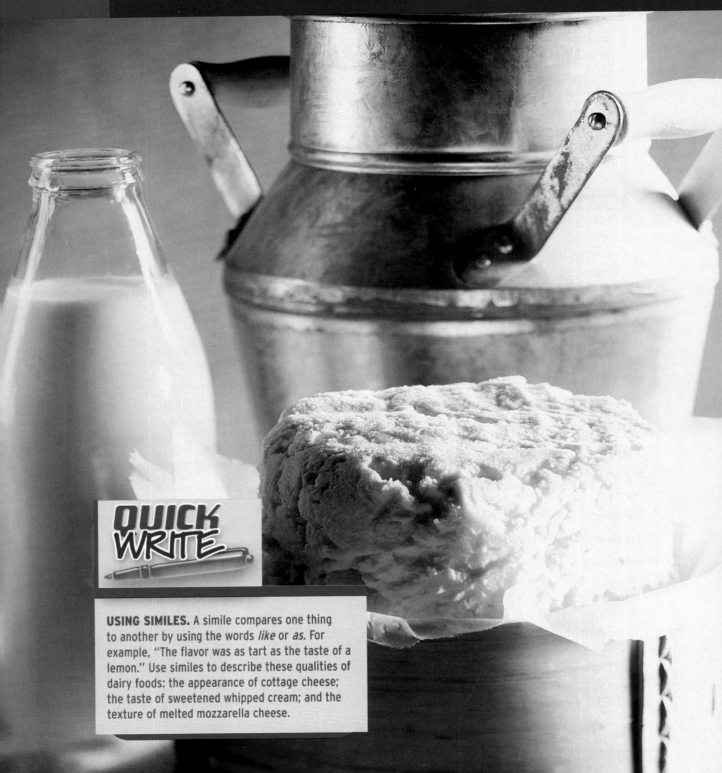

QUICK WRITE

USING SIMILES. A simile compares one thing to another by using the words *like* or *as*. For example, "The flavor was as tart as the taste of a lemon." Use similes to describe these qualities of dairy foods: the appearance of cottage cheese; the taste of sweetened whipped cream; and the texture of melted mozzarella cheese.

Objectives
- ▶ Identify dairy products and their uses.
- ▶ Explain the value of dairy products in the diet.
- ▶ Explain how to select and store dairy products.
- ▶ Describe and demonstrate methods for preparing, cooking, and serving dairy products.

Terms
- curdling
- curds
- foam
- fresh cheese
- homogenized
- nonfat milk solids
- pasteurized
- raw milk
- ripened cheese
- scalded milk
- scorching
- tempering
- whey
- yogurt

I N THE EARLY 1600S, THE FIRST DAIRY COWS were brought to the American colonies. The colonists could drink milk fresh from the cow and churn their own butter. After many years and lots of inventiveness, most people now visit supermarkets to choose from a huge array of creamy, refreshing foods and beverages called dairy foods. Milk, cream, butter, yogurt, frozen dairy desserts, and cheese are ready to eat. Many dairy products are also ready to use as ingredients in dishes.

NUTRIENTS IN DAIRY FOODS

Dairy foods are part of a healthful diet—for good reason. Dairy foods are rich in protein, vitamin A, riboflavin, vitamin B_{12}, calcium, phosphorus, and magnesium. Fortified milk is an excellent source of vitamin D. Health experts recommend three cups of dairy products each day. One cup equals 1 cup of milk or yogurt, $1\frac{1}{2}$ ounces of natural cheese, or 2 ounces of processed cheese.

Many dairy foods also contain saturated fat and cholesterol. Some, including cheese, are high in sodium. You can manage by reading labels and making careful choices.

MILK AND MILK PRODUCTS

According to federal law, all milk must be **pasteurized** (PAS-chuh-ryzd)—that is, heat-treated

Nutrition Connection

Low-fat dairy options. You can get nutrients with less fat and fewer calories by choosing low-fat or nonfat dairy products. Drinking a cup of fat-free milk instead of whole milk can save 8 grams of fat and 70 calories, yet the health benefits are virtually the same. Using plain, nonfat yogurt in place of sour cream saves 3 grams of fat for each tablespoon. With ice cream, a low-fat variety might have 4 grams of fat less per serving. Low-fat frozen yogurt is another idea.

 If a friend who wants to limit fat says, "But I don't want to give up 'real' ice cream," what's your advice?

to kill enzymes and any harmful bacteria. Pasteurization improves the keeping quality of milk but doesn't change the flavor or nutritional value. UHT (ultra-high temperature) milk is pasteurized at much higher temperatures than usual. As a result, it becomes a shelf-stable product that can be packaged in aseptic containers.

Milk that isn't pasteurized is called **raw milk**. Although some people believe lack of processing makes it more nutritious, raw milk may contain harmful bacteria.

Fresh milk from the cow contains about 87 percent water and 13 percent solids. Some of the solids are **nonfat milk solids**, which contain most of the protein, vitamins, minerals, and lactose (milk sugar) in milk.

Other solids are milk fat (sometimes called "butterfat"). The more milk fat a product has, the higher its calorie count. Because milk fat is lighter than other milk fluids and solids, it separates and rises to the top as cream. To prevent this from occurring, milk is **homogenized** (hoh-MAH-juh-nyzd). This process breaks down fat and distributes it in the milk, evenly and permanently.

If milk meets FDA or state standards, it is labeled "grade A," the highest quality. Only grade-A, pasteurized milk can be shipped between states for retail sale.

Kinds of Milk

To create some of the many kinds of milk on the market, fat is removed. The process also removes most vitamin A, which, by law, must be replaced. In addition, most milk producers voluntarily fortify milk with vitamin D. Which of these milk types have you tried? See **Fig. 34-1**.

- **Whole milk.** Has the highest amount of fat. By law, it must have 3.25 percent fat or more.
- **Reduced-fat milk.** Contains 2 percent fat.
- **Low-fat milk.** Contains either 2 percent or 1 percent fat.
- **Nonfat milk.** Contains less than ½ percent fat and is also called fat-free or skim milk.
- **Buttermilk.** Has a tangy flavor and smooth, thick texture. Despite its name, it isn't high in fat. Originally, it was the milk left after making butter. Today, special bacteria are added to pasteurized nonfat milk to produce the flavor and texture. Sometimes flecks of butter are added for flavor and visual appeal. Buttermilk is used in cooking and baking as well as for drinking.
- **Kefir** (keh-FIHR). Fermented milk with a slightly sour flavor, similar to yogurt. The authentic Middle Eastern product is made of fermented camel's milk. In the United States, kefir is made from cow's milk.
- **Chocolate milk.** Has chocolate or cocoa and sweetener added.
- **Nonfat dry milk.** Powdered form of nonfat milk, made by removing the fat and water from pasteurized milk. When rehydrated, dry milk is used like fresh milk and must be refrigerated. Dry milk may be added directly to recipes to

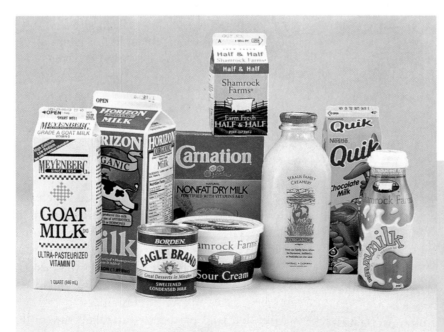

Fig. 34-1 Here you see some common forms of dairy products. Another product that you may see in supermarkets is carbonated milk, designed to promote milk as a replacement for soft drinks. You may also find milk in orange, strawberry, and caramel flavors, not just chocolate.

increase nutrients without adding fat. Although a convenient and inexpensive form of milk, the taste of nonfat dry milk differs slightly from regular milk.

- **Evaporated milk.** Canned, whole or nonfat milk that contains only half the amount of water in regular milk. It can be used as a cream substitute in beverages.
- **Sweetened condensed milk.** Concentrated form of milk with sweetener added; used to make candy and desserts. This product cannot be substituted for evaporated milk or diluted to use as regular milk.
- **Lactose-free or reduced-lactose milk.** Milk treated to break down lactose. It is used by people who can't digest lactose.
- **Acidophilus milk.** Has *lactobacillus acidophilus* (lak-toh-buh-SI-luhs a-suh-DAH-fuh-luhs) bacteria added to help aid digestion. Flavor and appearance are similar to regular milk.
- **Calcium-enriched milk.** Contains 500 milligrams of calcium in one cup. One cup of regular milk has about 300 milligrams.

Cream

Cream is the fatty part of whole milk. Many beverages, cereals, creamy casseroles, soups and sauces, ice cream, baked goods, and sweet syrups contain cream. Federal standards set minimum milk fat for each of these creams:

- **Half-and-half.** Homogenized mixture of milk and cream with 10½ to 18 percent milk fat. It is often used in coffee and other beverages.
- **Light, coffee, or table cream.** Contains 18 to 30 percent milk fat. Besides use as table cream, it is also a cooking ingredient.
- **Light whipping cream.** Has 30 to 36 percent milk fat. It is used in desserts.
- **Heavy whipping cream.** Contains over 36 percent milk fat. This cream whips easily and is frequently used in desserts.
- **Sour cream.** Contains 18 percent milk fat. Thick and rich with a tangy flavor, sour cream is made by adding lactic acid bacteria to light cream. Sour cream comes plain or with chives, fruit, or other foods added. You can also buy low-fat and nonfat products. Sour cream is often a topping on baked potatoes. Many recipes call for sour cream as an ingredient.

Butter

In colonial times, people made their own butter in large wooden churns. Mechanical means are used today, but churning still separates the fat from the liquid. Federal law requires butter to be at least 80 percent milk fat. The rest is buttermilk, which is left for flavor, texture, and appearance. Salt and coloring may also be added.

Butter is graded for quality by the USDA. Grade AA is superior quality. It spreads well and has a delicate, sweet flavor and smooth, creamy texture. Grade A butter is very good quality and has a pleasing flavor with a smooth texture. Grade B butter, made from cream that has gone sour, also has a pleasing flavor.

Butter comes in several forms. Unsalted (sweet) butter has no salt added. Some butter has salt, which adds flavor and acts as a preservative. Butter commonly comes in sticks, usually four to a 1-pound package. Whipped butter, generally unsalted and in tubs, is soft and spreadable. It isn't recommended for baking, however, because added air from whipping changes the density.

Yogurt

Yogurt is made by adding special harmless bacteria to milk. The result is a thick, creamy product that is like custard and has a tangy flavor. The bacteria added are believed to help keep the digestive system healthy. People eat yogurt from the container, combined with foods in dishes, and in cooking.

Yogurt contains similar nutrients to milk. Because it's more concentrated, however, yogurt has more nutrients than a similar amount of milk. For example, one cup of nonfat yogurt has 452 milligrams of calcium; like regular milk, a cup of nonfat milk contains about 300 milligrams of calcium.

Plain yogurt has no flavorings added. When eating yogurt, you might like a flavored version. Flavored yogurt contains added sugar or sugar substitutes and artificial flavors or real fruits. If you prefer, make your own flavored yogurt by stirring chopped kiwifruit, bananas, or other fruit into plain yogurt.

One cup of yogurt contains 120 to 250 calories, depending on the fat content of the milk used in production. Added sweeteners also affect calories. Check the label for calories and fat.

Frozen Dairy Desserts

According to one source, the largest ice cream sundae ever made was 12 feet tall and took over 4,600 gallons of ice cream. That's a sundae to be shared, for sure. A sundae is just one type of frozen dairy dessert you can enjoy. Some other options aren't ice cream at all.

- **Ice cream.** A whipped mixture of cream, milk, sugar, flavorings, and stabilizers. It must contain at least 10 percent milk fat. French ice cream has egg yolk solids added. In addition to regular ice cream, you can buy low-fat, nonfat, and no-sugar-added versions.
- **Frozen yogurt.** Varies in fat content depending on the yogurt and other ingredients used to produce it. Freezing destroys most of the beneficial bacteria.
- **Sherbet.** Made from fruit or juice, sugar, water, flavorings, and milk fat. It generally has less fat but more sugar than ice cream.
- **Sorbet (sor-BAY).** French word for "sherbet." Sorbet is a light dessert made with sweetened fruit, juice, and water, but never milk.

CHEESE

Scan a restaurant menu and you'll probably find cheese in many dishes. Cheese is a concentrated form of milk. When an enzyme such as rennin (REH-nuhn) is added to milk, the milk thickens and separates into solid clusters called **curds** and a thin, bluish liquid called **whey**. The whey is drained from the curds, which become the cheese. See **Fig. 34-2**.

Most cheeses originated in Europe centuries ago. They are made from the milk of such animals as cows, goats, and sheep. Cheeses made in the U.S. are usually made from cows' milk.

Cheese can be divided into two categories: fresh, or unripened, and aged, or ripened. Low-fat and nonfat types are often available.

Fresh Cheese

Fresh cheese has not ripened or aged. It is made from pasteurized milk and has a mild flavor. Fresh cheese, which is highly perishable, must be refrigerated and used within a few days. You can snack on fresh cheese or use it in salads, sandwiches, and cooking. These are some fresh cheese favorites:

- **Cottage cheese.** Contains large or small curds and has a bland flavor. Fresh cream is added to make creamed cottage cheese. Chives, pineapple, or other flavorings may be added. Cottage cheese doesn't melt. Both low-fat and nonfat products can be eaten plain or used in salads and other dishes.

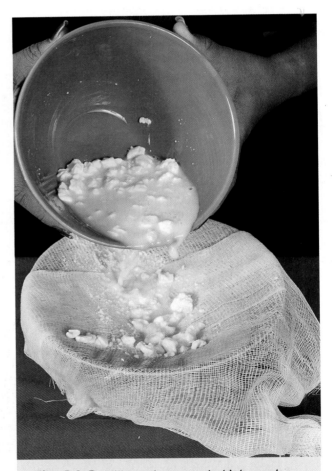

Fig. 34-2 Milk can be separated into curds and whey. The curds are used to make cheese, and the whey has many other uses in food processing.

- **Farmer's cheese.** Has a mild, slightly tangy flavor. It is similar to cottage cheese but drier and usually shaped in a loaf. This cheese can be crumbled or sliced and eaten plain or used in cooking.
- **Cream cheese.** Smooth, creamy, and spreadable cheese, with a mild, slightly tart flavor. Look for low-fat and nonfat varieties. Cream cheese is a spread and an ingredient in many dishes. Seasoned forms are available.
- **Ricotta (rih-KAH-tuh).** Similar to cottage cheese, with a small curd. Ricotta has a slightly sweet flavor and is traditional in Italian cuisine.

Ripened Cheese

Ripened cheese, also called aged, is made by adding ripening agents, such as bacteria, mold, yeast, or a combination of these, to the curds. The cheese is then aged under carefully controlled conditions. Aging time depends on the kind of cheese. For example, mild brick cheese ages for two weeks, but extra-sharp Parmesan takes as long as two years. Ripened cheese can be stored longer than fresh cheese.

Hundreds of ripened cheeses are available, each with distinctive flavor and texture. Flavors vary from mild to very sharp, or strong, and textures range from soft to very hard. **Fig. 34-3** on pages 482 and 483 describes ripened cheeses. They are grouped according to the following textures:

- **Firm.** Can be eaten plain or used in cooking. Most can be grated.
- **Semisoft.** Melts smoothly and is eaten plain or used in cooking.
- **Soft.** Has a soft texture with a hard, white crust that is edible. It's usually eaten plain.
- **Blue-veined.** Has certain molds added during the aging process to create veins or pockets of blue or green, edible mold. It can be eaten plain or used in salads, salad dressings, casseroles, and omelets.

Specialty cheeses are made by shredding and blending different ripened cheeses. Sometimes pimientos, pineapples, olives, or other foods are added. These cheeses are semisoft, with a smooth texture. They spread easily and melt quickly.

Specialty cheeses include cold pack cheese, a blend of ripened cheeses processed without heat, and pasteurized process cheese, a blend of ripened cheeses processed with heat. Examples of pasteurized process cheese are American cheese, cheese spread, and cheese food.

DAIRY SUBSTITUTES

What can you do if you're allergic to the protein in milk or can't digest lactose? What if you prefer foods that are free of saturated fats and cholesterol? Dairy substitutes provide options.

- **Margarine.** Made from hydrogenated vegetable oils and sold in sticks, similar to butter. Soft margarine blends hydrogenated and liquid vegetable oils to stay soft and spreadable. Liquid margarine is squeezed from pliable plastic bottles. Some margarines have no trans fats, and reduced fat and fat-free margarines are also available.
- **Soy milk.** The liquid pressed out of soybeans. Soy milk is high in protein, B vitamins, and iron and low in calcium, fat, and sodium. It contains no cholesterol. Choose a brand fortified with calcium and vitamins A, D, and B_{12}.
- **Soy cheese.** Made from soy milk. Low-fat and nonfat types are available.
- **Nondairy creamer.** Made with partially hydrogenated vegetable oil and corn syrup. Also called coffee lightener, it comes as a powder or liquid.
- **Whipped toppings.** Made from hydrogenated vegetable oils, sweeteners, and nonfat milk solids. You can choose from dry mixes, aerosol cans, or frozen tubs.

SAFETY ALERT

Good mold, bad mold. Molds are carefully selected and added to particular cheeses, including blue cheese, Roquefort, and Gorgonzola. This gives them their characteristic appearance and flavor. One type of mold added to cheese is related to penicillin. Because the process is carefully controlled, these cheeses are safe to eat. All cheeses may become moldy if stored improperly or for too long. This mold is not safe to eat.

Fig. 34-3

Ripened Cheeses

Cheese and Country of Origin	Description	Common Uses
Firm Ripened Cheeses		
Cheddar (England, United States, and Canada)	Pale yellow to deep orange in color; mild to extra-sharp flavor; melts well.	Eaten plain; ingredient in many recipes.
Parmesan/Romano (PAHR-muh-zahn/ruh-MAH-noh) (Italy)	Light yellow color; sharp flavor.	Grated; topping for pasta, pizza, vegetables; in cooking.
Swiss (Switzerland)	Pale yellow with large holes; nutty, slightly sweet flavor; melts well.	Eaten plain; sandwiches, salads; in cooking.
Provolone (proh-vuh-LOH-nee) (Italy)	Pale yellow with light brown rind; bland to sharp, smoky flavor; melts well.	Eaten plain; sandwiches; in cooking.
Semisoft Ripened Cheeses		
Gouda (GOO-duh) (Netherlands)	Creamy yellow with an inedible, yellow or red, wax coating; mild, nutlike flavor; similar to Edam in taste but richer; melts well.	Eaten plain; salads; in cooking.
Mozzarella (maht-suh-REH-luh) (Italy)	Creamy white; elastic texture; sweet, mild flavor; melts easily; also available fresh.	Eaten plain; on pizza; in dishes.
Brick (United States)	Light yellow in color; flavor ranges from mild to pungent.	Eaten plain; sandwiches.
Muenster (MUHNT-stuhr) (France)	Light yellow with orange rind; smooth texture with tiny holes; mild to pungent flavor.	Eaten plain; in cooking.
Monterey Jack (United States)	Creamy white; smooth texture and tiny cracks; mild flavor; melts well. Jalapeño Jack (hah-luh-PAY-nyoh) has a spicy-hot flavor.	Eaten plain; sandwiches; in cooking.

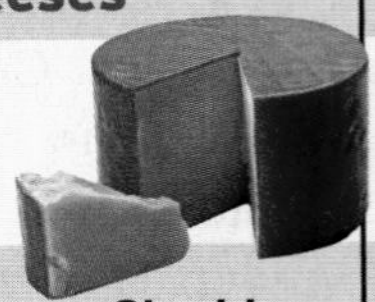

Cheddar

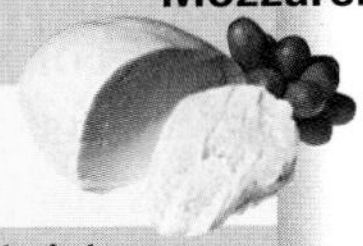

Mozzarella

- **Frozen desserts.** Nondairy ice cream made with cooked rice or tofu.

When you buy dairy substitutes, read labels carefully. The products may contain saturated fats, such as coconut or palm oils. As you know, those made with hydrogenated vegetable oils contain trans fats.

BUYING DAIRY FOODS

To be a smart consumer when buying dairy foods, consider fat amounts, container size, and product type. For instance, rich foods generally cost more than low-fat varieties. Large containers are usually a better buy than small ones. Foods with added ingredients, such as flavorings, fruit, and sugar, generally cost more than their plain counterparts.

Always check labels for nutrition and ingredient information. Containers should be tightly sealed and never opened. Also, look for the "sell by" date. Only buy quantities you can use in a relatively short time. Most dairy products must be used within a few days, although yogurt, butter, ripened cheese, and frozen desserts last longer when properly stored.

STORING DAIRY FOODS

Dairy foods are highly perishable, so take them home right after purchase and store them prop-

Fig. 34-3 (continued)

Ripened Cheeses

Cheese and Country of Origin	Description	Common Uses
Semisoft Ripened Cheeses		
Edam (EE-duhm) (Netherlands)	Creamy yellow with an inedible, red wax coating; mild, nutlike flavor; melts well.	Eaten plain; in cooking.
Feta (FEH-tuh) (Greece)	Pure white; crumbly texture; salty, sharp, and pickled flavor; must be stored in brine.	Crumbled in salads; in cooking.
Soft Ripened Cheeses		
Brie (BREE) (France)	Light yellow; buttery-soft texture; white, edible crust; mild to pungent flavor. When ripe, the interior should be soft enough to ooze.	Hors d'oeuvre or snack.
Neufchâtel (noo-shah-TEL) (France)	Mild, slightly salty flavor; creamy texture. American version is unripened and sold in bricks like cream cheese but with less fat.	Salads; sandwiches; in cooking.
Camembert (KA-muhm-behr) (France)	Similar to brie; creamy yellow; buttery texture; edible crust; mild to pungent flavor. When ripe, it should be soft enough to ooze.	Hors d'oeuvre or snack.
Blue-Veined Ripened Cheeses		
Blue cheese (Denmark)	Creamy white with blue vein; crumbly texture; salty, tangy flavor.	Salads; salad dressings; eaten plain.
Roquefort (ROHK-fuhrt) (France)	Creamy white with deep blue-green vein; strong, sharp, salty flavor.	Salads; salad dressings; eaten plain.
Gorgonzola (gawr-gun-ZOH-luh) (Italy)	Ivory-colored with blue-green vein; rich and creamy; flavor slightly to extremely pungent.	Eaten plain; salads; in cooking.
Stilton (England)	Pale yellow with blue-green vein; light brown, crusty rind; slightly cheddar flavor; mildest of all blue-veined cheeses.	Eaten plain.

Brie

Blue-veined

erly. It is best to refrigerate all dairy foods in original containers. Since dairy foods can pick up aromas from other foods and develop off-flavors, make sure containers are tightly closed.

After pouring milk, return the container to the refrigerator immediately. If milk has been sitting out in a serving pitcher, don't pour it back into the original container. Instead, if the milk has been at room temperature for less than two hours, refrigerate it in a separate container and use as soon as possible. Discard milk left at room temperature for more than two hours. Large amounts of harmful bacteria may have developed. Because light destroys the riboflavin in milk, store it away from light.

Keep ripened cheese tightly wrapped so it doesn't dry out. Firm and semisoft ripened cheeses can be frozen, but the texture changes. Freeze in $\frac{1}{2}$-pound portions and use it crumbled, shredded, or in cooked dishes.

You can refrigerate butter for several weeks and freeze it for up to nine months. Store frozen dairy desserts in tightly covered containers in the freezer.

USING DAIRY FOODS

Skillful cooks know how to use dairy products. Whether you make pizza with cheese or pudding with milk, certain knowledge promotes success.

Cooking with Milk and Cream

Milk isn't just for drinking and pouring on cereal. It's also used to prepare delicious cooked foods, including cocoa and soups. Since milk contains animal proteins, it is sensitive to heat. Therefore cook at moderate temperatures and for as short a time as possible. Several problems can occur when cooking milk.

Heat turns some milk solids and fat into a tough, rubbery skin that forms on the surface. The skin keeps steam from escaping. Pressure builds until the milk eventually boils over. To prevent skin from forming, cover the pan or stir the milk continuously as it cooks. If a skin does form, beat it into the milk; if you discard the skin, you throw away valuable nutrients.

Scorching can occur if milk overheats. When you heat milk, some solids settle on the sides and some fall to the bottom of the pan. If the milk overheats, the sugar lactose in the solids rapidly caramelizes and burns, or scorches. As a result, the milk develops an off-flavor. To prevent this, use low heat and stir the mixture to keep the solids from settling.

If you cook milk at a temperature that's too high, it separates into curds and whey. This is called **curdling**. Curdling may also occur when you add milk to hot foods, such as gravy, or to acidic foods, such as tomato soup. To prevent curdling, use a method called **tempering**. This technique brings one food to the right temperature or consistency before mixing it completely with another.

1. Pour a small amount of the hot or acidic mixture into the milk first, stirring constantly. Repeat, if needed. By doing this, you raise the temperature or acid level of the milk gradually, so there is less chance of curdling.
2. Slowly add the milk to the remaining mixture, stirring constantly. If you add the milk too quickly, the mixture may curdle.

If the mixture does curdle, you may be able to save it. Beat it vigorously until smooth.

To prevent the problems described, use a double boiler when heating milk. Place water in the bottom pan and milk in the upper one. The heat from the boiling water heats the milk without scorching or curdling.

Some recipes call for **scalded milk**, which is milk heated to just below the boiling point. Use low heat and cook only until bubbles appear around the sides of the pan.

Milk and milk-based recipes can be prepared easily in the microwave oven. Use a low setting to avoid overheating and curdling the milk, and make sure the container is large enough in case the milk foams up.

When choosing cream for whipping, look for heavy cream with a high fat content. This gives greater volume. When cream is whipped, a **foam** forms. See **Fig. 34-4**. As the cream is beaten, air is incorporated. At the same time, beating breaks down the protein, which then forms a fine film around pockets of air. This protein structure holds the air pockets and gives strength, or stability, to the foam. The fat in cream adds rigidity. As air cells multiply and become smaller with continued beating, the foam thickens. Don't overbeat, as cream will turn into butter. Add any other ingredients toward the end of whipping to avoid reducing the volume and overbeating.

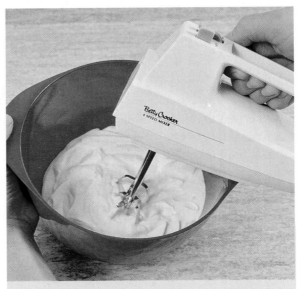

Fig. 34-4 When you whip cream, a foam is produced from the air and fat. The foam can be sweetened by gradually adding a little sugar at the end of the whipping process.

When you use cream in a recipe, follow the guidelines for cooking milk. Since cream is more sensitive to heat and acidic foods because it is richer, take extra care when using it in recipes.

Cooking with Yogurt

Yogurt works well as a low-fat substitute for sour cream, cream cheese, and mayonnaise. You can use yogurt in many recipes, including dips, soups, sauces, salads, and main dishes. During storage, the whey may separate from the curd. Stir the whey back into the yogurt before you use it. Cook yogurt at moderate temperatures for only the time needed. Yogurt is just as delicate as other dairy foods and curdles if overcooked.

Making Frozen Dairy Desserts

Special occasions—and even not-so-special occasions—offer a reason to make frozen dairy desserts. Treats like ice cream and mousse (MOOS) can be easily made at home.

- **Ice cream.** You can make ice cream with either a hand-operated or electric ice cream maker. Both work the same basic way. The inside container holds the ice cream mixture and a paddle that stirs the mix electrically or by hand. The outer container is filled with ice and salt, which freezes the ice cream mixture as the paddle rotates. (New models don't need ice and salt.) Stirring action prevents ice crystals, making the mixture light and airy.

- **Mousse.** A dessert mousse is a soft, creamy dish made with whipped cream and flavored, often with chocolate or fruit. Sometimes gelatin adds body and helps keep the mixture's shape. The dish is chilled or frozen in a decorative mold.

When making frozen dairy desserts, you need to keep ice crystals from forming. One way is to use enough fat since fat prevents crystal formation. The more fat a mixture has, the smoother it will be. That's why ice cream is smoother and richer than sherbet. Another method is to beat the mixture while making it. If frozen dairy desserts melt and refreeze during storage, ice crystals form, so keep frozen desserts solidly frozen at all times.

Serving Cheese

How many ways do people enjoy cheeses? Counting them isn't easy. Many cheeses are delicious plain, as a snack or hors d'oeuvre. Many dishes include cheese as an ingredient.

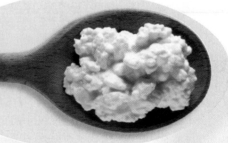

TRENDS in TECHNOLOGY

NEW DAIRY TECHNOLOGIES

Milk processors have found ways to keep milk products safer and more appealing as well.

- **Insulation.** A new container insulates milk. It resembles an insulated coffee carafe, but inside its plastic shell is a sealed layer of refrigerant, sandwiched with another layer of foam. After a night in the freezer, the container can hold a carton of milk at under 40°F for up to eight hours.

- **Electrification.** UHT milk may taste cooked. A new method of heating milk, called electroheating, uses electric currents to raise the milk's temperature within seconds, sterilizing the milk without producing the slightly stale flavor.

- **Carbonization.** The process that makes soft drinks bubbly also helps keep dairy foods safe. Carbon dioxide, which occurs naturally in milk, interferes with bacterial growth and may limit spoilage due to exposure to air. Adding carbon dioxide has been shown to add a week to the shelf life of milk and extend the three-week shelf life of cottage cheese to two months.

__**Think Beyond>>**__ If you were a dairy farmer, would you welcome these technologies? Why?

Because fresh cheese is highly perishable, serve it chilled. Its sweet, fresh flavor combines well with fruit in salads. Mixing with other foods works well too. You can put it in ham salad, salsa, and vegetable dishes. Making cheese dip is another possibility.

Cheddar and other ripened cheeses taste best when served at room temperature. Remove them from the refrigerator about 30 minutes before serving, or bring them to room temperature by microwaving. Follow the directions in the microwave oven owner's manual.

For an elegant dessert, serve assorted cheeses with fruit. An apple or berry pie can be topped with slices of sharp cheese. Warm the pie just long enough to melt the cheese before serving.

Cooking with Cheese

Cheese is a concentrated food, high in protein and fat, so cook with care. If you cook cheese for too long or use a temperature that's too high, the cheese becomes tough and rubbery. If fat separates into globules of grease, food will have an unappetizing appearance.

Cheese should be cooked just until it melts. To reduce cooking time, cut the cheese into small pieces or grate it. If you want to melt cheese by itself, use very low heat or a double boiler.

Cheese is a common ingredient in casseroles, soups, sauces, and other dishes. **Fig. 34-5** shows a recipe for a favorite casserole made with cheese. When other foods are combined with cheese, they should either be precooked or need only a short cooking time and moderate temperatures. Do you know why casseroles are often topped with bread crumbs or other topping? This layer not only adds crunch and flavor but also protects the cheese underneath from too much heat.

Some cheese varieties blend more readily than others during cooking. Process cheese mixes easily with other ingredients. Because cheddar blends well, it's a favorite for cooking. Fresh cheeses, such as cottage and cream cheese, don't blend well unless beaten into the mixture.

Be careful when microwaving dishes with cheese. The fat in the cheese attracts microwaves, so the cheese may be hotter than the rest of the food in the dish.

Career Prep

Technology in the Workplace

AT ONE TIME, THE BALLPOINT PEN was "high tech" in the office. Now workplace technology is so complex that some schools offer an associate's degree in the subject. What trends might you expect in technology on the job?

- **The virtual office.** In a manner of speaking, communication technology "breaks down office walls," enabling people to work together when thousands of miles apart. Instant messaging and videoconferencing are two examples. Telecommuting may become more common.

- **Self-employment.** Products of technology tend to grow more affordable and convenient over time, making it easier for would-be entre-

preneurs to start a business. A food stylist might invest in a digital camera and image-editing software to create and transmit photos of food displays to clients the world over.

- **Assistive technology.** Using technology to help people with disabilities function in an "able-bodied" world is an old practice. Newer technology is increasing their opportunities for challenging careers. For example, one computer program scans printed material and reads it aloud for visually impaired workers.

NEW CONCERNS

As always, changes in workplace technology have an impact beyond the workplace. Many

Fig. 34-5

Easy Macaroni and Cheese

Yield	Nutrition Analysis
4 servings	*Per Serving:* 420 calories, 10 g total fat, 6 g saturated fat, 0 g trans fat, 30 mg cholesterol, 610 mg sodium, 64 g total carbohydrate, 3 g dietary fiber, 14 g sugars, 18 g protein
	Percent Daily Value: vitamin A 15%, vitamin C 25%, calcium 35%, iron 15%

Ingredients

½ lb. cooked elbow macaroni
4 oz. process cheese spread (cut into cubes)
½ cup chopped green bell pepper
¼ cup finely chopped onion

1 tsp. butter or margarine
1 cup evaporated, fat-free milk
¼ tsp. ground pepper
½ cup dry breadcrumbs
1 tsp. butter or margarine, melted

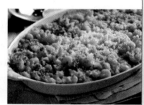

Directions

1. In a saucepan, sauté green bell pepper and onion over medium-low heat in 1 teaspoon butter or margarine, about 1 to 2 minutes, stirring constantly. Stir in milk and cheese.
2. Cook over medium-low heat, stirring constantly, until cheese melts. Stir in pepper.
3. Combine milk-and-cheese mixture with macaroni in 1½-qt. casserole. Mix gently.
4. Combine breadcrumbs and 1 teaspoon melted butter or margarine.
5. Sprinkle breadcrumb mixture over macaroni-and-cheese mixture.
6. Bake 20 to 30 minutes at 350°F until hot and bubbly.

---

people wonder whether schools can keep students current with rapid technological changes. Educators and business leaders may need to work more closely to decide what skills are most useful for which jobs and how and where the skills are best taught.

Social impact is another concern. For many people, work relationships are part of their social network. Will those who work from home feel isolated without the friendship and support of co-workers? Also, how will families handle the management of home and work life as the line separating the two areas blurs?

The emotional climate of the workplace could also feel the effects. Newer, faster technology may bring more opportunities to advance. Along with that, however, greater demands and higher expectations may come, plus continuing pressure to update skills. More job stress could be the result.

Potential problems are the price of advances in technology. Avoiding them is not always possible. Anticipating them and finding ways to cope is the solution.

Career Connection

Analyzing the impact. Research how technology has affected the workplace in one area of foods and nutrition.

Summarize Your Reading

▶ Dairy products are flavorful, rich, versatile, and nutritious. They include milk, cream, butter, yogurt, frozen dairy desserts, and cheese.

▶ Different kinds of milk may have different amounts of fat, milk solids, and/or water. Other kinds of milk may have such products as sugar, cocoa, or minerals added.

▶ When purchasing dairy foods, consumers should consider fat amounts, container size, and product type.

▶ Because dairy foods are perishable, they need to be refrigerated.

▶ Special care must be taken when cooking with dairy foods.

Check Your Knowledge

1. What nutrients do dairy foods provide?

2. To make a salad dressing that calls for 6 tablespoons of sour cream, how many fat grams could you save by substituting **yogurt** for the sour cream?

3. Why must **raw milk** be **pasteurized** before it's sold?

4. What is **homogenized** milk?

5. Compare these terms: whole milk, reduced-fat milk, low-fat milk, and nonfat milk.

6. What is the difference between evaporated milk and sweetened condensed milk?

7. How can each of these kinds of milk be used for health benefits: a) lactose-free; b) acidophilus; c) calcium-enriched?

8. What kind of cream is best for making whipped cream for a dessert? Which creams would most likely be added to coffee?

9. How is sour cream made?

10. Why is salt usually added to butter?

11. How is yogurt made, and why does it have more nutrients than milk?

12. What is the difference between sherbet and sorbet?

13. Explain how cheese is formed, using the terms **curds** and **whey**.

14. What is the difference between **fresh** and **ripened cheeses**?

15. Why do some people prefer to use dairy substitutes?

16. What advice would you give to a consumer who is considering dairy foods for purchase?

17. How would you store each of the following: a) milk; b) ripened cheese; c) butter?

18. **CRITICAL THINKING** During a brunch, the milk in a pitcher sat on the serving table for a little over two hours. What should be done with it? How might milk be served at a brunch to keep it safe?

19. What can you do to prevent skin from forming on milk when you heat it?

20. Describe two conditions, other than skin formation, that can occur when milk is overheated.

21. Describe the process that turns cream into whipped cream.

22. What should you do if you're about to use yogurt and you notice that the whey has separated from the curd?

23. In general, which cheeses should be served chilled and which should be served at room temperature?

24. What happens to cheese when it overcooks?

Apply Your Learning

1. **Calcium Amounts.** Look up the amount of calcium and vitamin D needed per day for teens. How much milk and other dairy foods would you need to get those amounts? Create menus for three days that would provide enough calcium and vitamin D.

2. **LANGUAGE ARTS** **Radio Spot.** Many teens don't get enough calcium. Write a radio spot that promotes milk drinking.

3. **Milk Taste Test.** Conduct a class taste test of these milks: whole; reduced fat; low fat; nonfat; buttermilk; and rehydrated dry milk. How do they compare?

4. **SCIENCE** **Effect of Acids.** Add 2 tablespoons of lemon juice to 1 cup of milk at room temperature. Let the milk stand for 10 minutes. Describe results. What is happening to the milk? Demonstrate a cooking technique that can prevent this from happening.

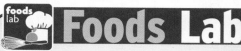

Foods Lab

Homemade Ice Cream

Procedure: Find recipes for homemade ice cream. Choose one to prepare in the lab, using a hand-crank ice cream maker. What food safety precautions need to be observed when making homemade ice cream?

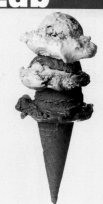

Analyzing Results

❶ How difficult was it to make the ice cream with a hand crank? How is an electric ice cream maker different?

❷ Evaluate your ice cream on taste, texture, and appearance.

❸ How do you think your ice cream compares with store-bought versions in quality and cost?

Food Science Experiment

Foam Comparison

Objective: To compare foam formation with different kinds of milk products.

Procedure:

1. Obtain one of the following milk samples, as assigned by your teacher: evaporated milk, half and half, coffee creamer, light whipping cream, and heavy whipping cream. All samples and bowls should be the same size. (Note: for added comparison, refrigerated and room temperature samples may be used.)

2. With an electric mixer at high speed, beat your sample until it forms a foam. Time and record when a foam is reached. Beat for no more than 15 minutes.

3. Use a skewer to measure the highest point of your foam. Record.

4. Observe your foam, recording its height and condition every 10 minutes for a half hour.

Analyzing Results

❶ Summarize the foaming results produced by your sample.

❷ How did the samples compare in forming a foam? What explains the variations?

❸ What do you think would happen if whole milk were used? Nonfat milk?

❹ Which milk products would you use in recipes that require a foam? Prepare and serve a recipe made with a foam.

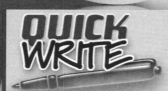

SENTENCE VARIETY. Good writing blends sentences that have different structures. For example: "Rosie gathered the eggs with a basket" and "Using a basket, Rosie gathered the eggs." In what other ways can sentence structures be varied? Write a paragraph that describes eggs or an egg dish you like, including at least three different sentence structures.

Objectives

▶ Describe the structure of an egg.

▶ Explain how to select and store eggs.

▶ Explain scientific principles related to egg cookery.

▶ Demonstrate how to separate and beat egg whites.

▶ Describe and demonstrate methods for cooking and serving eggs.

Terms

air cell	omelet
albumen	quiche
beading	shirred eggs
chalazae	soft peaks
coagulate	soufflé
custard	stiff peaks
emulsifier	weep
frittata	yolk
meringue	

SCRAMBLED, FRIED, OR POACHED, EGGS CAN be enjoyed in many ways, and not just for breakfast. Have you ever eaten a soufflé (soo-FLAY) or quiche (KEESH)? Both are delicious egg dishes that can be served for lunch or dinner.

Eggs are one of nature's most versatile, nutritious, and economical foods. Besides being tasty, they perform important functions in recipes. As you will see, eggs are star performers in many kitchens.

THE STRUCTURE OF EGGS

An egg has several parts. See **Fig. 35-1**. The hard shell is porous and lined with membranes. A pocket of air, also known as the **air cell**, lies between these membranes at the wide, round end. As an egg ages, this air cell gets larger. The shell also contains these three egg parts:

• **Albumen (al-BYOO-muhn).** The thick fluid commonly known as egg white is **albumen**. Albumen gets thinner as an egg ages. Cloudy white albumen indicates the egg is very fresh.

• **Yolk.** The round yellow portion of an egg is the **yolk**. It's encased in a thin membrane and floats within the albumen. The yolk flattens as the egg

ages. Yolk color depends on the hen's diet. Hens fed yellow cornmeal or marigold petals produce deeper yellow yolks than those fed white cornmeal. Artificial color additives are not allowed in chicken feeds.

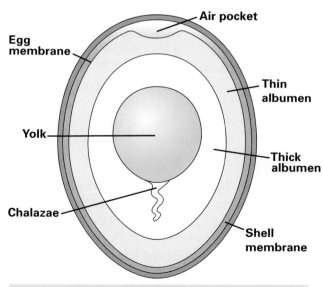

Fig. 35-1 These are the basic parts of an egg. What is the albumen commonly called? What is the purpose of the chalazae?

- **Chalazae (kuh-LAY-zee).** The two, thick, twisted strands of albumen that anchor the yolk in the center of an egg are called **chalazae**. They are not, as some people believe, the beginning of an embryo. The thicker and more prominent the chalazae are, the fresher the eggs.

NUTRIENTS IN EGGS

Eggs are an excellent source of protein and vitamin B_{12}. Both the white and the yolk contain proteins. In addition, eggs contain vitamin A, other B vitamins, vitamin D, iron, calcium, phosphorus, and other trace minerals. Eggs have only about 80 calories each.

In general, the yolk of an egg contains more vitamins and minerals than the white. Egg yolks are one of the few foods that are a natural source of vitamin D. Since eggs yolks also contain fats and cholesterol, however, health experts recommend eating them in moderation.

Are brown eggs more nutritious than white? Actually, the breed of hen determines shell color. The color isn't related to an egg's nutrients, flavor, or cooking qualities.

BUYING EGGS

When you buy eggs, select them from a refrigerated case. Open the carton to inspect them. The eggs should be clean and whole, without cracks. They should not be leaking or stuck in the carton. Buy them by the sell date.

Eggs are sold according to grade and size standards set by the USDA. The grade and size, which are clearly marked on the package, have no relationship to each other.

Grades

The USDA grade shield on a package means the eggs have been federally inspected for wholesomeness. The grade is determined by the inner and outer quality of the egg at the time of packaging. Workers examine egg interiors with bright lights in order to sort out unacceptable ones.

The three egg grades are AA, A, and B. All have the same nutritive value; however, appearances differ after cooking. Grade AA and A eggs have a thicker white, suitable when appearance is

important, as for fried and poached eggs. Grade B eggs can be used in baked goods, when appearance doesn't matter. Supermarkets typically carry grades AA and A.

Size

Eggs are classified into sizes by the minimum weight for a dozen, so sizes can vary slightly in the same carton. The sizes most commonly sold are medium, large, extra large, and jumbo. As a general rule, recipes assume that large eggs will be used. If you use eggs of another size, you may need more or fewer eggs for the same results.

The price of eggs depends on the size as well as the supply of various sizes. Check the unit price to determine which size is the best buy.

STORING EGGS

Since eggs are highly perishable, take them home right away after shopping and store them immediately. Handle eggs gently to prevent cracking them. Always discard dirty eggs and any that are cracked or leaking.

Don't wash eggs before storing them. Washing eggs at home removes the protective coating that prevents bacteria from getting inside the shell.

Refrigerate eggs in the original carton rather than the egg tray in the refrigerator door. Each time you open the door, the temperature drops, so eggs stored in the door may lose quality. In addition, since eggshells are porous, they pick up aromas from other foods if stored uncovered.

EGG LAYING TECHNOLOGY

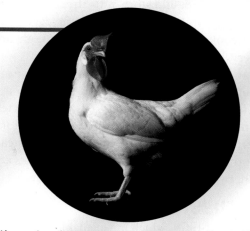

The egg may be nature's most nearly perfect food, but nature gets an assist from technology to keep commercial egg producers in business.

Laying hens are selectively bred, using modern genetics. The White Leghorn is the breed of choice in the United States. This breed matures quickly and produces large white eggs. The hens are fed a mash of corn and other grains, cottonseed meal, and soybean oil, plus antioxidants and mold inhibitors. The ration is carefully formulated to meet the birds' nutritional requirements and to produce the best quality eggs. Portions are dispensed through automated feeders set on timers.

The laying house is climate-controlled, with light, temperature, and humidity monitored to promote egg production. For example, the birds are exposed to about 15 hours of artificial light each day so that they regularly lay about one egg per day. By reducing light and food, egg farmers can influence the time when hens molt, or lose their feathers. This results in higher quality eggs and extended life for the hens.

Since heat and humidity affect quality, eggs are automatically gathered by conveyor belts that run beneath the bird's cage. The belt transports the eggs to refrigerated holding rooms. Within one or two days, they appear in your supermarket's dairy case.

__Think Beyond>> Why do you think light control has an impact on egg production?

Raw eggs stay fresh in the refrigerator for up to four weeks, depending on freshness when purchased and the refrigerator temperature. Refrigerate leftover cooked eggs and egg mixtures immediately and use them within three days. Use hard-cooked eggs in the shell within a week.

A recipe may call for only the yolk or the white. You can refrigerate leftover raw yolks (covered with water) for two days and whites for four days in a tightly covered container. For longer storage, freeze them.

A red spot in the egg means that one or more small blood vessels in the yolk ruptured, but the egg is safe to use. If an egg has an unpleasant odor when opened, it is spoiled, so discard it.

Freezing Eggs

To freeze raw whites, place each white in a separate compartment of an ice cube tray. After freezing, put the frozen cubes in a tightly sealed

Consumer FYI

Eggshells. The eggshell is obviously essential to the life of an egg. It plays a role in protecting your health as well.

An eggshell contains up to 17,000 pores, which are protected by a coating called the cuticle, or bloom. The pores grow larger with age, however, increasing the chance for bacterial contamination. To reduce this risk, eggs are gathered soon after laying. They're washed and lightly coated with mineral oil. This process also keeps oxygen from entering the shell, which helps maintain freshness.

Boiling eggs strips off the oil coat. That's why hard-cooked eggs must be eaten within a week, while fresh eggs keep much longer.

freezer container and store in the freezer. Use two thawed egg whites to equal one large egg. Don't freeze cooked whites since they get tough and rubbery.

Raw yolks need special treatment for freezing to keep them from getting thick and hard to mix after thawing. For every four yolks, beat in $\frac{1}{8}$ teaspoon of salt. If you plan to use the yolks for a dessert, beat in $1\frac{1}{2}$ teaspoons of sugar instead. Mark the container with the number of yolks and whether you added salt or sugar; then freeze.

EGG SUBSTITUTES

Egg substitutes, which are available frozen and in refrigerated liquid form, are an alternative to whole eggs. Most are made by combining egg whites with such ingredients as vegetable oils, tofu, nonfat dry milk powder, and chemical additives, including emulsifiers, stabilizers, antioxidants, and artificial colors. You can use egg substitutes much the same as whole eggs.

Since they contain no egg yolks, egg substitutes have no cholesterol or fat and are lower in calories. Therefore they are a healthy alternative for people who are watching their fat and cholesterol intake. Egg substitutes contain less protein and phosphorus than whole eggs, however, and they may lack some B vitamins. They are also more expensive than whole eggs.

EGG SCIENCE

An understanding of egg science can help you cook successfully with eggs. They have certain properties that result mostly from their high protein content.

Coagulation

The proteins in eggs are shaped like coils. When heated, the coils unwind and join loosely with other proteins. The new structures form pockets that hold water. When this happens, the egg **coagulates**, or becomes firm, changing from a liquid to a semisolid or solid state. This property is what helps eggs bind ingredients in foods like meatloaf and thicken such dishes as custards and fillings. See **Fig. 35-2**.

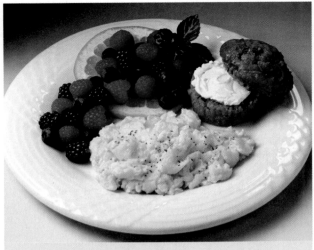

Fig. 35-2 A good example of coagulation is scrambling an egg. What happens to egg protein during this process?

High heat and overcooking cause the protein structure to tighten and push out the water. As a result, the protein becomes tough and watery. The cooked eggs may be dry and unappetizing. Gentle cooking helps prevents these problems.

Emulsifiers

Eggs are excellent **emulsifiers**, meaning they hold together two liquids that normally won't stay mixed, such as water and oil. Yolks do this quite well. As you recall, protein structures consist of many linked amino acids. In yolk protein, one end of an amino acid bonds with water, but the other end bonds with oil. This gives egg yolk the power to hold two ingredients together, whether it's vinegar and oil in a salad dressing or lemon juice and oil in mayonnaise. See **Fig. 35-3**.

Foams

When you beat egg whites, a foam forms, as occurs when you beat cream. Egg whites have large protein molecules. As the whites are beaten, air enters the mixture. Like cream, beating breaks down the protein, which then supplies a structure that gives the foam its strength. Continued beating thickens the foam.

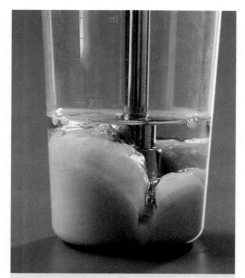

Fig. 35-3 Eggs serve as emulsifiers when making certain foods. How do eggs help when used in this way?

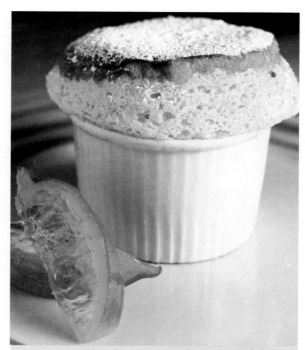

Fig. 35-4 Soufflés are baked in dishes with straight sides so the foam mixture can cling and "climb." The finished product typically rises above the edge of the dish.

An egg white foam adds volume and lightness to such baked products as angel food cake and soufflés. A **soufflé** is made by folding stiffly beaten whites into a sauce or puréed food. It is baked in a deep casserole until it puffs up. See **Fig. 35-4**. Beaten egg whites are also used to make meringues.

PREPARING EGGS FOR COOKING

For anyone who's new to the kitchen, even cracking an egg open can be a challenge. Hold the egg in the fingers of one hand. Then rap the center of the egg once firmly, but not too hard, against a clean surface. Some cooks use the edge of a clean bowl. Pull the two shell halves apart as though hinged at one side, allowing the egg to drop into the bowl. If you're not using the whole egg, you need to separate the parts.

Separating Eggs

Sometimes recipes call for only part of an egg. Yolks are used in custards, sauces, mayonnaise, and pastry. Because beaten egg whites are airy, they add lightness to many baked items.

To separate an egg, carefully break it into an egg separator. This small device allows the white to flow through, while leaving the yolk in the separator. See **Fig. 35-5** on page 496. Keep in mind that eggs separate more easily when cold. Refrigerate any unused yolk or white for later use.

Beating Egg Whites

Beaten egg whites are used in many dishes. When you beat whites, the foam should rise well. It should be stable and not collapse when folded with other ingredients and when baked. How can you make this happen?

First, make sure no trace of yolk is in the white. Even a drop of the yolk's fat can keep a foam from reaching full volume. If any yolk falls into the white, refrigerate it for later use and start again with another egg white. Be sure beaters and bowls are clean and free of fat. Use only glass or metal bowls since plastic and wooden bowls absorb fat and aluminum bowls darken the whites.

Another helpful technique is allowing egg whites to stand at room temperature for up to 20 minutes before beating. This helps the foam reach full volume. If the egg white is cold, the protein doesn't break down as readily to allow foam formation.

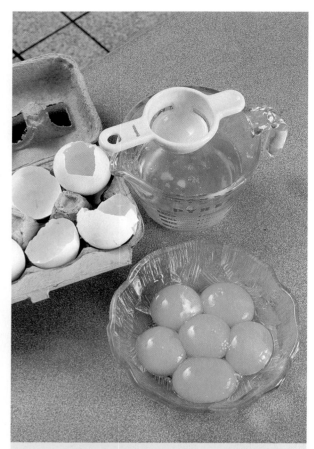

Fig. 35-5 Egg separators make it easy to separate whites from yolks. Why is this method recommended?

You can also add one or more substances to egg whites before or during beating to aid foam stability. An acidic ingredient, such as cream of tartar, may be added before beating. Some recipes call for vinegar or lemon juice, which adds flavor.

SAFETY ALERT

Separating eggs. The old standard method of separating the egg white from the yolk is no longer recommended. People used to pour the yolk back and forth between the two halves of the broken shell, letting the white fall into a bowl. Because bacteria on the egg shell can get into the egg, an egg separating tool should be used instead.

Sugar may be used along with cream of tartar for stabilization. Since sugar increases beating time, however, add it near the end of the beating process. Salt decreases foam stability. If a recipe calls for salt, add it to other ingredients rather than the whites.

As you beat whites, their texture and color change from thick, colorless, and transparent to fluffy, white, and opaque. The exact texture depends on how long they are beaten. Whites can be beaten to form soft or stiff peaks. When you lift the beaters from the mixture and the whites gently bend over like waves, these are **soft peaks**. **Stiff peaks** stand up straight when the beaters are lifted from the mixture. This is the maximum point to which egg whites should be beaten. See **Fig. 35-6**.

Stop beating egg whites as soon as they reach the stage called for in the recipe. Overbeating turns a foam dry, hard, and lumpy, making it fall apart. Once they lose air and moisture, the whites can't be used.

When you fold beaten egg whites into another mixture, do so gently. Stirring and beating cause loss of air and volume. Place the beaten whites on top of the mixture. Cut down through the whites with a rubber spatula to the bottom of the bowl. Drag some of the bottom mixture up the side, folding it lightly onto the whites in the middle. Turn the bowl and repeat just until the whites are incorporated.

COOKING WITH EGGS

Because eggs are a delicate high-protein food, they must be cooked carefully. Egg whites cook faster than yolks. Eggs should be cooked until the whites are firm. Yolks should be thickened, not runny.

Never eat raw or undercooked eggs and foods that contain them. Some eggs have been found to carry *Salmonella* bacteria. Therefore health experts recommend that all eggs be cooked thoroughly. Egg dishes should be cooked to 160°F in the center.

Egg cookery can be simple or complex. You can cook eggs alone or combine them with other ingredients in many recipes. Learning to cook them in the shell is a good place to start.

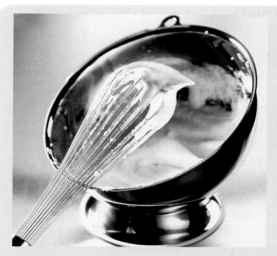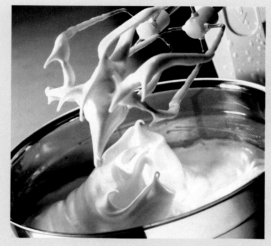

Fig. 35-6 A recipe tells whether to beat egg whites to soft or stiff peaks. Note how the white in the bowl on the right lifts into stiff peaks when the beater is removed. The white on the left, however, has soft peaks.

Eggs Cooked in the Shell

Since you can't see inside, knowing when an egg in the shell is cooked just right can be a challenge. Here's a method that works well. Place a single layer of eggs in a saucepan. Add water to a level at least 1 inch above the eggs. Cover the pan and bring the water to a boil. Turn the heat off as soon as boiling begins. On an electric range, remove the pan from the heating element to prevent further boiling. Let the eggs stand, covered, in the hot water. Allow 12 minutes for medium-size eggs, 15 minutes for large, and 18 minutes for extra large. Because eggs must be thoroughly cooked, don't use less time to make soft-cooked eggs. Harmful bacteria may survive.

When eggs are done, immediately pour off the hot water and run cold water over them or place them in ice water to stop the cooking process and cool them. Refrigerate them in their shells until needed.

Eggs sometimes crack as they cook because the air inside the eggs expands as it heats. This generally occurs when eggs are overheated or cooked for too long. Cooking them in more than one layer can also cause cracks when eggs bump together. An egg that cracks during cooking is safe for immediate use. Never prick the egg with a pin or thumbtack before cooking to release the air. Even a small hole can create hairline cracks that allow bacteria to enter after the egg has been cooled and saved for later use.

To peel a hard-cooked egg, gently tap the egg all over to crack the shell. Then roll the egg lightly between your hands to loosen the shell. Peel the shell away, starting at the wide end where the air cell is located. Hold the egg under cold running water to help ease off the shell. Fresh eggs are harder to peel. This is because the air cell enlarges and the egg contents shrink as eggs age.

SAFETY ALERT

Raw eggs. Thorough cooking destroys bacteria in egg-based foods. Raw eggs and foods that contain them are not safe to eat. This includes raw cookie dough, homemade dairy products that use raw eggs, protein shakes, traditional hollandaise sauce, traditional Caesar salad, and frosting made from raw egg whites. In recipes calling for whole raw eggs, you can cook them first or substitute a pasteurized egg product or pasteurized shell egg. The pasteurization process destroys harmful bacteria.

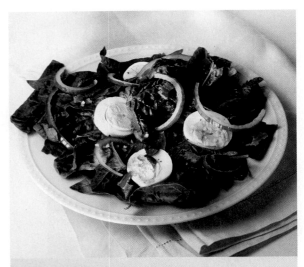

Fig. 35-7 Hard-cooked eggs can be a garnish or the main part of a dish. How are they used here?

Have you ever seen a hard-cooked egg yolk that has a gray-green surface? The color is a reaction between sulfur in the white and iron in the yolk. Cook eggs no longer than necessary to prevent this color change.

Once hard-cooked, eggs can be chopped, sliced, or cut into wedges. Add them to salads and casseroles, use in sandwiches or as a garnish, or make deviled or pickled eggs. See **Fig. 35-7**.

Poached Eggs

There are many ways to cook eggs out of the shell. Poaching cooks them in simmering water. This method adds no fat while cooking. Using fresh eggs and getting them to set quickly are keys to successful poaching.

To poach eggs, put water, milk, or broth in a saucepan to a depth of about 2 to 3 inches. Heat to boiling and then reduce to a gentle simmer. Break one egg at a time into a small dish. Hold the dish close to the surface of the liquid and slip in the egg. Cook until the white is completely set, about 3 to 5 minutes. The yolk should be thickened. Remove cooked eggs, one at a time, with a slotted spoon and drain for a few seconds.

Usually, poached eggs are served on toast. You can also spoon cooked vegetables onto toasted English muffins and top with poached eggs, or pour a flavored sauce, perhaps made with cheese, over the eggs.

Fried Eggs

Eggs can be fried in oil, margarine, or butter or in a nonstick skillet coated with vegetable oil cooking spray. Heat a small amount of fat in a skillet over medium-high heat until hot enough to sizzle a drop of water.

To avoid breaking the yolk, break one egg at a time into a small bowl or custard cup. Then gently slip the egg from the bowl into the heated skillet. Cook until whites are completely set and yolks thicken. To cook the tops, baste them with the hot fat, turn the egg over carefully, or cover the skillet with a lid for the last minute or two of cooking.

For an interesting variation on fried eggs, make a hole in a slice of bread or frozen waffle and place in a greased, heated skillet. Break the egg into the hole and fry. Fried eggs can also be served in a sandwich or on top of steak, hash, or vegetables.

Scrambled Eggs

To make fluffy scrambled eggs, beat eggs together with water or milk in a bowl. Use 1 tablespoon of liquid for each egg. Heat a small amount of fat on low in a skillet, or use a vegetable oil cooking spray.

Pour the egg mixture into the heated skillet. Then let it stand for 30 to 60 seconds. As the mixture starts to thicken, draw an inverted turner gently through the eggs. This forms large curds and allows uncooked egg to flow to the bottom of the skillet. Continue this process until the eggs are thickened and no visible liquid remains. Curds should be large and fluffy. Don't stir the eggs constantly. This beats out the air and moisture to produce small, tough curds.

You can also scramble eggs by breaking them directly into the skillet. When the whites begin to set, mix the eggs right in the pan and cook until they are thickened and no visible liquid remains. The eggs will be less fluffy and have streaks of white and yellow.

Baked Eggs

Baked eggs, also known as **shirred eggs**, are easy to prepare. Break the eggs into a small bowl.

Then slip them into a greased, shallow baking dish or large custard cup. You can use individual dishes or place several eggs in one dish. If you like, top the eggs with a small amount of milk.

Preheat the oven to 325°F. Bake the eggs until the whites are completely set and the yolks thicken, about 12 to 18 minutes.

You can also bake eggs in nests of cooked vegetables, cooked grains, or in hollowed-out rolls.

Basic Omelet

Unlike scrambled eggs, the eggs in an omelet are not stirred. Because of the cooking technique, an **omelet** holds the egg mixture together to form a large, thick pancake, which is filled and then folded over before serving. See **Fig. 35-8**. A basic omelet, also called a French omelet, is made as follows:

1. Mix 2 eggs, 2 tablespoons of water, and a dash each of salt and pepper with a fork or whisk until just blended.
2. Heat 1 tablespoon of butter or oil in an omelet pan or a skillet over medium heat until hot enough to sizzle a drop of water. Pour in the egg mixture all at once. Allow it to flow to the edge of the pan, but don't stir. The edge should begin to set right away.
3. With a turner, lift just a little around the firming edge so that uncooked portions flow beneath to the pan surface. Tilt the pan as needed. Be careful not to break the mixture that has already set. Continue until the top is thickened and no visible liquid egg remains.
4. Spread filling over half of the omelet.
5. Using the turner, fold the omelet in half or nearly so. Tilting the skillet slightly away from you and folding toward the low side may help.
6. Slide the omelet onto a plate and serve.

Your taste buds and your imagination can inspire ideas for omelet fillings. You can use cheese, sauces, yogurt, peanut butter, cooked vegetables, jam, diced or sliced fruit, or cooked diced meat, poultry, or fish. Small pieces are less likely to tear the omelet. Preheat cold fillings that are just out of the refrigerator and cook raw vegetables beforehand.

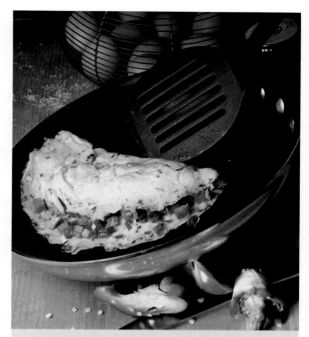

Fig. 35-8 An omelet can be folded in half or just part way over. What ingredients might you use to fill an omelet?

A **frittata** (free-TAH-tuh) is like an omelet, but the ingredients are stirred into the egg mixture, which is not folded after cooking. See **Fig. 35-9** on page 500 for a recipe to try.

Puffy Omelet

You can also bake an omelet in the oven. Beaten egg whites make it light and puffy. Separate the eggs and beat the whites and yolks separately. Fold the stiffly beaten whites into the yolks. Pour the mixture into a skillet with an ovenproof handle.

First, cook the mixture on top of the range, without disturbing, until it is puffed and lightly browned on the bottom, about 5 minutes. Then bake in a preheated oven at 350°F for 10 to 12 minutes or until a knife inserted in the center comes out clean.

You can serve the omelet folded or open-face. To serve folded, partially cut through the center of the omelet for ease in folding. Fill and fold.

To serve the omelet open-face, tilt the skillet over a warm plate. Slide the omelet onto the plate. Spoon filling, if desired, over the top. Cut in half or into wedges and serve immediately.

Fig. 35-9

Try This! **Recipe**

Italian Frittata

Yield	Nutrition Analysis
4 servings	***Per Serving:*** 190 calories, 14 g total fat, 6 g saturated fat, 0 g trans fat, 335 mg cholesterol, 230 mg sodium, 2 g total carbohydrate, 1 g dietary fiber, 1 g sugars, 14 g protein ***Percent Daily Value:*** vitamin A 15%, vitamin C 10%, calcium 15%, iron 10%

Ingredients
¼ lb. mushrooms, thinly sliced
2 green onions, minced
1½ Tbsp. butter or margarine
6 eggs

3 Tbsp. fresh parsley, chopped
½ tsp. dried basil, crumbled
¼ cup grated Parmesan cheese, divided in half
salt and pepper to taste

Directions
1. In large nonstick skillet with oven-safe handle, sauté mushrooms and green onions in butter or margarine over medium heat until tender-crisp.
2. Preheat oven broiler. Beat eggs in medium bowl. Add parsley, basil, half of the cheese, and salt and pepper to the eggs. Mix well.
3. Pour egg mixture over vegetables in skillet. Cook over medium heat, without stirring, until edges are lightly browned.
4. Sprinkle with remaining cheese.
5. Broil until top is golden brown. Cut into wedges and serve hot.

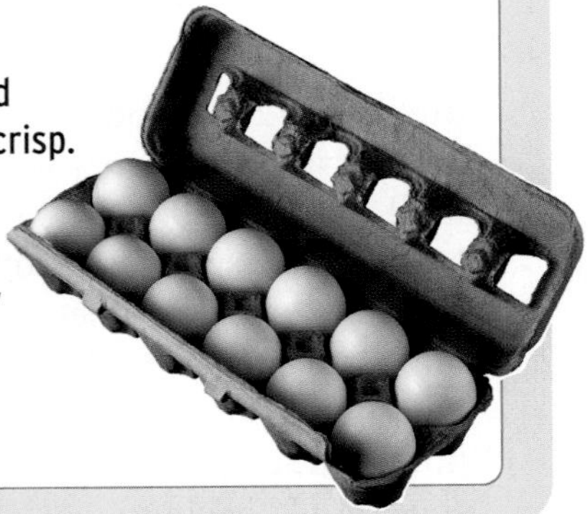

Microwaving Eggs

Cooking eggs in the microwave oven takes special care. First, never microwave eggs that are still in the shell. Heat and steam build up inside an egg, causing it to explode. Second, remember that microwave ovens cook unevenly. Make sure the egg or any egg dish is thoroughly cooked.

Since eggs overcook easily, start with the minimum time suggested and check them frequently. The yolk must be pierced before cooking to break the membrane and allow heat and steam to escape. Remove eggs from the microwave while still moist and soft. Standing time completes the cooking. Follow these cooking methods:

• **Fried eggs.** Break the eggs into a lightly greased dish. Gently pierce the yolks with the tip of a knife or a wooden pick. Cover and cook at 50 percent power until the eggs are done, about 2 to 3 minutes. Let stand, covered, until the whites are completely set and the yolks thicken, about 30 seconds to 1 minute.

• **Scrambled eggs.** Pour beaten egg mixture into a large custard cup. Cook on full power, stirring once or twice, until almost set, about 1 to 1½ minutes. Stir. If necessary, cover and let stand until eggs are thick and no visible liquid egg remains, about 1 minute.

• **Poached eggs.** Pour hot water into a large custard cup or small deep bowl. Break and slip in the eggs. Pierce the yolks with the tip of a knife or a wooden pick. Cook on full power for 1½ to 3 minutes. If necessary, let stand, covered, until whites are completely set and yolks thicken. Lift the eggs out with a slotted spoon, or pour the water off to serve in the custard cup.

Custards

A **custard** is a thickened blend of milk, eggs, and sugar. It can be a base for many main dishes. Custards are soft or baked.

Soft Custard

Soft custard, also known as stirred custard, is creamy and pourable. You can serve it as a pudding or as a sauce over cake or fruit. Soft custard is made by beating together eggs, sugar, and salt, if desired, then stirring in nonfat or low-fat milk. The amount of each ingredient determines the custard's thickness.

Cook the mixture over low heat, stirring constantly, until just thick enough to coat a metal spoon with a thin film. Remove from the heat to prevent overcooking. If soft custard is overcooked, it curdles. If undercooked, it is thin and watery. Cool quickly by setting the pan in a bowl of cold water. Stir for a few minutes, and then stir in vanilla. You may also prepare soft custard in a double boiler.

Baked Custard

Baked custard, which has a firm, delicate texture, is cooked in the oven. Many well-known desserts have a baked custard base, including custard pie. Another example is flan, Spanish custard topped with caramel sauce. If unsweetened, baked custard can become a main dish. **Quiche** is a pie with custard filling, containing such foods as chopped vegetables, cheese, and chopped, cooked meat. See **Fig. 35-10**.

To make baked custard, beat ingredients as you do for soft custard, but instead of stirring the mixture over the stove, pour it into lightly greased custard cups or a casserole dish. Set the cups or dish in a large baking pan. Add hot water to the pan up to $\frac{1}{2}$ inch below the top of the custard. This insulates the custard so it doesn't overcook.

Take care with baking time. If custard is overbaked, it curdles; if underbaked, it won't set. Bake the custard until a knife inserted near the center comes out clean. Promptly remove the custard from the hot water and cool on a wire rack for about 5 to 10 minutes. Serve warm or refrigerate.

Meringues

Lemon meringue pies are admired for the lightly browned, white topping that sits tall above a lemon base. Mastering meringue creation takes practice.

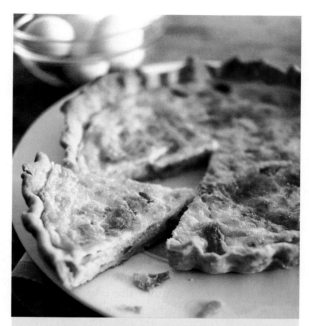

Fig. 35-10 Custard is often a dessert, but when baked with such ingredients as bacon and onions, it makes a delicious quiche. What other ingredients might be in a quiche?

Meringue (muh-RANG) is a foam made of beaten egg whites and sugar and used for baked desserts. Meringue can be either soft or hard. Soft meringue tops pies and tarts and is incorporated in rice and bread puddings. See **Fig. 35-11**. Hard meringue is made into cookies and dessert shells.

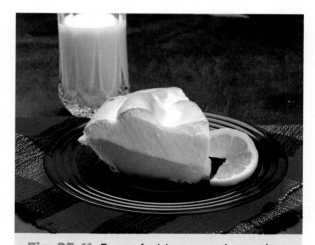

Fig. 35-11 For perfect lemon meringue pie, some cooks make the meringue before preparing the hot base. Spreading the meringue over the base when it's still hot helps prevent beading and weeping.

To make meringue, beat the whites along with cream of tartar until the mixture is foamy. Then gradually beat in sugar, one tablespoon at a time. Continue beating until the sugar dissolves. If the meringue feels gritty when a little is rubbed between your thumb and forefinger, not all the sugar has dissolved.

Soft Meringue

When making soft meringue, use 2 tablespoons of sugar to 1 egg white. You need about 3 egg whites to make enough meringue for a 9-inch pie. Beat the egg whites and sugar only until soft peaks form.

Spread soft meringue over hot, precooked pie filling or pudding. On a pie, the meringue should touch the crust all around the edge. Otherwise, the meringue may shrink during baking. Bake in a preheated oven according to recipe directions until the peaks are lightly browned. If you over-bake a meringue, a tough, chewy skin forms.

When liquid accumulates between the meringue and pie filling, the meringue is said to weep. This occurs because the meringue was spread on a cool filling. To avoid this, always spread the meringue on a hot filling. **Beading**, brown droplets on the surface of the meringue, may occur if the meringue is overcooked.

A soft meringue may also be poached to top puddings or be served with a fruit sauce. Soft custard topped with poached meringue is known as "floating island." To poach the meringue, pour milk or water into a large saucepan or skillet, just deep enough for the poaching process. Drop the meringue by spoonfuls into the liquid, leaving space between to allow the meringue to expand. Simmer uncovered until firm, about 5 minutes. You may need to turn larger spoonfuls over to cook completely. Remove with a slotted spoon and drain. Serve immediately or chill for later.

Hard Meringue

For hard meringue, use 4 tablespoons of sugar to 1 egg white. Beat the egg whites and sugar until stiff peaks form.

Career Prep

A Work Ethic

LISTEN THE NEXT TIME A SPORTS commentator describes a star athlete. You might hear about someone who "gives 100 percent," "comes ready to play," and "puts the team first." Those well-worn sports phrases also describe someone with a solid work ethic, someone who values doing a job—any job—well. Such people respect the job, its standards, and other employees in the field. They show professionalism in the truest meaning of the word, regardless of their education or the nature of the work.

What goes into a work ethic? These qualities help define it:

- **Responsibility.** Responsibility comes down to learning what you should do and doing it. It means taking blame if you let others down and not letting the situation happen again. Responsible workers treat things with care, whether it's a company's car or reputation.

- **Honesty.** Honesty starts with not lying or stealing, but it goes beyond words and things. Being honest with your talents means giving your best effort, instead of holding back and forcing others to carry the load. You show honesty with time by arriving ready to work and giving "an honest day's work for an honest day's pay." Honest workers can be counted on to give supervisors sincere opinions, whether good or bad, when asked.

- **Loyalty.** Like loyal friends, loyal workers stick with an employer and co-workers through bad

To make meringue shells, line a baking sheet with parchment paper or foil. Using a spoon, spatula, or pastry tube, spread the mixture on the baking sheet to the desired size. Build up the edges to form rims. You can shape small individual shells or a large one. You can also shape meringue in a pie plate to make a meringue pie crust.

The characteristic crispness of a hard meringue is achieved by baking at a low temperature for a long time. This allows the water to evaporate slowly, leaving the meringue light and crisp. Bake the meringue in a preheated oven at 225°F for 1 to 1½ hours. Turn off the oven and allow the shells to dry out in the oven for at least one hour. If it doesn't dry well, the meringue may be sticky and chewy. Cool completely and then fill the shells just as you would a pastry shell. See **Fig. 35-12** for an idea.

To shape meringue cookies, you can either drop the meringue onto a lightly greased or lined baking sheet with a spoon or pipe it from a pastry bag. When baked, the cookies should be crisp and dry but not browned.

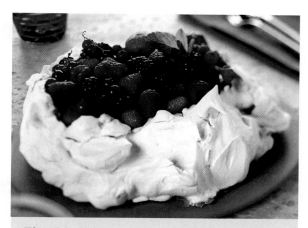

Fig. 35-12 This shell was made with hard meringue, which takes more sugar than a soft meringue. The sugar removes water from the foam, making the meringue crisp and dry.

times as well as good. They give extra when needed. They avoid speaking poorly of supervisors, spreading rumors, and other actions that undermine morale. They consider more than just the money when thinking about a job change.

- **Initiative.** Initiative is the willingness to start a task or take on a project without being asked. Showing initiative at work might mean offering to organize an office picnic, update the company Web site, or simply help get a task done.

- **Teamwork.** Showing teamwork is not just getting along with others. It's putting goal achievement above personal recognition. It's bringing out the best in others, inspiring them to contribute their talents, and seeing that others get the credit they deserve.

- **Enthusiasm.** Enthusiastic workers bring an energy and freshness to the job. They look at problems as challenges and challenges as chances to succeed. They enjoy what they do and are dedicated to it.

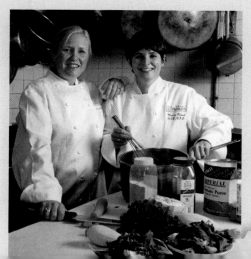

Career Connection

Teen work ethic. In writing explain how a teen can start showing a strong work ethic before taking on a job. Consider efforts at school, at home, and in community activities. Refer to the traits listed and any others that apply.

Summarize Your Reading

▶ Eggs contribute to health as well as to a huge array of dishes that can be prepared with them. Egg science shows why eggs are such versatile performers in the kitchen.

▶ Eggs are sold according to grade and size standards set by the USDA.

▶ Since eggs are highly perishable, care is needed when handling and storing them.

▶ Eggs can be cooked in many different ways, using methods that range from simple to complex. Just beating the whites provides a foam used to make many desserts.

Check Your Knowledge

1. Describe the three egg parts inside the shell.

2. Why do health experts say that **yolks** are nutritious but recommend eating them in moderation?

3. What qualities should you look for when purchasing eggs?

4. Compare the three egg grades and how they are used.

5. Why should eggs be stored in their original cartons?

6. What is the procedure for freezing eggs?

7. What are egg substitutes and why do some people prefer them?

8. What happens when an egg **coagulates**?

9. How do eggs act as **emulsifiers**?

10. Why does beating egg whites cause them to foam?

11. How should you separate an egg?

12. What are tips for beating egg whites?

13. Compare **soft peaks** with **stiff peaks.**

14. What is the basic procedure for cooking each of these eggs: a) in the shell; b) poached; c) fried; d) scrambled?

15. How are **shirred eggs** made?

16. What is the basic difference between cooking an **omelet** and making scrambled eggs?

17. What is the difference between making a basic omelet and a puffy omelet?

18. How would you cook each of these in a microwave oven: a) fried eggs; b) scrambled eggs; c) poached eggs?

19. What is a **quiche**?

20. What is the difference between a soft and a baked **custard**?

21. Compare soft and hard **meringues**.

22. **CRITICAL THINKING** Predict what could happen in these situations: a) an unmarked container of frozen yolks is used in a cake; b) an egg is cracked on the edge of a bowl that contains other ingredients; c) three eggs are broken directly into other ingredients; d) eggs are cooked in the shell for 20 minutes; e) scrambled eggs are cooked over high heat; f) a chocolate pie filling is made one day and topped with meringue the next day.

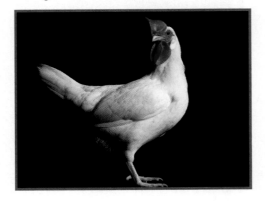

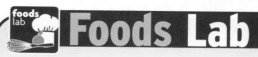
Apply Your Learning

1. **MATH** **Protein Foods.** Compare the protein in eggs with other protein sources. Which foods have the most protein per serving? Compare cost per serving of protein. Which protein sources are least expensive?

2. **Egg Examination.** Crack two or more eggs purchased in different weeks onto separate plates. Identify the parts of an egg. Evaluate the eggs' freshness. How can you tell?

3. **SCIENCE** **Experiment Ideas.** Create and conduct a simple experiment based on one of the following: a) what happens when cooked egg whites are frozen; b) how various cooking times affect hard-cooked eggs; c) how egg freshness affects peeling shells from hard-cooked eggs; d) use of egg substitutes; e) how temperature affects egg coagulation; f) how yolk affects foaming ability.

4. **Brunch.** Plan and serve a brunch that includes an egg dish as the main course. Write the menu, the shopping list, and a preparation work plan.

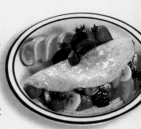

Foods Lab

Making an Omelet

Procedure: Make an omelet, either basic or puffy. Choose ingredients for the filling and seasoning. Review the procedure before you begin and make a list of criteria that you think the finished omelet should meet—even browning, for example. Evaluate the omelet on taste, appearance, and texture.

Analyzing Results

❶ Did the ingredients you added work well in the omelet? Describe the results.

❷ How well did the omelet meet the criteria you listed?

❸ What was the biggest challenge in preparing the omelet? What could you do to make preparation easier in the future?

Food Science Experiment

Making Meringue

Objective: To observe how the addition of sugar affects egg protein foams.

Procedure:

1. Make a meringue, following the assigned variation below:

   Variation 1: Place one egg white in a clean glass bowl. Beat constantly on high speed with an electric mixer until the foam reaches the stiff peak stage. Record the total time it takes.

   Variation 2: Follow variation 1, but add 2 Tbsp. of sugar when you start beating.

   Variation 3: Follow variation 1, but when the foam reaches the soft peak stage, gradually add 2 Tbsp. of sugar as you beat.

2. Set out your foam for comparison. Label the variation number and the recorded time.

Analyzing Results

❶ Which variation produced a foam with the greatest overall volume? Which had the least?

❷ Which variation produced the most stable foam? The least?

❸ What was the relationship, if any, between when sugar was added and the time needed to reach stiff peak stage? Between when sugar was added and foam stability and volume?

❹ What do you conclude?

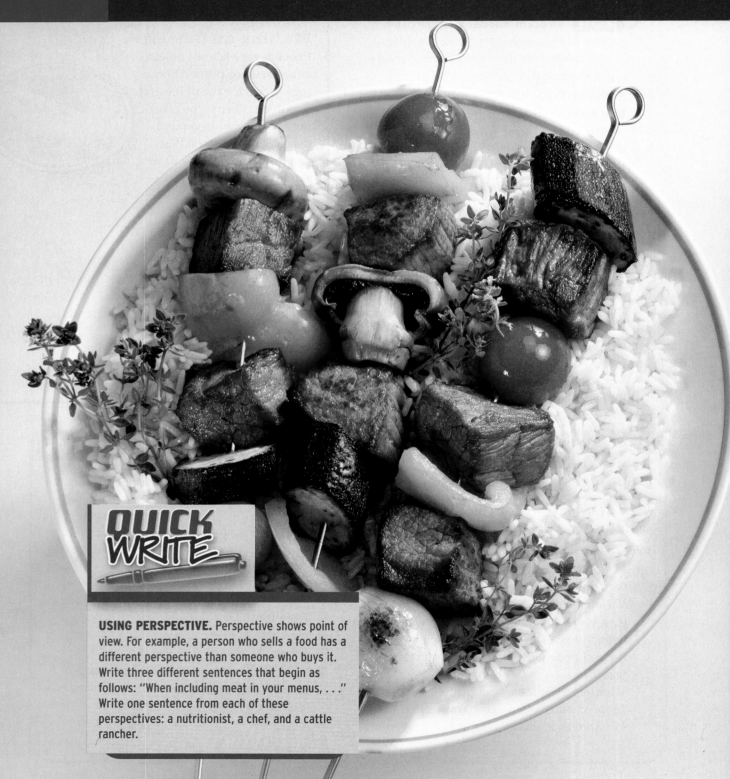

QUICK WRITE

USING PERSPECTIVE. Perspective shows point of view. For example, a person who sells a food has a different perspective than someone who buys it. Write three different sentences that begin as follows: "When including meat in your menus, . . ." Write one sentence from each of these perspectives: a nutritionist, a chef, and a cattle rancher.

Objectives
▶ Explain the nutritional role of meats in the diet.

▶ Explain the makeup of meat.

▶ Describe cuts and other forms of meat.

▶ Explain how to select and store meats.

▶ Describe and demonstrate methods for preparing and cooking meats.

Terms
cold cuts	meat
collagen	muscle
connective tissue	processed meats
cut	retail cuts
doneness	variety meats
elastin	
grain	wholesale cuts
marbling	

FAMILIES OFTEN PLAN MAIN MEALS AROUND meat and then select accompaniments. Pot roast with potatoes, carrots, and onions and ham with sweet potatoes and broccoli are traditional combinations in many homes. Meat is flavorful, versatile, and highly nutritious, but it can also be one of the most expensive items in the food budget.

To prepare meat successfully, you need to understand the physical makeup of meat, shop wisely, store meat properly, and select the right cooking methods.

NUTRIENTS IN MEAT

Meat is an excellent source of protein. It's also a major source of iron, zinc, phosphorus, thiamin, riboflavin, niacin, and vitamins B_6 and B_{12}. Because meat can be high in saturated fat, however, choose lean meats when possible.

Meat belongs to the same food group as poultry, fish, dry beans, eggs, and nuts. On a 2,000-calorie diet, a person needs 5½ ounces of these protein foods each day. Two to 3 ounces of cooked meat is about the size of your palm.

MAKEUP OF MEAT

Meat is the edible muscle of animals, typically cattle, sheep, and pigs. Meat has muscle, connective tissue, and fat. The tissue of a **muscle** is made of long, thin cells, sometimes called muscle fibers. These fibers are bound into bundles with thin sheets of protein material, known as **connective tissue**. In turn, as bundles group together, they form individual muscles. See **Fig. 36-1.**

Muscle Tissue

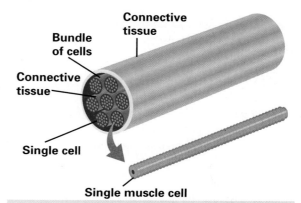

Fig. 36-1 The long cells that bundle together to form muscle tissue in meat are sometimes called fibers. Why are they strong?

Connective tissue not only holds fibers together but also anchors muscle to bone. Meat has several types of connective tissue, including collagen and elastin.

- **Collagen** (KAH-luh-juhn). **Collagen** is the thin, white, transparent tissue found in tendons, between muscle cells, and between muscles. When cooked in moist heat, collagen softens and turns into gelatin.
- **Elastin** (ih-LAS-tuhn). The connective tissue called **elastin** is very tough, elastic, and yellowish and is found in ligaments and blood vessel walls. It cannot be softened by heat and is therefore usually cut away before cooking. To tenderize elastin, you must pound, cut, or grind it.

Meat contains both visible and invisible fat. A layer of visible fat sometimes surrounds the muscle. In addition, small white flecks of fat, called **marbling**, may appear within the muscle tissue. Invisible fat is part of the chemical composition of meat.

The lengthwise direction of muscle is called the **grain**. If you cut meat across the grain, you break up the muscle fibers, making it easier to chew. Most meats sold in retail stores are cut across the grain.

IDENTIFYING MEAT CUTS

The four most common meats sold in the United States are beef, veal, lamb, and pork. In some areas, meat from goats is also available. **Fig. 36-2** shows the source and characteristics of different types of meat.

A **cut** is a specific, edible part of meat, such as a steak, chop, or roast. Meat is first divided into large **wholesale cuts**, also called primal cuts, which are sold to retail stores. **Fig. 36-3** shows the wholesale cuts of beef, veal, lamb, and pork.

The retailer divides wholesale cuts into **retail cuts**, which are the smaller cuts you find for sale. For example, one wholesale cut of beef is chuck, from the shoulder area. Retail cuts from chuck include blade roast, short ribs, and arm pot roast. Meat cuts from the same location in beef, veal, lamb, and pork are usually similar in shape but vary in size.

The price label on a meat package identifies the cut. The meat type, which might say beef or pork, is listed first. The wholesale cut is second, for instance, chuck, rib, or round. This tells you which part of the animal the meat came from. The retail cut is listed third. Examples are spareribs, chops, and steak. See **Fig. 36-4**.

Fig. 36-2

Types of Meat

Meat	Source	Characteristics
Beef	Cattle more than one year old.	Hearty flavor; firm texture; bright, deep red color with firm, creamy white fat.
Veal	Calves (young cattle), usually one to three months old.	Mild flavor; firm texture; light, gray-pink color with very little fat.
Baby beef	Calves between six and twelve months old.	Pink-red color; stronger flavor and coarser texture than veal.
Lamb	Sheep less than a year old.	Unique, mild flavor; bright, pink-red color; white brittle fat. Sometimes covered with a fell, a thin membrane under the hide, which helps retain juices during cooking.
Mutton	Sheep over two years old.	Less tender than lamb; stronger flavor.
Pork	Pigs less than a year old.	Tender texture; mild flavor; gray-pink color; soft white fat. Older animals have a darker pink color.

Fig. 36-3 Wholesale Cuts of Meat

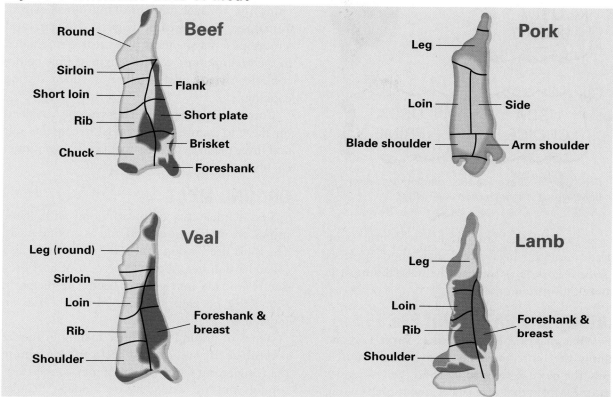

Beef
- Round
- Sirloin
- Short loin
- Rib
- Chuck
- Flank
- Short plate
- Brisket
- Foreshank

Pork
- Leg
- Loin
- Side
- Blade shoulder
- Arm shoulder

Veal
- Leg (round)
- Sirloin
- Loin
- Rib
- Shoulder
- Foreshank & breast

Lamb
- Leg
- Loin
- Rib
- Shoulder
- Foreshank & breast

INSPECTION AND GRADING

The Federal Meat Inspection Act requires that all meat shipped across state lines be inspected for wholesomeness. States have similar laws that apply to meat produced locally and sold within a state. Meat products that pass federal inspection standards are marked with a round, purple stamp. Since the inspection stamp appears in only a few places on the animal, you probably won't see it on retail cuts.

The USDA may also grade meat. Grading is a voluntary program available to the meat industry, which pays for the service. Meat is graded according to standards that include amount of marbling, age of the animal, and texture and appearance of the meat. The grade is stamped on the meat, like the inspection stamp. See **Fig. 36-5** on page 510. Both inspection and grade marks are stamped with a harmless vegetable dye, so they don't have to be cut off before cooking.

These are the most common grades of beef:

- **Prime.** This is the highest and most expensive grade. The meat is well marbled, tender, and flavorful.
- **Choice.** As the most common grade sold in supermarkets, choice beef has less marbling than prime but is still tender and flavorful.
- **Select.** This grade contains the least amount of marbling and is the least expensive. It is sometimes sold as a store brand.

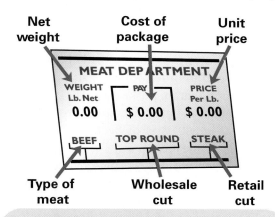

Net weight

Cost of package

Unit price

MEAT DEPARTMENT

WEIGHT Lb. Net	PAY	PRICE Per Lb.
0.00	$ 0.00	$ 0.00
BEEF	TOP ROUND	STEAK

Type of meat

Wholesale cut

Retail cut

Fig. 36-4 The label on a meat package looks something like this. What is the difference between wholesale and retail cuts?

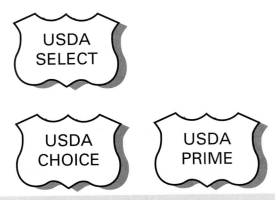

Fig. 36-5 These are the common grades of beef. Which is most expensive? Why?

Lamb and veal are graded with the same grades used for beef except that "good" replaces "select." Pork is not graded because the meat is more uniform in quality.

JUDGING MEAT TENDERNESS

What makes meat tenderness vary? For one thing, the more movement an animal's muscle gets, the more developed it is and the less tender the meat from that area is. Because muscles along the backbone get very little movement, meat from that area is more tender than meat from other parts.

The amount of marbling also affects tenderness. Fat in marbling melts during cooking, releasing juice and flavor. As fat melts, it penetrates the muscle tissue and helps separate muscle fibers. This makes the meat easier to chew.

Bone shapes, which are nearly identical in beef, veal, lamb, and pork, give clues about where the meat comes from on the animal and how tender it is. **Fig. 36-6** shows the seven common bone shapes. The rib and T-shape bones, which are part of the backbone, indicate the meat is tender. The meat on a blade bone, which is part of the shoulder, is not as tender.

Less tender cuts can be tenderized before cooking by one of several methods. Mechanical methods, which include grinding, pounding, and cutting, tenderize meat by breaking down elastin. Less tender cuts of beef, for instance, can be ground into hamburger or pounded with a meat pounder to make cube steaks.

Acids also tenderize meat by chemically softening the collagen and breaking down elastin. Tomatoes, sour cream, yogurt, vinegar, and lemon juice may be used. The meat is marinated in the mixture for a certain length of time before cooking, or the acid mixture is added during cooking.

Commercial meat tenderizer may be sprinkled on meat to increase tenderness. It contains salt and three papaya enzymes that break down muscle fibers.

GROUND MEAT

Less tender cuts of meat, along with trimmings, are often ground and sold as ground meat. The most used ground meat is ground beef, also called hamburger. About 45 percent of beef produced is made into ground beef. The recipe in **Fig. 36-7** on page 512 uses ground beef as an ingredient.

Types of ground beef differ mainly in the fat percentage. By law, ground beef can't have more than 30 percent fat by weight. It may contain seasonings but no extenders or binders. Regular ground beef has the most fat, is least expensive, and shrinks most when cooked. Ground chuck contains 15 to 20 percent fat, which makes for flavorful and juicy hamburgers. Ground round and ground sirloin have the least fat but are the most expensive. Ground meat that is labeled "lean" must have less than 10 grams of total fat, less than 4.5 grams of saturated fat, and less than 95 milligrams of cholesterol per 3½-ounce serving. Lean ground beef usually costs more than regular ground beef.

You can buy ground beef already packaged or have it ground to order. You may also find packages of ground lamb, pork, and veal. If not, you can ask to have the meat ground for you. A combination of equal parts of beef, pork, and veal works well for meatloaf.

Prepackaged ground beef is often red on the outside and slightly bluish on the inside. When meat is exposed to air, oxygen causes it to turn red. The interior of the ground beef doesn't get enough oxygen to turn the meat red, resulting in the bluish color.

Fig. 36-6 Bone Shapes: The Clue to Tenderness

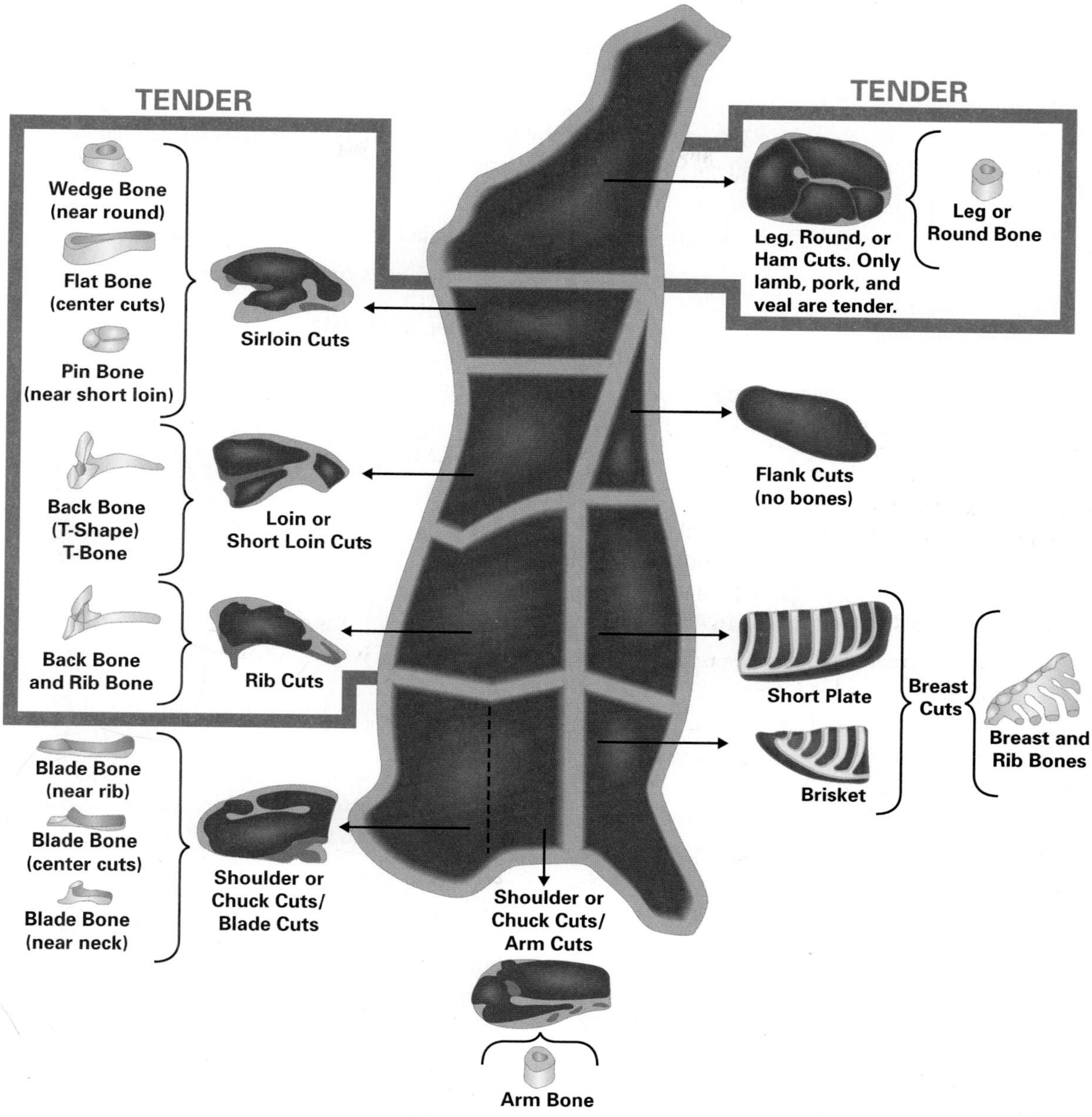

TENDER

Wedge Bone (near round)

Flat Bone (center cuts)

Pin Bone (near short loin)

Sirloin Cuts

Back Bone (T-Shape) T-Bone

Loin or Short Loin Cuts

Back Bone and Rib Bone

Rib Cuts

Blade Bone (near rib)

Blade Bone (center cuts)

Blade Bone (near neck)

Shoulder or Chuck Cuts/ Blade Cuts

Shoulder or Chuck Cuts/ Arm Cuts

Arm Bone

TENDER

Leg, Round, or Ham Cuts. Only lamb, pork, and veal are tender.

Leg or Round Bone

Flank Cuts (no bones)

Short Plate

Brisket

Breast Cuts

Breast and Rib Bones

VARIETY MEATS

Variety meats are the edible organs and extremities of beef, veal, lamb, and pork. They are used extensively in Europe and other parts of the world. Andouille (ahn-DOO-ee), for instance, is a French sausage made with chitterlings (pig intestines) and tripe (the stomach lining of cattle). The Cajun version is spicy and usually made from pork shoulder. It's a major ingredient in jambalaya and gumbo. Because variety meats are used less in the United States, most of those produced in the U.S. are exported.

Variety meats include the following: liver, kidney, pig's feet, brains, heart, tongue, oxtails, and sweetbreads (thymus gland). Because variety meats are highly perishable, they must be fresh when purchased and cooked within 24 hours.

Fig. 36-7

Chili

Yield	Nutrition Analysis
8 to 10 servings	***Per Serving:*** 360 calories, 18 g total fat, 7 g saturated fat, 1 g trans fat, 125 mg cholesterol, 680 mg sodium, 9 g total carbohydrate, 3 g dietary fiber, 3 g sugars, 41 g protein ***Percent Daily Value:*** vitamin A 40%, vitamin C 15%, calcium 6%, iron 35%

Ingredients

3 lbs. ground beef
1 medium chopped onion
3 small garlic cloves, finely chopped
15-oz. can tomato sauce
5½ cups water

6 Tbsp. chili powder, or to taste
1 Tbsp. paprika
1 Tbsp. crushed cumin seeds
1 tsp. salt
½ tsp. ground black pepper

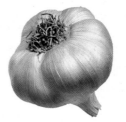

Directions

1. Combine ground beef, onion, and garlic in a 2-qt. saucepan. Brown over medium heat, stirring to crumble.
2. Drain off pan drippings. Add remaining ingredients. Mix well.
3. Cook over low heat for 3½ to 4 hours, stirring occasionally.

PROCESSED MEATS

Meats that have been changed by various methods to add flavor and to help preserve them are **processed meats**. About 35 percent of the meat produced in the United States is processed. About 75 percent of all meat processed is pork; the remainder is beef. Processed meats include ham, bacon, sausage, and cold cuts. **Cold cuts** are processed slices of cold meat and poultry.

Three methods are used to process meats: curing, smoking, and cooking. Often, several methods are used on one product.

Cured meat can be pickle-cured or dry-cured. Pickle-curing involves soaking the meat in a solution of salt, sugar, sodium nitrate, potassium nitrate, ascorbic acid, and water or pumping the solution into the meat. In dry-curing, no water is added to the mixture. The mixture is rubbed onto the surface of the meat.

Originally, smoking meat meant exposing it to wood smoke to preserve and flavor it. Today, only liquid smoke is used for flavoring.

Many processed meats are cooked, providing a ready-to-eat product. Pasteurization increases the shelf life of the meat.

CONVENIENCE FORMS

When you need a quick meal, canned meat entrées may be the answer. Options include beef stew, spaghetti and meatballs, and many others. Frozen entrées often have accompaniments. Roast beef, for example, might have side servings of peas and mashed potatoes.

Most supermarkets carry ready-to-cook meats. Ready-made meatloaf just needs baking. As you might guess, convenience products cost much more than the same foods prepared from scratch at home.

BUYING MEAT

If you know how to shop for meat, you can get the best value for your money. First, decide how much meat you need based on the number of people to be served and whether you want leftovers. Buy only the amount you need.

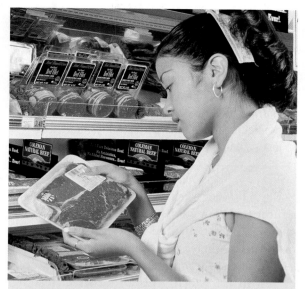

Fig. 36-8 When you buy meat, how can you tell whether it's lean? What about tenderness?

Choose the cut that looks the leanest. You'll save money because you won't have to trim off excess fat. See **Fig. 36-8**. Look for these lean cuts: for beef roasts and steaks—round, loin, sirloin, and chuck arm; for pork roasts and chops—tenderloin, center loin, and ham; for veal cuts—all except ground veal; for lamb roasts and chops—leg, loin, and foreshank. Remember that tender cuts are usually more expensive than less tender ones. By learning to cook less tender cuts, you can save money.

Always compare the cost per serving of different cuts. If you find a bargain that isn't on your shopping list, why not change plans? Even small savings add up over time.

STORING MEAT

Meat must be refrigerated. Place meat in a plastic bag to keep the juices from dripping on other food. Variety meats should be used within one day and ground meat within two days. Other fresh meats keep in the refrigerator for three to five days. For longer storage, freeze the meat.

If you are refrigerating unopened packages of processed meat, refer to the date on the label for length of storage. If the package has been opened, use the meat within a few days. Read label directions for storing canned meats.

COOKING MEAT

Cooking affects meat in several ways. When properly cooked, meat becomes more firm, fat melts, and connective tissues soften. As a result, the meat is tender, juicy, and flavorful.

Because protein is sensitive to heat, cooking temperatures and times must be carefully controlled. Lengthy cooking at high temperatures can cause meat to shrink significantly, whether you use dry or moist heat. If you overcook meat, it becomes tough and dry and may be difficult to cut and digest. See **Fig. 36-9**.

Heat doesn't usually destroy nutrients in meat; however, water-soluble vitamins, such as B vitamins, may be lost in the meat juices or cooking liquid. To recapture the vitamins, these liquids can be added to soups, sauces, or gravies.

Preparation

The USDA requires that safe handling instructions be on all packages of raw and not fully cooked meat. Before cooking meat, rinse it under cold water and pat dry with a paper towel. Trim any visible fat, using a sharp knife and cutting board. With that done, you won't have to skim off excess fat from any drippings you use. Fat is easier to trim when meat is very cold or partially frozen.

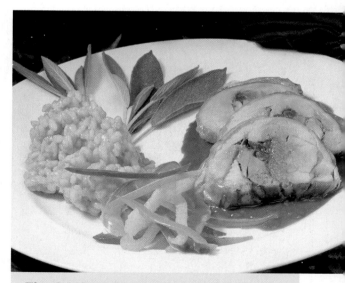

Fig. 36-9 Well-prepared meat isn't dry or tough. How can you cook meat to keep it moist and tender?

Thaw frozen raw meat before cooking to save time and preserve quality. If you wish to cook frozen meat, increase the cooking time by about 50 percent. For example, if normal cooking time is 40 minutes, cook a frozen cut for 60 minutes.

Before cooking meat, you can marinate it for added flavor and tenderizing. To make a marinade, choose at least one acidic ingredient. Vinegar, yogurt, or fruit juice can be used. Add a little cooking oil and season with herbs and spices. Pour the marinade over the meat, cover, and refrigerate. Don't marinate for more than 24 hours or the meat will get mushy. Marinating works best on thin cuts of meat. Since acid pits aluminum, an aluminum pan shouldn't be used for marinating. Marinades can pick up contaminants from raw meat, so don't use them for basting unless boiled first for one minute.

The tenderness of a meat cut determines cooking method. Tender cuts—for instance, steaks, chops, and roasts—can be cooked with dry heat methods. Roasting and broiling work well. Less tender cuts, such as arm shoulder chops and short ribs, must be cooked in moist heat. This breaks down the collagen in the meat, making it tender.

To Test for Doneness

Doneness is the point at which meat has cooked enough to make it flavorful and safe to eat. If any part is not cooked, foodborne illness is a risk.

Since doneness is hard to judge visually, using a meat thermometer is the safest method. When you roast cuts more than 2 inches thick, insert the meat thermometer into the thickest part. Be sure the tip of the thermometer does not touch bone or rest in fat, which gives an incorrect reading. You can use an instant-read or oven-safe thermometer. If you use the oven-safe type, leave it in place for the entire cooking period. For thin cuts, check the temperature with an instant-read thermometer near the end of the cooking time. See **Fig. 36-10**. Some instant-read thermometers have a dial and some, a digital display.

Meat can be cooked to these basic stages of doneness: medium rare, medium, and well done. Each stage is indicated by a specific internal temperature, as shown in **Fig. 36-11**.

Cooking times depend on the cooking method and the cut of meat. The cooking time in the recipe is just a guide. Begin testing the meat for

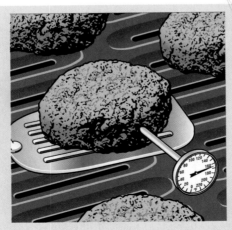
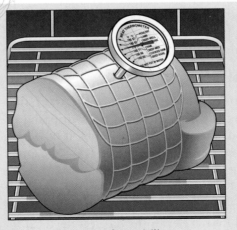

Fig. 36-10 Use an instant-read thermometer to test thin cuts of meat like hamburger. An oven-safe or instant-read thermometer can be used with large cuts of meat. An oven-safe thermometer is shown on the right.

Fig. 36-11

Internal Doneness Temperatures for Meat	
Food	**°F**
Ground Meat and Meat Mixtures	
Beef, pork, veal, lamb	160
Fresh Beef, Veal, Lamb	
Medium rare	145
Medium	160
Well done	170
Fresh Pork	
Medium	160
Well done	170
Ham	
Fresh (raw)	160
To reheat precooked ham	140
Leftovers and Casseroles	165

doneness about 10 minutes before the end of the expected cooking time.

Broiling Meat

Steaks, chops, ham slices, liver, bacon, ground beef, and other tender meat cuts can be broiled. Steaks and chops should be at least ½ inch thick. Thinner pieces dry out if broiled.

When fat cooks, it melts and shrinks, pulling up the meat. Before broiling, make slashes through any fat left on the edges to help keep the meat from curling. Add flavor, if you wish, by brushing a sauce on the meat.

Place the broiler pan so the meat is 2 to 5 inches from the heat. The thicker the meat, the farther it should be from the heat because it needs more time to cook. Broil until the top is brown and the meat is slightly more than half done inside. Season if desired. Turn and complete the broiling on the other side.

Grilling Meat

Tender cuts of meat can also be grilled. For a different way to grill meat, try kebabs. To make them, thread cubes of meat onto skewers, alternating with tomato quarters, mushrooms, green pepper chunks, or other vegetables. Brush with oil, melted butter, or a sauce to keep the foods from drying out.

Heat the grill. Place the meat or kebabs on the grate and turn regularly to cook through. Brush the meat occasionally with a sauce. Sauces that contain a large amount of sugar cause meat to char. This happens easily with barbecue sauce. When you use sweet sauces, limit basting to the last few minutes of cooking.

Roasting Meat

Roasting works best with large tender cuts of meat. These include loin, rib, and leg roasts. Follow these steps to roast meat:

1. Place the meat fat side up on a rack in an open, shallow roasting pan. As the fat melts, it automatically bastes the meat. The rack should hold the roast out of the drippings. For standing rib roasts or crown of pork, the ribs form a natural rack, so the meat can be placed directly on the pan bottom.
2. Season the meat as desired.
3. Insert an oven-safe meat thermometer so the tip is centered in the largest muscle.
4. Don't add water or cover the pan. This cooks the meat with moisture rather than dry heat.
5. Roast at 325°F without preheating the oven. If you wish, add whole small potatoes, onions, and carrots around the roast about an hour before it's done.
6. Remove the roast from the oven when the meat thermometer registers five degrees lower than the desired internal temperature. The meat continues to cook as it stands.
7. Let the roast stand for 15 to 20 minutes after removing it from the oven. This allows the juices to set and makes the roast easier to carve.

Frying Meat

Chops, hamburgers, ham slices, bacon, liver, and other thin pieces of tender meat can be fried in a small amount of fat. Lean cuts of meat or cuts that are floured or breaded need more fat.

Cook uncovered in a skillet preheated to medium, turning occasionally so that both sides brown. If you cover the skillet, the meat cooks in moist heat and loses crispness and flavor. Season the meat after browning.

Pan-Broiling Meat

Pan-broiling is a fast, convenient way to cook tender cuts of meat that are too thin to broil. Thickness should be 1 inch or less. To pan-broil meat, preheat a heavy skillet. Most cuts have enough fat to prevent sticking. For lean cuts, brush or spray the cooking surface with oil. If you're using a nonstick skillet, you don't need to add oil.

Use medium heat and do not cover. Turn the meat occasionally and pour off fat as it accumulates. Cook until brown on both sides, and then season if desired.

Braising Meat

Braising is used to cook large, less tender cuts of meat, such as pot roast and Swiss steak. See **Fig. 36-12.** It also gives flavor to tender cuts like pork chops.

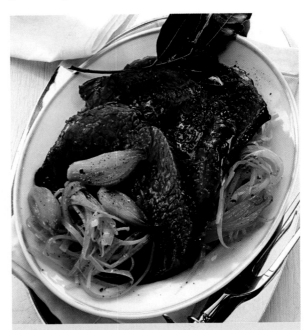

Fig. 36-12 Braised meat is tender because it cooks to well done. The meat is done when a fork is inserted and removed easily. What might be done with the liquid in the pan?

First, pat the meat dry so it browns easily. Brown the meat slowly on all sides in a large heavy pan, using a little fat as needed to prevent sticking. After browning, drain off excess fat. Add just enough liquid—water, tomato juice, meat stock, or other seasoned liquid—to cover the bottom of the pan about ¼ inch deep. The liquid must flow under the food to keep it from sticking to the pan. Add seasonings and cover the pan with a tight-fitting lid.

Simmer on low heat until the meat is tender, or cook in the oven at 325°F. About halfway through the cooking time, you can add carrots, potatoes, and onions.

Pressure-Cooking Meat

Large, less tender cuts of meat can be pressure cooked. This cooks the meat in moist heat and tenderizes it under high pressure within a relatively short time. Refer to the owner's manual for directions on using the pressure cooker.

Slow-Cooking Meat

Because a slow cooker uses a low temperature for a long cooking time, it's ideal for less tender cuts of meat. In the morning, simply combine the meat, seasonings, and liquid—perhaps broth, water, or barbecue sauce—in the slow cooker. The meat is ready by the evening meal. Become familiar with using the slow cooker before you leave it unattended for a long time. Remember that if you open the lid, cooking time lengthens.

Microwaving Meat

When buying meat to microwave, choose cuts of uniform size. Even with a turntable, microwave ovens don't cook evenly. Follow recipe directions exactly to be sure the meat cooks through.

During standing time, cover the meat loosely with foil to hold in the heat. After standing time, check the meat in several spots with an instant-read thermometer to be sure it has reached the proper internal temperature throughout.

Since microwave ovens cook with moist heat, meat won't have the crisp, dark brown crust and characteristic flavor of meat cooked in dry heat. It may look unappetizing. You can add a sauce or gravy, brush it with a dark sauce before cooking, or broil briefly.

Executive Director

DINA CHACÓN-REITZEL: If Dina Chacón-Reitzel isn't in her office at the New Mexico Beef Council representing the interests of beef ranchers, she may be out on horseback, tending to the health of beef cattle. Personally and professionally, the council's executive director embodies the entire industry, from the herd to the halls of legislature. Her career intertwines a solid education, diverse experiences, and love for a way of life.

Roaming from the Range. Dina's roots in New Mexico go back some 400 years, when her ancestors arrived with Spanish colonists. Farmers and ranchers fill the family tree. She grew up on a cattle ranch in the state's north central mountain range and attended New Mexico State University, also a family tradition. "Your education is what gives you the choices that you want to have in life," she says, a conviction that her parents instilled in her and her three brothers. It was there that Dina learned about the home-economics-in-business major. It seemed ideal preparation for a career in any of her interests: home economics, business, and journalism. After graduation, an internship in the state senator's office in Washington, D.C., gave her a view on public policy-making.

Dina returned to the university, working as a community leadership educator with its Cooperative Extension Service. At the same time she earned a master's degree in business administration, hoping it "would open new doors to me." It did, first to a job in business development, then in marketing computers. Eventually she returned to the cattle industry as well, as director of community affairs for the New Mexico Beef Council. When the council's executive director left, she applied for the position. Of the 180 other applicants, none could match Dina's experience in educating consumers, forming policy, promoting a product—and working cattle. It was, she says, "a perfect fit."

Ensuring a Legacy. As executive director, Dina oversees all of the council's work in promoting New Mexico beef. She authorizes research and analyzes results. She maps a strategy to spread the word about the industry and its products through ad campaigns, school programs, and exhibits at the state fair. She discusses economic ranching issues with lawmakers and reports on accomplishments to cattle producers.

Dina brings more to her job than professional expertise. She brings a sense of mission. "I strongly believe that committing myself to agriculture is the best way to maintain my rural roots and my Spanish heritage." Societal changes have convinced her that "what I grew up with would be lost to *my* children if I don't actively work to preserve it." Dina and her husband and children return to the family ranch during spring and fall roundups. They lend a hand as they brand cattle, doctor sick animals, clear brush, and plant pastures. Says Dina: "The kind of juggling you have to do to keep your family happy and healthy, your work life happy and productive, and finally your personal being happy and healthy can be monumental. The ranching families I work for inspire me."

On-line Connections

1. To learn more about topics in this article, search the Internet for these key words: Cooperative Extension Service; beef industry.

2. To learn about related careers, search the Internet for these key words: lobbyist; ranch management.

Summarize Your Reading

▶ Meat is made of muscle, connective tissue, and fat.

▶ The four most common meats sold in the United States are beef, veal, lamb, and pork. Cuts vary according to location on the animal and how the retailer cuts the meat.

▶ Some meats are processed to add flavor and help preserve them.

▶ Meats are perishable and must be stored properly for health safety.

▶ Meat cuts vary in tenderness, which influences cooking methods.

▶ Different cooking methods yield a different taste and flavor, giving variety to ordinary meat cuts.

Check Your Knowledge

1. Compare **collagen** with **elastin**.

2. Describe the two kinds of fat in meat.

3. Compare beef with veal.

4. How are **wholesale cuts** and **retail cuts** of meat different? Give examples of each.

5. Compare the prime, choice, and select grades of meat.

6. **CRITICAL THINKING** Why is meat from the loin more tender than meat from the chuck?

7. **CRITICAL THINKING** While buying meat, a consumer was trying to figure out which cuts might be the most tender. How might this be determined?

8. How does **marbling** affect tenderness?

9. How can less tender pieces of meat be tenderized before cooking?

10. Explain the fat percentages in different kinds of ground beef.

11. What are **variety meats**? Give examples.

12. Describe three ways that meats are processed.

13. Are all processed meats ready to eat? Explain.

14. How does pasteurization affect meat?

15. Name three different kinds of convenience meats.

16. How can a cook save money when shopping for meat?

17. How long can each of these meats be stored in the refrigerator: a) liver; b) ground meat; c) pork chops?

18. How does meat change when cooked?

19. Why should cooks avoid overcooking meat?

20. How should meat be prepared for cooking?

21. How is meat marinated?

22. How does a cook know when meat is done and ready to eat?

23. What is the difference between broiling and grilling meat?

24. How do you roast meat?

25. Describe three ways to prepare less tender cuts of meat.

26. Why doesn't meat cooked in a microwave oven develop a brown crust?

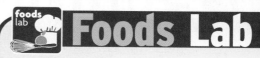
Apply Your Learning

1. **MATH** **Nutrition Comparison.** Compare protein and fat amounts in different cuts of beef and pork. Chart your results. Which cuts provide the least amount of fat?

2. **Meat Cut Identification.** Tour a butcher shop or the meat cutting department of a supermarket. Learn to identify meat cuts by bone shape. Practice reading meat labels to identify cuts and probable tenderness. How does tenderness relate to cooking methods?

3. **SCIENCE** **Ground Beef Comparison.** Prepare a ground meat patty from regular ground beef and one from lean or extra-lean ground beef. Cook by the same method. Weigh the meat before and after cooking. What conclusions can you draw?

4. **Doneness Demonstration.** Demonstrate how to use meat thermometers to test the doneness of a hamburger and a roast. Use oven-safe and instant-read thermometers.

Foods Lab

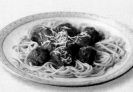

Meatball Comparison

Procedure: Choose a recipe for meatballs. Prepare the recipe. Also prepare ready-made meatballs purchased as a convenience food. Follow package directions. Conduct a taste test to sample and compare both products.

Analyzing Results

❶ How did the products compare in taste, texture, and appearance?

❷ How did the products compare nutritionally? Did the meat you used for the recipe have any impact?

❸ How did the products compare in cost per serving?

❹ Would you use the recipe or the convenience food again? If so, in what situations? How would cost influence your decision?

Food Science Experiment

Tenderizing Meat

Objective: To compare the effectiveness of different methods of meat tenderizing.

Procedure:

1. Cut three portions, about ½ inch thick, from one cut of less tender meat.

2. Prepare the first piece of meat by applying lemon juice liberally to both sides. Rub salt (or meat tenderizer) into both sides of the second piece. Pound the third piece with a mallet on both sides.

3. Cover and refrigerate the meat overnight, labeling the containers with the preparation method.

4. The next day, rinse the lemon- and salt-treated meat and pat dry. Broil all three pieces until a temperature check shows doneness. Evaluate the meat on taste and mouthfeel. Compare your evaluation with that of other lab teams.

Analyzing Results

❶ Which piece of meat was the most tender and juicy? The least?

❷ How did each method tenderize the meat? Why do you think one was more effective than the others?

❸ Did other lab teams reach the same conclusion? What might explain differing results?

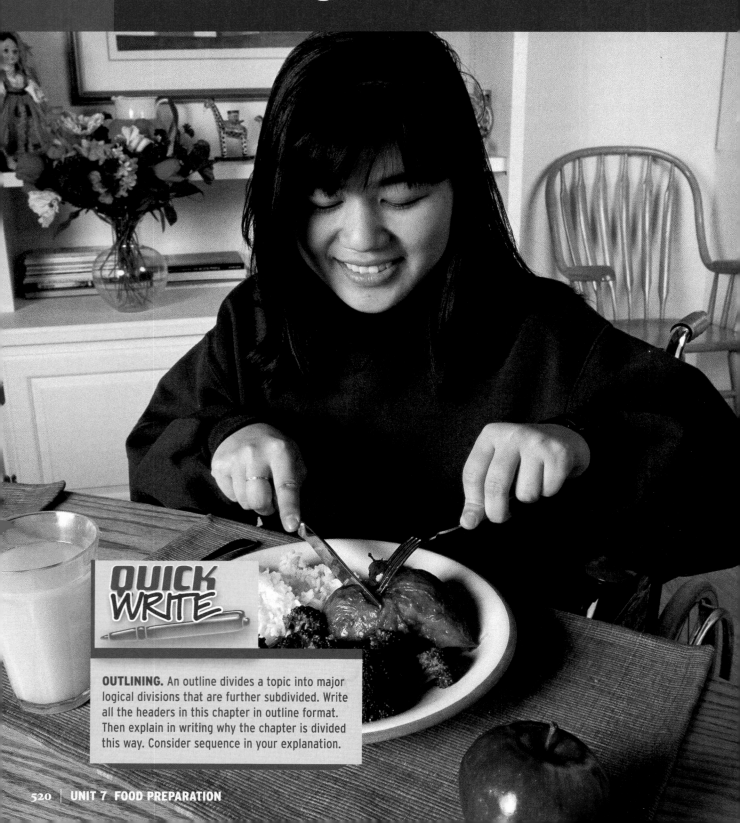

QUICK WRITE

OUTLINING. An outline divides a topic into major logical divisions that are further subdivided. Write all the headers in this chapter in outline format. Then explain in writing why the chapter is divided this way. Consider sequence in your explanation.

I F YOU SURVEYED THE STUDENTS IN YOUR CLASS, chances are you'd find that many of them eat poultry several times a week. Poultry has become a favorite in the United States. This nutritious food is easy to prepare in many different ways.

NUTRIENTS

Poultry is a good source of protein. It also provides niacin, vitamins B_6 and B_{12}, calcium, phosphorus, iron, and other trace minerals.

Poultry is generally lower in fat and calories than red meat, making it a nutritious protein option. Of the types of poultry, turkey and chicken are relatively low in fat and duck and goose are higher. Most of the fat in poultry is stored under the skin. If you remove the skin before eating, you substantially decrease the fat you eat, including saturated. See **Fig. 37-1**.

Poultry belongs to the same food group as meat, fish, dry beans, eggs, and nuts. On a 2,000-calorie diet, a person needs 5½ ounces of these protein foods each day. Two to 3 ounces of cooked poultry is about the size of your palm.

TYPES OF POULTRY

Any bird raised for food is called **poultry**. The four most common types of poultry eaten are chicken, turkey, duck, and goose.

Most people realize that chicken and turkey have both light and dark meat, but they might not know why. This coloring depends on the amount of exercise a muscle gets while the bird is alive. Muscles

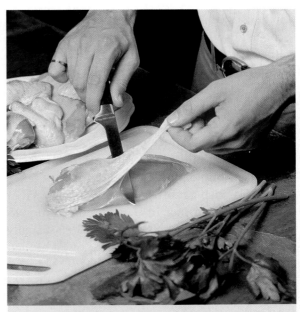

Fig. 37-1 If you remove the skin from poultry, you reduce the amount of fat in a dish.

that get frequent, strenuous exercise need more oxygen than others. The oxygen is stored in a reddish protein pigment called **myoglobin** (my-uh-GLOH-bun). The more myoglobin the muscle tissue has, the darker the color of the meat.

Because domesticated breeds of chickens and turkeys don't fly, their breast and wing muscles don't need as much oxygen to function. These tissues contain less myoglobin, making the breast meat a lighter color. Dark meat is in the chicken and turkey parts that get the most exercise, such as the legs. Legs include the drumstick and thigh. Ducks and geese have all dark meat, which is tender and more flavorful but contains more fat than light meat.

A bird's size and age determine meat tenderness and the cooking method needed. Like beef and other meats, if poultry is cut across the grain it is more tender and easier to chew.

Chicken

Chickens vary by age and weight. The following types are available:

- **Broiler-fryer chickens.** Sold at about 7 weeks of age and 3 to 4 pounds in weight, these are the most tender and most common. They don't have as much meat as other types. They can be cooked using almost any method.
- **Roaster chickens.** Slightly larger at 4 to 7 pounds and 3 to 5 months old, roasters are raised to be roasted whole. They yield more meat per pound than broiler-fryers.
- **Stewing chickens.** These large, mature birds are less tender than younger birds, so they must be cooked in moist heat. They are best in such dishes as soup or chicken and dumplings.
- **Rock Cornish game hens.** This special breed of young, small chicken has less meat in relation to size than other chickens. One hen usually equals one serving. Game hens can be broiled or roasted.
- **Capons (KAY-pahns).** Desexed roosters under ten months old, capons are tender and flavorful. They are best roasted.
- **Free-range chickens.** Most chickens are mass-produced and kept in coops with 1 square foot of space allowed for each bird. Free-range chickens have more space in the coops and are allowed space to roam outdoors. Some free-range chickens can be labeled organic since they are not exposed to pesticides, artificial fertilizers, growth hormones, or antibiotics when raised. Free-range chickens are considered to be more flavorful but usually have more fat and are more expensive than mass-produced birds.

Turkey

The several types of whole turkeys available differ mainly in size. See **Fig. 37-2**.

- **Fryer-roaster turkeys.** With an average weight of 5 to 9 pounds, these small turkeys are not always available.
- **Hen turkeys.** Hens are female turkeys weighing about 8 to 16 pounds.
- **Tom turkeys.** These male turkeys can weigh up to 24 pounds.
- **Self-basting turkeys.** When self-basting, turkeys are injected with broth, oil, or butter and seasonings to make them more moist and flavorful. The label identifies self-basting turkeys by such terms as "basted," "marinated," or "added flavoring."

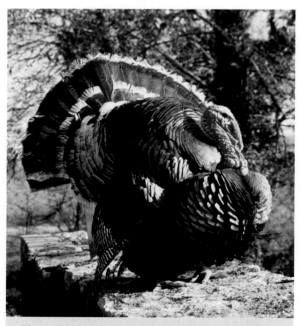

Fig. 37-2 A turkey is larger than a chicken and has a stronger flavor.

Duck

Duck has dark meat and a delicious flavor and is high in fat. Most ducks are young and tender.

- **Broilers and fryers.** The smallest ducks are less than eight weeks old and weigh an average of 3 pounds.
- **Roasters.** Larger birds are no more than 16 weeks old and weigh up to 5½ pounds.
- **Long Island ducks.** This type of duck has a dark, succulent flesh. About half the ducks raised for food are Long Island ducks.

Goose

Geese weigh from 5 to 18 pounds. Meat from a young goose, or gosling, is the most tender. Cooked goose is high in fat but flavorful. Because of its high fat content, it is best roasted.

FORMS OF POULTRY

Besides whole poultry, you can purchase parts or pieces, ground poultry, internal organs, processed forms, and convenience forms.

Parts

An entire cut-up chicken costs more than a whole bird because processing adds to the cost. By buying a whole bird and cutting it up yourself, you can save money. See **Fig. 37-3**.

Cut-up chicken is sold in halves, quarters, or parts, such as breasts, wings, thighs, and drumsticks. Breasts and thighs are sold bone-in, boneless and skinless, or as cutlets, which are small thin slices that are more costly. Meat on the bone is more tender and flavorful than boneless. Breasts, drumsticks, and thighs contain more meat than wings and backs. What would you buy to prepare the recipe in **Fig. 37-4** on page 524?

Fig. 37-3

How to Cut Up a Whole Chicken

To cut up a whole chicken, use a sharp knife and large, solid cutting board that won't slip.

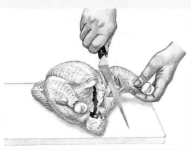

1. With chicken breast-side up, remove legs and wings. For legs, slice skin between body and thigh. Bend leg to crack the joint. Then cut through the joint and remove leg. Remove wings by cutting inside the wing joint. Cut from the top down through the joint.

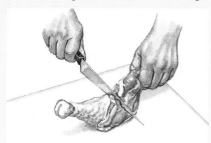

2. If desired, separate the drumstick and thigh by cracking the joint and cutting through it.

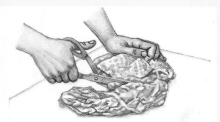

3. Use kitchen shears to cut along the backbone on both sides, separating the breast from the back.

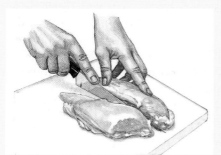

4. Beginning at the V of the wishbone, cut the breast in half. Leave the breastbone on one of the halves.

Fig. 37-4

Chicken with Pasta and Horseradish Cream Sauce

Yield
4 servings

Nutrition Analysis
Per Serving: 570 calories, 21 g total fat, 12 g saturated fat, 0 g trans fat, 100 mg cholesterol, 240 mg sodium, 68 g total carbohydrate, 3 g dietary fiber, 5 g sugars, 28 g protein

Percent Daily Value: vitamin A 40%, vitamin C 110%, calcium 8%, iron 20%

Ingredients
2 split chicken breasts (4 pieces)
1 cup reduced-sodium chicken stock
1 cup whipping cream
white horseradish to taste, prepared
  or grated

12 ounces cooked linguine
salt (if desired) and pepper
red and yellow bell peppers, cut into
  small pieces
Parmesan or Asiago cheese, grated

Directions
1. Grill or sauté chicken.
2. Bring chicken stock and cream to boil in large, heavy skillet over high heat.
3. Reduce heat and simmer until mixture thickens enough to coat spoon, whisking occasionally, about 10 minutes.
4. Gradually whisk in horseradish in small additions. Taste for hotness. Add linguine and toss to coat.
5. Remove skillet from heat. Slice cooked chicken and add to skillet. Toss to combine. Season to taste with salt and pepper.
6. Top with a confetti of bell peppers and sprinkling of cheese.

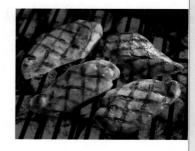

Turkey parts include breasts, drumsticks, thighs, wings, and necks. Turkey breasts are sold bone-in, boneless, and as tenderloins and cutlets. Because turkeys are so large, small families and singles may prefer parts.

Ground Poultry

Ground chicken and turkey are found in many meat departments. When buying either product, read the label carefully. If it says "ground turkey breast" or "ground chicken," both the flesh and skin were used. If the word *meat* is part of the description, as in "ground turkey breast meat" and "ground chicken meat," the poultry was ground without the skin and is leaner.

You can substitute ground poultry for ground beef in many recipes, but it results in a drier, blander product. Add a little more liquid and seasonings to the recipe to increase the flavor.

Giblets

Giblets (JIB-luhts) are the edible internal organs of poultry. They include the liver, gizzard (stomach), and heart. Giblets are usually included in a package stuffed inside the whole, cleaned bird. Chicken livers and gizzards are also sold separately.

Processed Poultry

Turkey is cured and smoked to make turkey ham and turkey bacon. Turkey and chicken are also processed into frankfurters and others types of sausage. You can also buy such smoked turkey products as legs and wings. Some are ready to eat but others need to be cooked, so read the label.

Convenience Forms

If you're looking for a quick meal made with poultry, you can choose from a wide assortment of convenience foods. Canned, boneless chicken or turkey is ready to use in salads, sandwiches, and casseroles. Many frozen dinners feature chicken or turkey as the entrée, from roast turkey to curried chicken. Supermarket deli sections offer ready-to-eat barbecued, roasted, and fried chicken as well as sliced, cooked turkey and chicken, often used for sandwiches.

INSPECTION AND GRADING

Poultry is inspected and graded by the USDA. Inspection is mandatory; grading is a voluntary program. The inspection and grade marks may appear on the package label or on a wing tag attached to the bird. See **Fig. 37-5**. In addition, the USDA requires that labels on all raw or partially cooked poultry products include safe handling instructions for storing and cooking.

Grade A poultry is the most common grade sold in stores. It indicates that the poultry is practically free of defects, has a good shape and appearance, and is meaty.

BUYING POULTRY

Chicken, turkey, and duck are available fresh or frozen. Goose is always sold frozen. "Fresh" indicates that the poultry has never been chilled below 26°F. "Frozen" poultry has been chilled to below 0°F.

When you buy poultry, look for plump, meaty birds with smooth, soft skin. The color of the skin may vary from creamy white to yellow, depending on the food eaten by the bird.

Avoid poultry with tiny feathers or skin that is bruised or torn. Don't buy packages that are leaking or have an off-odor. Frozen poultry should be frozen solid, with no off-odor.

Always check the sell-by date on the package. Unless you plan to cook the poultry soon, avoid buying packages close to the sell-by date.

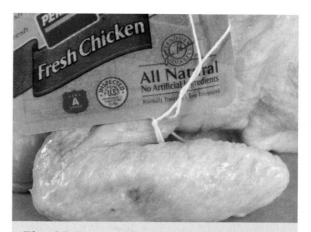

Fig. 37-5 Grading and inspection stamps are either attached to the wing of the bird or placed on packaging. This tells you the poultry has been inspected and is safe for consumption.

STORING POULTRY

Refrigerate poultry immediately after purchase. If prepackaged in plastic, poultry can be stored in the original wrapper, but put it in a plastic bag to keep juices from dripping onto other food. Use fresh poultry within one or two days.

Already-frozen poultry can be stored in the freezer in the original wrapping. Never thaw frozen poultry at room temperature, as this may allow dangerous bacteria to grow. Instead, leave it in the freezer wrapping and thaw in a container in the refrigerator or in cold water. Refrigerator thawing may take several hours to several days, depending on the bird's type and size. Soaking in cold water to defrost takes less time. Poultry can also be defrosted in the microwave oven but must be cooked right after thawing.

To prevent bacterial growth, poultry and stuffing should be refrigerated separately, both before and after cooking. Use leftover cooked poultry and stuffing within a day or two. For longer storage, freeze them.

COOKING POULTRY

Because *Salmonella* bacteria can be present in raw poultry, handle poultry with care. Follow the cleanliness procedures you've learned both before and after preparing raw poultry.

When you cook whole poultry, first remove the giblets and neck from the body and neck cavities. Also remove any foreign matter in the cavities. Then rinse the cavities several times. Before you cook poultry, rinse it well under cold running water. Allow the poultry to drain, or pat it dry with paper towels.

Poultry is cooked at a moderate temperature until well done. If cooked for too long or at a temperature that's too high, poultry dries out and becomes tough.

To cut down on fat, remove the skin when cooking poultry in moist heat. When you use dry-heat methods, however, leave the skin on to keep the poultry from drying out. Most fat melts and drips away during cooking. You can remove the skin just before eating to avoid eating any remaining fat.

Sometimes the bones in cooked poultry turn a dark color. This is common in poultry that was frozen before cooking. The blood cells in the bones break down during freezing, causing the discoloration. This has no effect on flavor or food safety. You might also notice a pink color to the meat after cooking. This does not necessarily mean the meat has not been thoroughly cooked. Sometimes a chemical reaction occurs between the poultry and gases in the oven, and this causes the pinkish tinge to the meat.

Testing for Doneness

Because poultry may carry *Salmonella* bacteria, never eat raw or partially cooked poultry. Always cook it until well done. See **Fig. 37-6**.

Cook whole poultry and chicken and turkey thighs, legs, and wings to an internal temperature of 180°F. Cook chicken and turkey breasts to an internal temperature of 170°F. Stuffing and ground poultry should be cooked to an internal temperature of 165°F. Use an instant-read thermometer to test thin pieces. Pieces that are too thin or small to test should be tender, with the juices running clear.

Broiling Poultry

Broiling is one of the quickest cooking methods. Choose a broiler-fryer chicken and split it

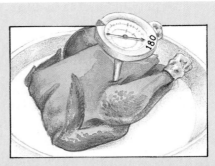

Fig. 37-6 For cooking whole poultry, insert a meat thermometer into the inner thigh, near the breast. The tip of the probe should reach the thickest part of the meat without touching the bone.

in half lengthwise or cut it into quarters or pieces.

Place the chicken pieces skin-side down on the broiler pan. Brush with oil or melted butter. Place the broiler pan so the top of the chicken is about 6 to 7 inches below the heat, depending on the thickness of the pieces. Broil about 15 minutes.

Turn the chicken and brush with oil or melted butter. Continue broiling until the chicken is browned and crisp. Test for doneness with an instant-read thermometer.

When you add barbecue sauce or any other sweetened sauce, brush it on about two minutes before the chicken is done. If applied sooner, the sauce chars due to its high sugar content.

Grilling Poultry

Chicken is a grilling favorite. Choose a broiler-fryer chicken cut into halves, quarters, or pieces.

Chicken should be grilled until the outside is browned, but not charred, and the inside is well done. To do so, cook it slowly over moderate heat. Begin by brushing the grate lightly with oil so the chicken doesn't stick. Place the chicken skin-side up on the grate and then brush with oil or melted butter. Turn the pieces often and brush frequently with oil or melted butter.

Grilling time depends on size, but a chicken half may take 50 to 60 minutes. Test for doneness with an instant-read thermometer. Boneless and skinless chicken pieces, such as breasts and cutlets, cook faster and more evenly. Brush them with oil or melted butter to keep them moist.

Chicken can be marinated for added flavor. You can also make kebabs by threading cubes of chicken and assorted vegetables onto skewers. Brush with oil or melted butter to keep them from drying out. To add flavor with a sweetened sauce, brush it on during the last few minutes of cooking.

Roasting Poultry

Turkey, duck, and goose are best roasted. To roast a chicken, choose a whole broiler-fryer or roaster.

You can roast poultry with or without stuffing. Because stuffing placed inside raw poultry is a breeding ground for harmful bacteria, experts recommend cooking stuffing separately. Place the stuffing in a greased casserole, cover, and bake during the last 45 minutes or so of the bird's roasting time.

To roast a bird without stuffing, season the cavity with salt, pepper, herbs, and spices. For more flavor, insert carrots, onions, celery, or other aromatic vegetables.

If you do stuff the bird, guard against bacterial growth by packing the stuffing loosely in the cavity. This usually takes about ¾ cup of stuffing per pound of bird. Also, wait until roasting time to stuff the bird. Never stuff a bird and refrigerate it to roast on the following day. Because a stuffed bird is thick and compact, the inside takes a long time to chill, and harmful bacteria will flourish.

To prepare a bird for roasting, **trussing** is an option. This procedure closes the cavity and binds the legs and wings to the bird to make it more compact, easier to handle, and attractive to serve. Trussing methods vary. See **Fig. 37-7**.

After preparing the bird, follow these steps for roasting:

1. Place the bird breast-side up on a rack in a roasting pan large enough to hold the bird and drippings.
2. If roasting a chicken or turkey, brush the skin with oil or melted butter. Duck and goose have enough natural fat.
3. Insert a meat thermometer so the tip is in the center of the inside thigh muscle or the thickest part of the breast meat. Be sure the tip doesn't touch bone or fat. If the bird is stuffed, also insert a thermometer into the center of the stuffing.
4. If you wish, baste the bird occasionally. Add any vegetables about 1 hour before the bird will be done.
5. Roast uncovered at 325°F until the meat reaches 180°F. An unstuffed turkey weighing 12 to 14 pounds takes about 3 to 3½ hours to cook. A stuffed bird the same size takes about a half hour longer overall. If the bird is stuffed, be sure to cook until the center of the stuffing reaches 165°F. Note that the meat may cook to 180°F before the stuffing is safe. Cook until both temperatures are reached.
6. Allow the bird to stand about 15 minutes after cooking for easier carving. If the bird is stuffed, remove the stuffing immediately after the standing time.

In addition to whole poultry, you may also roast a turkey breast or chicken pieces. Place the breast or pieces in a shallow baking pan skin-side up and season as desired. For turkey breast, insert a meat thermometer into the thickest part and roast at 350°F until the meat reaches a temperature of 170°F. Roast chicken pieces at 400°F for 45 to 55 minutes. Test for doneness with an instant-read thermometer.

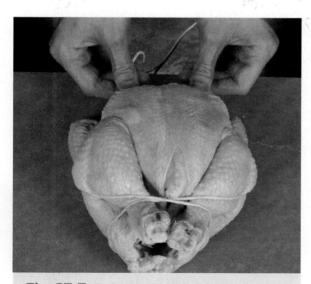

Fig. 37-7 To truss a bird, twine can be wrapped around the legs and then pulled to the opposite side of the bird. Doing this secures the bird and keeps the openings closed.

Frying Poultry

Cut-up chicken may be fried, deep-fried, or oven-fried. It is usually floured or breaded first to keep it from drying out.

- **To fry chicken.** Pour cooking oil into a large, heavy skillet to a depth of about $\frac{1}{2}$ inch. Heat until a cube of bread sizzles. Place chicken pieces skin-side down in the skillet. Fry uncovered over low heat so that the outside does not overcook before the inside is done. If you fry too many pieces at once, they steam and lose crispness. The chicken cooks in about 30 to 45 minutes, depending on the size of the pieces. Test for doneness with an instant-read thermometer. Remove pieces as they are done, and drain on paper towels. Keep warm in the oven.

- **To deep-fry chicken.** Heat a deep pan of oil to 350°F. Fry three to four pieces at a time for 10 to 15 minutes or until browned and cooked through. Test for doneness with an instant-read thermometer. Drain on paper towels.

- **To oven-fry chicken.** Place in a shallow baking pan skin-side up and drizzle with oil or melted butter. Bake uncovered at 350°F until tender, about 35 to 45 minutes. Test for doneness with an instant-read thermometer.

Braising Poultry

Any bird that is too tough to cook in dry heat can be braised. You can also braise young, tender birds in a seasoned sauce to give them flavor. See **Fig. 37-8**.

To braise poultry pieces, brown them first and drain off any excess fat. Add seasonings and a small amount of liquid, such as water, tomato juice, stock, or other seasoned liquid. You can also add vegetables if you wish. Cover the pan tightly and simmer until tender, either on top of the range or in the oven.

Pressure-Cooking Poultry

Pressure cooking is usually used for tough, mature birds that cannot be cooked in dry heat.

Career Prep

Responsible Leadership

IF YOU WERE HIRING WORKERS, would you be more impressed by the student with good grades or the student who organized and ran a study group aimed at helping students get good grades? Wise employers know that just as technical skills get the job done, leadership skills keep the job on track.

What makes a good leader? The following list describes a few of the qualities an effective leader displays:

- **Management.** Leadership has been summed up as "get good people; then get out of their way." In other words, leaders don't try to do it all themselves. They encourage participation from everyone, respecting and channeling each person's talent to its best use.

- **Problem solving.** Leaders look for creative solutions but don't overlook the obvious. They welcome suggestions from others.

- **Decision making.** Everyone makes decisions. Leaders make good decisions. They gather information from different sources, carefully reason through the pros and cons, and stay focused on the ultimate goal.

- **Communication.** Leaders are equally skilled speakers and listeners. They hear people's needs, concerns, and questions and respond in ways that are understandable, honest, and meaningful to others.

- **Character.** Like any kind of power, leadership is dangerous unless put toward honorable goals. A responsible leader focuses on improv-

Young, tender birds fall apart in a pressure cooker. Refer to the owner's manual for recipes and instructions for using the pressure cooker.

Slow-Cooking Poultry

An almost unlimited combination of poultry pieces, liquid, seasonings, and vegetables can be prepared in a slow cooker. Because the food cooks slowly at a low temperature, the flavors have time to develop and blend.

Microwaving Poultry

Be sure to thaw frozen chicken thoroughly before microwaving. Then follow recipe directions for cooking. Chicken pieces are usually microwaved in a sauce, which adds flavor and color. They may be coated instead with either plain or seasoned crumbs. Avoid coating with flour, as it becomes gummy in the microwave.

Remember that poultry won't brown in a microwave oven. For more appeal, brush a dark sauce on the poultry, use a browning dish, or broil the meat for a few minutes after microwaving.

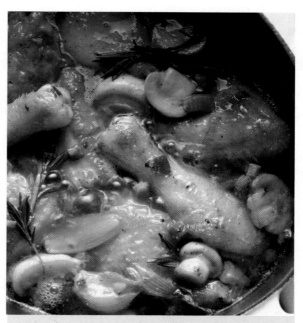

Fig. 37-8 Braising is used to make many delicious dishes with poultry. How is braising different from roasting?

ing life for others by making positive changes that reap long-lasting rewards. Leaders see their ability to motivate others and to change their world as a call to service.

DEVELOPING LEADERSHIP

Whether leaders are born or made is often debated, but leadership skills develop with practice. Where are your opportunities to practice leadership? They are anywhere you have the chance to extend positive influence. Do you belong to a sports team or volunteer group? Ask a coach or committee chairperson what jobs you can take on. Maybe you could help with younger siblings at home. Children always need role models who demonstrate kindness, fairness, and positive values. Even suggesting a movie to watch is a chance to be a constructive influence. Don't forget that the "L" in FCCLA stands for "Leaders." Learn how FCCLA can help you develop leadership skills.

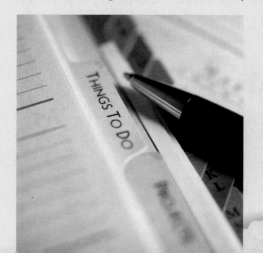

Career Connection

Life of a leader. Research the early life of someone who became a constructive leader in the community or the world. Look for signs of leadership potential, such as activities and events the person took part in when young. Compare life stories in class. Suggest similar opportunities for young people today.

Summarize Your Reading

▶ Poultry, which has become a common meal choice in many homes, includes chicken, turkey, duck, and goose.

▶ Several types of each kind of poultry are available.

▶ Because poultry is perishable, it needs to be refrigerated or frozen.

▶ For safety, poultry must be cooked until well done and tested for doneness.

▶ Because poultry can be cooked in so many different ways, it's a versatile ingredient in the kitchen.

Check Your Knowledge

1. Why is **poultry** often chosen for meals instead of red meat?

2. What advantage is there to removing the skin from poultry?

3. Why does poultry have both light and dark meat?

4. **CRITICAL THINKING** Predict what could happen if a stewing chicken is cut up and grilled.

5. What makes Rock Cornish game hens different from other chickens?

6. How do free-range chickens compare with chickens that are mass-produced?

7. Describe each of the following: a) hen turkey; b) tom turkey; c) self-basting turkey.

8. Which types of poultry are highest in fat?

9. How do you remove legs and wings when cutting up a whole chicken?

10. If the word *meat* is part of the description for ground poultry, what does that mean?

11. What are **giblets**?

12. **CRITICAL THINKING** What kinds of poultry would you recommend for the following: a) casseroles; b) soups; c) barbecue? Explain your choices

13. What does "grade A" mean on poultry?

14. What should you look for when purchasing fresh poultry?

15. How should frozen poultry be thawed, and why?

16. How do you prepare whole poultry for cooking?

17. What temperatures indicate doneness in poultry?

18. Why do many people prepare stuffing in a dish separate from the bird?

19. Why do cooks often **truss** a bird before roasting?

20. How is an oven-safe thermometer placed in a whole turkey?

21. How do you fry chicken?

22. When would you pressure-cook and slow-cook poultry?

23. Why should microwaved chicken not be coated with flour?

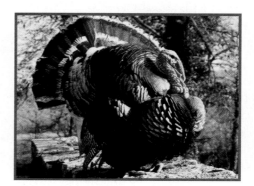

Apply Your Learning

1. **SCIENCE** **Serving Size.** Weigh 3 ounces, a serving size, of cooked chicken meat. Then trim the meat from a cooked chicken drumstick of average size. Weigh the poultry and compare to the first portion. What do you conclude?

2. **MATH** **Cost Comparison.** Boneless meat generally contains four servings per pound. Compare the cost of boneless chicken with boneless beef and boneless pork. What did you discover?

3. **Low-Fat Alternatives.** Poultry is used to make low-fat alternatives to some foods. Turkey bacon and turkey sausage are examples. What others are available? Prepare one for the class to sample and evaluate.

4. **Cross-Contamination.** Demonstrate how a cook should work with poultry in order to prevent cross-contamination.

5. **Trussing.** Research and demonstrate one way to truss a chicken for roasting.

6. **Oven-Fried.** Find and make a recipe for oven-fried chicken. How does this dish compare to regular fried chicken?

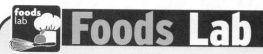 **Foods Lab**

Cutting Up a Chicken

Procedure: Using a whole chicken, cut it into separate parts, including breast halves, wings, thighs, and drumsticks. Use a sharp knife and large, solid cutting board that won't slip. Place a damp dishcloth under the board if necessary. Study the directions in the chapter before you begin. Also, review the knife safety material in Chapter 21.

Analyzing Results

❶ Were some steps in the process more difficult than others? If so, how?

❷ How does the cost of the parts compare to the cost of the whole bird?

❸ What if you only needed certain parts for a meal? What would you do?

❹ Would you use this process at home? Why or why not?

 Food Science Experiment

Meat and Poultry Comparison

Objective: To compare how fat in meat and poultry affects sensory qualities.

Procedure:

1. Weigh a 4-oz. portion each of ground poultry and ground beef. Shape each portion into a patty.

2. Cook each patty in a nonstick skillet, turning once, until done. Test with an instant-read thermometer.

3. Remove and weigh each patty. Measure any drippings in the skillet.

4. Sample and evaluate the patties.

Analyzing Results

❶ Which patty retained more of its weight after cooking? What might explain that result?

❷ Compare the patties on taste, texture, and appearance. What might account for any differences in these qualities?

❸ How might you change a ground beef recipe if you wanted to use ground poultry instead?

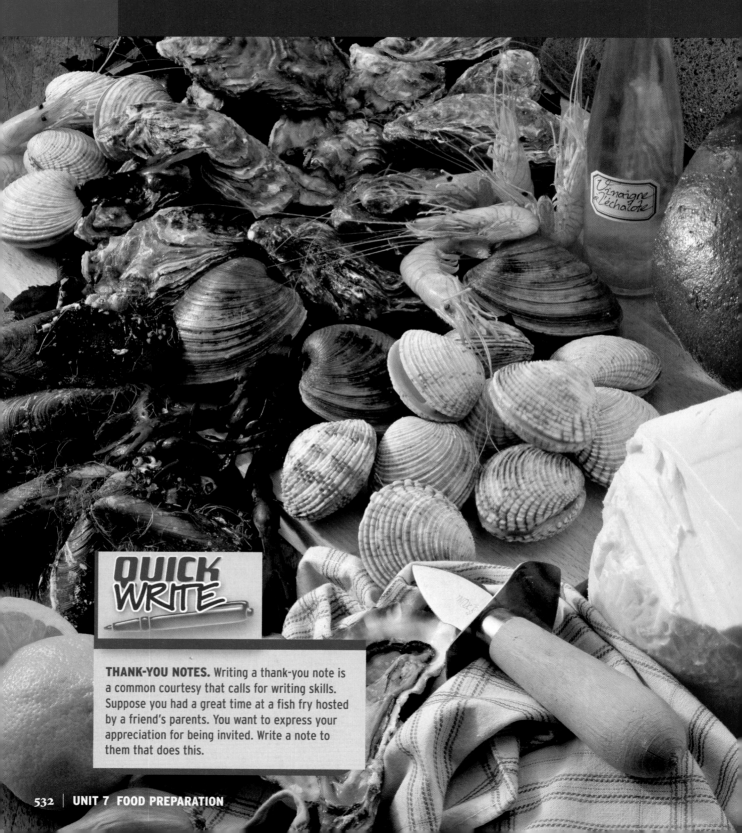

QUICK WRITE

THANK-YOU NOTES. Writing a thank-you note is a common courtesy that calls for writing skills. Suppose you had a great time at a fish fry hosted by a friend's parents. You want to express your appreciation for being invited. Write a note to them that does this.

IN COASTAL REGIONS AND NEAR LAKES AND rivers, people have always enjoyed a plentiful supply of fish. Through today's technology, people almost everywhere can eat fish and shellfish from around the world. Have you ever eaten smoked salmon and cream cheese on a bagel? Clam chowder? Crab cakes? These are just a few of the hundreds of delicious and nutritious dishes made with fish and shellfish.

FISH AND SHELLFISH NUTRITION

Fish and shellfish are high in protein, some B vitamins, iron, phosphorus, selenium, zinc, and copper. Saltwater fish are high in iodine. Fish are one of the few natural sources of vitamin D. They are also good sources of omega-3 fatty acids, particularly salmon. Fish and shellfish are low in saturated fat and, except for shrimp and squid, are also low in cholesterol.

Fish belong to the same food group as meat, poultry, dry beans, eggs, and nuts. On a 2,000-calorie diet, a person needs 5½ ounces of these protein foods each day. Two to 3 ounces of cooked fish is about the size of your palm.

Mercury in Fish

Studies have shown that fish and shellfish can contain mercury. When mercury settles to the bottom of waterways, it's absorbed by **plankton**, minute animal and plant life in the water. Small fish eat the plankton plus the mercury. In turn, the small fish are eaten by larger fish, which are eaten by still larger fish, ending with deep-sea fish like tuna. The most mercury accumulates in the largest fish. Albacore (AL-buh-kohr), or white tuna, is larger than the smaller tuna sold as "chunk light." Therefore albacore tuna may have up to three times the amount of mercury.

Other fish that have high mercury levels include shark, swordfish, king mackerel, and tilefish. Fish that contain low levels of mercury and are safe for most people to eat include canned chunk light tuna, salmon, pollock, catfish, sardines, and herring.

Even low levels of mercury are harmful to humans in the early years of their life. As a result, the FDA and EPA advise women of childbearing age, pregnant and nursing women, and young children to eat no more than 12 ounces of fish per week. Of that amount, no more than 6 ounces should be albacore tuna.

TYPES OF FISH AND SHELLFISH

Some fish and shellfish come from freshwater lakes, rivers, streams, and ponds, where water is not salty. These fish are known as freshwater varieties. Saltwater fish come from oceans and seas. Some freshwater and saltwater fish and shellfish are raised on fish farms. **Seafood** technically means saltwater fish and shellfish. The term is often used, however, to cover all fish and shellfish.

What is the difference between fish and shellfish? **Fish** have fins and a center spine with bones. **Shellfish** have a shell but no spine or bones.

Types of Fish

Fish can be divided into two categories. **Low-fat fish** have less than 5 grams of fat in 3½ ounces. The flesh is white or pale, with a delicate texture and mild flavor. Low-fat fish include bass, carp, catfish, cod, haddock, halibut, pike, perch, pollock, red snapper, and whiting. Some of these are described in **Fig. 38-1**.

Fatty fish have more than 5 grams of fat in 3½ ounces. The flesh is firm, with a deeper color and a stronger flavor than low-fat fish, and is higher in calories. Fatty fish include shad as well as the fish in **Fig. 38-2**.

When preparing fish, you can usually substitute one low-fat fish for another and one fatty fish for another.

Types of Shellfish

Shellfish generally have a mild, sweet flavor. Almost all shellfish come from oceans and seas, but a few come from freshwater. There are two types of shellfish. **Crustaceans** (krus-TAY-shuhns) have long bodies and jointed limbs and are covered with a shell. Examples are crabs, crayfish, lobsters, and shrimp. **Mollusks** (MAH-lusks) have soft bodies covered by a rigid shell. Clams, mussels, oysters, scallops, and squid are all mollusks. See **Fig. 38-3**.

INSPECTION AND GRADING

The FDA's food safety system, Hazard Analysis and Critical Control Point (HACCP), includes identifying and preventing hazards that could cause foodborne illness during stages of fish processing. A voluntary inspection and grading program is also carried on jointly by the FDA and the National Marine Fisheries Service of the U.S.

Fig. 38-1

	Low-Fat Fish	
Type	**Characteristics**	**Common Cooking Methods**
Carp	Dark flesh. Moderate flavor.	Baked, fried, poached.
Catfish	White flesh; firm yet slightly flaky. Mild flavor, with touch of sweetness.	Fried with cornmeal coating; can be grilled, broiled, baked.
Cod	Opaque flesh; large flakes. Mild, delicate flavor.	Boiled, baked, sautéed, broiled, steamed, deep-fried.
Haddock	White flesh; firm, tender texture, with fine flake. Delicate, slightly sweet flavor.	Sautéed, poached, pan-fried, smoked.
Halibut	Firm flesh. Mild flavor.	Grilled, baked, sautéed, steamed, poached, broiled.
Perch	Opaque flesh; tender but somewhat firm texture. Mild flavor.	Sautéed, broiled, steamed, baked, poached.
Pike	Somewhat firm flesh; dry. Moderate flavor.	Grilled, baked, broiled, sautéed, poached.
Pollock (Alaskan)	Opaque flesh; small flakes; slightly tender. Mild, delicate flavor.	Baked, broiled, steamed, sautéed, poached.

Carp

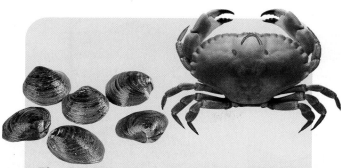

Fig. 38-3 Here you see clams on the left and a crab on the right. Which basic type of shellfish is each of these?

Department of Commerce. This program attempts to focus on parts of fish processing that may carry risks to consumer safety. Some state and local fish inspection services are also available.

BUYING FISH AND SHELLFISH

Fish and shellfish retain quality only when properly handled from the time they are caught to the time they are cooked. Therefore start with the freshest fish possible, purchased from a reliable source.

Notice the way fish and shellfish are displayed. If several layers are piled on ice, the top layer may be too warm for safekeeping. Don't buy fish or shellfish displayed under hot lights. Ready-to-eat fish and shellfish should not be piled next to fresh varieties. Harmful bacteria from the fresh items can transfer to the ready-to-eat products.

Fish and shellfish naturally have a slight fish smell, but a strong "fishy" or ammonia odor should make you suspicious. This indicates that protein in the fish or shellfish—along with quality—has begun to deteriorate.

Buying Fish

You can purchase several market forms of fish, including **whole**, **drawn**, **dressed**, **fillets** (fih-LAYS), and **steaks**. See **Fig. 38-4** on page 536.

Use appearance, aroma, and touch to judge the quality of fresh fish. Look for shiny skin and glistening color. Whole or drawn fish should have clear, full eyes and bright red or pink gills. Any fish should have a mild, fresh aroma like cucumbers or seaweed. Skin should spring back when pressed.

Fig. 38-2

Fatty Fish		
Type	**Characteristics**	**Common Cooking Methods**
Herring	Semi-moist flesh; fine, soft texture. Medium flavor.	Baked, grilled, sautéed.
Mackerel	Off-white, firm flesh; flaky. May be mild or strong and fishy flavor.	Best grilled or broiled; also baked or poached.
Salmon	Orange, pink, or red flesh; large, moist flakes. Delicate flavor.	Baked, grilled, broiled, poached.
Sardines	*Sardines* is a general term for variety of small fish with varied characteristics. Strong flavor.	Grilled, broiled, fried. In U.S. generally canned, salted, or smoked.
Tuna (Albacore)	Off-white flesh; firm texture. Mild flavor.	Grilled, broiled, braised.
Tuna (Bluefin)	Off-white flesh; firm. Distinctive flavor.	Grilled, baked, broiled.
Trout (Rainbow)	Pale white, pink, or orange flesh; flaky. Mild, delicate, slightly nutty flavor.	Grilled, broiled, baked, poached, sautéed, deep-fried.

Trout

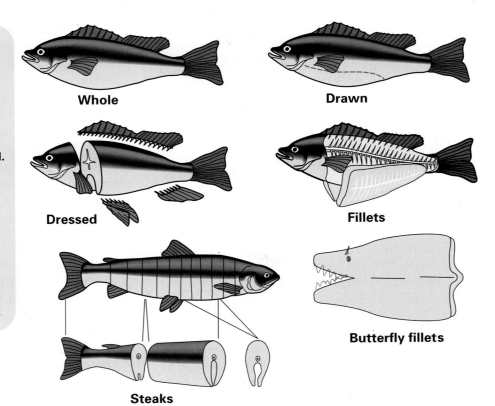

Fig. 38-4

- **Whole** fish: sold as caught and the most perishable; scales and internal organs must be removed.
- **Drawn** fish: whole fish with scales, gills, and internal organs removed.
- **Dressed** fish: drawn fish with head, tail, and fins removed.
- **Fillets:** sides of fish, usually boneless, cut lengthwise away from bones and backbone.
- **Steaks:** cross sections cut from large, dressed fish; may contain bones from backbone and ribs.

Whole

Drawn

Dressed

Fillets

Butterfly fillets

Steaks

Buying Shellfish

Some shellfish are sold live because they deteriorate so quickly. Look for these signs of quality in shellfish:

- **Live clams, oysters, and mussels.** Shells should be tightly closed, moist, and intact, with no cracks, chips, or breaks. If shells are slightly open, tap them with a knife. They should close. If they don't, discard them. These mollusks are also sold without the shell (shucked). Shucked oysters should have a slightly milky or light gray liquid around them.
- **Scallops.** Scallops are usually sold without shells. They should look moist but not be in liquid or in direct contact with ice, and they should have a fresh sea smell.
- **Live lobsters and crabs.** Lobsters are dark bluish-green until cooked, when they turn bright red. Look for lobsters and crabs that are active, with legs moving. A lobster's tail curls under when picked up.
- **Raw shrimp.** Shrimp vary in size and color, and they are sold with or without the shell. If they are in the shell, look for translucent shells without black spots. If unshelled, the meat should be firm. Shrimp should be moist but not in liquid.

Convenience Forms of Fish and Shellfish

For convenience, you can buy fish and shellfish in several forms. Included are cooked and ready to eat, canned, frozen, and cured.

Lobster, crab, and shrimp are sold cooked and ready to eat. You can usually buy them by the pound in the fish department.

Canned fish and shellfish are usually ready to eat and are generally used in recipes. Tuna, for instance, is often an ingredient in salads and casseroles. Fish packed in water has fewer calories than fish packed in oil. If you purchase oil-packed fish, drain and rinse it well before using. Salmon and sardines are good sources of calcium when eaten with the bones.

Many frozen forms of fish are available, including ready-to-cook fillets. Frozen, breaded, fish fillets and fish sticks are generally precooked and only need reheating. Follow the instructions on the label.

Cured fish can be salt-dried, smoked, or pickled. Cod is often salted and dried. Salmon and herring are the most common smoked fish, and herring is often pickled.

STORING FISH AND SHELLFISH

Since fish is highly perishable, refrigerate it immediately after purchase and use within a day or two. Place it in a plastic bag to keep juices from dripping on other foods. For longer storage, freeze fish. Leave already frozen fish in the original wrapping and store in the freezer immediately. Never store fish that hasn't been gutted, because organs deteriorate faster than flesh.

Refrigerate live shellfish in containers covered with a clean, damp cloth. They need breathing space to stay alive, so don't seal them in a plastic bag. Don't put saltwater shellfish in fresh water—they won't live. Properly stored, shellfish live for a few days. If they die in storage, discard them.

Put leftover cooked fish and unused portions of canned fish in a covered container and refrigerate. Use within three or four days.

COOKING FISH

Fish flesh is more tender than meat and poultry flesh and cooks much faster because the muscles are arranged differently. In contrast to the long fibers in meat and poultry, fish has very short fibers arranged in layers. The layers are separated by sheets of very thin, fragile, connective tissue. See **Fig. 38-5**. When heated, the connective tissue turns into gelatin and the muscle fibers separate. This is why the flesh flakes, or separates into small pieces, when fish is cooked.

Fish must be properly prepared before cooking. Inspect fillets carefully to be sure all bones have been removed. If any remain, remove them with clean tweezers. To be sure the fish is clean, wash it under cool, running water and wipe dry. Thaw frozen fish in the refrigerator and cook within 24 hours.

Because fish is tender, both moist heat and dry heat cook it effectively. Since low-fat fish tends to dry out when cooked, however, moist-heat cooking methods are better. If cooked in dry heat, the

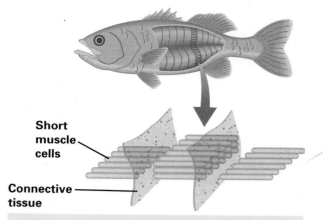

Short muscle cells

Connective tissue

Fig. 38-5 How does the muscle structure of fish explain why fish flakes easily when cooked?

fish must be basted generously with oil, melted butter, or a sauce for moisture. Dry-heat methods—broiling, grilling, and baking—are ideal for fatty fish, although moist heat can be used.

Like other high-protein foods, fish must be cooked at low temperatures just until done. If overcooked in dry heat, fish toughens and becomes rubbery. If overcooked in moist heat, the fish falls apart.

Fish leaves an unpleasant odor while cooking. Since acidic foods help eliminate fish odors, many fish recipes include an acidic liquid, such as vinegar or a citrus juice. (This is why lemon is often served with fish.) If fish leaves an odor on your hands, rub them with a piece of lemon or rinse them in vinegar.

Testing for Doneness

Since fish is tender, it cooks in a short time. With conventional cooking methods, remember the 10-minute rule. Cook fish 10 minutes for every inch of thickness, measured at the thickest part. For example, cook a fish fillet that is 1 inch thick for 5 minutes on each side, a total of 10 minutes. There are a few exceptions. If fish is baked in a sauce, add about 5 minutes to the cooking time. Also increase cooking time for frozen fish. Some moist-heat recipes may call for longer cooking times to allow flavors to blend.

Begin to check for doneness about 2 or 3 minutes before the cooking time is up. When lifted gently with a fork, the flesh should flake easily.

Another cue is opaqueness. Raw fish is translucent due to light's ability to pass through individual proteins. When fish is cooked, however, the proteins coagulate and light can't pass through, making the flesh opaque. See **Fig. 38-6**.

Never eat fish or shellfish undercooked or raw. It may be contaminated with harmful bacteria. For example, sushi is a traditional Japanese dish that has become popular in the United States. It's made with various foods, including raw fish. Raw fish may carry harmful parasites, bacteria, and viruses that can cause serious illness.

Broiling Fish

Fish should be at least 1 inch thick for broiling. You can broil drawn and dressed fish under 3 pounds as well as steaks and fillets.

To broil fish, oil the grid of the broiler pan. Place the fish skin-side down in a single layer on the grid, making sure the pieces don't touch each other. Brush with seasoned oil, melted butter, or a sauce to prevent drying.

Turn the fish halfway through the cooking period. Continue broiling just until done, and then baste as needed.

Grilling Fish

Fish must be turned while grilling. Thick cuts, such as salmon and tuna steaks, hold their shape well and can be turned easily. Firm, drawn, and dressed fish also grill well, including pompano and red snapper, but avoid grilling a fish that is too large to turn. Thin fillets and small, low-fat, drawn and dressed fish fall apart if you try to turn them. Instead, grill them in a fish basket.

To grill fish, oil the grate lightly. Brush the fish with oil or melted butter to keep moist. Add seasonings and lemon juice if you wish. Place skin-side down on the grate. Grill for about half the cooking time, basting frequently with oil or melted butter. Turn and grill until done, basting frequently.

Baking Fish

Drawn and dressed fish, large steaks, and fillets bake well. For added flavor, season the oil or melted butter for basting. Generally you don't need to turn fish while it bakes. When you pre-

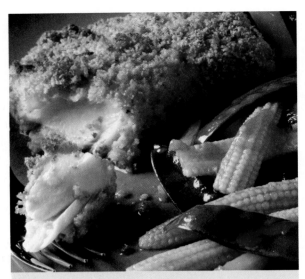

Fig. 38-6 When fish is done, the flesh turns opaque and separates easily with a fork.

pare fish **en papillote**, it is wrapped, often in parchment paper, and baked. See the recipe in **Fig. 38-7**.

- **Drawn and dressed fish.** Stuff, if desired. Oil a large, shallow baking pan. Place the fish in the pan and brush with oil or melted butter. Bake uncovered at 400°F, basting as needed to keep the fish from drying out.
- **Large steaks and fillets.** Oil a large, shallow, baking pan. Arrange the fish in a single layer, making sure the pieces don't touch each other. Brush with oil or melted butter. Bake at 350°F, basting as needed.

Poaching Fish

Fish is commonly poached. Many people consider poached fish to be a delicacy, and it's often served in fine restaurants.

You may poach a drawn or dressed fish, fillets, and steaks. The liquid used for poaching may be water, fish or vegetable stock, or milk. Usually the liquid is seasoned to add more flavor to the fish. For example, you can add lemon juice or grapefruit juice. You might also experiment with such herbs and spices as dill or grated fresh ginger or add sautéed aromatic vegetables—onions and green peppers, for example.

Fig. 38-7

Fish and Vegetables en Papillote

Yield	Nutrition Analysis
2 servings	**Per Serving:** 200 calories, 5 g total fat, 1 g saturated fat, 0g trans fat, 85 mg cholesterol, 270 mg sodium, 9 g total carbohydrate, 3 g dietary fiber, 4 g sugars, 29 g protein
	Percent Daily Value: vitamin A 160%, vitamin C 70%, calcium 8%, iron 10%

Ingredients

8 oz. fish fillet, ½ inch thick
lemon pepper seasoning
½ green bell pepper, cut into strips
2 medium carrots, cut into julienne
   strips

2 tsp. margarine, diced
2 tsp. lemon juice
2 Tbsp. chopped fresh parsley
4 lemon slices
salt to taste (optional)

Directions

1. Preheat oven to 450°F. Place fish on a sheet of heavy-duty aluminum foil or parchment paper for baking, large enough to fold around fish. Sprinkle fish with lemon pepper.
2. Arrange green pepper and carrots around fish. Top with margarine, lemon juice, parsley, lemon slices, and salt.
3. Wrap foil around fish and vegetables and fold to seal.
4. Place packet on cookie sheet. Bake for 18 minutes at 450°F or until fish flakes easily with a fork.

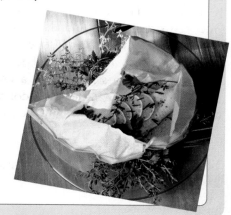

You can serve hot poached fish with a sauce made from the cooking liquid. After removing the fish from the pan, boil the cooking liquid to reduce the amount and reach the desired flavor.

- **Poaching fish fillets.** Pour the cooking liquid into a large, deep skillet. Bring to a boil and reduce the heat to a simmer. Place the fillets in a single layer in the pan. Add more liquid, if necessary, to cover the fish by at least 1 inch. Cover the pan and simmer gently until the fish is opaque throughout and flakes easily. Do not turn the fillets while poaching.

- **Poaching drawn and dressed fish.** For easier handling and to help keep the shape of the fish, wrap it in cheesecloth. Allow enough length at the ends so you can twist and knot the cloth. Use the ends as handles to lower and raise the fish easily. Place in simmering liquid in a large pan, making sure the fish is covered by at least 1 inch of liquid. Cover the pan and simmer gently until the fish is opaque and flakes easily.

Steaming Fish

Drawn and dressed fish, steaks, and large fillets can be steamed. Use a steamer or a large, deep pot fitted with a steaming rack. Pour water into the pot so it is about 1 inch deep but below the level of the rack.

Oil the rack and place the fish on it. Then cover the pot tightly. Heat the water to boiling. Steam the fish over boiling water until the flesh turns opaque and flakes easily.

Braising Fish

Although braising is typically used for less tender cuts of meat and poultry, it adds flavor and color to fish. The challenge is to cook the fish just long enough for the flavors to blend without overcooking the flesh.

Braising is best used with small or medium, drawn or dressed fish. To braise, use a large skillet with a tight-fitting lid. Flour the fish and brown it in the skillet. Add a small amount of liquid, seasonings, and vegetables. Cover and simmer gently just until the fish turns opaque and flakes easily.

Frying Fish

You can fry fillets, small steaks, and small drawn or dressed fish, such as trout, in oil, butter, or a mixture of half oil and half butter. The fish is usually floured or breaded first.

To fry fish, heat a small amount of fat in a large, heavy skillet over moderate heat. Place the breaded fish in the pan in a single layer, making sure the pieces don't touch. If the pan is crowded, the fish steams and loses crispness. Fry on one side for half the cooking time; then turn and fry on the other side until the flesh flakes easily. Drain on paper towels. You may keep the fish warm in the oven until serving.

Breaded fish may also be oven-fried. Grease a large, shallow baking pan. Arrange fish in a single layer, making sure pieces don't touch each other. Drizzle with oil or melted butter and bake, uncovered, at 500°F. Contrary to the general rules for cooking protein, fish is oven-fried at a high temperature. The fish doesn't dry out or toughen because the crumb coating and high temperature combine to create an attractive, brown crust that holds in juices. Bake without turning or basting until the flesh is golden brown and flakes easily.

Deep-Frying Fish

You can deep-fry small fillets and fish cut into sticks or squares. Bread the pieces first. Then heat a large pot of oil to 375°F and place one layer of breaded fish in a deep-fry basket. Lower it slowly into the fat and fry the fish until golden brown. Remove and drain on paper towels. Keep warm in the oven while you continue to fry remaining pieces in small batches.

Career Prep

Setting Priorities

SETTING PRIORITIES MEANS MAKING decisions about what tasks you need to do and when. It's a time management tool that only gets more valuable in the world of work.

The steps to prioritizing are fairly simple. Set aside a time each day to make a to-do list of the tasks you want to accomplish on the following day. Rank and complete each task in order of importance. For instance, you may need to finish some research before writing a paper that's due next week. On the other hand, if you have a quiz tomorrow, studying for that may be a higher priority.

The plan that looks so good on paper, however, faces real-life obstacles. Many people overschedule by underestimating the time a task

will take. Others procrastinate. Due to a lack of clear goals or a fear of failure, they put off tasks they know are important. Some people have trouble just making a decision.

To control your time better, try keeping a "time diary." For three days, write down your activities and the time spent on each one. Include even minor activities. These are often the time wasters. Also note whether an activity was related to work, health, or family; planned or unplanned; and urgent or trivial.

Review your diary. How much time did you spend on things that were very important? If you didn't accomplish all you wanted, what stopped you?

You may need to cut down on wasted time. If interruptions are a problem, tell people when

Be careful not to cook too many pieces at a time because the oil may bubble over and ignite. In addition, the oil temperature may go down quickly when several pieces are added, allowing the fish to absorb a great deal of fat.

COOKING SHELLFISH

Shellfish are naturally tender and need to be cooked for only a short time at moderate temperatures. If overcooked, they dry out and toughen.

Since each type of shellfish is different, cooking methods vary. The cooking method and the size of the shellfish influence cooking times. Lobsters and crabs are usually cooked in moist heat. They are often boiled or steamed. Some recipes call for boiling or steaming until partially done and then following up by grilling, baking, or broiling. Shrimp can be poached, baked, broiled, grilled, or fried. Mollusks can be steamed, poached, baked, or sautéed. Follow the instructions in the recipe you're using.

How can you tell when shellfish is done? The shells of crustaceans turn bright red, orange, or pink and the flesh becomes white and opaque. If mollusks are cooked in their shells, they're done when the shells open. Shucked mollusks become plump and opaque when cooked.

MICROWAVING METHODS

Microwaving is ideal for cooking fish and shellfish in moist heat. Cook small amounts at a time, preferably less than a pound, to make sure the flesh is thoroughly cooked. Place the fish or shellfish in a microwaveable dish. A sauce can be added for flavor. Cover with a lid or plastic wrap.

Because fish and shellfish are tender and the microwave oven cooks quickly, it's easy to overcook them. Remove from the oven when the outer edges are opaque and the center is still slightly translucent. Let stand for five minutes to complete the cooking; then check for doneness.

you need to be undisturbed. If you're easily distracted by the television, try turning it off, going to another room, or allowing yourself a limited amount of time for watching.

Some tasks might be delegated, or assigned to other people. The job is still your responsibility, however, so follow up to make sure it's done right.

Look for ways to combine or double up on tasks. You could plan what to pack for lunch while working out. Mowing the grass could count as a workout. As a precaution, however,

put this suggestion in perspective. Stress can come from trying to do too much. Everyone needs time for relaxation too.

Finally, accept that some things can't be done when or as well as you would like. Look for compromises. Remember that setting priorities starts with deciding what is genuinely important.

As your time management improves, beware of using "found" time to take on more jobs. The real benefits of sticking to your priorities are more energy, less stress, and better balance between work, family, and personal life.

Career Connection

Tools for prioritizing. Learn about the tools used to manage time and priorities in the workplace, such as day planners, erasable wall calendars, personal digital assistants (PDAs), and handheld organizers. Demonstrate how to use one of these items for the class.

Summarize Your Reading

▶ Although seafood technically refers to salt-water fish and shellfish, it is often used to cover freshwater fish and shellfish as well.

▶ Fish can be divided into two categories, low-fat fish and fatty fish. Shellfish can be divided into crustaceans and mollusks.

▶ Fish can be purchased in several different forms.

▶ Since fish is perishable, it needs to be refrigerated or frozen.

▶ Because fish is more tender than meat and poultry, it cooks much faster.

▶ Although fish cooks quickly, it must be checked for doneness before serving.

Check Your Knowledge

1. Why do nutrition experts recommend that people eat fish and shellfish?

2. How does mercury accumulate in large fish?

3. What is the difference between **fish** and **shellfish**?

4. How are **low-fat fish** and **fatty fish** different? Give examples of each.

5. Compare **crustaceans** and **mollusks**. Give examples of each.

6. What assurances do consumers have that fish and shellfish are safe to eat?

7. What should you note about the display when buying fish and shellfish?

8. Explain each of the following: a) **drawn**; b) **dressed**; c) **fillets**; d) **steaks**.

9. How do you judge quality when purchasing the following: a) fish; b) live clams, oysters, and mussels?

10. What should you notice when buying live lobster?

11. What should you do before using fish that is packed in oil?

12. How should you store fish after purchase?

13. How should you store live shellfish after purchase?

14. Why does fish flake?

15. What should you do to prepare fish before cooking it?

16. How do the following affect the cooking of fish: a) moist heat; b) dry heat; c) cooking temperature?

17. Why do you think the recipe, "Fish and Vegetables en Papillote," includes lemon juice?

18. Explain the 10-minute rule when cooking fish.

19. How would you broil a salmon fillet?

20. How do you prepare fish **en papillote**?

21. What is the basic difference between poaching and steaming fish?

22. How can you tell when shellfish is done?

23. **CRITICAL THINKING** Why do you think microwaving works well for cooking fish?

24. **CRITICAL THINKING** Which do you think are the most healthful ways to prepare fish and why?

Apply Your Learning

1. **MATH** **Cost per Serving.** Compare the cost per serving of various fish and shellfish. Based on your results, recommend how these foods can be economically included in an eating plan.

2. **SCIENCE** **Mercury.** Learn about mercury in the environment and report your findings. How harmful is mercury? How can mercury levels be reduced in waters?

3. **SOCIAL STUDIES** **Fishing Industry.** Research and report on the fishing industry. Where is it centered? What bodies of water are included? How is aquaculture involved? What issues are faced?

4. **SOCIAL STUDIES** **Eating Etiquette.** Learn the appropriate ways to eat such shellfish as lobster, crab legs, oysters, and clams. Teach these techniques to the class.

5. **Menu Ideas.** Create menus that include fish and shellfish. Choose recipes that focus on economy and ease of preparation.

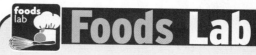

Foods Lab

Cooking Methods for Fish

Procedure: Choose two simple recipes for cooking a fish fillet, one that uses a moist-heat method and one that uses a dry-heat method. Obtain two low-fat fish fillets of the same type and prepare the two recipes. Be sure the fish is done in each recipe. Compare results.

Analyzing Results

❶ How did the fish look and taste after each recipe was prepared?
❷ Compare the effects of the two cooking methods.
❸ What do you conclude?
❹ What recommendations do you have for cooking fish?

Food Science Experiment

Evaluating Fish Doneness

Objective: To observe changes in fish flesh as it cooks and determine doneness.

Procedure:

1. Obtain an uncooked white fish fillet at least 1 inch thick. Determine its likely cooking time by measuring the thickest part of the fish. Record the appearance of the fish flesh, noting color and translucence or opaqueness.

2. Begin to cook the fillet in a skillet with a small amount of oil, using moderate heat.

3. At 2-minute intervals, examine the flesh of the fish. Use a fork to expose the flesh carefully for observation. Record your observations at each inspection, noting color, translucence or opaqueness, moisture, and flakiness. Turn the fish half way through cooking.

4. Record the time and condition when you believe the fish is done cooking. Continue cooking the fish for an additional 6 minutes. Continue to record your observations.

Analyzing Results

❶ What changes did you see as the fish cooked?
❷ How did you decide when the fish was done? Was timing accurate?
❸ What happened to the fish as it continued to cook after it was done?
❹ What do you conclude about cooking fish and determining doneness?

39 Beverages

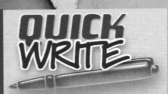

PARAPHRASING. To paraphrase is to restate something in different words. The ability to paraphrase concisely can help you take notes and learn new material. Paraphrasing can be done to shorten or add clarity. It might also be done to add interest or to be creative. Choose a paragraph from the chapter. Read it carefully. Then rewrite the ideas in the paragraph, using your own words.

To Guide Your Reading:

Objectives

- Identify types of beverages.
- Explain how various beverages fit into a healthy eating plan.
- Explain how to select and store beverages.
- Describe and demonstrate methods for preparing and serving beverages.

Terms

bloom
caffeine
carbonated
cocoa
cocoa butter
cocoa powder
coffee bean
decaffeinated coffee
fruit-flavored drinks
herb teas
juice
juice drinks
mulled
punch
smoothie
steep
tea

No meal seems complete without a beverage. Of course, many beverages are satisfying and refreshing by themselves. They are also an important source of fluid. If beverages are made with nutritious ingredients, they supply the nutrients in those foods. For example, fruit juices contain vitamins, minerals, and phytochemicals.

Some beverages are **carbonated**. In other words, they've been combined with carbon dioxide to make them bubbly. Many beverages contain **caffeine**, a natural stimulant that affects the nervous system, heart, and kidneys. Although caffeine isn't considered harmful, it produces unwanted side effects in some people. Coffee, tea, chocolate, cocoa, and cola drinks contain differing amounts of caffeine. **Fig. 39-1** shows the approximate amounts in certain beverages.

WATER

When you've worked up a good thirst, nothing beats a refreshing glass of cold water. Since water is one of the main nutrients needed by your body, it is one of the most healthful beverages to drink. Although tap water is readily available in most places, bottled water is also very popular. Of the two, tap water is probably more convenient, more

Fig. 39-1

How Much Caffeine?

Beverage	Approximate Amount of Caffeine
Coffee (8 oz.)	
Brewed	80–150 mg
Instant	65–100 mg
Decaffeinated	2–5 mg
Espresso (1.5–2 oz.)	60–140 mg
Tea (8 oz.)	
Brewed	40–100 mg
Instant	25–30 mg
Iced (12 oz.)	30–75 mg
Caffeinated soft drinks (12 oz.)	
Regular	40–60 mg
Diet	35–45 mg
High-energy drinks (12 oz.)	40-120 mg
Chocolate milk (8 oz.)	2–7 mg
Hot chocolate or cocoa (8 oz.)	3–10 mg

economical, and often the safest. Tap water must meet EPA regulations, while bottled water is subject to FDA standards that are not as strict.

If you like to carry bottled water with you, save money by buying several reusable sports bottles and filling them with tap water. You can add a little lemon juice, if you like, for flavor. To minimize the growth of harmful bacteria, wash the bottle thoroughly every day in hot sudsy water. Rinse well and let air dry.

Bottled Water

Several kinds of bottled water are sold.

- **Spring water.** This comes from underground formations.
- **Mineral water.** This water contains such minerals as calcium, magnesium, sodium, and bicarbonates.
- **Naturally sparkling water.** Often from a spring, this is naturally carbonated water.
- **Purified drinking water.** This water is processed to remove minerals and impurities. It is often made with ground water or tap water.
- **Enhanced water.** This may contain sugar, vitamins, minerals, and herbs.

When buying bottled water, read the label and cap carefully. Some bottled water is actually tap water, which may or may not have been treated further. If the bottled water comes from a tap, the label will say "from a municipal source or from a community water system."

If you're eating a wide variety of foods or taking multivitamin and mineral supplements, avoid enhanced water. It could lead to an overdose of nutrients, which may be harmful to your health.

Remember to recycle bottled water containers, but don't reuse them by refilling them with tap water. They are intended for one-time use only. Over time, the plastic could break down and develop cracks or leaks, allowing harmful bacteria to contaminate the water.

JUICES

Fruits and vegetables are converted into a wide array of beverages. Some contain all fruit or vegetable juice; others may have large amounts of added sugar and other ingredients. The label helps you determine how much actual juice a drink contains and whether or not it has been pasteurized.

To be labeled as a **juice**, a product must be 100 percent fruit or vegetable juice. The most common fruit juices are orange, apple, grape, pineapple, and grapefruit. Favorite vegetable juices include tomato, carrot, and mixed vegetables.

Juices contain all the nutrients found in fruits and vegetables except dietary fiber, and some are fortified with such nutrients as vitamins A and D and calcium. Some juices, however, are less nutritious than others. For example, apple and white grape juice are not as nutritious as orange juice.

Keep in mind that fruit juices are concentrated forms of fruit. As a result, even though fruit juices are nutritious, they are high in natural sugars and therefore high in calories. Choosing fresh fruits and vegetables more often than juices gives you nutrition without extra calories. See **Fig. 39-2**.

Juice drinks, also called "juice cocktail," contain about 10 to 50 percent juice. The remainder is water, sweeteners, flavorings, and other additives. The percentage of juice must be listed on the label.

Fruit-flavored drinks, although often fortified with vitamins and minerals, don't contain any juice. They are usually made with water, sweeteners, and flavorings that give a fruitlike flavor.

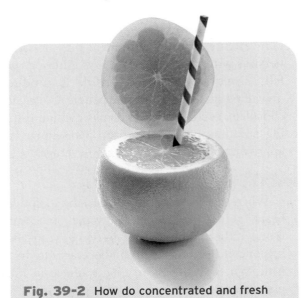

Fig. 39-2 How do concentrated and fresh juices compare?

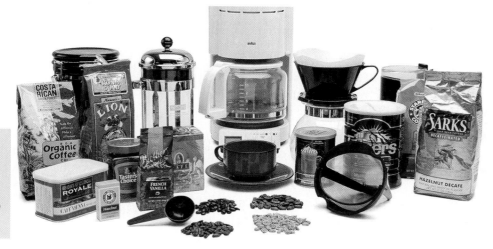

Fig. 39-3 High interest in coffee among consumers has brought a huge range of products to the market.

Buying Juices

Juices and drinks are available in the refrigerated section, in cans and bottles in grocery aisles, and as frozen concentrates. Some come in powdered form or as liquid concentrates, which must be reconstituted by adding water.

Juices must be pasteurized to destroy harmful bacteria. If a juice is not pasteurized, the label must carry a warning stating that it wasn't and may contain harmful bacteria that could cause serious illness.

Making Your Own Juice

It's easy to make your own juice with a juicer or blender. The simplest juicer is a hand-operated reamer, which extracts juice from such citrus fruits as oranges, grapefruits, and lemons. You can also buy electric juicers that turn almost any fruit or vegetable into juice.

COFFEE

People have been drinking coffee for centuries, and although many colorful tales surround its origins, Arabian people were the first to cultivate and trade it. As coffee spread throughout the world, coffee houses sprang up, dating back to the middle ages. They provided places for people to gather, drink coffee, and socialize. Eventually European colonists introduced coffee to the New World. Today the top coffee producers are Central and South America, Indonesia, Africa, and Hawaii. Coffee, in many flavor combinations, is widely consumed today. See **Fig. 39-3**.

Coffee is made from the **coffee bean**, actually the twin seeds of a deep-red fruit produced by the tropical coffee plant. See **Fig. 39-4**. The seeds are fermented, dried, and graded according to size. The beans are then roasted.

Two main types of coffee beans are used in coffee production. Arabica (uh-RA-buh-kuh) beans produce the finest flavor. Best grown in semitropical climates at high altitudes, they are often labeled "mountain-grown." In contrast, robusta (roh-BUHS-tuh) beans grow at low altitudes in tropical climates. They have less flavor than arabicas but twice as much caffeine. Supermarket coffees usually blend robusta varieties with a little arabica for flavor. Beans sold in specialty coffee shops are generally all arabica.

Hundreds of varieties of these two main beans exist. Usually the region where they are grown

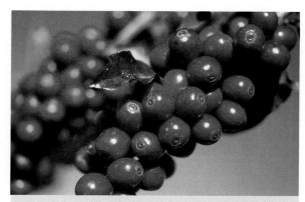

Fig. 39-4 Coffee trees produce berries that contain the beans used to make the beverage. Each berry contains two beans.

gives coffees their name, such as Colombian, Brazilian, or Mocha (after a town in Yemen on the Red Sea).

Buying and Storing Coffee

Coffee beans are roasted to bring out the flavor. The most popular roasts are these:

- **American or regular roast.** This medium roast produces a moderate flavor and color.
- **French roast.** This produces a stronger coffee with a dark color.
- **Italian roast.** This produces strongly flavored beans used to make espresso (eh-SPREH-soh) coffee. This strong coffee is made in a special coffeemaker that creates a thin layer of creamy foam on the surface of the coffee. Note that there is no *x* in espresso.

Coffee is sold as beans or already ground. You can have coffee beans ground to order where you buy them. The ground coffee is then poured into a paper bag. Since grinding the beans just before brewing ensures freshness, some people prefer to buy the beans and grind them themselves with a coffee grinder.

Ground coffee may be finely or coarsely ground. When finely ground, coffee has a greater surface area exposed to water. As a result, the water takes longer to run through the ground coffee as it brews. When coffee is coarsely ground, less surface area is exposed to water, and the water passes through the ground coffee more quickly.

The grind you select depends on the coffeemaker you have. Regular grind is recommended for electric coffeemakers and percolators. Choose drip grind for automatic drip coffeemakers. Fine grind is used in vacuum coffeemakers, but the drip grind may also be used. Ground coffee comes in cans of various sizes. The label shows the roast and grind, so check to find the right one for your coffeemaker.

Instant coffee is prepared coffee in powdered form. Only hot water needs to be added. One of the two available types is instant coffee powder, which is made by heat-drying freshly brewed coffee. Freeze-dried coffee is made from freshly brewed coffee that is first frozen and then dried. It's more expensive than coffee powder. Instant and freeze-dried coffees come in jars. **Decaffeinated coffee**, which has had the caffeine removed, is available in both ground and instant.

You can store unopened cans of vacuum-packed coffee at room temperature for about a year. Once opened, refrigerate fresh coffee, whether ground or whole beans, in an airtight container. Use within a week or freeze for longer storage. Instant coffee can be kept at room temperature. If you have purchased ground coffee in a paper bag, transfer it to an airtight container.

Making Coffee

The most-used appliance for making coffee is the automatic drip coffeemaker. Most automatic coffeemakers have four parts—a water reservoir, a basket that holds a filter and the coffee, a carafe (kuh-RAF) that catches the coffee as it brews, and a hot plate that keeps the carafe and coffee warm.

Automatic drip coffeemakers are easy to use. First, put the filter in the coffeemaker basket and place the ground coffee in the filter. Then fill the carafe with the amount of cold water needed and pour that into the reservoir. Set the carafe in place to catch the coffee, and turn on the controls. You can experiment with the amounts of water and coffee to get the strength you want. Usually 1 to 2 tablespoons are recommended per 6-ounce cup. Coffeemakers usually have convenient markings on the carafe or sides of the reservoir so that you can measure the water easily.

Coffee is enjoyed to its fullest when served piping hot, right after it's made. If held at a high temperature for too long, or reheated, coffee loses it flavor and aroma and may turn bitter. Some people like iced coffee. The coffee is made double strength and poured over ice cubes.

Clean the coffee carafe and basket in hot sudsy water after every use. Coffee contains oils that cling to the inside of the carafe and basket, and they can give the next batch of coffee an unpleasant flavor.

TEA

Although tea has been used as a beverage in China for centuries, it wasn't introduced in Europe until the early seventeenth century. Eventually it became the favored beverage among the British, who now drink three times as much tea as the Japanese. Tea is also a popular beverage all around the world, including such countries as Russia, India, and Morocco. Tea drinkers savor its soothing qualities, and studies show that it may have health benefits.

Buying and Storing Tea

Tea is made from the leaves of a shrub grown in tropical areas. See **Fig. 39-5**. The method of processing determines the variety of tea.

- **Black tea.** The leaves are fermented, then heated and dried, producing a dark brew with a well-developed flavor.
- **Green tea.** The leaves are steamed, rolled, and dried but not fermented. This produces a light, greenish-yellow tea with a slightly bitter flavor.
- **Oolong tea.** The leaves are partially fermented, resulting in a color and flavor between black and green teas.

Tea lovers have many options. Specialty teas, made from black tea, may be flavored with spices, jasmine blossoms, or such fruits as orange or lemon peel. See **Fig. 39-6** on page 550.

Tea contains caffeine, although not as much as coffee. It is also available decaffeinated.

Brewing Tea

Tea can be brewed in a pot or cup. An automatic hot tea maker works much the same way as

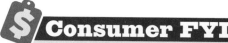

Consumer FYI

Tea and health. Can tea prevent cancer? Some studies suggest that. Black and green tea (though not herbals) contain antioxidants called polyphenols. Antioxidants, you'll recall, are substances that may protect cells from the normal wear of aging. This protection, it is thought, lowers the risk of some diseases. Laboratory tests and scientific surveys of tea drinkers suggest that polyphenols are especially effective against the growth of cancer tumors.

The findings are promising but not yet conclusive. While the latest research may not be reason enough to start a tea habit, it gives tea lovers one more reason to enjoy their favorite beverage.

automatic coffeemakers. After preheating the teapot and brewing the tea, this appliance holds the tea at serving temperature.

When brewing tea yourself, use a ceramic or glass teapot rather than metal. Pigments in tea react with metal to give a bitter flavor. They also create a light film over the surface of the tea. As you drink, the film clings to the inside of the cup.

Preheat the teapot or cup by rinsing it out with hot water. Then add the tea—1 teaspoon of tea or one tea bag for each serving. To make loose tea easier to use, put it in an infuser. This small con-

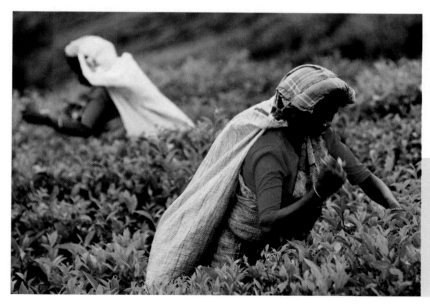

Fig. 39-5 The quality of tea varies, depending on where it's grown. The best teas come from tropical areas in high altitudes, with good soil and water. Tea leaves are picked by hand and processed into one of the three varieties.

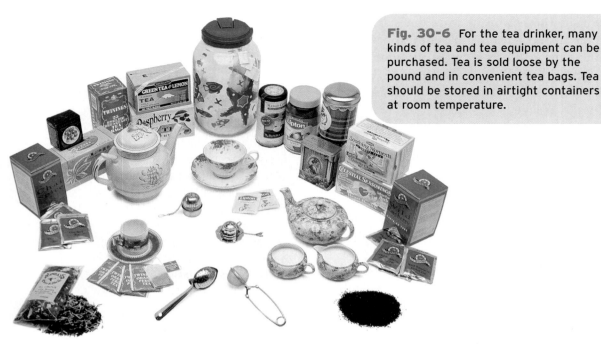

Fig. 30-6 For the tea drinker, many kinds of tea and tea equipment can be purchased. Tea is sold loose by the pound and in convenient tea bags. Tea should be stored in airtight containers at room temperature.

tainer has tiny holes that let water in without allowing the tea leaves to float out into the water. Like tea bags, the infuser is easy to remove at the end of the brewing time.

For black or oolong tea, heat fresh, cold water in a teakettle to a rolling boil. Pour the boiling water over the tea and let the tea **steep**, or brew, in the hot water for about 3 to 5 minutes, depending on the kind of tea and the strength you prefer. If you like strong tea, use more tea rather than lengthen the steeping time. Tea becomes bitter when cooked.

The method for making green tea is a little different. The water should be close to, but not at, the boiling point. Steep green tea for a shorter time than other teas, usually about 1½ minutes. If you use boiling water or allow the tea to steep longer, it turns bitter.

The color of brewed tea does not necessarily indicate strength. Some varieties have a light color and strong flavor; others brew to a very dark color that has a light flavor.

Stir tea before pouring or drinking to be sure it's uniformly strong. If the brewed tea is too strong, you can add a little hot water. Tea may be served with sweetener and milk or lemon.

To make iced tea, brew as for hot tea but use 50 percent more tea. For example, put 9 teaspoons of tea in the pot to get six servings. This allows for ice that melts when hot tea is poured into ice-filled glasses. After brewing, remove the tea from the pot and pour over ice, stirring until chilled. To prevent tea from turning cloudy, cool it to room temperature before refrigerating. Adding a little boiling water may remove cloudiness.

To make spiced tea, add 6 to 8 whole cloves and a cinnamon stick to the teapot when you add the tea.

Herb Teas

Herb teas are made not from tea leaves but from the flowers, leaves, seeds, and roots of herbs and other plants. They are caffeine-free. Although usually sold in tea bags, they may be purchased loose. Some well-liked herb teas include mint, chamomile (KA-muh-meel), and lemon verbena (vuhr-BEE-nuh). Many packaged teas are blends.

To brew herb tea, use 1 tea bag or 1 teaspoon loose tea for each cup of boiling water. Let steep for no more than 5 minutes. If brewed too long, the tea becomes bitter. Herb tea can be flavored with lemon or honey.

For some people, certain plants used in herb teas can cause allergic reactions. Buy herb teas only from reliable sources. Most supermarkets carry major brands. Avoid teas that make health claims, such as weight loss.

DAIRY-BASED BEVERAGES

Since milk provides protein, calcium, phosphorus, and vitamins D and A, it's a wholesome beverage by itself. As a special treat, you can make beverages that combine milk, yogurt, or other dairy products with fruit or flavorings. These beverages are delicious and also contain the nutrients of milk; however, they may have more sugar, fat, and calories.

Smoothies

A **smoothie** is a blend of milk or yogurt and fresh fruit, as in the recipe in **Fig. 39-7**. You can also add such other foods as peanut butter, wheat germ, or pieces of candied ginger. Ice is sometimes added to chill and thicken the mixture, but too much melting ice can dilute the smoothie. Instead of ice, an alternative is to freeze the fruit first or use commercially frozen fruit.

Smoothies are not only nutritious but also versatile. They're quick and easy to make for a snack or a quick breakfast.

Almost any fruit works in a smoothie. Try combining several fruits. Which of these sounds most appealing to you: kiwifruit and honeydew melon; bananas, strawberries, and frozen orange juice concentrate; or bananas and peanut butter?

To make a smoothie, you need a blender. Small fruits like berries and pitted cherries can be put in the blender whole. Cut larger fruits—cantaloupe, bananas, and peaches, for example—into chunks. Use about $3\frac{1}{2}$ cups of fruit for every cup of liquid.

Pour milk or yogurt into the blender and add the fruit. If you're not using frozen fruit, add a little ice or frozen fruit juice concentrate to chill and thicken the mixture. Blend just until the fruit is puréed and the mixture is thick. Serve immediately. If you wish, garnish with fruit slices.

Hot Chocolate and Cocoa

Long ago in ancient civilizations, people harvested cacao (kuh-KAY-oh) beans, the seeds in pods on cacao trees. Upon grinding the beans, they produced a liquid called chocolate. For many

---

Fig. 39-7

Try This! Recipe

Strawberry Yogurt Splendor

Yield	Nutrition Analysis
8 servings	**Per Serving:** 90 calories, 1.5 g total fat, 0.5 g saturated fat, 0 g trans fat, 5 mg cholesterol, 45 mg sodium, 18 g total carbohydrate, 3 g dietary fiber, 12 g sugars, 4 g protein
	Percent Daily Value: vitamin A 2%, vitamin C 100%, calcium 15%, iron 2%

Ingredients

4 cups sliced strawberries, plus
  additional for garnish
2 cups yogurt, plain or vanilla
2 bananas, peeled and sliced

16 ice cubes
1 vanilla bean, slit and insides
  scraped
Sliced strawberries for garnish

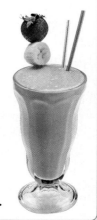

Directions

1. In a food processor or blender, combine the strawberries, yogurt, banana, ice cubes, and vanilla.
2. Process until smooth.
3. Pour into glasses and garnish each serving with fresh strawberries. Serve immediately.

Variation: Use other fruits, such as peaches or kiwifruit, in place of strawberries.

centuries this liquid was the basis for chocolate beverages. In the 1700s English chocolate houses, much like coffee houses, provided places to enjoy the beverage.

During the nineteenth century, people learned to separate a fat called **cocoa butter** from the chocolate liquid, leaving solids known as **cocoa powder**. This opened the door to making many chocolate products besides beverages.

Today people enjoy two tasty beverages that contain chocolate and milk. One is hot chocolate, made with solid, unsweetened chocolate. To make it, you combine chopped, unsweetened chocolate with milk in a saucepan. This is stirred constantly over low heat until the chocolate melts. Sugar and a pinch of salt are added. The mixture simmers for a few minutes without boiling. Cocoa butter adds richness to this beverage.

The other beverage is hot cocoa. It's made with **cocoa**, a product of cocoa powder. Since it has less fat, the cocoa blends easily with hot liquid and is less likely to separate than solid chocolate. Cocoa comes in different forms—powder, syrup, and sweetened instant. The powder and syrup forms are mixed with milk. Instant cocoa mixes are combined with milk or water to make hot and cold beverages.

To make hot cocoa, use 1 tablespoon cocoa, 1 tablespoon sugar, and 1 cup of milk for one serving. In a saucepan, mix the cocoa with sugar first for a smooth mixture. Gradually add the milk, stirring well, and cook over low heat. Stir constantly until bubbles appear at the sides, but don't boil. Using a double boiler prevents scorching.

Cocoa and chocolate should be stored in a cool, dry place in original containers. Cocoa usually keeps better than chocolate. If stored in a hot area, chocolate may show patches of white, called **bloom**. This is cocoa butter that has come to the surface. Flavor is unaffected.

Chocolate beverages may be served plain or topped with marshmallows, whipped cream, or ground nutmeg. Add flavor by stirring with a cinnamon stick. To make mocha, substitute brewed coffee for the milk.

Career Prep

A Positive Attitude

"LOOK ON THE BRIGHT SIDE." WHEN you have a problem, this old advice may not sound very helpful—and it isn't by itself. By combining a positive attitude with problem-solving skills, however, you create a winning combination. A positive attitude is an asset in everyday living, whether you have a problem or not. It can help you build strong relationships at home, with friends, and on the job.

A positive attitude sees the best in others. It isn't scornful or hateful. It's reflected in what you say and how you act. Having a positive attitude makes taking positive action possible. Consider these benefits:

- **A focus on assets.** Looking at what you have instead of what you lack can reveal a solution that otherwise remains hidden. One teen who planned to be a chef was frustrated at not finding a job in a restaurant. She decided to offer her skills as a soup kitchen volunteer instead. There she learned much about kitchen management and nutrition—and social responsibility as well.

- **A sense of humor.** Looking at the light side helps keep difficulties in perspective. It saves you from spending too much time and mental energy on one problem at the expense of solving others. You may discover that some things aren't worth the worry.

- **Good relations.** Do you like being around people who are continually complaining? Co-workers, friends, and family members—those

PUNCH

A **punch** is generally a mixture of fruit juices and tea or a carbonated beverage such as ginger ale or seltzer water. Sherbet, ice cream, or fruit may be added. To serve the punch, ladle it from the bowl into small glasses or cups.

If you are serving punch cold, combine all liquids except the carbonated beverage ahead of time and chill well. Chill the unopened carbonated beverage separately and add just before serving the punch. If added too early, the carbonation is lost.

Punch may also be **mulled**, or served hot and flavored with such spices as cinnamon, nutmeg, or cloves. This is a delicious way to serve cider.

SOFT DRINKS

Soft drinks—carbonated beverages—have wide appeal. They have few nutrients, if any, and are best consumed sparingly. Many are available with and without caffeine and sugar.

Flavored soft drinks are made with water and additives that may include artificial flavorings and colorings, sweeteners, acidifiers for tartness, and sodium. Diet soft drinks are made with sugar substitutes. Cola beverages contain caffeine.

Club soda is carbonated water with added salts and minerals. Seltzer water is carbonated water with no added salts.

MICROWAVING BEVERAGES

Beverages can be prepared and reheated in the microwave oven. Always stir them before placing in the oven. When a beverage stands for even a short time, it develops a very smooth surface that acts almost like a film or skin. When you stir it, you break up the film. If you heat a beverage without stirring it, the smooth surface could keep steam from escaping and allow it to build up, causing the beverage to spurt out of the container.

---

individuals who are best able to help—are more inclined to support someone who acts hopeful about finding a solution. In contrast, spreading gloom and anger to co-workers and customers only creates another problem.

- **The unexpected answer.** You may have heard stories about the waitress who treats a shabby-looking customer with kindness and respect

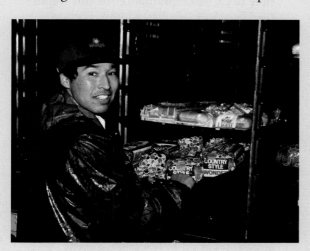

and is later rewarded when the customer turns out to be a millionaire. Tales like that may belong in the movies, but they're based on a truth. When you stay positive and cheerful, you open yourself to others and their needs. They, in turn, can open doors to a world of possibilities.

- **A better alternative.** Even if it brings no practical benefit, a positive attitude makes life more enjoyable for you and for others. It helps you cope with the relatively few things that go wrong and helps you appreciate all the things that go right. Can you say that about a negative attitude?

Career Connection

Finding examples. Interview workers to find real-life examples of how a positive attitude improved a difficult situation on the job. Compile these stories to create a class bulletin board.

Summarize Your Reading

▶ Beverages come in many variations. Depending on their ingredients, they may contribute nutrients to the diet. On the other hand, some contribute little more than sugar.

▶ Some beverages are served hot, and others are served cold.

▶ Water is one of the most healthful beverages to drink.

▶ You need to read labels on beverages in order to learn about the contents. Too much caffeine can produce unwanted side effects. Too much sugar adds calories that can contribute to weight gain.

▶ Coffee, tea, and cocoa have been consumed by people for many centuries.

▶ To create new beverages with interesting flavors, you can blend beverages.

Check Your Knowledge

1. What are **carbonated** beverages?

2. Compare the **caffeine** in coffee, tea, caffeinated soft drinks, high-energy drinks, chocolate milk, and cocoa.

3. Compare tap water with bottled water.

4. Why should you avoid enhanced water if you're taking multivitamin and mineral supplements?

5. How do **juice**, **juice drinks**, and **fruit-flavored drinks** differ?

6. Why is juice pasteurized?

7. How can you make watermelon juice with a blender?

8. What is the difference between arabica and robusta **coffee beans**?

9. Describe American, French, and Italian coffee bean roasts.

10. How do fine and coarse grinds affect coffee preparation?

11. What is **decaffeinated coffee**?

12. How do you make coffee using an automatic drip coffeemaker?

13. How are black, green, and oolong **teas** different?

14. How does making green tea differ from making black tea?

15. What precaution should be taken when buying **herb teas**?

16. **CRITICAL THINKING** Why do you think **cocoa**, coffee, and tea have been popular beverages throughout history?

17. How do you make a **smoothie**?

18. What is the difference between hot chocolate and hot cocoa?

19. What is **punch**?

20. Describe **mulled** punch.

21. **CRITICAL THINKING** Statistics show Americans consume more carbonated beverages than ever before. What are some possible negative consequences of this trend?

22. Why should beverages be stirred before heating in a microwave oven?

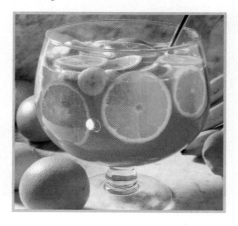

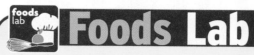

Apply Your Learning

1. **Caffeine.** Research and report on caffeine in the diet. What concerns have been raised about caffeine and pregnancy?

2. **MATH Cost and Quality.** Compare the cost per ounce and nutritional quality of several beverages. Include milk, juices, soft drinks, and coffee beverages. Chart your results and make recommendations.

3. **Label Check.** Read labels on "fruit" beverages. Study the ingredients and the statements on the labels. What do you conclude?

4. **SOCIAL STUDIES High Tea.** Research "high tea," which was enjoyed in Victorian England. Invite someone to your house or classroom for high tea. How will the tea be prepared? What variety of tea will you serve? What foods will be served with the tea?

5. **Punch Preparation.** Choose a punch recipe. Make and serve it at a school function or for the class. Evaluate the results.

Foods Lab

Smoothie Recipes

Procedure: Develop a recipe for a smoothie. Consider ways to make your smoothie unique. How could you add extra nutrition? Prepare and evaluate your smoothie. Offer samples for a taste test and sample the recipes made by different lab groups.

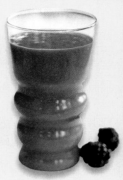

Analyzing Results

❶ How did your smoothie turn out in appearance, texture, and taste?
❷ Calculate the nutritional value of one 8-oz. serving of your smoothie.
❸ What modifications would you make in your recipe?

Food Science Experiment

Solar Water Purifier

Objective: To harness solar power to purify water.

Procedure:

1. Measure 1 cup of water into a clean, dry bowl with high sides. Add 1 teaspoon of salt and stir to dissolve. Use a clean spoon to taste the water. Record your observation.

2. Place a short glass in the center of the bowl. The rim of the glass must be below the rim of the bowl.

3. Cover the bowl with plastic wrap so that the bowl rim is completely sealed but the plastic is slightly loose.

4. Place a rock or similar weight in the center of the plastic so that it forms a funnel-shape

just above the glass but without touching the glass.

5. Leave the bowl in a sunny spot for several hours or the rest of the day. Then examine the bowl.

Analyzing Results

❶ What changes have occurred?
❷ Taste a small sample of the water inside and outside the glass. What difference can you taste?
❸ Based on the results you described in questions 1 and 2, identify the process that was at work. How did it affect the water?
❹ In what situations or parts of the world would this technology be especially useful? Why would it be so useful?

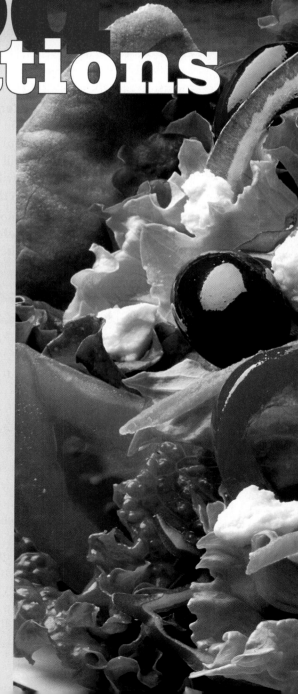

UNIT 8

Food Combinations

CHAPTER 40   **Sandwiches & Pizza**

CHAPTER 41   **Salads & Dressings**

CHAPTER 42   **Stir-Fries & Casseroles**

CHAPTER 43   **Soups, Stews & Sauces**

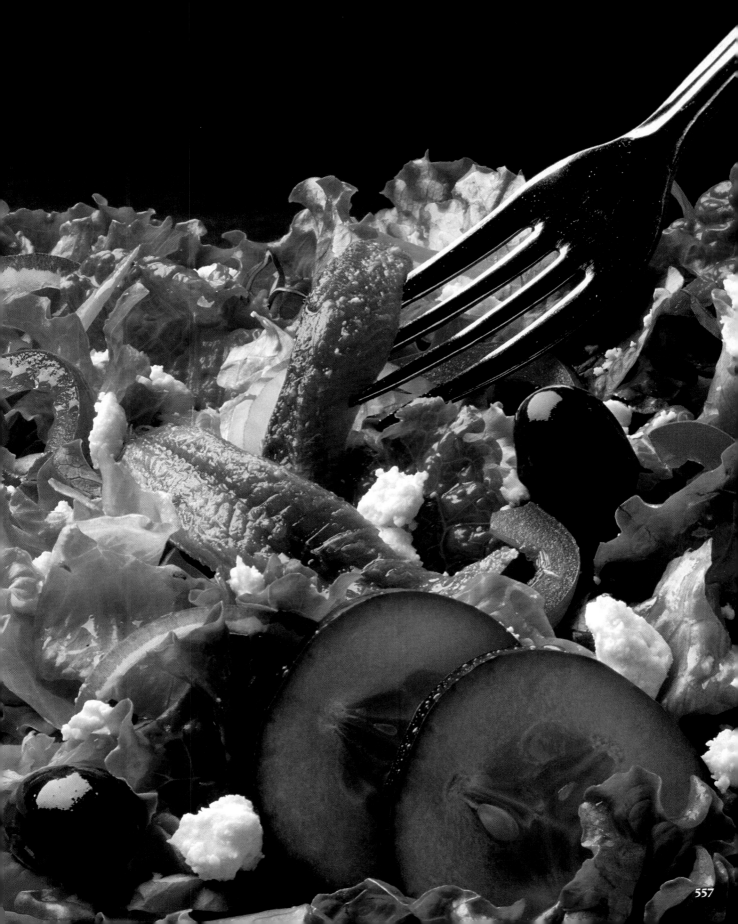

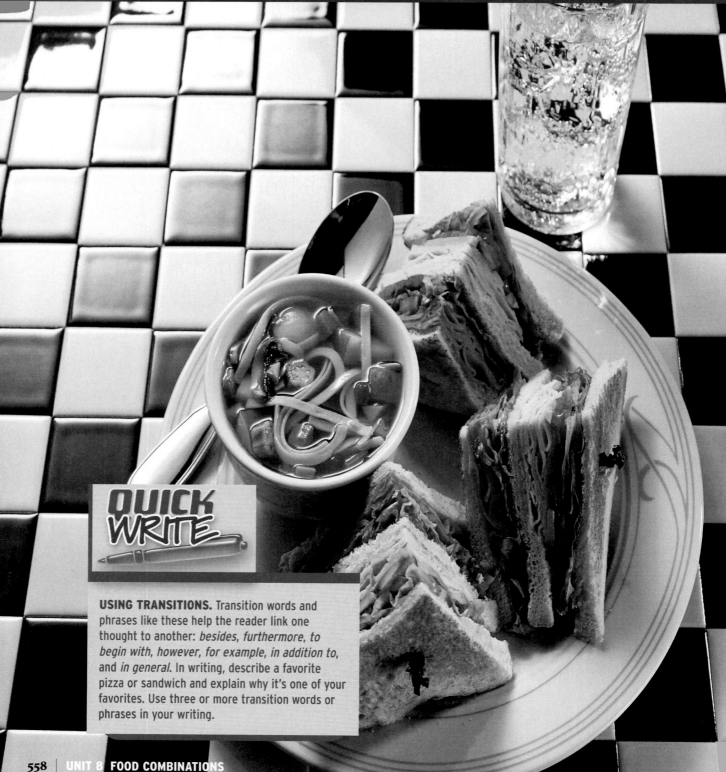

QUICK WRITE

USING TRANSITIONS. Transition words and phrases like these help the reader link one thought to another: *besides, furthermore, to begin with, however, for example, in addition to,* and *in general.* In writing, describe a favorite pizza or sandwich and explain why it's one of your favorites. Use three or more transition words or phrases in your writing.

Objectives

▶ Compare types of sandwiches.

▶ Suggest ingredients for sandwich fillings.

▶ Describe and demonstrate how to make different sandwiches.

▶ Describe how to make pizzas.

Terms

basic sandwich	lahvosh
calzone	open-face sandwich
club sandwich	pita
fajitas	pizza sandwich
falafel	tea sandwich
focaccia	tortilla
guacamole	wrap
gyro	
hero	

JOHN MONTAGU, THE FOURTH EARL OF Sandwich, was intent on his game of cards one day around 1762, too involved to even stop to eat. Instead, he had his servant bring a piece of salt beef between two pieces of bread. The hand-held meal allowed him to play uninterrupted—and without getting grease on the cards. Impressed, his friends declared, "We'll have the same as Sandwich!" That, according to legend, is how the sandwich got its name.

While the Earl may have contributed the name, the sandwich itself was not his invention. Some 2,000 years ago, the Jewish people began a Passover custom of eating chopped apples, nuts, and other symbolic ingredients between two pieces of unleavened bread. Even then, the bread-and-filling concept in some form was already familiar in other civilizations.

Wrapped, rolled, or layered into a tidy bundle, the sandwich may be the original fast food. Convenience is still one of its advantages today, but culinary innovators have also taken the sandwich, literally, to new heights.

WHAT IS A SANDWICH?

As you've just seen, a **sandwich** is filling between slices of bread. In contrast to this short definition, the sandwich has many variations. A sandwich can be a simple combination, quickly assembled and ideal for packed lunches and picnics. It can also be an elaborate main dish that's prepared in an oven and eaten with a knife and fork. It's no wonder that the sandwich is one of the best-liked foods in the United States, especially as each cultural group has added its specialty to the table.

Nutrition Connection

Nutrition checkup. A sandwich is as nutritious as the foods that go into it. Read Nutrition Facts panels and ingredient lists to compare the fat, sodium, and sugar content of different bread and filling choices. If a spread is high in fat and calories, balance it with a low-fat filling. Look for fresh foods with less processing, including whole-wheat and multigrain breads.

 How does one of your favorite sandwiches fare nutritionally?

Basic Sandwiches

The **basic sandwich** (like the one the Earl enjoyed) consists of just two slices of bread with a filling in between. It is always served cold. The inside is often thinly coated with a fat-based spread, such as butter, margarine, mayonnaise, or cream cheese. The fat adds flavor and keeps moist fillings from soaking into the bread. It also helps hold the filling in place.

While a basic sandwich is simple to make, there are still guidelines for making one successfully.

- Start with firm bread that is easy to cut, handle, and eat. Options include whole wheat, multi-grain, rye, and sourdough. You can also use hard rolls, bagels, English muffins, and sandwich buns and rolls. Soft breads can be toasted first to add body.
- If you prefer the fluffy texture of soft breads, choose a firm filling. If the filling is soft, spread it carefully to avoid squashing the bread.
- If you plan to use butter, margarine, or cream cheese, soften it to room temperature for easier spreading. You can also use whipped varieties.
- Put the filling on one slice of bread only. To make cutting and eating neater, use several thin slices of meat or cheese rather than one thick slice. For soft, chunky fillings like egg salad or baked beans, spread thinly just to the edge of the bread to keep them from oozing out.
- Add condiments, such as mustard, pickles, tomato slices, and lettuce, just before eating or serving the sandwich. If added too early, they can make the bread soggy.
- Use a sharp, serrated knife to cut sandwiches without smashing or tearing.

For filling a sandwich, the first ingredient that comes to mind is often cold cuts. You can use almost any food, however, including tuna, shrimp, chicken, or egg salad; cheeses; cooked or raw vegetables; baked tofu; and even leftovers. **Fig. 40-1** uses black olives to make a sandwich spread.

Club Sandwich

A **club sandwich** is an expanded basic sandwich made with three slices of toasted bread and

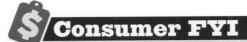

Consumer FYI

Creative condiments. To reduce the fat and sodium of some store-bought condiments, add fresh and flavorful ingredients to create your own blends. Try mixing mustard with cranberry relish, honey, or maple syrup for a sweet-and-sour tang. For extra heat, blend mustard with a little salsa or horseradish.

Mayonnaise's mild flavor lends itself to a variety of cooking styles. Stir in Parmesan cheese and powdered garlic for an Italian seasoning or chili powder for a taste of the Southwest. A dash of low-sodium soy sauce and ginger gives an Asian flair.

Are you considering catsup? Add a few drops of liquid smoke or hot sauce to create a customized barbecue flavor. Toss with chunks of tomato, chopped onion, and diced pepper to make a garden vegetable medley.

two layers of different fillings. The classic club has mayonnaise, lettuce, tomato, bacon, and turkey, but you can mix and match ingredients to suit your taste. For example, ham, mustard, and Swiss cheese could be one layer, with sliced roast chicken and tomatoes as the next. See **Fig. 40-2**.

To keep the layers stacked while cutting, secure them with four wooden picks placed in the four corners about an inch from the crust. Cut the sandwich in halves or quarters. Cutting diagonally provides triangular sections. Place the picks accordingly. For a garnish, spear olives or thickly sliced pickle onto the wooden picks.

Open-Face Sandwich

You can take a different approach by making an **open-face sandwich**, which has just one slice of bread and a topping. Most any filling can be used, but the bread should be firm enough to support it.

Heroes

If you and a friend decide to share a sandwich in an area sandwich shop, do you order a hoagie, sub, grinder, poor boy, or muffeletta? As a filling, do you ask for meatballs, corned beef and pastrami, or fried shrimp? Your choices depend on

Fig. 40-1

Italian Sandwiches

Yield	Nutrition Analysis
4 servings	*Per Serving:* 250 calories, 12 g total fat, 5 g saturated fat, 0 g trans fat, 15 mg cholesterol, 770 mg sodium, 24 g total carbohydrate, 2 g dietary fiber, 3 g sugars, 12 g protein
	Percent Daily Value: vitamin A 6%, vitamin C 4%, calcium 30%, iron 15%

Ingredients

1 cup black olives, pitted and drained
2 cloves garlic, peeled
2 tsp. olive oil
2 tsp. lemon zest

1 Tbsp. capers, or more, drained
4 slices mozzarella cheese
8 slices white bread

Directions

1. To make a spread, place olives and garlic in a blender or food processor. Process to desired texture, either coarse or smooth, adding enough olive oil to make the mixture dense.
2. Scrape the spread into a clean bowl. Mix in lemon zest and at least 1 Tbsp. of capers. Capers are the tiny, pungent, pickled buds of a shrub native to the Mediterranean.
3. Cover the bowl and refrigerate.
4. Slice the mozzarella cheese.
5. Place bread slices flat and trim off crusts. For each sandwich, put the spread on both slices of bread. Add cheese to one slice of bread and top with the other spread-covered bread.

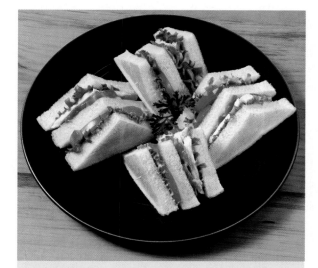

Fig. 40-2 A club sandwich is a common item on many restaurant menus. It is often cut into triangular shapes. How could you hold the layers together?

where you live. These are all regional variations of a **hero**, a very large sandwich made on a loaf of Italian or French bread or a large hard roll. The sandwiches are layered with an assortment of thinly sliced, cooked and cured meats and cheeses and seasoned to taste with onions, peppers, mushrooms, and olives. The spread is usually mayonnaise or salad dressing.

Your own hero recipe is limited only by your imagination and the food in your refrigerator. You can make a Tex-Mex hero with leftover chili, chopped onions, tomatoes, and Cheddar cheese. Try a fruit salad hero with any fruit on hand: whole berries or sliced bananas, kiwifruit, pears, or cantaloupe. Stick the fruit onto a thin layer of peanut butter, top with yogurt, and then sprinkle with nuts, wheat germ, or granola.

Unlike the basic sandwich, some heroes improve with "aging." Wrap the hero tightly in foil or plastic and refrigerate for up to four hours to let the flavors blend.

Wraps

Breads don't need to be thick and spongy to hold a filling. The world's oldest and most popular breads are flat. Sandwiches made by wrapping or rolling a filling in flatbread are descriptively called **wraps** or rollups. These sandwiches have been known for thousands of years, from the Mediterranean to Mexico. Several flatbreads, and their sandwich-making possibilities, have found their way into meals in the United States.

Pita

Pita, which originated in the Middle East, is a round, leavened flatbread that can be used to make a rollup. Since it forms a pocket when split, it's also called pocket bread. Pita comes in different sizes and types, including whole wheat.

To make a rollup, spread a filling down the center of a pita or over the entire bread, leaving about 1 inch free around the edges. Fold one side partially over the filling and roll the other side over to close the pita. For easier and neater handling, wrap the roll in foil. Peel back the foil as you eat the sandwich.

To use the pita's pocket, cut the bread in half. Gently pull apart the two sides at the cut end to form a pocket. This method makes two sandwiches. As an alternative, you can partially slit a whole pita along the seam to make one large pocket.

A favorite Middle Eastern filling for pita is **falafel** (fuh-LAH-fuhl). These small, deep-fried patties are made with highly seasoned, ground garbanzo beans. Several falafel are placed in each pocket, along with pickled vegetables and hummus, a spread made with mashed, cooked garbanzo beans and ground sesame seeds. Another filler idea is chopped vegetable salad, which combines such chopped foods as fresh mint, tomatoes, bell pepper, radishes, onion, celery, and lettuce, as well as shredded cheese. Use yogurt as the dressing.

A **gyro** (YEE-roh) is a Greek specialty made with minced roasted lamb, grilled onions, sweet peppers, and a cucumber-yogurt sauce, all wrapped in a pita.

Lahvosh

Lahvosh (LAH-vohsh) is an Armenian flatbread that is larger and thinner than pita. It's available crisp or soft and in various flavors, such as spinach. The soft version is used for wraps and pockets. Since it doesn't have its own pocket, you can spread on the filling and then fold the bottom up and the sides over.

Tortillas

A Mexican staple, the **tortilla** (tawr-TEE-yuh) is a thin, round, unleavened flatbread made with either corn or wheat flour and baked on a griddle. Like the pita, this bread is the base for several different sandwiches. A tortilla rolled around a filling is called a burrito. Folded in half, a tortilla forms a soft-shell taco. For a crisper wrap, heat the tortilla for a few minutes in a 400°F oven before filling. You can also deep-fry them briefly and fold them immediately so they hold their shape, or you can buy taco shells ready to use. See **Fig. 40-3**.

In the traditional style, tortillas are filled with combinations of chopped, cooked meat or poultry, refried beans, sour cream, shredded cheese, chopped lettuce and tomatoes, and salsa. Some tastes, however, could run from peanut butter and honey to spinach and cheese sauce.

Fajitas (fuh-HEE-tuhs) are made with grilled meat or poultry that is rolled up in a warm tortilla. They are generally served with other foods to mix in: refried beans, salsa, and **guacamole** (gwah-kuh-MOH-lee), a Mexican dish made with mashed avocados, lemon or lime juice, and seasonings.

Hot Sandwiches

You can also turn almost any sandwich into a hot sandwich by warming it in a conventional, microwave, or toaster oven. You can also press the sandwich in a waffle maker brushed with oil or sprayed with cooking spray. To keep any fresh vegetables or fruits from wilting, add them after heating.

When you microwave a sandwich, wrap it in a paper towel first. The towel absorbs extra moisture. Time will vary according to the sandwich, but usually 30 seconds or less on high is enough.

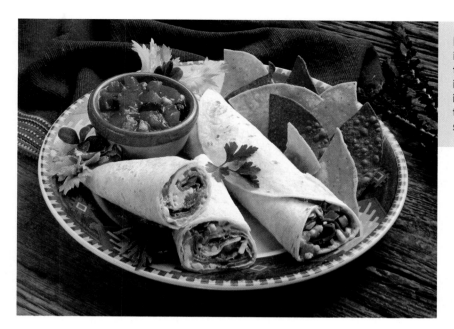

Fig. 40-3 Tortilla bread is very versatile. Here this unleavened flatbread is rolled around the ingredients. How else can tortillas be used to make sandwiches?

For certain sandwiches, cooking is part of the recipe. In some, only the filling is hot. In others, the whole sandwich is grilled.

Cooked Fillings

You may not think of hot dogs and hamburgers as sandwiches, yet they are the most popular cooked sandwiches in the United States. Served on a bun or roll, they can be topped with condiments ranging from the standard ketchup, mustard, and pickles to sauerkraut, salsa, or chutney. Chutney is a sauce from India made with fruits, sugar, vinegar, and spices.

Hot dogs are already cooked but should be heated until steaming for safety. Topped with chili and cheese, they become chili dogs.

The traditional hamburger is a ground beef patty seasoned with salt and pepper, but ground poultry is an alternative. See **Fig. 40-4**. To cook the patty by broiling or grilling, make it at least 1 inch thick. Make it thinner to pan-broil or sauté. For a cheeseburger, top the cooked patty with the sliced cheese of your choice and remove from the heat when the cheese starts to melt.

In a barbecue sandwich, flavor comes in liquid form. Shredded pork or sliced roast beef is heated in a tangy, tomato-based sauce that is seasoned with onions and garlic and sweetened with brown sugar or molasses. For a Sloppy Joe, ground beef is cooked loose-style with chopped onions, chili

sauce, ketchup, Worcestershire sauce, and various spices, according to the cook's tastes. The mixture is "slopped" over a split bun. These and other substantial hot sandwiches may be served open-face and eaten with a knife and fork—and plenty of napkins.

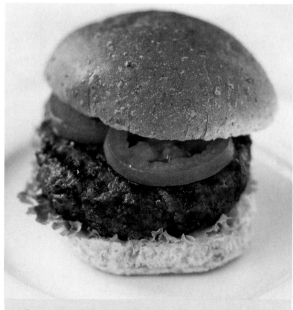

Fig. 40-4 You can liven up hamburgers by seasoning the meat mixture with herbs, dry mustard, chopped onions and bell pepper, bacon bits, and grated cheese. How could you add spice?

Meat is not the only hot filling for sandwiches. Scrambled eggs on toast or an English muffin is a natural pairing. If you scramble the egg with diced ham, chopped onion, and bell pepper, you have a Western or Denver sandwich.

Hot vegetarian fillings are another choice. You can pan-broil patties made of cooked, mashed beans or lentils. Add egg, breadcrumbs, cooked grains, ground nuts, or peanut butter for flavor, body, and nutrition. Explore the increasing variety of frozen soy burgers on the market, or invent your own from textured soy protein (TSP). Try a barbecue sandwich with crumbled tofu.

Grilled Sandwiches

Not every "grilled" sandwich is grilled. Some have grilled fillings—grilled chicken, for example. In contrast, a true grilled sandwich is made by sautéing the filled bread. See **Fig. 40-5**.

To grill a sandwich, first spread both slices of bread on the outside with softened butter or margarine, or melt a little butter or margarine in a heavy skillet. Assemble the sandwich and sauté on both sides until nicely browned. If the filling includes cheese, sauté until the cheese is just melted. Cut the sandwich in half for easier eating.

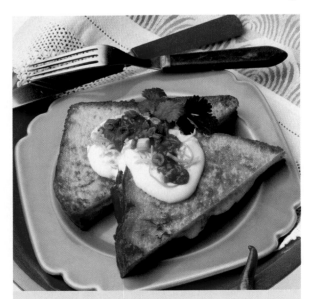

Fig. 40-5 A Monte Cristo sandwich is typically made with ham, chicken or turkey, and Swiss cheese. It is dipped in a mixture of beaten egg, milk, and salt and then sautéed in butter.

To keep butter off your hands and the cutting board, you can carefully build the sandwich right in the skillet. Put one slice of bread in the skillet, buttered side down. Add the filling, top with the other slice, buttered side up, and grill.

Grilling has produced many sandwich favorites. Grilled cheese is enjoyed by children and adults alike. Adding sliced tomatoes, crisp cooked bacon, or thinly sliced ham before grilling makes a heartier dish. In a Reuben sandwich, a stack of thinly sliced corned beef, sauerkraut, and sliced Swiss cheese is pressed between rye bread that is spread with Russian or Thousand Island dressing.

Broiled Sandwiches

Many sandwiches that can be grilled can also be broiled. Place the sandwich on the broiler pan and brush with oil or melted butter or margarine. Broil until lightly browned. Turn the sandwich over and repeat with the other side, or sprinkle the second side with grated cheese and broil until the cheese melts.

Open-face sandwiches called melts are also made in the broiler. Top the filling with sliced or shredded cheese to keep it from drying out. Broil just long enough to melt the cheese. If you want any ingredients to stay crisp, add them afterward. You can make a tuna melt, tomato melt, and even a peanut butter melt. For variety, build a broiled sandwich on **focaccia** (foh-KAH-chee-uh), a round, herbed, Italian bread that is brushed with olive oil. **Fig. 40-6** has another idea for a broiled sandwich that uses pizza ingredients.

Tea Sandwiches

The name "tea sandwich" may make you think of people in fancy clothes nibbling dainty sandwiches at a formal affair, yet tea sandwiches can make any gathering more festive. **Tea sandwiches**, also called finger sandwiches, are small, attractive, cold sandwiches often served at receptions and parties.

In tea sandwiches, appearance means as much as taste. You should allow six to eight sandwiches per guest, depending on what else will be served. Each sandwich is a chance to show your creativity in choosing shapes and fillings. Remember, however, that neatness counts too—people at parties want to focus on socializing, not eating.

Fig. 40-6

Pizza Snacks

Yield	Nutrition Analysis
4 servings	**Per Serving:** 80 calories, 2.5 g total fat, 1 g saturated fat, 0 g trans fat, 5 mg cholesterol, 210 mg sodium, 11 g total carbohydrate, 2 g dietary fiber, 2 g sugars, 6 g protein
	Percent Daily Value: vitamin A 6%, vitamin C 6%, calcium 15%, iron 4%

Ingredients

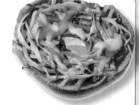

2 English muffins, split into halves
½ cup prepared pizza sauce
1 Tbsp. chopped, green bell pepper

1 Tbsp. sliced mushrooms
1 Tbsp. chopped onion
½ cup shredded, low-fat, mozzarella cheese

Directions

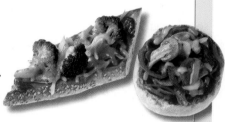

1. Place English muffin halves, crust-side down, on broiler pan.
2. Spread each muffin half with 2 Tbsp. pizza sauce.
3. Top with green pepper, mushrooms, and onion.
4. Sprinkle each muffin half with 2 Tbsp. cheese.
5. Position broiler pan so muffins are about 4 inches from the heat.
6. Broil until cheese is bubbly, about 2 to 4 minutes. Remove immediately and serve hot. (Broiling time may vary.)

Begin with firm, thinly sliced bread or day-old, soft bread that is well chilled. For variety, combine contrasting bread in one sandwich, such as white with whole wheat or pumpernickel.

Choose spreadable fillings—deviled ham, perhaps, or egg, chicken, or seafood salad. Softened cream cheese also works well. Vary the flavor by adding mixed herbs, grated sharp cheese, drained crushed pineapple, sweet relish, chopped dates, crisp bacon bits, or honey.

To make a basic tea sandwich, trim off the crusts and cut out shapes, using a sharp knife or cookie cutters. Spread the slices of bread lightly with butter, margarine, or mayonnaise. Then spread a thin layer of filling on half of the slices all the way to the edges. You need just enough to flavor the sandwich. Too much filling oozes out the edges. Top with a second slice. See **Fig. 40-7**.

Tea sandwiches can be prepared several hours ahead of time. Cover them with wax paper and a damp dish towel. Refrigerate until serving.

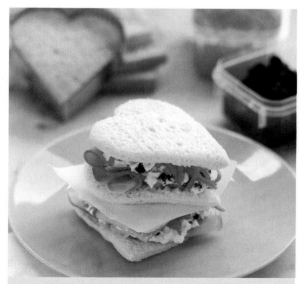

Fig. 40-7 With a little creativity, you can come up with lots of ideas for interesting tea sandwiches. They are as tasty as they are attractive. **How would you make an open-face tea sandwich?**

PIZZA

Although the word **pizza** is Italian for "pie," it is also a sandwich—an oversized, baked sandwich with a yeast-bread base, usually served open-face with assorted toppings. It can be round or square, shallow or deep, and modestly topped or piled with ingredients.

Pizza is one of the few sandwiches that often inspire people to make their own bread. Pizza crust is made with basic yeast dough. Water is used rather than milk for a crispy texture. After punching down and resting the dough, roll it out on a floured surface to fit the shape of the pan. Place the ball of dough in the center of the pan and alternately press it gently and stretch it to the rim with your fingers.

The thickness of the dough depends on personal preference. Thin crusts have added crispness and crunch. Thick crusts are softer and chewier. Leave the crust thick to make a deep-dish pizza, which needs the body to support the added filling. Bake deep-dish pizza in a pan that's 2 inches deep.

You can also make a stuffed-crust pizza. Roll out the dough so it extends about 1 inch beyond the rim of the pan. About 1 inch from the edge of the dough, place a 1-inch band of cheese, shredded or cut into strips. Fold the overhanging dough over the cheese and press firmly to seal. Fill the pizza as desired. Mozzarella is most commonly used, but you might experiment with other cheeses that go with the filling.

If you don't want to make dough from scratch, choose a convenience form that is partially or fully prepared. Packaged mixes require oil, water, and kneading. Unbaked frozen dough needs to be thawed. Refrigerated tubes of dough are unrolled and pressed into a pan. Preformed pizza shells are ready to be filled and baked.

You're probably familiar with traditional pizza ingredients: a spicy, tomato-based sauce; meats that include pepperoni and Italian sausage; such vegetables as sliced mushrooms, bell peppers, olives, and onion; and mozzarella and Parmesan cheese. That basic formula is standard, but imagination can take you to new taste sensations. A seafood pizza might feature cooked shrimp, crab, tuna, or salmon in a light white sauce. For a vegetarian pizza, brush the crust with oil, scatter with your favorite vegetables and fresh herbs, and top with shredded cheddar or soy cheese.

After assembling the pizza, bake it in a preheated oven at 450°F for 20 minutes or until the crust is golden brown. Let it cool for a few minutes to set the toppings. To serve, cut the pizza into wedges or squares with a pizza cutter, kitchen shears, or sharp knife.

Calzone

A **calzone** (kahl-ZOHN) is a double-crust, semicircular pizza. Any dough and fillings that you would put in a pizza can also become a calzone. See **Fig. 40-8**.

Roll the pizza dough out to make a circle about 10 inches in diameter. Spread the filling over one half of the circle to within 1 inch of the edge. Fold the other half of the dough over the filling. Press with your fingertips or the tines of a fork to seal the edges tightly.

Place the calzone on a lightly greased baking sheet and brush with olive oil. Bake in a preheated oven at about 400°F for 30 minutes or until golden brown. Cut into wedges and serve immediately.

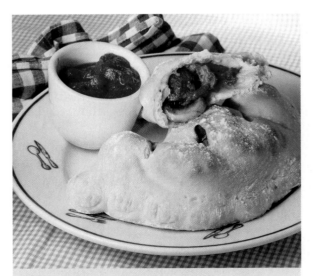

Fig. 40-8 Even though a calzone is like a pizza, you could make one with other fillings. What would you use?

Marketer

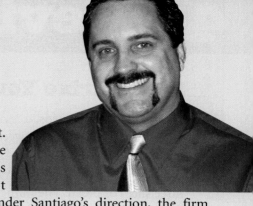

SANTIAGO OGRADÓN CORTÉS: As executive vice-president for a major Hispanic advertising firm, Santiago Ograndón Cortés knows that selling food to the United States' Hispanic market means more than knowing how to say "french fries" in Spanish. It means knowing your potential customers and respecting their culture.

Just the Right Words. Spanish-born and Los Angeles-raised, Santiago earned a bachelor's degree in Hispanic studies and a graduate degree in translation and interpretation. His first professional "interface" between Spanish and American cultures came on a big stage, as an interpreter at the 1984 Olympics in Los Angeles. That role remains a point of pride. He calls it "that 'grain of sand' toward mutual understanding, and the whole world had its eyes on it." It also led to a job in sales with a local television station, the first affiliate of the Spanish-language television network Telemundo.

Selling commercial time for the station taught Santiago a frustrating reality: to many advertisers, selling to Hispanic consumers consisted of just translating an English ad into Spanish. They did not see that what appealed to a mainstream audience might fall flat with Hispanics. Santiago recalls: "I realized how little was known about the Hispanic market—how to talk to it, cultural insights, motivators."

By the 1990s, Santiago was himself creating ads for a global advertising firm when the general manager of an agency dedicated to Hispanic marketing offered him a job. Today the agency, Castells & Asociados, includes Santiago Ogradón as one of its driving forces.

Ads and Understanding. Santiago's responsibilities include developing new accounts and maintaining current ones. His personal and professional insight into Hispanic tastes is a definite asset. Consider the McDonald's restaurant campaign. Under Santiago's direction, the firm helped the fast-food chain design a "fiesta menu," with foods like beef *tortas* (sandwiches on crisp, round rolls) and a new McFlurry shake, *dulce de leche*, based on a traditional, caramelized milk dessert. Television and print ads featured vibrant colors and Latin-inspired rhythms.

Santiago's expertise sells causes as well as things. An anti-smoking campaign for the state of California uses the importance of family in Hispanic culture, especially the father, to discourage teen smoking. His work on the firm's *pro bono* projects—done for free—includes Recording Artists Against Drunk Driving (RADD) and AIDS education.

The sense that advertising can serve a greater purpose also makes the job "a thrill." Santiago explains: "Possibly the best is when we bridge the cultural gap between a U.S. company and the Hispanic market, waking up Anglo understanding to a culturally different market. You can do advertising with total integrity, and have fun, and make money."

On-line Connections

1. To learn more about topics in this article, search the Internet for these key words: Hispanic consumers; multicultural marketing.

2. To learn about related careers, search the Internet for these key words: specialty food producer; foreign language specialist.

Summarize Your Reading

▶ A sandwich—from tacos, to gyros, to roast beef on rye—is a filling between slices of bread.

▶ Sandwiches can be made from one, two, or three slices of bread. The fillings used and the methods for putting sandwiches together result in many variations.

▶ Sandwiches can be served hot or cold.

▶ A pizza is essentially an oversized, baked sandwich.

▶ Sandwiches can cross category lines and be made with uniqueness and experimentation.

Check Your Knowledge

1. How do you make a **basic sandwich**?

2. **CRITICAL THINKING** What could happen if a sandwich maker forgets to put spread on the bread before adding the filling?

3. How is a **club sandwich** different from a basic sandwich?

4. Why is firm bread often preferred for an **open-face sandwich**?

5. What is a **hero** sandwich?

6. What are regional names for a hero sandwich?

7. How is a **wrap** different from a basic sandwich?

8. How do you make a **pita** rollup?

9. What is **lahvosh**?

10. What is a **tortilla**?

11. How do you use a tortilla to make a burrito and a taco?

12. What foods might be eaten in a **fajita**?

13. If you make a hot sandwich in a waffle maker, how can you keep vegetables from wilting?

14. What is chutney?

15. Suggest ingredients for a vegetarian burger.

16. How do you make a grilled cheese sandwich and a broiled, open-face cheese sandwich?

17. What is **focaccia**?

18. What are **tea sandwiches**, and when are they usually served?

19. What fillings would you most likely find on a tea sandwich?

20. **CRITICAL THINKING** Why do you think sandwiches are so well liked in society?

21. How do you make a stuffed-crust pizza?

22. Compare **calzones** with pizza.

23. **CRITICAL THINKING** Analyze the nutritional role of sandwiches and pizzas in the diet.

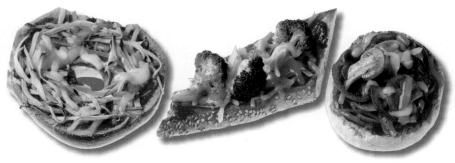

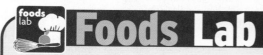
Apply Your Learning

1. **Broiler Use.** Demonstrate the use of the broiler for making sandwiches. Include safety hints and preparation tips.

2. **MATH Bread Comparison.** Using such breads as potato, whole wheat, 7-grain, rye, and raisin, compare the following: price per serving, calories per serving, nutritional value, taste, and uses. Chart your results.

3. **LANGUAGE ARTS Hot Dog History.** Research and write a paper about the history of the hot dog.

4. **Tea Sandwiches.** With your lab team, make one version of a tea sandwich. Serve all lab versions of the sandwich in class or at a special event.

5. **MATH Pizza Cost Comparison.** Compare the cost of delivered pizza, frozen pizzas, and pizza made from scratch. Chart the cost per serving of each. In what situations would each be most suitable?

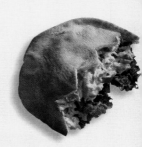

Foods Lab

Making Sandwiches

Procedure: Choose one of the following sandwich types to make to: a) basic; b) club; c) open-face; d) hero; e) flat-bread; f) grilled; g) broiled. Use or modify a recipe or put together ingredients to make your own creation. Prepare and evaluate your sandwich.

Analyzing Results

❶ How did your sandwich rate on taste, texture, and appearance?

❷ If you did something original in making your sandwich, what was it and how effective was it?

❸ What improvements would you make in your sandwich or your technique?

Food Science Experiment

Baking Pizza

Objective: To identify conditions for successful pizza baking.

Procedure:

1. Cut an unbaked cheese pizza into six equal slices. Preheat the oven according to package directions.

2. Place one slice on a small baking sheet. Set it on the oven's upper rack. Set a second slice next to it directly on the oven rack. Place aluminum foil on the oven bottom to catch any drips. Bake the pizza as directed. Examine the slices when cool enough to handle. Compare the appearance, taste, and texture of each crust and topping and record results.

3. Repeat Step 2, placing two slices on the middle rack.

4. Repeat Step 2, placing two slices on the lowest rack. (Note: for further comparison, you can bake additional slices on a pizza stone.)

Analyzing Results

❶ Which position gave the best crust results for baking on a sheet? On a rack?

❷ Which method and position gave the best topping results?

❸ How did placing the slices on a sheet affect the method of heat transfer? How might this difference explain your findings?

❹ Based on this experiment, how would you bake a pizza? Why?

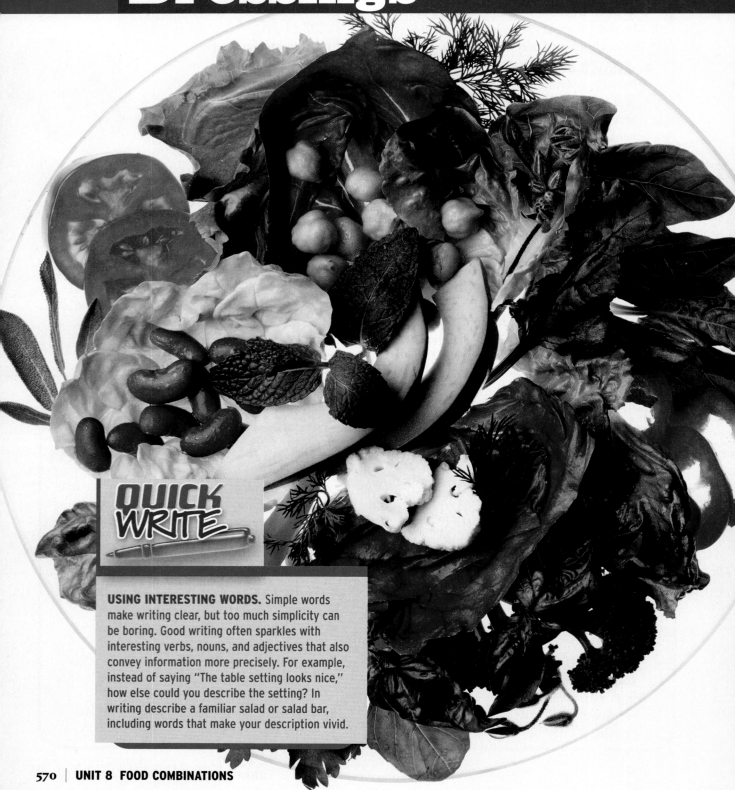

QUICK WRITE

USING INTERESTING WORDS. Simple words make writing clear, but too much simplicity can be boring. Good writing often sparkles with interesting verbs, nouns, and adjectives that also convey information more precisely. For example, instead of saying "The table setting looks nice," how else could you describe the setting? In writing describe a familiar salad or salad bar, including words that make your description vivid.

As the first Roman emperor, Augustus Caesar spent 20 years rebuilding a civilization that was about to collapse from years of turmoil and corruption. He reunited people, built highways and canals, reformed the government, and promoted the arts and sciences, all while in poor health.

After one particularly bad bout of illness, Augustus reportedly raised a statue to the food that he believed cured him, a food said to have medicinal powers—lettuce. The Romans typically prepared lettuce with olive oil and salt. The Latin word for salt is *sal*, a derivative of the word salad. Although salads aren't said to cure illnesses today, they do make a healthful contribution to the diet.

TYPES OF SALADS

A **salad** is a mixture of raw or cooked vegetables and other ready-to-eat foods and is usually served with a dressing. With their great flexibility, salads can be appetizers, entrées, side dishes, and desserts. See **Fig. 41-1**. Salads are made with foods from all of the food groups. You can often substitute ingredients to take advantage of the freshest, most nutritious foods available.

A salad may brim with complex carbohydrates, protein, vitamins, minerals, phytochemi-

cals, and dietary fiber. On the other hand, it can be laden with fat and calories, depending on what goes into the salad.

For all of their versatility, salads are usually built around one or two main types of food, and that's the basis for categorizing them.

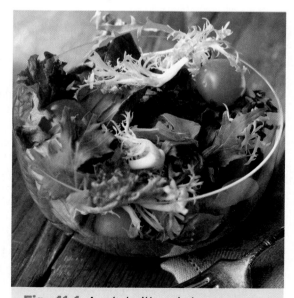

Fig. 41-1 A salad with varied greens makes a nutritious, tasty meal accompaniment. Chilling the bowl or plate beforehand helps the salad stay cold for serving and eating.

Vegetable Salads

Vegetable salads include any salad made exclusively with vegetables, whether raw, cooked, or canned. They usually accompany a meal.

A well-known example is coleslaw. One vegetable, shredded cabbage, is mixed with an oil-and-vinegar or creamy dressing. See **Fig. 41-2**. Likewise, potato salad is made with sliced or cubed, cooked potatoes and mayonnaise. To add crunch or color, either recipe may be accented with various vegetables.

Another version of a vegetable salad is the Caesar salad, named not for the emperor, but for another Italian who created it, Caesar Cardini. In the classic recipe, romaine lettuce is tossed with a dressing of olive oil, lemon juice, salt, pepper, Worcestershire sauce, soft-cooked eggs, and Parmesan cheese. **Croutons**, small pieces of bread made crisp by baking or sautéing, are added last. For food safety, Caesar salads today are made with eggs that are pasteurized or hard-cooked and crumbled.

Fruit Salads

For some people, fruit salad simply means canned "fruit cocktail" in syrup. Homemade fruit salads can be a more interesting balance of flavors. Ambrosia salad, for example, combines the sweetness of mandarin oranges, bananas, cherries, miniature marshmallows, and flaked coconut with the sharpness of pecans and tang of pineapple chunks and sour cream. Waldorf salad mixes diced apples, sliced celery, chopped walnuts, and mayonnaise. A refreshing, light dressing can be made with fruit vinegars or spiced citrus juice. Fresh mint adds coolness.

On the other hand, a rich, sweetened dressing turns fruit salad into a dessert. You can mix fruit with cream cheese thinned with evaporated milk, or pudding cooked with juice. Frozen fruit salads are usually made with assorted fruits, gelatin, and mayonnaise, cream cheese, or cream. The mixture is frozen and then sliced into serving pieces. These are tasty ways to include fruit in your diet.

Fig. 41-2

Try This! **Recipe**

Homestyle Coleslaw

Yield	Nutrition Analysis
About 10 servings	**Per Serving:** 60 calories, 0 g total fat, 0 g saturated fat, 0 g trans fat, 0 mg cholesterol, 30 mg sodium, 15 g total carbohydrate, 1 g dietary fiber, 6 g sugars, 2 g protein
	Percent Daily Value: vitamin A 35%, vitamin C 90%, calcium 8%, iron 6%

Ingredients
1 head cabbage
1 cup onion, diced
2 carrots, shredded
1 large bell pepper, cut into strips

½ cup cider vinegar
2 Tbsp. honey
2 Tbsp. caraway seeds

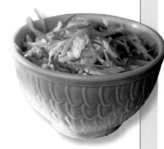

Directions
1. With a large knife, cut the cabbage in half. Make a V-shaped slit at the bottom of each half to remove the hard white core. Discard the core.
2. With the cut-side down, cut each cabbage half into ¼-inch-wide slices. With your hands, separate each slice into thin strips.
3. Add the cabbage strips to a large mixing bowl. Add the onion, carrots, and bell pepper.
4. In a small mixing bowl, combine the cider vinegar and honey. Use a wire whisk to combine.
5. Pour the dressing over the cabbage mixture. Add the caraway seeds. Stir to combine.

SALADS IN SPACE

One sacrifice that astronauts make is foregoing fresh fruits and vegetables for most of their stay in space. Fresh produce that arrives with supply crafts must still be eaten within a few days.

If recent trials fulfill their promise, fruit and vegetable salad bars on space travels could be a reality. In 2002, one experiment on the International Space Station involved growing soybean seeds. For about three months, the plants thrived in a special growth chamber under conditions monitored and controlled by scientists on earth. The soybeans returned on the Atlantis space shuttle as the first crops to be sprouted, raised to maturity, and harvested entirely in outer space. Researchers ran chemical and biological tests on the seeds to determine the effects of growing in low or no gravity. They found the space-bred crops similar physically and biologically to their earthly counterparts.

The information the experiment provides can be applied not only to growing other produce in space

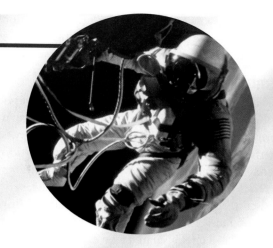

but also to improving soybean strains on earth. If "space farming" causes positive changes in soybeans, for instance, scientists will investigate whether those changes could be passed genetically to future generations. As soybeans are one of the most consumed crops in the world and the leading source of protein in the human diet, the results could have great impact on soybean farming and nutrition worldwide.

_Think Beyond>> Astronauts currently choose all meals before their flight. How might having access to fresh produce affect this practice?

Cooked Grain Salads

If you think rice casserole tastes better cold, why not serve it that way? Rice, bulgur, barley, or pasta—whatever grain you choose—may be equally as appealing as a cooked, chilled salad.

As in casseroles, grains in salads lend themselves to any number of preparations. You can dress them lightly with oil, vinegar, salt, and pepper. Grains go well with a creamy dressing, sharpened with lemon juice or mustard. For color and texture contrast, add diced bell pepper, sliced olives, or parsley. Macaroni is a standard that can be made with any of these ingredients. Rice mixed with pineapple chunks and orange juice sweetened with honey is very Polynesian. **Tabbouleh** (tuh-BOO-lee) is a Middle Eastern salad of cooked bulgur, chopped tomatoes, onions, parsley, mint, olive oil, and lemon juice.

Grain salads tend to be more flavorful if prepared warm and then chilled for serving. Hot

grains absorb dressings and seasonings better. To dry drained, cooked pasta, spread it onto a paper-towel-lined baking sheet and roll gently.

Dry Bean Salads

Almost every supermarket deli seems to feature a three-bean salad, a mix of common types of beans in oil and vinegar. Bean salads, however, can have less common combinations and different flavoring ingredients. For example, you might combine navy and pinto beans with diced tomatoes, sourdough croutons, rice vinegar, and basil.

Cooked Meat, Poultry, Fish, and Egg Salads

Chopped salads are made with cooked meat, poultry, fish, or eggs. Preparation is basically the same for all. After the main ingredient is chopped, it is mixed with seasonings and diced vegetables. Onions, celery, and bell peppers are common additions. For the dressing, sour cream or mayonnaise is traditional. Updated and ethnic recipes may use light dressings, including lime juice and honey or rice vinegar and sesame oil.

Combination Salads

What do you do when you have leftover servings of pasta, ham, and peas? You could turn them into a combination salad, which puts together several different foods. Combination salads are easily converted from side dishes to entrées. Greens, tomato wedges, and slices of hard-cooked egg make a filling side salad. Adding strips of ham, turkey, and cheese makes a main dish salad—a chef's salad, to be exact.

Similarly, a wilted salad starts out as leafy dark greens and crumbled bacon, which is then drizzled with a dressing of hot bacon fat, sugar, and vinegar. To expand this recipe, you can add hard-cooked eggs, tomatoes, mandarin oranges, or cashews.

Molded Salads

At one time, molded salads were a dish for the wealthy. **Molded salads** are made with gelatin that thickens and conforms to the shape of a container called a mold. Extracting gelatin, a protein from animals, was a costly process. Today, purified gelatin is readily found as an unflavored powder and also in sweetened, dry mixes with many fruit flavors. Molded salads are now as common as they are varied. Colorful, cool, and shimmering, they brighten many meals.

Plain or flavored, gelatin works when dissolved by water and heat. Do you recall how eggs coagulate, or thicken? Like egg protein, gelatin is made of long amino acid chains. Adding hot water breaks the bonds that hold the chains together. As the water and gelatin chill in the refrigerator, these chains reunite in a new structure. Water is trapped in this new protein network that thickens to hold your salad together. Through this process, gelatin can "tie up" as much as 100 times its weight in water. One tablespoon of unflavored gelatin can set 2 cups of liquid.

Before it sets, this gelling mass can also lock up other foods, whether fruits, vegetables, cooked shrimp, chopped nuts, cottage cheese, or salsa.

Lightweight foods, including bananas, apples, pears, and celery, tend to float to the top. Most meats, poultry, and fish drop to the bottom, as do grapes, citrus fruits, canned fruits, and many vegetables. This can create an attractive layered look. If you would rather distribute foods evenly, fold them in as soon as the mixture has chilled to slightly thickened, about the consistency of cold egg whites.

A few fruits produce unwelcome results in gelatin salads. Fresh and frozen pineapples, mangoes, kiwifruit, and papayas contain the enzyme bromelin, which digests proteins and keeps the mixture from setting. Cooked or canned forms of these fruits and juices will work because the heat of cooking or processing deactivates the enzyme.

After all ingredients are added, the gelatin mixture is ready for the mold. You can choose a ring mold or one with a tiered design or intricate details. First, lightly oil the inside of the mold or rinse it with cold water so the salad will be easier to remove later. Then pour in the gelatin mixture. Refrigerate to set. Once the salad is completely set, follow these steps to release it from the mold:

1. Dip the mold almost to the rim in warm water, not hot, for about ten seconds. Watch the timing so the gelatin doesn't melt. Lift it from the water and shake slightly to loosen the gelatin.
2. Run the tip of a small, pointed knife between the salad and the rim of the mold.
3. Place a serving plate upside down on top of the mold. Invert the plate and mold together so the plate is on the bottom. Shake gently again and lift off the mold. If necessary, repeat the steps until the salad is released.
4. Slide the salad carefully to center it on the plate. This is easier if you rinse the plate in cold water first.

CHOOSING SALAD GREENS

Many salads include greens. See **Fig. 41-3** on pages 576 and 577. They may be in the body, the main part of the salad, or make up a base, a foundation on which other ingredients are placed. Chopped salads, for example, look attractive on a bed of greens.

Iceberg lettuce has long been the most commonly used salad green, but many other varieties are enjoyed as well. Each green contributes its own flavor, texture, and nutrients. Mixing different kinds adds interest.

In the supermarket, greens may be sold either in bulk or premixed and packaged. If you keep a home garden, check what varieties grow well in your area.

When you buy salad greens, keep in mind that color is the key to nutrition. The greener the greens, the more vitamin A they have. Examine greens for brown spotting, called rust, or other signs of disease or spoilage. If you buy packaged greens, look for the sell-by date to get the freshest product.

Cleaning Greens

Even greens from the supermarket may hide soil, especially spinach, since it grows in sandy conditions. Wash, drain, and refrigerate salad greens as soon as you get them home. In addition to dirt, washing greens rinses away harmful bacteria that might multiply in the refrigerator. Once washed, the greens will be ready when you need them. Washing and chilling also helps greens stay crisp.

To clean most greens, pull the leaves away from the bunch and wash them individually under cold, running water. You may want to soak them for about ten minutes to rehydrate their cells and restore crispness. Drain the leaves well, placing each one, stem-side down, in a colander so the water drains off easily. You may also need to pat the greens dry before storing.

Iceberg lettuce takes a different technique. Hold the head of lettuce in your hands, core-side down. Strike the core firmly on a counter to loosen it. Pull out the core and let cold water run into the cavity for a minute until it pours out between the leaves. Let the head drain in a colander, core-side down. See **Fig. 41-4**.

Packaged greens may or may not have been washed. Look for the words "washed" or "ready to eat" on the label. Washing the greens eliminates any doubt. Be sure to always wash mixed greens bought in bulk.

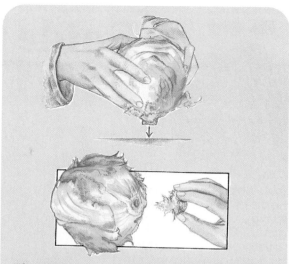

Fig. 41-4 To core lettuce, strike the core end of the head against the countertop. This loosens the core for easy removal. To wash the lettuce, pour water into the opening and let it drain.

Drain salad greens as thoroughly as possible. Water left on the leaves dilutes the dressing and hastens spoilage. A salad spinner makes it easy to wash and drain greens. This kitchen tool has an inner, spinning basket that holds the separated leaves. As you pour water in from a faucet, an outer bowl catches the water that spins off. The water drains into the sink from holes in the outer bowl.

Keep washed and drained greens wrapped in a dry paper towel and refrigerated in a plastic container or a large plastic bag. Most greens are best used within one week. Iceberg lettuce holds its quality for about two weeks. If greens look limp, immerse them for a few minutes in ice water and dry them just before making the salad. To prevent enzymatic browning, tear greens or cut them with a plastic lettuce knife rather than metal.

CHOOSING SALAD DRESSINGS

Some salads are so flavorful that you could eat them with just a splash of lemon juice and a sprinkling of herbs or seeds. On the other hand, some people believe a salad is best with **salad dressing**, a seasoned mixture of oil and vinegar used to flavor a salad. Salad dressing also acts as a

Fig. 41-3

A Guide to Salad Greens

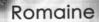

Romaine

(roh-MAYN). Long, narrow head of loosely packed leaves. Outer leaves are dark green. Center leaves are pale green. Crisp texture with a sharp, nutty flavor. Most nutritious lettuce.

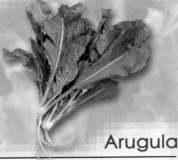

Iceberg Lettuce

Large, round, compact head with pale green, crisp leaves. Mild flavor. Low in nutritional value.

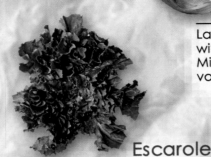

Escarole

(ES-kuh-roh). Flat, loose head of broad, slightly curved, green, outer leaves with yellow center leaves. Firm texture with a slightly bitter flavor.

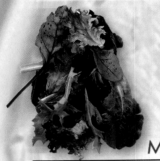

Mesclun

(MEHS-kluhn). A popular mix of various types of young, small greens. Sold in bulk or prepackaged.

Arugula

(uh-ROO-guh-luh). Small, bright green, smooth leaves. Sold in small bunches. Highly perishable. Tender texture with a pungent, peppery, nutty flavor.

binder, holding the ingredients together. Some dressings are mixed in, as in potato or chicken salad. For a tossed or chef's salad, they are added just before serving to avoid wilting the greens.

Besides flavor and color, dressings add almost all of the fat and most of the calories in many salads. Read labels when buying salad dressings. Look for reduced-fat or fat-free varieties of bottled dressing. Packaged mixes, which require you to add oil and other ingredients, often give directions for low-fat options. For instance, you might use buttermilk in place of sour cream. If you make dressings ahead of time, the seasonings can blend, adding flavor with less fat. It's thoughtful to offer a variety of dressings separately at the table so people can add just the amount of the type they want.

Which dressing should you serve with which salad? If any rule exists, it's that the dressing should complement the other flavors in the salad. Tart fruits are usually served with a sweet dressing. Use a tangy dressing for such mild-flavored foods as potatoes and whitefish.

Homemade Dressings

Making your own salad dressing gives you more control over flavor and ingredients. It also confronts you with one of the oldest challenges in food preparation: getting oil and water—or vinegar, which is acidic, flavored water—to mix.

Making Vinaigrettes

The simplest salad dressing is vinaigrette (vi-ni-GREHT), sometimes called French dressing. **Vinaigrettes**

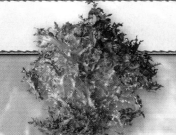

Curly Endive

Sometimes called chicory. Loose head of curled, lacy leaves with bright green edges and off-white center. Coarse texture with bitter flavor. Best mixed with other greens.

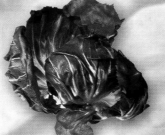

Radicchio

(ra-DIH-kee-oh). Small, loose head, either round or long and narrow. Colors vary from deep red with white ribs to streaked with pink, red, or green. Firm texture with slightly bitter flavor.

Butterhead Lettuce

Small head with loosely packed leaves. Sweet flavor with tender, buttery texture. Wash and handle gently to avoid leaf damage. Bibb and Boston are two varieties.

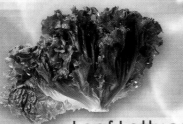

Leaf Lettuce

A loose bunch of crinkly leaves. Crisp texture with a mild flavor. Usually medium to dark green color. Some varieties have red-tipped leaves.

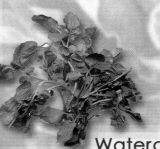

Watercress

Grows in running streams. Small, dark green leaves. Crisp texture with a slightly bitter, peppery flavor.

are a mixture of vegetable oil, vinegar or lemon juice, and seasonings. To make vinaigrette, whisk the oil steadily into the other ingredients, using a ratio of 3 parts oil to 1 part vinegar or juice. The mixture thickens as the liquids are evenly dispersed in very fine drops. What you have made is technically known as an **emulsion**, a mixture of two liquids that normally don't combine.

From this basic recipe you can prepare dozens of variations. Vinaigrette made with ketchup, sugar, and grated onion is called Catalina dressing. Italian dressing uses an Italian seasoning blend and Romano cheese.

If a simple vinaigrette dressing stands for a while, you'll see that it is only a **temporary emulsion**. As soon as you stop mixing them, the oil and vinegar droplets start to rejoin others of their own kind. Eventually, the two liquids separate.

Nutrition Connection

Quantity awareness. When you're watching fat and calories, a few tablespoons of salad dressing make a big difference. On a salad dressing label, 2 grams of saturated fat per tablespoon may not seem like much, but if you pour on 5 tablespoons, that's nearly half a day's limit of saturated fat. Paying attention to the quantity you use helps. To many people, salads that aren't drenched in dressing taste better. You can also ask to have dressings served on the side.

 What is the fat and calorie count for salad dressings that you typically use? How do the numbers translate to the amount you put on a salad?

You'll need to mix them before using the vinaigrette again.

Making Mayonnaise

To make other types of dressing, you need to make a **permanent emulsion**, one that won't separate. You need an emulsifier, a substance that stabilizes an emulsion. That is, it keeps the oil and vinegar blended.

As you know, a common emulsifier in foods is egg yolk. By adding egg yolk to the vinaigrette, you can make **mayonnaise**, a thick, creamy dressing that is an emulsion of oil, vinegar or lemon juice, egg yolks, and seasonings. The oil is very gradually drizzled and blended into the other ingredients. Each addition must be broken down into tiny droplets and coated with yolk before more is added. Mustard, both the spice and the condiment, is a secondary emulsifier in many mayonnaise recipes and in some vinaigrettes.

Due to concerns about *Salmonella* contamination, some new recipes for making mayonnaise call for cooking the egg mixture before adding the oil. To make recipes that call for raw eggs, use egg substitutes or pasteurized eggs, which are safe to eat uncooked.

Making Cooked Dressings

If you've made gravy, you've seen how starches can also hold an emulsion together. Fat and water don't separate when they're cooked with a dissolved starch like flour or cornstarch. This is how a **cooked dressing** is made. Instead of using eggs, the dressing is thickened by cooking a starch paste. Traditional German potato salad, for instance, is made with a cooked dressing of bacon drippings, flour, sugar, and cider vinegar.

Commercially prepared mayonnaise and cooked dressings, which by law are called salad dressings, are emulsified with both proteins and starches. Starches are useful as egg yolk replacers in reduced-fat varieties. They appear on ingredient lists as cellulose gel, maltodextrin, xanthan (ZAN-thuhn) gum, and gum arabic.

Career Prep

Business Etiquette

IN LARGE PART, BUSINESS ETIQUETTE is simply everyday politeness and respect applied to workplace situations. For example, you respect a classmate's right to privacy by not looking into the person's locker or listening in on conversations. Likewise, you would not look in a co-worker's desk or read someone else's e-mails.

Some work situations take slightly different rules. Gender matters less in business than in a social setting. Whoever opens a door first holds it for the person who follows, male or female. On the other hand, a person's position is significant. When making introductions, you address the higher-ranking employee and introduce the lower-ranking worker to that person.

Other situations that commonly crop up in the workplace have their own rules of etiquette. Some are described here:

- **Watch and learn.** If you're new to the job, learn how things are done and follow the routine. Later, when you've learned more and earned the respect of co-workers, you can suggest improvements or try a new way.

- **Sharing space.** Co-workers who share an office, lunchroom, or refrigerator are all responsible for keeping things clean and keeping noise levels in work areas reasonable. Office supplies may not always be distinguishable from personal supplies, so don't remove anything from a desk or refrigerator unless invited.

Making Dairy Dressings

Dairy dressings are based on buttermilk, yogurt, sour cream, or cottage cheese, with seasonings added. They are enhanced with herbs, spices, sharp mustard, grated cheese, honey, or lime or lemon juice. Ranch dressing includes chopped green onion, ground pepper, thyme, and garlic. Blue cheese and Worcestershire or steak sauce go into blue cheese dressing. A blend of brown sugar, cinnamon, and frozen juice concentrate makes a creamy dressing for fruit salad.

MAKING AND SERVING SALADS

When you put salads together, your imagination can spark endless combinations and ways of presenting them. Choose ingredients that complement each other and the rest of the meal in flavor, color, texture, and nutrients.

In general, salads can be tossed, arranged, or layered. A **tossed salad** is usually a mixture of greens and a dressing, often mixed with other vegetables. For an arranged salad, ingredients are placed in an attractive pattern—for example,

wedges of tomato fanned around a scoop of chicken salad on a bed of lettuce. A layered salad has ingredients added one on top of the other, ideally in a glass bowl for greatest visual effect. See **Fig. 41-5**.

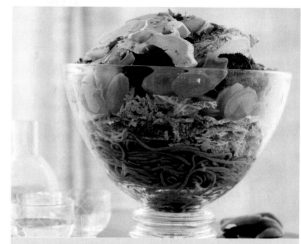

Fig. 41-5 A layered salad looks best in a glass bowl. Well-chilled ingredients are crisper and taste better.

• **Gossip.** Gossip is especially destructive on the job, where teamwork is essential. Would you respect a co-worker who spreads stories about you or anyone else? Ignoring gossip is one good response. Tactfully defusing it is another. You might ask: "Where did you hear that? Did you talk to the people involved? I'll wait until I know for sure." If you hear something genuinely disturbing, get the facts from a supervisor, rather than from "the grapevine."

• **Extra jobs.** Doing an occasional personal or professional favor for a supervisor or co-worker is part of the give-and-take of relationships. No one, however, should be expected to run errands or do another employee's work, regardless of position, unless it's part of the job description. A polite reminder or explanation that the added work interferes with assigned tasks may be in order.

Career Connection

Parliamentary procedure. A particular type of business etiquette is parliamentary procedure, a set of rules for running a formal meeting. Learn about parliamentary procedure. Watch it in action, perhaps at the next school board or local government meeting. In class, discuss the rules and processes used. What are the advantages of using parliamentary procedure?

Summarize Your Reading

▶ Salads are as varied as the ingredients used to make them.

▶ Salads can be served as appetizers, a meal accompaniment, main course, or even dessert.

▶ Many salads are filled with complex carbohydrates, protein, vitamins, minerals, phytochemicals, and dietary fiber.

▶ Salad greens must be selected, stored, and used properly to remain fresh.

▶ Although some salads need very little extra flavoring, many salads are enjoyed with salad dressing.

▶ Some salad dressings form either temporary or permanent emulsions.

Check Your Knowledge

1. Define **salad**.

2. Are all salads healthful? Explain your answer.

3. How can salads be categorized?

4. What common salad is made with shredded cabbage? How is it made?

5. Why has the method for making Caesar salad changed?

6. What are **croutons**?

7. What ingredients go into an ambrosia salad?

8. What ingredients make up a Waldorf salad?

9. What are grain salads?

10. Describe a bean salad that could be made with navy and pinto beans.

11. **CRITICAL THINKING** A cook mixes canned tuna with onions, chives, olives, walnuts, mayonnaise, and herb seasoning powder. Has the cook made a salad or a sandwich filling? Explain.

12. How does the gelatin in a **molded salad** cause the salad to thicken?

13. Which fruits should not be used in a molded salad, and why?

14. Explain how to release a molded salad from its mold.

15. Are all salad greens green? Explain.

16. What should you look for when purchasing salad greens?

17. Why should salad greens be washed?

18. How should greens be washed and stored?

19. What may happen if you cut greens with a metal knife?

20. If salad greens are limp, how can you restore their crispness?

21. What is **vinaigrette**, and how can you turn it into **mayonnaise**?

22. Define **emulsion**, and explain the basic difference between **temporary** and **permanent emulsions**.

23. What is a **cooked dressing**?

24. Compare the following salad presentations: **tossed**, arranged, and layered.

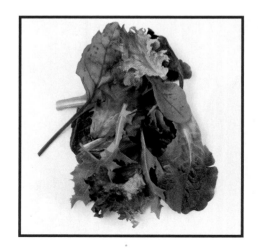

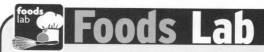
Apply Your Learning

1. **LANGUAGE ARTS** **Greens Speech.** Prepare and present a talk about the different greens used in salads. How can you incorporate visuals to make your talk more interesting?

2. **Greens Sampling.** Taste a variety of greens and compare their nutritional value. Which ones would you use in salads? Why?

3. **Unmolding Gelatin.** Demonstrate how to unmold a gelatin salad. Include tips for easier unmolding.

4. **MATH** **Greens Cost Comparison.** Compare costs of several different greens. Include iceberg lettuce; other greens; ready-to-eat packaged greens; and bulk greens. Chart the results and make recommendations to the class.

Foods Lab

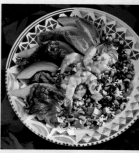

Ethnic Salads

Procedure: Find ethnic salad recipes and choose one to prepare. You might select a recipe from your own heritage. Prepare the recipe and share samples in class. Evaluate the salad on taste, texture, and appearance.

Analyzing Results

❶ What is the ethnic background for the salad you prepared?

❷ Do you think the salad is authentic, or has it been modified to suit American taste?

❸ How did your salad turn out? What improvements would you make in ingredients or preparation method?

Food Science Experiment

Making Emulsions

Objective: To compare different types of emulsions.

Procedure:

1. In a clear jar with a lid, mix 3 Tbsp. vegetable oil and 1 Tbsp. lemon juice. Close the jar tightly and shake vigorously for 15 seconds. Record the results.

2. Let the jar stand. Observe for five minutes, recording any changes you notice at one-minute intervals.

3. In a bowl, lightly beat an egg yolk. Slowly add the oil mixture, pouring in a steady stream and beating constantly. Continue beating until all ingredients are well blended.

4. Let the bowl stand, and observe for five minutes. Record any changes at one-minute intervals.

Analyzing Results

❶ How did the oil-and-juice mixture appear immediately after you stopped shaking the jar? What, if anything, occurred over the next five minutes?

❷ How did the addition of egg yolk affect the mixture? What do you think created this result?

❸ Which mixture was a permanent emulsion? A temporary emulsion? When might you use each type of emulsion in cooking?

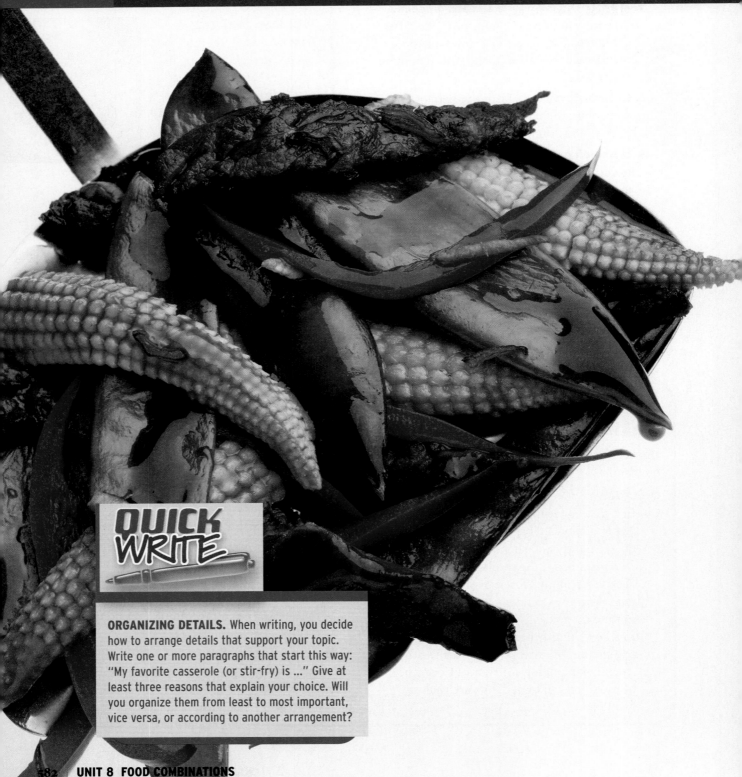

QUICK WRITE

ORGANIZING DETAILS. When writing, you decide how to arrange details that support your topic. Write one or more paragraphs that start this way: "My favorite casserole (or stir-fry) is ..." Give at least three reasons that explain your choice. Will you organize them from least to most important, vice versa, or according to another arrangement?

Objectives

- ► Compare stir-fries with casseroles.
- ► Describe how to prepare ingredients for a stir-fry dish.
- ► Demonstrate how to cook a stir-fry dish.
- ► Explain the roles of basic ingredients in a casserole.
- ► Demonstrate how to make a casserole.

Terms

- au gratin
- binder
- casserole
- mise en place
- stir-fry

I N SOME WAYS, STIR-FRIES AND CASSEROLES ARE opposites. Stir-fries are quickly sautéed and served right away. Casseroles bake for up to an hour and can be prepared ahead and reheated—in fact, some people say they're better that way.

Both dishes, however, share something in common: they were born of necessity. Stir-fries developed in China about 2,000 years ago, when firewood and cooking oil were scarce. Casseroles arose from the age-old need to turn scraps and leftovers into an appealing meal. Both circumstances led to similar results—economical dishes, easily prepared, that make scant amounts of food go a long way.

Thrift is still an advantage to these dishes today, but convenience and versatility are what make them most appreciated. Both lend themselves to pre-preparation tasks that can be done in advance. Both invite the cook's creativity. You may literally never prepare the same recipe twice.

STIR-FRIES

A **stir-fry** is just that: a combination dish of bite-size pieces of food that are stirred constantly while frying in a small amount of oil over high heat. When done successfully, vegetables are tender on the outside yet remain crisp inside. See

Fig. 42-1. High temperatures and quick cooking—between 30 seconds and 5 minutes, depending on the ingredients—help foods retain nutrients while absorbing little fat.

Stir-fries tend to be equally based on vegetables and protein foods. Meat, poultry, or seafood is one ingredient among others, rather than the center of the recipe. These dishes include a light, flavorful sauce. If you serve them with cooked

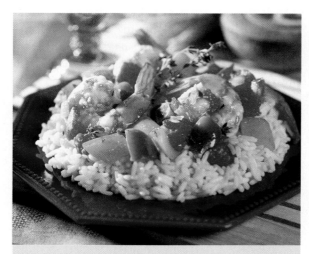

Fig. 42-1 Here's one example of a stir-fried dish. What ingredients would you like in a stir-fry?

grain and possibly a salad, you have a complete, balanced meal.

While ingredients vary, the process for combining them is always the same. The keys to a good stir-fry are preparation, organization, coordination, and speed.

Pre-preparation

When you start a stir-fry, you should be prepared. The grain must be cooked, the ingredients cut, the sauce mixed, and all ingredients arranged in the proper order. Once you begin, you won't have time to hunt for a missing spice or to slice another carrot. Review the recipe steps several times before you start cooking.

Cooking the Grain

The grain should be ready and waiting when the stir-fry is finished. Coordinate tasks so the grain cooks while you prepare the other foods. Rice is a traditional accompaniment, but you might try barley, brown rice, couscous, millet, or pasta. To save time, you can reheat precooked grain or use packaged chow mein noodles.

Remember that each grain adds a characteristic flavor and texture. Choose one that complements the meal. Also, different grains have different cooking times. Adjust your timetable as needed.

Preparing the Vegetables

When you stir-fry a medley of vegetables, from carrots to spinach, they cook in the same pan at the same time. They can come out colorful, flavorful, and tender-crisp or as charred chunks in a sea of soggy greens. Part of the difference lies in proper preparation.

Each vegetable should be cut into pieces of similar size to promote even cooking. Slice large vegetables into pieces no thicker than ¼ inch. Those that tend to be dense or fibrous—green beans, green onions, and carrots, for example—should be cut on the diagonal. This exposes a larger area to the heat, while adding interest.

Remove the midrib—the "backbone"—and the stem ends from cabbage and leafy greens before slicing. Finely chop these parts separately. Greens, bell peppers, and onions can be cut into strips or coarsely chopped.

Different kinds of vegetables may be added to the stir-fry at different times, so keep them separate after cutting them.

Preparing Protein Foods

If you use raw meat or poultry, cut it across the grain into very thin strips about 1½ inches long. Use a large, sharp knife and a secure cutting board. This task is easier when the food is slightly frozen.

Fresh fish should also be cut into strips. Choose a firm-fleshed variety like tuna, halibut, mahi-mahi, or bass. Fresh shrimp and scallops are naturally sized for stir-frying. Cut tofu or tempeh into cubes. To add flavor and to protect against drying out, marinate protein foods before cooking.

You can also use slices or cubes of cooked meat, poultry, and seafood, either canned or left-over. These foods are usually the last added since they only need to be heated through. What protein food is used in the recipe in **Fig. 42-2**?

Mixing the Sauce

Sauce is the finishing touch in a stir-fry. A base of water, broth, or juice is seasoned with soy, tamari, or Worcestershire sauce, as well as herbs and spices. You might also add rice vinegar, sugar, nut butters, or toasted sesame seeds. Put the mixture you choose, along with cornstarch, into a small jar, shake to blend, and set aside until needed.

Later, when the sauce is added to the stir-fry, heat thickens it. In the next chapter, you'll read more about making sauces. Some recipes call for additional water or broth to cook vegetables that need more moisture. Have this close by as well.

Arranging the Ingredients

In stir-frying, the sequence for adding ingredients is important. The goal is thorough, even cooking. Foods are added according to the time needed to cook them, starting with those that take the longest and ending with those that cook most quickly.

To add one ingredient while focusing on those already cooking, chefs use a practice called **mise en place** (MEE-zahn-plahs). This French term

Fig. 42-2

Fresh 'n' Fast Fried Rice

Yield
6 servings; about 1 cup each

Nutrition Analysis
Per Serving: 240 calories, 7 g total fat, 1.5 g saturated fat, 0 g trans fat, 105 mg cholesterol, 85 mg sodium, 35 g total carbohydrate, 2 g dietary fiber, 2 g sugars, 9 g protein

Percent Daily Value: vitamin A 20%, vitamin C 40%, calcium 4%, iron 15%

Ingredients
3 eggs
2 tsp. vegetable oil
2 tsp. additional vegetable oil
4 cups cooked rice, chilled
1 cup reduced-sodium chicken broth

1 cup frozen green peas, thawed
⅓ cup diced, red bell pepper
1 cup canned bean sprouts, drained
⅓ cup chopped green onions

Directions
1. In a small bowl, beat the eggs until well combined.
2. In a large, nonstick skillet or wok, heat 2 tsp. vegetable oil over medium heat. Add the eggs and cook, stirring occasionally, for 2 to 5 minutes or until eggs are set. Put eggs in a bowl and set aside.
3. Heat the additional 2 tsp. oil over medium-high heat. Add rice and stir-fry 5 minutes.
4. Add remaining ingredients and cooked eggs, and stir-fry a final 2 minutes.
5. Season as desired, or serve with soy sauce.

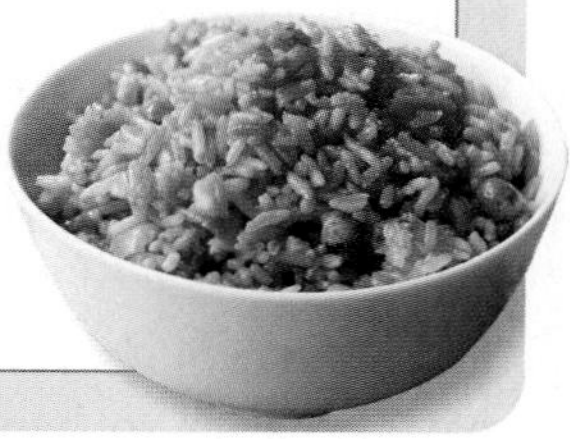

means "put in place." In other words, all ingredients are prepared and arranged ahead in cooking order. A large tray or cart is handy for placing all ingredients close to the cooking location. Otherwise, assemble them on a counter. Either way, make sure they are easy to reach and in this order:

1. **Oil.** Any oil with a smoking point of about 400°F can take the heat of stir-frying. That includes almost all commercially available types. Peanut oil is noted for its flavor.
2. **Seasonings.** Fresh ginger and minced garlic are usually added at the beginning to flavor both the oil and meat. Other seasonings may be added at different stages.
3. **Raw meat, poultry, and seafood.** Meat, poultry, fish, and most shellfish are cooked before other ingredients. Scallops may be added with the vegetables to avoid toughening their delicate protein.

4. **Vegetables.** Check the recipe to see whether different vegetables should be added in a certain order. Place sturdy vegetables like carrots and broccoli stems before easily wilted cabbage and spinach.
5. **Cooked meat, poultry, and seafood and tofu.** These and other ready-to-eat foods are added near the end of the cooking time since they only need to be heated.
6. **Fruits.** Stir-fry recipes occasionally include such tropical fruits as pineapples and mangoes. These may be cooked with the tender vegetables or added without cooking just before serving.
7. **Sauce.** The sauce is added a few minutes before cooking is complete.

Cooking the Stir-Fry

A stir-fry is traditionally prepared in a wok. This roomy, bowl-shaped pan is well designed for

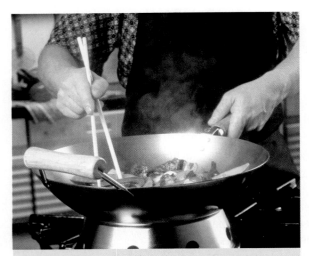

Fig. 42-3 A wok is the traditional pan for stir-frying. What advantages does it have over a skillet?

the technique. Food placed in the rounded bottom is nearest to the heat, where it cooks quickly, while other foods pushed onto the deep sides stay warm without overcooking. The curved sides also let you briskly stir and lightly toss food without tossing it out of the pan. See **Fig. 42-3**.

Using a wok skillfully takes practice. A flat-bottomed wok is more similar to a skillet and may be easier to handle. To get the most from either model, you might invest in special equipment. A stir-fry spatula has an angled edge that conforms to the wok's sloping sides, where food might escape a straightedge spatula. A shallow, wide-mesh strainer helps drain oil when removing food. If you feel more comfortable with conventional cookware, use a large, deep skillet and a wide spatula.

Whatever equipment you choose, work quickly and in small batches. In order to fry rather than steam, foods must contact the pan. The water released by cooking needs room to evaporate. At the same time, be ready to add a tablespoon of water at any point if the pan or food seems to be burning.

Compared to the pre-preparation, stir-frying itself goes quickly. You will find some variation among recipes, but most follow these basic steps:

1. Heat the wok on high until a few water drops sizzle and evaporate immediately.

2. Add 1 to 2 tablespoons of oil. Tilt the pan to coat the entire surface. In some recipes, half the oil is used to brown the meat, and the other half is added before cooking the vegetables.

3. Add seasonings as directed in the recipe.

4. Add raw meat, poultry, or seafood. Stir constantly, and gently tumble the food to brown all sides. Some recipes call for these foods to be completely cooked and then removed or pushed up the side of the wok. Others tell you to let them finish cooking with the vegetables.

5. Add the vegetables according to cooking time. To prevent burning, stir continuously until they are softened on the outside but still firm inside. Undercook rather than overcook. Undercooked food can always be returned to the heat.

6. Return or add cooked meat, poultry, seafood, or tofu to the pan, if needed.

7. Shake the sauce to recombine the ingredients. Stir in and cook until the mixture thickens.

8. Cover the pan briefly, if needed, to steam the vegetables until done. Some vegetables have enough natural moisture to create sufficient steam. Others may need an extra spoonful or two of hot broth or water.

9. Serve immediately on a bed of hot grain.

CASSEROLES

The **casserole**—a flavorful combination of precooked or quick-cooking foods in a one-dish meal—has a multicultural past. It draws from the Asian one-pot meal and medieval pies made with a mashed rice crust. "Casserole" is a French word for a baking dish. Around 1700, English-speaking people began using the word to refer to both the dish and the recipe. They still do.

Casseroles gained popularity in the United States in the mid-twentieth century. With the Depression, two World Wars, and women in the workforce, families needed nourishing, easy-to-prepare meals that made use of whatever ingredients were on hand. That hasn't changed.

Casseroles have an image as a "second chance" for leftover cooked meat, poultry, grains, dried beans, and vegetables. If a recipe sounds tasty and nutritious, however, you may want to buy the ingredients you need. Then the casserole itself can become a leftover.

Like stir-fries, casseroles consist of certain types of ingredients. Within this basic outline are almost limitless choices.

Main Ingredients

The main ingredient in a casserole provides the dominant flavor. Main-dish casseroles may include cooked meat or poultry, canned fish or shellfish, or tofu. Cooked ground meat is first drained of fat. Browning, which brings out flavor, helps seared or roasted meat and poultry stand out when combined with other foods.

A main ingredient can also be a vegetable, grain, or legume. A casserole based on sweet potatoes, brown rice, or lentils makes a hearty side dish or a meatless entrée. See **Fig. 42-4**.

Vegetables

Any cooked or canned vegetables can go into a casserole. You can also use fresh or frozen vegeta-

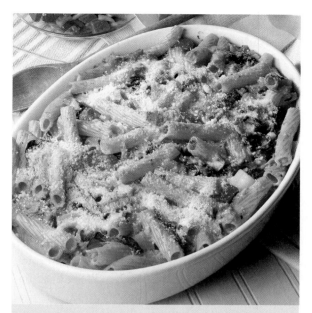

Fig. 42-4 Casserole ingredients are open to variation. Once you learn the basics, like the ratio of liquid to starches, you can apply some creativity. **How could you revise this dish?**

bles that cook quickly, like peas and mushrooms. Include aromatic vegetables, such as celery, onions, bell peppers, and garlic, and others that bring color and flavor to the dish.

Casseroles are an economical way to stretch vegetables while dressing them up as side dishes. Broccoli, sliced mushrooms, and toasted almonds baked in a cream soup serve more people than broccoli alone. You can add ingredients that go well with other dishes. The brown sugar and apples in a sweet potato casserole, for instance, complement the flavor of baked ham.

Starches

Starches thicken the mixture by absorbing liquids while adding flavor and nutrients. They include cooked dry beans, potatoes, and such cooked grain products as pasta, rice, and barley. You might try something less common: for example, high-protein quinoa or wild rice.

Bread is a typical starch in casseroles. In one favored brunch casserole, cubes of bread, cheese, and ham are baked in a custard of beaten eggs and milk. Poultry stuffing uses coarse, fresh or dry bread cubes.

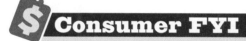

Consumer FYI

"Casseroles" to go. Consumers' demand for convenience has taken one-dish meals to the next stage: one-hand meals. Foods traditionally served as a sit-down meal can now be eaten on the run.

For example, some combination dishes come frozen as dough-wrapped turnovers. Varieties range from broccoli and cheese to gingered pork with water chestnuts. Stuffed pizza slices are also fully enclosed in crust. Ham and egg in a split biscuit, the breakfast in a bun made popular by fast-food restaurants, also appears in the grocer's freezer case. Another breakfast standard, a bowl of cereal and milk, has evolved into milk-and-cereal bars.

Meal replacement bars, especially those sold as part of special diet plans, also feed the "grab-and-go" trend. By some estimates, Americans spent nearly $2 billion on these products in 2003. Before choosing them often, read labels to check their nutrition impact.

Binders

A **binder** is a liquid that helps hold a mixture together. Binders, with different textures and flavors, range from milk, to yogurt, to pasta sauce. They sometimes help thicken the casserole as well. A baked macaroni and cheese casserole, for example, gets body from both eggs and cheese.

Seasonings

Seasonings used in casseroles vary with the ingredients and with other parts of the meal. Herbs and spices like oregano, basil, tarragon, black pepper, and marjoram bring out a food's savory qualities. For a sweet accent, try ginger, nutmeg, cinnamon, or allspice. In casseroles, dried herbs are preferred to fresh. Fresh herb flavors "flatten" during long cooking times.

Seasoning also comes in bottled sauces—soy, Worcestershire, tamari, barbecue, or hot pepper—and in mustards and other condiments.

Some binders add seasonings as well. Canned, condensed soups are often highly salted. A pasta sauce may contribute garlic or Romano cheese. Adjust the seasonings accordingly.

Toppings

Like dressings on salads, casserole toppings add flavor, color, and texture and keep the mixture from drying out. Crunchy toppings include croutons, cracker crumbs, and chow mein noodles. A casserole described as **au gratin** (oh GRAH-tun) is topped with buttered breadcrumbs or grated cheese. It may be browned under the broiler after baking. Mashed potatoes and unbaked biscuits provide a fluffy topping texture. See **Fig. 42-5**. You might mix ingredients like crushed cereal and wheat germ or mashed sweet potatoes and carrots.

A casserole may be topped before it goes in the oven or a few minutes before it comes out, depending on the ingredients. Some brown too quickly to last through the baking time. Frozen onion rings need to bake with the casserole, while cheese strips only need to melt.

Career Prep

Positive Work Relationships

GOOD WORK RELATIONSHIPS SHARE important qualities with friendships and family relationships yet are substantially different. Understanding the demands particular to work relations can help you enjoy your job and succeed in your future career.

AUTHORITY

Unless you're an entrepreneur your entire life, you'll deal with authority figures. If you do your job without causing problems, you will probably get along with your boss, but the relationship offers much more.

Most bosses want to foster enthusiasm and help employees learn and advance in their careers—after all, your success reflects directly on your supervisor. Show that you want to be an exceptional employee. Ask for specific goals—and then work to surpass them. Learn your boss's preferred way of doing things. Appreciate that he or she has other responsibilities and expects you to solve some problems yourself. If you must bring up a problem, try to offer a solution as well. If you make a mistake, accept responsibility and explain how you'll do things better the next time.

DIVERSITY

As American society grows more diverse, so does the workplace. It's natural to feel hesitant about approaching people who differ from you. The less you understand about someone's ethnicity, age, or abilities, the more you may worry about saying or doing something offensive.

Baking Casseroles

A casserole dish is about 2 to 4 inches deep and usually has a matching lid. Most are designed for baking and serving.

Often casserole ingredients are mixed together, placed in the dish, and covered with topping. In some recipes, layers are repeated and then topped. Lasagne, for example, has several layers of cooked noodles, cooked ground meat or vegetables, ricotta or cottage cheese, and tomato sauce. Grated cheese is the topping.

Casseroles are typically baked for 30 to 45 minutes in an oven preheated to about 350°F. They may be covered at the beginning and uncovered toward the end of the cooking time to thicken the mixture or brown the crust. They should rest for about 10 minutes before serving to set the ingredients.

Casseroles can be microwaved too. Combine all ingredients except the topping in an ungreased baking dish. Cover and cook at 100 percent power for 6 to 18 minutes, depending on the ingredients.

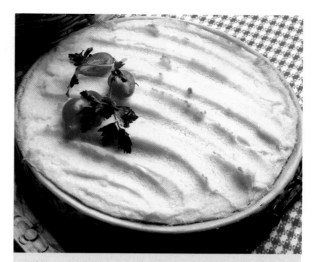

Fig. 42-5 For a shepherd's pie, mashed potatoes cover a blend of ground meat, onion, corn, green beans, and seasonings.

Stir once or twice during cooking, or rotate layered casseroles through the cooking time. Add the topping and brown under the broiler.

Stop and think, though: that person may feel the same about you. That's one thing you have in common. Focusing on other things is a start toward overcoming awkwardness. Everyone needs acceptance and approval. Everyone needs respect. As co-workers, moreover, you share the goals of your workplace.

Oddly, finding similarities helps you appreciate differences. It's an antidote to stereotypes, oversimplified and distorted assumptions about a certain group of people.

Stereotypes narrow thinking. They can be an excuse for poor relationships. People who don't get along conveniently blame it on being "too different."

Stereotypes are also ridiculous. If any single quality did determine someone's entire personality, the world would be a very boring place.

Whatever the makeup of your workplace, strive for an atmosphere of respect. Silently going along with demeaning remarks and jokes is not the sign of a team player. Such intolerance only stifles individual talents on which teamwork depends.

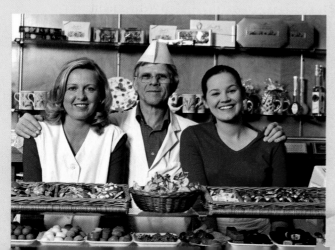

Career Connection

Bosses' wish list. Ask this question of a supervisor, your own or any other: "What is one thing employees could do to make your job easier?" Compare answers in class. Identify the most frequent requests.

Summarize Your Reading

▶ Both stir-fries and casseroles are economical dishes that are easily prepared and make scant amounts of food go a long way.

▶ The main ingredients in a typical stir-fry include a choice of meat, poultry, seafood, or tofu along with vegetables. With seasonings and sauce, these are cooked in a certain order.

▶ A main-dish casserole usually combines a protein food, vegetables, starch, binder, and seasonings.

▶ A variety of ingredients add color, flavor, and texture to stir-fries and casseroles.

Check Your Knowledge

1. In what ways are stir-fries and casseroles opposites?

2. Why were stir-fries and casseroles first developed?

3. What is a **stir-fry**?

4. What pre-preparation should be done before cooking a stir-fry?

5. For a stir-fry, why should you cut vegetables into pieces of similar size?

6. When preparing vegetables to stir-fry, why should dense or fibrous vegetables be cut on the diagonal?

7. **CRITICAL THINKING** A cook stir-fries leftover chicken and then adds vegetables. When eaten, the chicken tastes rubbery and dry. How could this have been prevented?

8. What ingredients might be combined to make a stir-fry sauce?

9. Explain the French term **mise en place**.

10. In what order should foods be added to a stir-fry?

11. Why does a wok work well for stir-fries?

12. What should you do if you are cooking a stir-fry and the pan or food seems to be burning?

13. Describe the steps to follow when cooking a stir-fry.

14. **CRITICAL THINKING** How are taste, color, and texture balanced in these stir-fry combinations: a) pork loin, carrots, broccoli, bean sprouts, and pineapple chunks in a sweet-and-sour sauce; b) tofu, carrots, broccoli, and red bell peppers in a peanut butter sauce?

15. What is a **casserole**?

16. What role do starches have in casseroles? Give examples.

17. How are **binders** used in casseroles?

18. Why are dried herbs preferred over fresh herbs in casseroles?

19. Describe some casserole toppings.

20. How is a casserole prepared for baking?

21. **CRITICAL THINKING** Why might you want to add water chestnuts to a casserole that contains couscous, black beans, roasted peppers, and ricotta cheese?

Apply Your Learning

1. **MATH** **Vegetable Comparison.** Is it less expensive to cut up fresh vegetables for stir-fries or to purchase ready-to-use vegetables? After checking prices, make recommendations for economical cooking.

2. **Wok Poster.** Make an educational poster about the wok and the utensils used with it. Be sure your poster teaches basic concepts about wok cooking.

3. **Stir-Fry Sauces.** Find recipes for stir-fry sauces. Choose one that sounds tasty. Try it out in a stir-fry dish.

4. **Planning Ahead.** Find recipes for main-dish casseroles that can be prepared a day ahead. Write a work plan for preparing one of the casseroles.

5. **Casserole variations.** Choose a vegetable or fruit that is often used in side dishes for a meal. Apples, sweet potatoes, and green beans are examples. Find and compare recipes for casseroles that use the food as a main ingredient. Which ones are the most nutritious? Prepare one dish and evaluate.

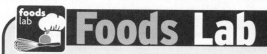

Foods Lab

Stir-Fry Recipes

Procedure: Develop a recipe for a stir-fry. Use vegetables, herbs, spices, or condiments that you think will work well together. Include meat, poultry, or other protein food 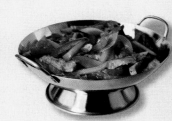 if you wish. The recipe must serve four people and be nutritious. Prepare the recipe and ask other lab teams to help evaluate the flavor, texture, and appearance.

Analyzing Results

❶ Were all the foods cooked to the desired texture? Explain.

❷ How well did the flavors blend? Did the flavors of different ingredients work well together? Explain.

❸ What was the biggest challenge in making a stir-fry? What tips would you give on making stir-fry dishes?

Food Science Experiment

Comparing Extenders

Objective: To compare qualities of different extenders. Extenders are ingredients that increase the size of a dish, sometimes to make it serve more people.

Procedure:

1. Measure enough of each of the following dry foods to make 2 servings: instant rice; mashed potato flakes; and stuffing mix. Weigh each food. Record these figures.

2. Prepare the foods according to package directions. Measure and weigh each one again. Record the figures.

3. Sample the foods, comparing them on texture and consistency.

Analyzing Results

❶ Which food gained the most in weight? In volume?

❷ Did the heaviest food also have the greatest volume? What might explain this result?

❸ How did the qualities of water absorption and volume affect the texture and consistency of each food? Why are these factors important when choosing an extender for a casserole?

Soups, Stews & Sauces

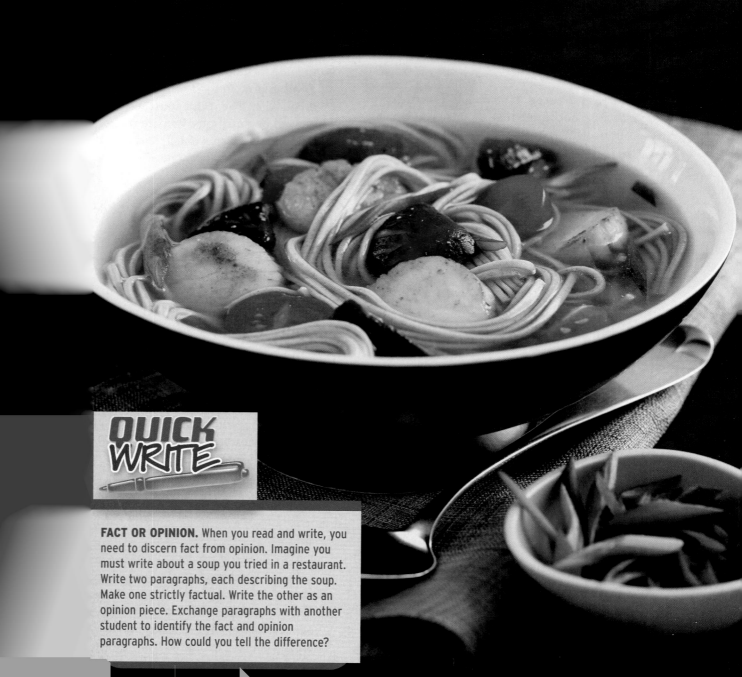

QUICK WRITE

FACT OR OPINION. When you read and write, you need to discern fact from opinion. Imagine you must write about a soup you tried in a restaurant. Write two paragraphs, each describing the soup. Make one strictly factual. Write the other as an opinion piece. Exchange paragraphs with another student to identify the fact and opinion paragraphs. How could you tell the difference?

Objectives

▶ Identify various soups, stews, and sauces.

▶ Explain ways to thicken a liquid.

▶ Describe and demonstrate how to make soups, stews, and sauces.

▶ Explain how to store soups, stews, and sauces.

Terms

au jus	reduction
bisque	roux
bouillon	sauce
broth	soup
consommé	stew
cornstarch	stock
gelatinization	

WHAT DO THESE FOODS HAVE IN common: a peppery shrimp gumbo served at a New Orleans restaurant; a homemade chicken gravy passed at a family dinner table; and tomato soup ladled out in a school cafeteria? Each one—a stew, a sauce, and a soup—starts from one basic formula: a liquid plus something to thicken it. Their differences come from the proportion of one ingredient to the other and from the ingredients added by imaginative chefs.

LIQUIDS

To make soups, stews, and sauces, you need a liquid. The choice depends on the other ingredients in the recipe. For a hearty vegetable beef stew, already filled with a variety of flavors, you could use just water. A mild soup based on one vegetable benefits from fruit juice or broth. **Broth**, also called **stock**, is the flavorful liquid made by simmering meat, poultry, fish, or vegetables in water. A pumpkin soup might start with chicken broth, and tomato soup might begin with tomato juice. Lemon juice sharpens a sauce for a baked potato.

Making Broth

Making broth can be time-consuming, but many people like the results better than store-bought versions. The flavors are more distinct and can be tailored to personal preferences.

A broth is also a worthy end for food scraps—seafood shells, vegetables or their peels, and animal bones, usually with some meat attached. Any combination of these ingredients is placed in a large pot with assorted herbs and covered with cold water. The gelatin in bones from raw meat and poultry adds richness. Very ripe, aromatic vegetables quickly release their flavors.

A broth in the making simmers for several hours. Added water replaces what evaporates so the ingredients remain submerged. The broth is then strained and the ingredients discarded.

As it cools, broth is a prime breeding place for bacteria, especially when made from fat- and protein-rich meat stock. Pour the broth into shallow containers and chill quickly. Chilling encourages any fat to rise to the surface. After the fat sets, you can suction it off with a baster or skim it off with a spoon. Homemade broth should be used

---

SAFETY ALERT

Safe stock. Before using homemade stock in a recipe, bring it to a full boil for a few minutes to destroy any lingering microorganisms. Throw out any stock that bubbles in the refrigerator. That's a sign of fermentation and spoilage.

within about four days or frozen in recipe-size portions for up to three months.

When making broth isn't practical, you can choose from convenience forms. Canned, ready-to-use broth comes in several varieties, including reduced-sodium, fat-free, and vegetarian. Concentrated cubes or granules are dissolved in hot water. This form is often labeled **bouillon** (BOOL-yahn), which is yet another name for broth. Convenience broths may be flavored with animal fat and dehydrated meat, poultry, or vegetables, but a main ingredient is usually salt.

THICKENING METHODS

In many soups, stews, and sauces, the liquid is thickened. One thickening method decreases the amount of liquid. A starchy or protein food is used in other thickening methods.

Whatever method you use for thickening, cook the mixture over low heat. High heat speeds evaporation, and the mixture may get too thick or burn. Evaporation continues as the mixture cools, often leaving an unsightly skin of concentrated proteins on the surface. To prevent this, lightly press a piece of wax paper or plastic wrap onto the surface until serving.

Reduction

A simple thickening technique is **reduction**, or simmering an uncovered mixture until some of the liquid evaporates. The liquid cooks until reaching the desired volume and consistency. Interestingly, this method sometimes starts by increasing the liquid. You might add fish stock to flavor the liquid used to poach fish and then simmer it down into a sauce.

Reduction concentrates flavors. Therefore you should season liquids after reducing them so that flavors won't be unpleasantly strong.

Grain Products

As you know, the starch in grain products makes an excellent thickener. The grain product chosen for thickening brings different qualities to the dish you make.

Prepared Grain Products

Whole grains and baked products thicken soups and stews by absorbing water and releasing starch as they cook or dissolve. They also contribute texture and nutrients. Their use is a tradition in many European cuisines. Oats are found in some Irish stews. The German beef dish *sauerbraten* is served with gravy thickened by gingersnap cookies.

Such grains as barley and rice are added with other ingredients in a soup or stew according to their cooking time. Bread slices or crumbs are thoroughly soaked with water or vinegar to make a paste and stirred in during the last 5 to 10 minutes of cooking. The stew in **Fig. 43-1** is thickened with bread crumbs and also with tapioca, a starch extracted from the root of the cassava plant.

Flour and Cornstarch

Flour is a standard thickener for soups, stews, and sauces. Any flour can be used, but all-purpose flour has more starch than other types. A mixture thickened with flour turns opaque, as in gravy.

Cornstarch is a fine, white powder that is pure starch made from the endosperm of the corn kernel. Cornstarch is often chosen to thicken desserts and Asian stir-fries. It adds a clear, glossy finish. Since cornstarch has twice the thickening power of flour, you need only half as much to thicken the same amount of liquid.

If you try to add flour or cornstarch directly to a hot liquid, lumps form. If caught in time, these pasty lumps can be mashed against the pan sides or strained to remove them. Otherwise, they cook in the liquid, leaving a lumpy—and unappetizing—product.

An easy solution is to mix the starch with cold water before adding it to the liquid to be thickened. Begin by mixing one part starch with two parts cold water in a jar or small bowl. This separates the starch granules so they won't clump together when they contact the hot liquid.

How much starch do you need to thicken a liquid? **Fig. 43-2** shows what to use to get different consistencies. A medium thickness is enough to coat the back of a spoon. To thicken 1 cup of liquid to medium thickness, you need 2 tablespoons of flour. Mix that amount with twice as much cold water, or 4 tablespoons (¼ cup).

Next, slowly pour and stir the cool starch mixture into the hot liquid. Simmer over medium

Fig. 43-1

French Oven Beef Stew

Yield	Nutrition Analysis
8 servings	*Per Serving:* 420 calories, 10 g total fat, 3.5 g saturated fat, 0 g trans fat, 90 mg cholesterol, 1020 mg sodium, 50 g total carbohydrate, 5 g dietary fiber, 13 g sugars, 32 g protein
	Percent Daily Value: vitamin A 100%, vitamin C 40%, calcium 15%, iron 30%

Ingredients

2½ pounds lean beef stew meat (trimmed and cut into cubes)

1 can diced, seasoned tomatoes (28 ounces)

½ cup beef broth

¼ cup balsamic vinegar

¼ cup water

1 pound small white onions, peeled

5 medium-size carrots, peeled and cut into bite-size pieces

2 pounds small potatoes, peeled

4 or 5 stalks celery, cut into bite-size pieces

4 Tbsp. tapioca

¼ cup fine bread crumbs

bay leaf

1 tsp. salt

pepper to taste

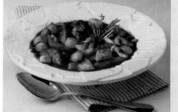

Directions

1. Preheat oven to 250°F.
2. Place all prepared ingredients in a large casserole dish or Dutch oven and stir well.
3. Bake for 5 to 6 hours, stirring occasionally. End cooking time when meat is thoroughly cooked and vegetables are tender. If needed to reduce liquid, cook uncovered for the last half hour.

heat until thickened, stirring constantly to keep starch granules separated. A flour mixture must be simmered for several minutes to prevent a raw flour taste.

This thickening process is called **gelatinization** (juh-LA-tun-uh-ZAY-shun). Energized by heat, the starch granules absorb water and slowly swell, although you don't see this while you stir. Eventually, the granules burst and the starch that rushes out thickens the liquid very quickly. Wait for this thickening process to occur before deciding you need extra starch mixture. Adding more starch too soon might make your product too thick.

Acids interfere with the thickening process, but they don't undo prior thickening. For this reason, an ingredient like lemon juice is added after a liquid has thickened.

Thickened mixtures are rather sensitive. Overcooking and prolonged stirring can cause

them to revert to a runny state. Freezing the mixture gives the same result. To avoid these problems, add starches during the last minutes of cooking and simmer gently. Freeze soup or stew unthickened, and stir in the starch when you reheat it for serving.

Fig. 43-2

Starch Amount for Thickening Liquids

Desired Thickness of Liquid	Starch Amount Per One Cup of Liquid	
	Flour	Cornstarch
Thin	1 Tbsp.	1½ tsp.
Medium	2 Tbsp.	1 Tbsp.
Thick	3 Tbsp.	1½ Tbsp.

Making a Roux

Another way to use flour to thicken a liquid is to make a roux (ROO). A **roux** is a mixture of equal amounts of flour and fat. The fat might be butter, margarine, or fat drippings from cooked foods. Base the fat and flour amount on how thick you want the liquid to be. As you saw in **Fig. 43-1**, a medium thickness takes 2 tablespoons of flour for every cup of liquid. Use an equal amount of fat. Remember the ratio 2:2:1, and adjust it for thickness.

To make the roux, measure the fat. If necessary, melt the fat over medium heat to liquefy it. Then stir in an equal amount of flour. As a smooth paste forms, the fat coats the starch granules. Cook and stir the roux only until it bubbles.

To use the roux, gradually stir in the liquid that you want to thicken. Stirring constantly, continue cooking over low heat until the mixture is smooth and thick. The coated starch granules prevent lumps from forming.

Some recipes call for a roux that is beige to dark brown in color. Longer cooking—as much as 20 minutes or more—creates a nutty flavor and a deeper color but lessens the roux's thickening power. You need more flour in proportion to fat, depending on the degree of browning.

If you want to save a roux for later use, you can refrigerate or freeze uncooked roux by the tablespoon. It's often added to correct a runny sauce.

Legumes and Vegetables

Cooked legumes and vegetables thicken in the same way that grain products do. Beans, split peas, and other high-starch foods are most effective. Broccoli, squash, and carrots have less starch but more color and flavor. Mash or purée the ingredients and stir them into the soup or stew. Simmer a few minutes to let them blend, release starch, and heat through.

You can thicken 1 cup of liquid with 3 tablespoons of grated raw potato. Add the potato about 15 to 20 minutes before the end of the cooking time.

Eggs

Eggs are less effective than starch at thickening, but they add richness and flavor. Generally, 1 large egg or 2 yolks thicken 1 cup of liquid, depending on the other foods in the mixture.

Since eggs curdle easily when added to a hot liquid or an acidic food, they must be tempered. First beat the eggs lightly. Then stir in a small amount of the hot or acidic liquid. Pour the diluted egg mixture a little at a time into the rest of the liquid, stirring constantly. If the mixture does start to curdle, strenuous beating and straining can sometimes save it.

SOUPS

What comes to mind when you think of soup? Whether you picture a simmering kettle of homemade soup, a can of soup for lunch, or a container of steaming soup from the deli, all share a common definition. **Soups** are basically dishes of solid foods cooked in liquid. They often contain broth as the liquid, along with meat, poultry, seafood, or vegetables. See **Fig. 43-3**.

Soups have been enjoyed throughout history. Records show that ancient Greeks sold soup on the streets of Athens, perhaps white beans in beef broth or garbanzo beans with spinach, two early recipes.

Soups can be highly nutritious. Long cooking destroys some B vitamins and vitamin C, but other water-soluble vitamins remain in the liquid.

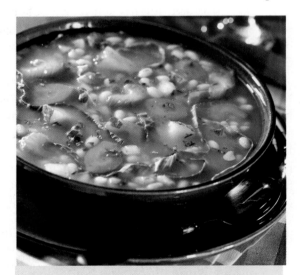

Fig. 43-3 Soup has universal appeal. For centuries it has appeared on tables, enjoyed by royalty and peasantry, old and young, and every nationality.

As a rule, one quart of soup serves six as an appetizer or three as an entrée.

Soup Types

Soup recipes cover an amazing array of combinations. Nevertheless, they all fall into five basic groups.

Clear Soups

Besides providing a base for more complex soups and sauces, broth can be served as a clear, thin soup. **Consommé** is a clarified broth, completely strained of all particles and sediment. It may be served warm as an appetizer. A favorite breakfast food in Japan is a clear soup made from *miso* (MEE-soh), a fermented soybean paste.

Cream Soups

A smooth cream soup typically begins with vegetables and seasonings that are cooked in a liquid like broth. The mixture is puréed in a blender, food processor, or food mill and thickened with flour and milk or cream. Low-fat recipes use evaporated milk or nonfat dry milk powder.

Broccoli, squash, and asparagus—almost any vegetable—can be used as the base for a cream soup. **Bisque** (BISK), however, is a rich cream soup that uses shellfish as the base.

Soups made with starchy foods like potatoes and legumes don't need additional thickening. See **Fig. 43-4**. Split pea soup, for instance, is made by cooking green split peas in liquid with seasonings and puréeing the mixture. You can make black bean soup by cooking black beans in water, puréeing the mixture, and adding seasonings, including hot pepper sauce and liquid smoke.

Chunky Soups

Chunky soups brim with chunks of vegetables, meat, poultry, seafood, legumes, and pasta in assorted combinations. A chunky soup, some crusty bread, and a salad make a simple but nourishing meal. Here are a few of these hearty soups:

- **Chowder.** Chowders are fish, meat, or vegetable soups thickened with potatoes or cream. The classic New England clam chowder is thick with

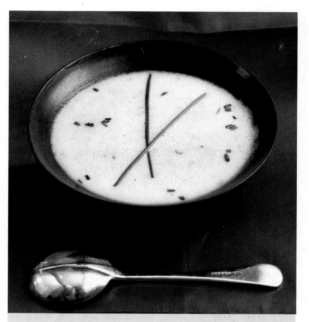

Fig. 43-4 Potato soup is creamy. How is it thickened?

cream, chunky with potatoes, and flavored with bacon. Manhattan clam chowder is lighter and features chunks of both potatoes and tomatoes.

- **Mulligatawny** (muh-lih-guh-TAW-nee). Mulligatawny means "pepper water" in southern India, where this soup originated. It starts with a chicken broth, highly seasoned with chiles, curry powder, and other spices. Its many versions include poultry or meat, a variety of vegetables, rice, eggs, shredded coconut, and coconut milk or cream.

- **Minestrone** (mih-nuh-STROH-nee). This hearty Italian soup is made with vegetables, beans, and pasta and topped with grated Parmesan cheese.

Fruit Soups

Fruit soups, a Scandinavian and Eastern European import, have gained interest in the United States. Served hot or cold, they can be another healthful way to take advantage of seasonal fruits. Out of season, dried, canned, or frozen varieties work well. Fruits are puréed, flavored with spices or grated peel, and thickened with cornstarch, gelatin, buttermilk, or yogurt. Dry fruits, and sometimes fresh, are simmered first in water or juice. Richer recipes call for light or sour cream.

Cold Soups

Fruit soups are not the only ones served cold. In hot weather especially, cold vegetable soups make a refreshing beginning to a meal. See **Fig. 43-5**. Not surprisingly, some classic recipes originated in hot climates. *Vichyssoise* (vi-shee-SWAHZ) was named for its inventor's home in southern France. The soup is an elegant purée of cooked leeks and potatoes in heavy cream, garnished with chives. *Gazpacho* (guz-PAH-choh) is a well-seasoned, uncooked soup of southern Spain. Dry bread is soaked and puréed with fresh tomatoes, bell peppers, onions, celery, cucumbers, olive oil, and vinegar.

Making Soup

How you start a soup depends on what you want in the end. Chicken vegetable soup is a basic model for a hot, simmered soup. Begin by sautéing chopped onions, carrots, celery, garlic, and other aromatic vegetables in a pot or slow cooker.

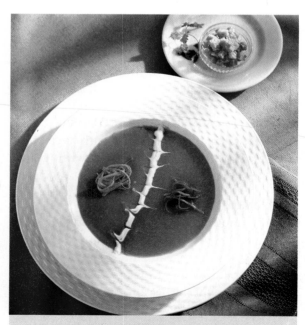

Fig. 43-5 This cold soup is actually two soups in one. Why might someone serve a cold soup?

To this mixture, add the liquid and main ingredients. Using three or four different vegetables adds flavor and color—tomatoes, potatoes, carrots, and corn, perhaps. Remember to add ingredients at different times, if needed, depending on how long each one takes to cook. Raw chicken nuggets go in first, followed by rice, sliced fresh vegetables, and cooked vegetables. As an alternative, you can sauté the chicken first to bring out the flavor. You can also put in whole pieces of chicken, remove it from the bones after cooking, and return the chicken to the pot.

Season and simmer the soup until all ingredients are tender. Thicken the broth if needed. Finally, taste the soup and adjust the seasonings before serving.

Soup can be garnished to enhance appearance, complement the flavor, and add texture. See **Fig. 43-6**. You might top a thin onion soup with crisp croutons or sprinkle chopped, fresh parsley on a seafood chowder. Toppings can be placed in each bowl before serving or arranged as an assortment to let guests choose their own.

Soups with Convenience

As you can see, homemade soups are not whipped up on a moment's notice. A microwave oven can help with some steps, but not with the slow simmering needed to tenderize meats or bring out flavors. That's why many people make a

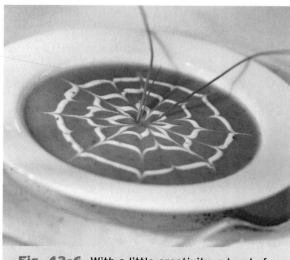

Fig. 43-6 With a little creativity, a bowl of soup can become a work of art.

large pot of soup when time permits and refrigerate or freeze servings for later meals. If stored in individual containers, they are easily reheated in the microwave.

Packaged soup starters are available, but you can make your own. Stir together the dry ingredients—grains, legumes, seasonings, and bouillon granules—and store in a cool place. To prepare, add liquid and fresh ingredients to the mix and simmer until done.

STEWS

It may sound obvious, but a **stew** is any dish prepared by stewing, or simmering small pieces of food in a tightly covered pan. See **Fig. 43-7**. Most stews include vegetables and meat, poultry, or fish. Stews tend to contain less liquid than soups. Water is the usual liquid, but broth, tomato or vegetable juice, or fruit juice can be used. The method and the dish are simple and ancient, tracing back to open-fire cooking.

Like broth, stew goes by other names, with subtle differences in meaning. A ragout (ra-GOO) is thick, meaty, and highly seasoned. Fricassee (FRIH-kuh-see) usually refers to a chicken stew. To fricassee is to sauté in butter without browning, which is the first step in the recipe.

Some stews have become points of pride in cuisines around the world. A sampling of ethnic stews includes these:

- **Goulash.** This Hungarian national dish is made with beef cubes, onions, bell peppers, water, vinegar, and paprika. It's served over buttered noodles.
- **Irish stew.** A traditional stew in Ireland's history was made with lamb, water, potatoes, onions, and parsley. When available, turnips, carrots, and barley were also added. Many variations are in recipes today.
- **Dovi (doe-vee).** For this stew from Zimbabwe, tomatoes, sweet potatoes, okra, and other vegetables simmer with chicken in a stock thickened with peanut butter. It's traditionally scooped from a communal pot with flatbread or served with cornmeal mush.
- **Israeli wheat berry stew.** Seasoned with garlic and onions, this hearty vegetarian stew uses the

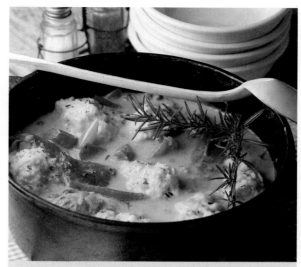

Fig. 43-7 Dumplings are added to some stews. These balls of dough cook as they simmer and steam in the liquid.

entire wheat kernel, or berry, along with beans and potatoes.
- **Posole (poh-SOH-leh).** This pork stew is a Christmas season tradition in Mexican homes. Authentic recipes use posole corn, kernels that have been soaked and dried. Hominy, the flaked inner kernel, is a common replacement. The stew is seasoned with chilies, garlic, and cilantro. It's topped with thinly sliced lettuce, cabbage, or radishes.
- **Burgoo (BUHR-goo).** The meat for this stew, made famous in Kentucky, traditionally included "whatever you catch," meaning such game as squirrel or deer. Modern versions include beef and chicken along with carrots, tomatoes, potatoes, cabbage, celery, and onions.

Making a Stew

One reason for stew's long-lasting popularity is that it's an ideal way to prepare inexpensive cuts of meat and poultry. The slow simmering tenderizes them while juices from the foods flavor the liquid. This is the basic method:

1. Cut meat for stewing into 1- to 2-inch cubes. Cut chicken into parts. Since the chicken cooks in liquid, removing the skin reduces fat.

2. Dredge the meat in flour and brown it in a small amount of fat in a large pot or skillet. Chicken may be browned or not, as you like.
3. Transfer the meat to a clean plate. Drain any excess fat from the pan.
4. Sauté aromatic vegetables in remaining fat.
5. Return the meat to the pan. Add seasonings and enough liquid to cover the meat. Cover the pan and simmer until the meat is tender. Beef may simmer for 2 to 3 hours. Poultry may cook in less than an hour. Fish may need as little as 10 minutes and is often added after other ingredients.

Due to the long simmering involved, stew vegetables usually include chunks or quarters of carrots, potatoes, parsnips, and other root vegetables and tubers. More delicate vegetables like baby corn can be added later during cooking. To vary the flavor, consider adding fruit or juice. Some suitable combinations include pork with fresh apples, beef with dried plums or apricots, and poultry with pineapple or orange juice.

You can make a vegetarian stew by cooking virtually any vegetables with seasonings in vegetable broth. You might try carrots, tomatoes, bell peppers, leeks, turnips, okra, acorn squash, Brussels sprouts, or green beans.

Stews can also be prepared in a slow cooker or oven. The meat or poultry may be browned or simply added with other ingredients. The stew cooks at a low temperature, usually around 300°F, for up to 5 hours.

A stew can be served over noodles, hot biscuits, mashed potatoes, or brown rice. Many people feel a good stew needs a hearty bread to "sop up" the juices.

SAUCES

Sauces go back to the days before refrigeration. They literally covered up the taste of foods that were going bad. Inspired by Italian chefs, the French elevated sauce making to an art by the 1800s. In fact, one principle of French cuisine states that "the sauce is everything."

Today a **sauce**, a flavored liquid that is often thickened, is served to enhance the flavor of another food, not to hide it. See **Fig. 43-8**. This

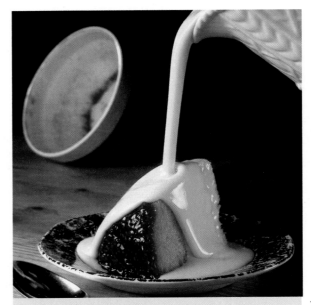

Fig. 43-8 Dessert sauces are sweet. Some use cornstarch to thicken a fruit juice. The sauce may be seasoned with a flavoring like vanilla.

sweeping definition includes both the ketchup squirted on french fries and the cream-rich diplomat sauce served with shellfish.

In sauce cookery, several basic types are the source of many variations. These are hollandaise; basic white sauce; light and brown, stock-based sauces; and tomato-based, or red, sauce. Another sauce is a salad dressing—oil and vinegar.

Hollandaise

To make hollandaise sauce, egg yolks are whisked with melted butter and lemon juice over a double boiler. The yolks are the emulsifier that holds the mixture together. Hollandaise sauce turns poached eggs, ham, and an English muffin into eggs Benedict. The sauce is also a favorite on asparagus or fish.

Hollandaise is the foundation for béarnaise (BAY-ahr-nayz) sauce, which features white vinegar, green onions, and tarragon. Puréed tomatoes turn hollandaise into Choron (show-RAWN) sauce.

Basic White Sauce

White sauce is also called cream sauce or béchamel (bay-shuh-MEL). See **Fig. 43-9**. It is milk or cream thickened with a butter-and-flour roux. Make the roux as described earlier according to the sauce thickness you want. Cook the roux only until it bubbles, without browning. Gradually stir in the milk and cook over low heat, stirring constantly until thickened. Season as desired.

This mild sauce is easily converted into classic recipes. Using heavy cream and adding Parmesan cheese makes Alfredo sauce to toss with pasta. With cream and paprika, white sauce becomes a rich Newburg sauce for lobster. White sauce is also the base for that American classic, macaroni and cheese.

Stock-Based Sauces

A stock-based sauce is made like a white sauce, with animal fat and meat juices replacing the butter and milk. Poultry drippings and a white roux produce a light sauce. Brown sauces are made from red meat juices and a brown roux.

The pan or "country" gravy served with roast beef or chicken shows how a stock-based sauce is made. First remove the cooked meat or poultry from the pan and pour the juices that remain into a measuring cup. Skim off and reserve the fat. Make a roux in the roasting pan, using 2 tablespoons each of flour and reserved fat for each cup of juice. Add beef or chicken broth if you don't have enough juice. For a richer flavor, scrape the bottom of the pan to loosen browned bits of meat or poultry.

Like white sauce, stock-based sauces are expanded into different recipes. When chicken gravy is reduced with heavy cream it's called supreme sauce. Deviled sauce is a brown sauce made with vinegar or Worcestershire sauce and cayenne pepper.

Tomato-Based Sauces

A basic tomato sauce takes nothing more than sautéed aromatic vegetables and some kind of

---

Fig. 43-9

Try This! Recipe

White Sauce

Yield
About 2 cups (6 servings)

Nutrition Analysis
Per Serving: 140 calories, 9 g total fat, 7 g saturated fat, 0 g trans fat, 30 mg cholesterol, 290 mg sodium, 9 g total carbohydrate, 0 g dietary fiber, 5 g sugars, 4 g protein

Percent Daily Value: vitamin A 10%, vitamin C 0%, calcium 10%, iron 2%

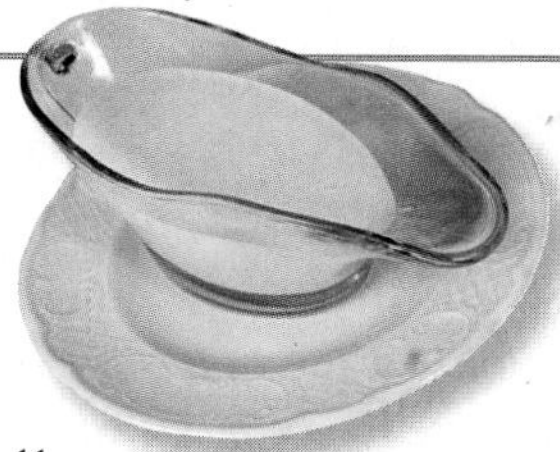

Ingredients
4 Tbsp. butter
4 Tbsp. flour
2½ cups 2% milk, heated

½ tsp. salt (or to taste)
¼ tsp. pepper (or to taste)
nutmeg (if desired)

Directions
1. In a heavy-bottomed, medium saucepan over medium-low heat, melt butter.
2. Stir in flour and cook, stirring constantly until paste bubbles, about 2 minutes. This makes a roux. For traditional white sauce, do not let the roux brown.
3. Add hot milk, continuing to stir while the sauce thickens.
4. Bring mixture to a boil. Add salt and pepper to taste. Reduce heat to low and continue stirring for 2 to 3 minutes. Remove saucepan from heat.
5. If saving sauce for later use, pour a film of milk over the top or top with plastic wrap or wax paper to prevent skin from forming.

Variation: Add cheese or herbs for different flavors.

tomato product. The thickness, flavor, and color depend on the ingredients you choose.

Traditional Italian sauces start with onions and garlic in olive oil or butter. To maintain a smooth texture, stir in canned tomato paste or purée, diluted with hot water or broth. Simmer and reduce to the desired thickness, adding herbs and spices in the last 10 minutes of cooking.

Tomato sauces are usually associated with pasta, but they complement other dishes as well. Slices of eggplant are breaded, fried, and covered with tomato sauce for eggplant Parmesan. You can serve rice with a hot Creole tomato sauce made with celery and bell pepper. Barbecue sauce is also a tomato-based sauce, sweet with brown sugar or molasses and tangy with mustard, onions, and garlic. See **Fig. 43-10**.

Oil-and-Vinegar Sauces

A recipe for an oil-and-vinegar sauce might remind you of a vinaigrette salad dressing. The two mixtures use the same ingredients—oil, acidic liquids, and seasonings. Sauces, however, tend to use more liquid compared to oil. An Asian sweet and sour sauce, for example, might use a few tablespoons of peanut oil to a cup of rice vinegar, along with garlic, ginger, and ketchup.

Marinades also belong to the oil-and-vinegar class. Besides adding flavor, marinades tenderize less costly cuts of meat by breaking down connective tissue. To prevent eating contaminants picked up from raw meat, poultry, or fish, marinades should be discarded after use. You can make extra to serve as a sauce. To make marinades, use any type of cooking oil and substitute other acidic ingredients for the vinegar, including cider and buttermilk. For seasonings, try such aromatic vegetables as onions and garlic along with your choice of herbs and spices.

To use a marinade, shake the ingredients in a tightly closed jar. Place the food in a glass, stainless steel, or enamel pan. Pour the marinade over the food and refrigerate. You can also marinate food in a plastic bag that zips securely closed. Place it in a container to catch leaks. For even coverage, turn or stir the food at least once while marinating.

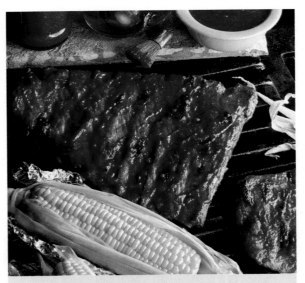

Fig. 43-10 You can make your own barbecue sauce or buy one of many different sauces that are ready to use. Which suits you, mild or firehouse hot?

Marinating time depends on the food. Fish fillets may get mushy after 30 minutes. Some meats can be marinated for up to 24 hours.

Quick Sauces

When time or other resources are short, you can make sauces by diluting cream soups with a little milk or stock. Yogurt is a common sauce base in Mediterranean cuisines. Tailor convenience sauces to fit your recipe by adding seasonings, mustard, honey, citrus juice, or relishes. The simplest, lightest option when preparing roasts is to serve them **au jus** (oh-ZHOO), with the natural meat juices, unthickened and skimmed of fat. For a quick marinade, try a salad dressing.

STORAGE

Refrigerate leftover soups, stews, and sauces immediately. Many people feel that soups and stews taste better "the next day," but use them within three or four days. For longer storage, freeze soups and stews for up to three months. Some sauces may be frozen, but remember that mixtures thickened with flour or cornstarch may separate when thawed.

Television Co-Host

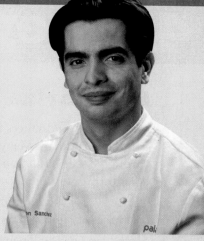

AARON SANCHEZ: Aaron Sanchez should be tired. Still in his thirties, he has already found success as a chef, television personality, and cookbook author. It's all part of a career that he describes as "a great ride that I hope never ends."

"Always in a hurry." Aaron's passion for foods comes naturally. His mother, noted Mexican chef Zarela Martinez, brought the family from El Paso, Texas, to New York City in 1984. Soon she was impressing sophisticated diners with authentic tastes of her native southwestern Mexico, with eleven-year-old Aaron helping in the pantry. At age sixteen, he worked with New Orleans chef Paul Prudhomme for a year after high school. Next came a culinary arts degree from Johnson and Wales University in Rhode Island. His training came full circle with a return to New York City in 1994. "I was always in a hurry," he says, "to grow up, to accomplish, to live."

Making the Cuisine Scene. In New York, Aaron joined the forefront of *nuevo Latino*—new Latin—cuisine. Nuevo Latino is dramatic and innovative. Fresh ingredients and bold flavors show off the depth and variety of traditional Latin and Caribbean cooking. Lamb is rubbed with a paste of chilies, garlic, and allspice. Salads feature cactus leaves. Desserts include coconut ice cream with caramelized pineapple.

Aaron became one of the cuisine's bright young stars. After earning glowing reviews as a sous chef and executive chef, he and a partner opened their own restaurant, Paladar, in 2001. A *paladare* in Cuba is a small restaurant run from the owner's home. Despite the "funky but chic" atmosphere, Paladar's menu is based on Latin home cooking that might be served in such a place—but with a flair. A *paladare* might serve grilled corn. Paladar's grilled corn comes with chile-lime butter.

New Food in the Neighborhood. As this exotic trend gained momentum, the Food Network asked Aaron to join the cast of co-hosts on *The Melting Pot*, a show that explores ethnic cuisines of the United States. He followed that success with his first cookbook, *La Comida del Barrio: Latin-American Cooking Across the United States.* That makes him a third-generation cookbook author, "which is very cool."

Like his other ventures, the book is a way to share his beloved Latino traditions and culture. "I felt it important for people to know more about the people who cook this food and the kind of places where Latin Americans seek comfort food. I wanted to make a clear statement that this is a new kind of American food."

Aaron's prediction for nuevo Latino could be a forecast for his career as well: "Look to the past to find the answers to what lies ahead." He balances his mother's example to "keep reinventing myself and finding new passions" with his own advice: "Find one thing that you do well and let it shine."

On-line Connections

1. To learn more about topics in this article, search the Internet for these key words: Zarela Martinez; culinary arts degree; nuevo Latino cuisine.

2. To learn about related careers, search the Internet for these key words: restaurant manager; sous chef.

Summarize Your Reading

▶ Soups, stews, and sauces are all made from a liquid ingredient. Many are thickened through either reduction or the use of a starchy or protein food.

▶ Broth is a flavorful liquid that is often used as a base for soups, stews, and sauces.

▶ Soups can be clear, creamy, or chunky. They can also be made with fruit and served cold.

▶ The stewing technique is basically simple and dates back to ancient times, when open-fire cooking was common.

▶ With all their variety, sauces enhance the flavors of food, often turning them from simple to elegant.

Check Your Knowledge

1. What are **broths** and **stocks**?

2. How should broth be stored, and why?

3. Why should **soups**, **stews**, and **sauces** be thickened over low heat?

4. What can you do to prevent the unsightly skin that forms on the surface of soups, stews, and sauces when cooling?

5. How does **reduction** thicken a sauce?

6. **CRITICAL THINKING** While using cornstarch to make a sauce for a fruit dessert, a cook dropped two tablespoons of cornstarch into hot juice. Predict what may happen. What do you suggest?

7. To make 2½ cups of sauce with medium thickness, how much flour do you need and what do you do with the flour before adding it to hot liquid?

8. Explain **gelatinization**.

9. How do you make a **roux** and use it to thicken a liquid?

10. How are legumes and vegetables used to thicken a soup or stew?

11. What is **consommé**?

12. **CRITICAL THINKING** Compare the following soups: clear, creamy, and chunky.

13. Describe these chunky soups: chowder, mulligatawny, and minestrone.

14. How do you make a fruit soup?

15. Why is the order of adding ingredients important when making soup?

16. How is a stew different from a soup?

17. Describe these stews: goulash, Irish stew, and burgoo.

18. How is a basic beef stew prepared?

19. What are the five sauces that are basic to making all sauces?

20. How do you make and use a hollandaise sauce?

21. Compare white sauce with stock-based sauce.

22. Is a roux used to make a tomato-based sauce? Explain.

23. Why is **au jus** a quick sauce?

24. How should soups, stews, and sauces be stored?

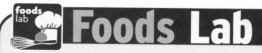
Apply Your Learning

1. **Menu Development.** Develop a menu for a soup and sandwich shop. What kinds of soups will you sell? Include at least one ethnic soup.

2. **MATH** **Menu Pricing.** Determine pricing for the menu planned in activity 1 above. Remember that ingredient costs, overhead expenses, employees' wages, and profit need to be factored into prices.

3. **MATH** **Cost Comparison.** Compare costs of soups, including broths, bouillons, soups made with starters, soups made from scratch, canned and dried soups, soups from a deli, and organic soups. Report findings and recommend soups for different situations, such as a buffet for 50, a family supper, a fancy gourmet meal, and an after-game party.

4. **Demonstration.** Demonstrate how to make one of the following: a) roux; b) white sauce; c) lemon sauce with cornstarch; d) homemade stock; e) cold fruit soup.

Foods Lab

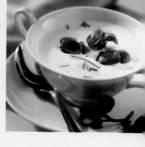

Comparing Thickeners

Procedure: Prepare a potato soup recipe provided by your teacher. Complete the recipe using one of these assigned methods:

Method 1: Purée half the soup in a blender. Return to the saucepan and heat through.

Method 2: Dissolve 2 Tbsp. cornstarch in ¼ cup water. Gradually whisk into the hot soup. Cook and stir until thickened, about 1 minute.

Sample and compare each recipe.

Analyzing Results

❶ How did each method affect the soup's appearance, taste, and texture?

❷ Which method do you think gave better results? Why?

Food Science Experiment

Simmering a Sauce

Objective: To observe how simmering affects a sauce.

Procedure:

1. Prepare 8 ounces of spaghetti and set aside.
2. Prepare a tomato-based sauce. In a medium saucepan, sauté ½ cup chopped onions and 4 chopped garlic cloves in 3 tablespoons of olive oil. Add one 28-ounce can of Italian-seasoned, crushed tomatoes and ½ cup of water. Stir. Heat to simmering.
3. Remove ½ cup of sauce and place it on a small serving of spaghetti. Wait for 1 minute

and record your observations on appearance, consistency, and taste.

4. Using a clean wooden skewer, measure the height of the sauce in the pan.
5. Simmer the sauce, stirring occasionally. Every 10 minutes, measure the sauce and record its height and appearance. After measuring at 30 minutes, repeat Step 3.

Analyzing Results

❶ What process did you observe as you cooked the sauce?

❷ How did simmering affect the sauce's appearance, consistency, and taste over time?

❸ What do you conclude?

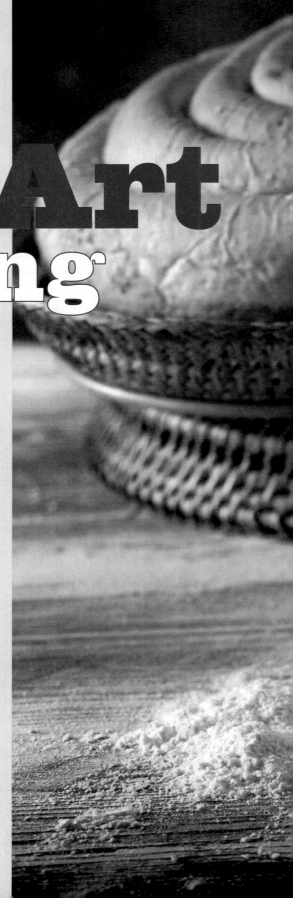

The Art
of Baking

CHAPTER 44   **Baking Basics**

CHAPTER 45   **Quick & Yeast Breads**

CHAPTER 46   **Cakes, Cookies & Candies**

CHAPTER 47   **Pies & Tarts**

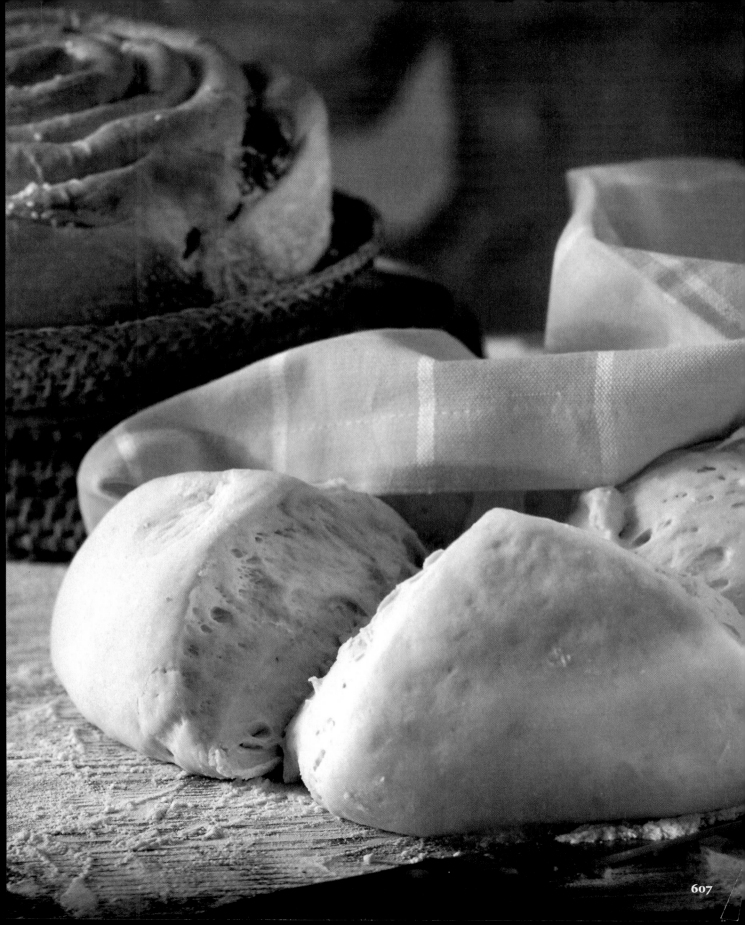

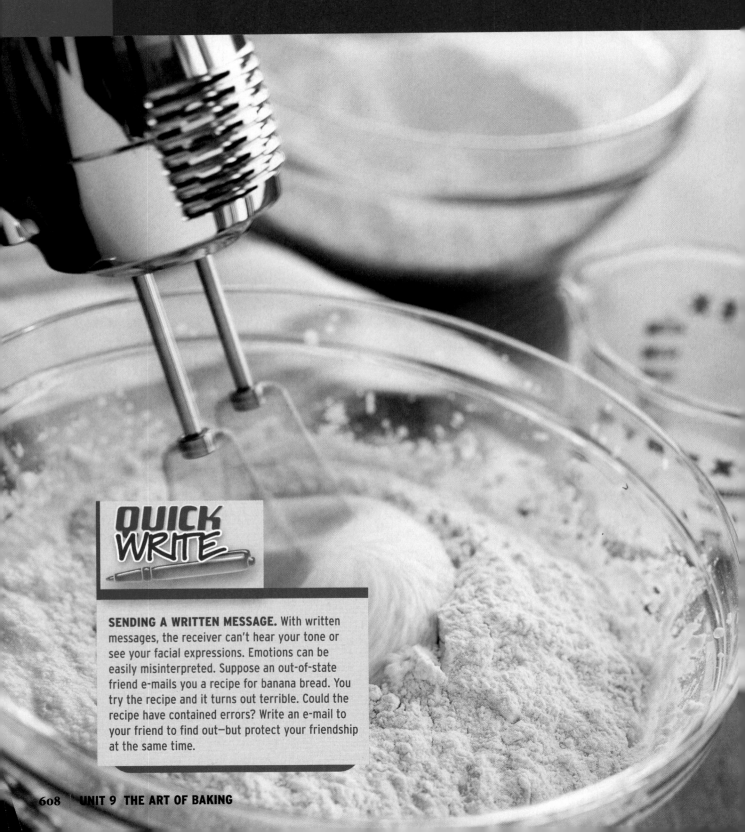

QUICK WRITE

SENDING A WRITTEN MESSAGE. With written messages, the receiver can't hear your tone or see your facial expressions. Emotions can be easily misinterpreted. Suppose an out-of-state friend e-mails you a recipe for banana bread. You try the recipe and it turns out terrible. Could the recipe have contained errors? Write an e-mail to your friend to find out—but protect your friendship at the same time.

Objectives
▶ Describe basic baking ingredients.
▶ Explain the effects of different baking ingredients.
▶ Explain how to choose and store baking ingredients.
▶ Suggest ways to lower fat and sugar in recipes for baked goods.
▶ Describe and demonstrate basic techniques that are part of the baking process.

Terms
active dry yeast
bleached flour
brown sugar
compressed yeast
confectioners' sugar
gluten
granulated sugar
hot spot
leavening agent
preheat
proofing
quick-rising yeast
self-rising flour
unbleached flour

L IKE A MAGICIAN, A SKILLED BAKER CAN transform a few basic ingredients into a galaxy of delights: hearty rye bread, fudgy brownies, or an airy angel food cake. Still, baking "tricks" are fairly simple when you see how they work. With this understanding and some practice, you can perform your own kitchen magic.

INGREDIENTS FOR BAKING

Basic baking ingredients are among the oldest and simplest of foods—flour, liquid, leavening agents, fat, sweeteners, eggs, and flavoring—yet they play multiple, complex roles in a recipe. You can combine them in numerous ways to create different effects in taste, texture, appearance, and nutrition.

Flour

Most flour is made by milling wheat kernels after the bran and germ are removed. The remaining portion, the endosperm, contains starch and proteins, both of which help give structure to baked items. Starch absorbs some of the liquid in the recipe. Certain proteins in wheat flour combine with liquid to create an elastic sub-stance called **gluten** (GLOO-tun). Gluten affects the texture and the rising of baked products.

The Role of Gluten

Gluten develops as flour is mixed with liquid. It forms strong, elastic strands that crisscross in a springy mesh, or weave, of tiny cells. The cells trap air or gas in the baked product. As the product bakes, cells expand with heated air or gas, much like bubble gum stretches to hold air without bursting. Eventually the heat sets the proteins and starch into the framework that becomes the food's final shape.

The longer the mixing time, the stronger the gluten will be. In cakes, where ingredients are quickly combined, gluten remains weak and the cells remain small. The result is a silky, melt-in-the-mouth texture.

For yeast breads, on the other hand, the dough may be worked for ten minutes to develop the gluten. This very elastic framework expands easily. Air cells can grow larger, giving yeast breads a chewy texture. See **Fig. 44-1** on page 610.

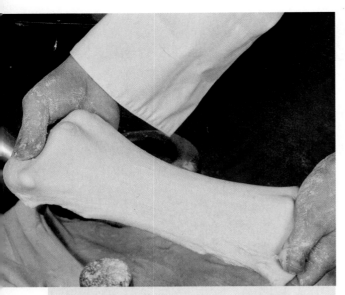

Fig. 44-1 Gluten has an amazing ability to stretch without breaking and resume its former shape.

Kinds of Flour

Flour used in baking is milled from two basic varieties of wheat. High-protein, hard wheat forms very strong gluten. Commercial bakers prefer it for making bread. Since soft wheat is lower in protein, it forms weak gluten. It's ideal when a tender, delicate texture is desired. A third kind of wheat, durum, is the hardest type grown—too hard for making baked products. Durum is milled into semolina, a grainy flour that gives pasta its sturdy structure.

The main quality that distinguishes the different flours used in baking is protein content, which affects gluten strength. See **Fig. 44-2**. These flours include:

- **All-purpose flour.** This is the most-used flour in American kitchens. Blended from hard and soft wheat, its moderate protein content gives good results for most recipes. All-purpose flour is routinely **bleached**, or chemically treated to neutralize the yellow pigment. **Unbleached flour** adds a slight beige tone to the final product. **Self-rising flour** contains added baking powder and salt.
- **Whole-wheat flour.** This whole-grain flour includes the germ and the bran. Bran limits gluten formation, so products are more dense and heavier than those made with all-purpose flour. Recipes using whole-wheat flour typically include an equal or greater amount of all-purpose flour.
- **Bread flour.** Bread flour blends hard-wheat, unbleached flour with barley flour. With high gluten potential, bread flour is favored for making yeast bread.
- **Cake and pastry flours.** These soft-wheat products create less gluten, producing baked goods with a fine, tender texture. Cake flour is bleached. Pastry flour is available as whole wheat.
- **Gluten flour.** This high-protein flour is made from hard wheat, with protein solids added and most starch removed. The added protein makes the flour a strong gluten producer. Gluten flour is never used alone. Instead, it is often added to doughs made with low-protein flour, like rye. Bagels and hearty breads, including those that are heavy with nuts or dried fruit, may be strengthened with gluten flour.

Flour is made from other grains as well, including buckwheat, oats, and rice. Nuts and legumes can also be milled. These plants lack the needed proteins in the right amounts to form gluten, however, and must be mixed with wheat flour to bake products that rise.

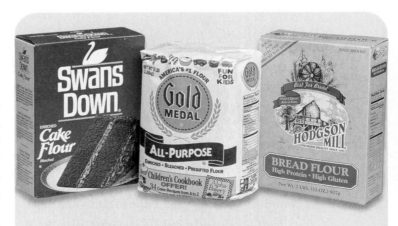

Fig. 44-2 These are three common flours. How are they different? What other types of flour are there?

Buying and Storing Flour

For the average home baker, a 5-pound bag of flour is the most practical choice. Larger sizes are available, as well as smaller bags of specialty types. Read labels carefully to be sure you buy the kind you want. Check that the bag is well sealed and undamaged. Handle bags carefully—they tear easily.

Flour should be stored in a cool, dry place. Transfer it from an opened bag to a tightly covered container to keep it free from dirt, moisture, and pests. Refrigerate opened packages of whole-grain flour, which contains oils that could turn rancid at room temperature.

Liquids

Besides their role in developing gluten, liquids make possible many of the physical and chemical changes that add structure and texture to baked goods. Water and milk are the most commonly used liquids. Some recipes call for fruit juice, buttermilk, sour cream, or yogurt. All liquids supply moistness, but their individual qualities affect recipes differently. The proteins in milk, for instance, add richness and increase browning.

Proportion of Liquid and Flour

The amount of liquid in relation to the amount of flour also affects the qualities of the finished product, especially texture and rising ability. Baked goods are made from either batters or doughs, batters having the higher proportion of liquid. See **Fig. 44-3**. Each type of mixture includes two categories.

- **Pour batters.** Mixing nearly equal amounts of liquid and flour creates a thin, flowing pour batter. Cakes, pancakes, and waffles are examples.
- **Drop batters.** These thicker mixtures contain twice as much flour as liquid. They are usually dropped by the spoonful onto baking pans or sheets for quick breads and cookies, thus the name.
- **Soft doughs.** A ratio of one part liquid to three parts flour makes a soft dough that is sticky but moldable. This dough is the basis for many yeast breads and rolled biscuits.
- **Stiff doughs.** With a ratio of one part liquid to six to eight parts flour, stiff doughs are the easiest to handle. They include piecrusts and some rolled cookies.

Leavening Agents

A **leavening agent**, or leavener, is a substance that triggers a chemical reaction that makes a baked product grow larger, or rise. Most often, a combination of leaveners is at work in one recipe, adding volume and height.

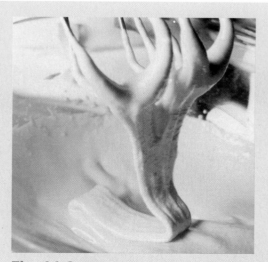
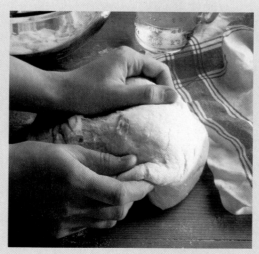

Fig. 44-3 Here you can compare batter and dough. Which one is the batter? What makes them different?

Kinds of Leavening Agents

Some leavening agents are as common as air. Others are chemical formulas. Still others are living organisms. See **Fig. 44-4**.

- **Air.** Air is added while ingredients are combined and beaten, as when sifting flour, creaming fat and sugar, and beating a batter. When the mixture is heated, the trapped air expands and raises the product. Angel food cake, in fact, is leavened mainly by the air in beaten egg whites.
- **Steam.** Steam leavens products that contain large amounts of liquid. The heat of baking turns the liquid into steam. As the steam expands and rises, so does the product. Popovers and cream puffs are steam leavened.
- **Baking soda.** Baking soda is the chemical opposite of an acid. It reacts chemically with an acidic liquid in the recipe, such as buttermilk, to produce carbon dioxide gas, which expands when heated. Baking soda reacts with the liquid instantly. Therefore it's mixed first with dry ingredients and then with the liquid, which prevents the gas from escaping before baking.
- **Baking powder.** Baking powder is a combination of baking soda and a dry acid like cream of tartar. Thus no acidic liquid is needed for it to work. The most common type, double-acting baking powder, releases some carbon dioxide when first mixed with liquid. More releases during baking.
- **Yeast.** Yeast is a fungus that thrives on moisture and warmth. It feeds on the simple sugars in flour and sweeteners. As it grows, yeast gives off carbon dioxide, while other by-products lend a distinctive flavor and aroma. Yeast is readily found in packets or jars as **active dry yeast**, in which partially dormant yeast is contained in flour granules. Regular and quick-rising varieties are available. **Quick-rising yeast** works in about half the time as regular. **Compressed yeast**, a combination of yeast and starch, is moist and comes in small, individually wrapped cakes that are very perishable.

Sometimes a recipe calls for both baking powder and baking soda. That usually happens when buttermilk, yogurt, or another acidic liquid is one of the ingredients. As a balanced mix of baking soda and dry acid, the baking powder leavens the product. The extra acid ingredient, however, upsets the chemical balance. Therefore baking soda is added to neutralize the excess acid.

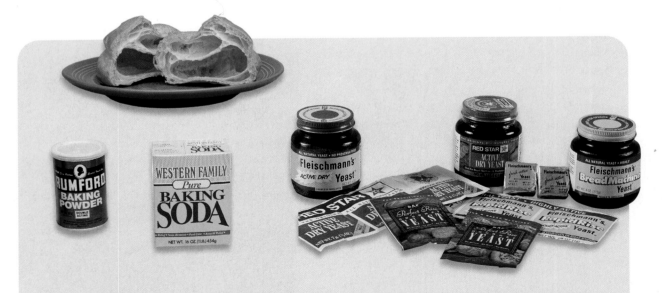

Fig. 44-4 Baked products are leavened differently. The cream puff shows the action of air and steam. Baking soda and baking powder leaven chemically by producing carbon dioxide. Yeast is an organism that produces carbon dioxide for leavening.

Buying and Storing Leavening Agents

Baking soda and powder and active dry yeast are found with baking supplies in the supermarket. Store these ingredients in a cool, dry cabinet. Keep the baking powder container tightly sealed. Otherwise moisture may get in and trigger a reaction, leaving it useless for baking.

Compressed yeast, found in the refrigerated section of the supermarket, should be refrigerated at home. This yeast is a light, creamy gray when fresh but turns brown as it ages.

Even carefully kept leaveners lose their potency over time. Observe the sell-by and use-by dates on labels. To test baking soda for freshness, add 1 teaspoon of soda to 2 tablespoons of white vinegar. Fresh baking soda will fizz and froth.

To test baking powder, mix 1 teaspoon of powder with ⅓ cup of hot water. It should bubble energetically.

Yeast is tested by a process called **proofing**. Place the yeast in a small bowl with a pinch of sugar and enough warm water to dissolve. Set it aside for 5 to 10 minutes. If the mixture puffs and foams, the yeast is alive.

Fats

Fats add richness and flavor to baked goods. They make brown crusts and tender textures possible. The exact effect varies with the makeup of each fat.

Common solid fats used for baking are butter, margarine, and vegetable shortening. All add volume by trapping air. Butter and margarine bring a particular flavor and sometimes include such additives as salt and coloring. Vegetable shortening is an oil that has been hydrogenated, or chemically altered to make it solid. It adds neither flavor nor color. Lard—purified pork fat—makes very flaky piecrusts and biscuits but is used in commercial more than home baking.

Generally, you can replace one solid fat with another, either completely or in part. Some bakers blend butter and margarine, for example, to get a buttery flavor but less saturated fat and cholesterol. The results are different in color and texture, yet successful. *Solid* is the key word. Unless the recipe calls for it, don't substitute whipped butter and soft margarines for solid fats. They are

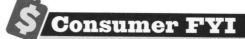

Consumer FYI

Fats for baking. Recipes that call for margarine leave some consumers wondering "which margarine?" More varieties are available now than ever, but not every margarine is suited for every recipe. A vegetable spread used for baking should be at least 60 percent fat. The legal definition for margarine is that it must contain at least 80 percent vegetable oil. Thus, while you won't see the exact percentage on the package, any item labeled margarine should be suitable for baking.

Depending on fat content, diet and light margarines may not produce the same browning and texture in baked goods. Low-fat spreads also contain more water. Cookies may spread and run together. Pastry dough will be sticky and hard to handle. If limiting fats is a concern, look for specially formulated, low-fat recipes.

useful in other ways—to brush on rolls before baking, for example.

Since solid fats and oils work differently in baking, the two aren't interchangeable. If a recipe calls for oil, always use it. Oils add moistness and density rather than volume. Any mild-flavored cooking oil can be used, and one can be substituted for another. Corn, canola, and vegetable oil blends are common choices. Olive oil has a distinctive flavor, so it isn't usually used for baking.

Buying and Storing Fat

Keep butter and margarine in the coldest part of the refrigerator, usually toward the rear of the middle shelf. Be sure they are well wrapped, as they tend to absorb flavors and aromas from other foods. Use butter within one month and margarine within two months, or freeze them in their original containers for up to four months.

Vegetable shortening and oils usually keep well in a cool, dry area. They may need refrigeration, especially if not used within one month. Check the label on each product.

Sweeteners

Like fats, sweeteners add the same qualities—flavor, tenderness, and browning—but to different degrees. This is due to the different types of sugar and amounts of liquid they contain. Due to this varying makeup, substituting sweeteners in recipes often requires other changes as well. Compare the contributions of these common sweeteners:

- **Sugar. Granulated sugar** is highly refined sucrose crystals derived by boiling the juice of sugarcane or sugar beets. When creamed with a solid fat, it adds air and volume. **Confectioners' sugar**, or powdered sugar, is pulverized granulated sugar with a trace of added cornstarch. It dissolves easily and is most often used for frostings. **Brown sugar** is granulated sugar coated with molasses. Molasses adds moisture and a caramel flavor but reduces the ability to trap air. A light or dark color reflects the amount of molasses and intensity of flavor.
- **Honey.** Honey is produced by bees from flower nectar. Different flowers impart different colors and flavors. Mild clover honey is most popular in baking. The sugar in honey, fructose, is much sweeter than sucrose. It also attracts and holds more moisture, so baked goods stay fresh longer. See **Fig. 44-5**.
- **Molasses.** When sugarcane juice is boiled to make sugar, crystallized sugar is removed at different stages. At each stage, a syrup by-product that is less sweet than sugar forms. These are the different grades of molasses. Light molasses, which is extracted first, is highest in sugar and sweetness. Dark molasses is taken after further boiling has extracted more raw sugar.
- **Corn syrup.** Corn syrup is made by breaking down the starch in corn into dextrose and water. The dark variety has added caramel flavoring. Small amounts of corn syrup help make baked goods soft and chewy, but it's used most commonly in cooked frostings and candies.

Buying and Storing Sweeteners

Most sweeteners keep best in tightly sealed containers in a cool, dry area. Check the label to be sure. After using liquid sweeteners, wipe the containers with a damp cloth to remove drips. Traces of sugars on jars and shelves attract insects.

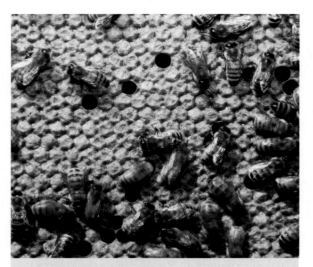

Fig. 44-5 Worker bees add enzymes to nectar and reduce the moisture to make honey. After making a wax comb in the hive, the bees store honey in the cells and cover them with wax caps.

Even when properly stored, confectioners' sugar often cakes. To remove lumps, sift it before using. Likewise, brown sugar can harden. To soften, put a piece of bread or cut raw fruit—apples work well—in the container, or microwave the sugar with a few drops of water in a glass bowl. Use 100 percent power for 10 to 15 seconds.

Crystallization can occur in honey, especially when refrigerated. To liquefy crystallized honey, remove the lid and set the container in about 2 inches of warm water.

Eggs

Eggs are another "multitasker" in baked products. Fats in eggs add flavor, color, richness, and tenderness. Certain fats in the yolk create an emulsion, binding liquids and fats in the recipe to keep batters from separating. Beating egg white proteins adds air and volume. Heating them helps set the structure.

Flavorings

Seasonings and flavorings add variety to baked products. Recipes often include spices or liquid extracts, such as maple, almond, or vanilla. Some use dried fruit, chopped nuts, citrus peel, or flavored syrups. Chocolate flavor may be added with baking chocolate, which is an unsweetened

CRYOGENICS IN THE KITCHEN

Successful baking takes proper preheating—in your oven, not your ingredients. Ingredients that get too hot in storage or mixing can frustrate pastry chefs. Butter quickly becomes unworkable. Overheated flour can change the consistency and even damage the quality of dough. The results are cracked crusts and poor pastries.

To cool things down, chefs may add ice to the recipe, sometimes as part of the liquid ingredients. That's more work and means adjusting the other ingredients to make up for extra moisture.

A better solution may be found in cryogenics, a technology that uses extremely low temperatures. Professional kitchens can be fitted with a system of cryogenically cooled storage, delivery, and mixing equipment. Cryogenic cooling systems run on the same principle as a home refrigerator. They change liquids (and sometimes solids) to gases, a process that absorbs heat and lowers the surrounding temperature. They use liquid nitrogen and solid

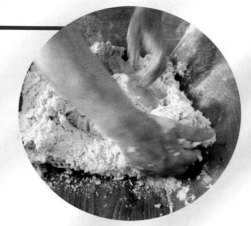

carbon dioxide (dry ice), however, which change to gases at remarkably low temperatures. Liquid nitrogen, for example, boils at -320ºF. Thus they cool more efficiently than conventional refrigeration systems.

Cryogenically chilled ingredients not only stay cool, but they also stay more consistently cool. Computerized and self-monitoring, these systems automatically adjust to maintain the desired temperature.

__Think Beyond>> Would cryogenic cooling be useful to a home baker? Why or why not?

product. Adding some of these ingredients to a recipe that doesn't call for them may change the texture and color as well as the flavor.

THE BAKING PROCESS

Choosing ingredients is just one skill in baking. You also need to learn some basic techniques that are part of the baking process.

Choosing Oven Temperature

To bake even a humble buttermilk biscuit properly takes precise timing. As the biscuit bakes, the surface absorbs the heat while moisture evaporates, forming a crust. The crust temperature rises and the crust begins to brown. At the same time, heat penetrates the inside, activating leavening agents that push against the still-soft crust to raise the biscuit. This small feat is repeated in every leavened item.

The right oven temperature is the key that keeps this balancing act in balance. If the oven is too hot, the crust forms too quickly. The biscuit struggles to expand, sometimes cracking the crust. The crust may look nicely browned, while the inside is only half baked.

On the other hand, if the temperature is too low, rising may outpace structure setting. The leavening gas escapes before the gluten and starch in the flour can form the framework. Your biscuit comes out dry and fallen.

To avoid these mishaps, always use the temperature given in the recipe. Before you turn the oven on, make sure the oven racks are properly positioned. For most baked goods, that means near the middle of the chamber. Unless the recipe states otherwise, **preheat** the oven. Turn the oven on about 10 minutes before using so it will be at the desired temperature when the food is placed inside.

Choosing Pans

As with oven temperature, recipes are developed for certain pans. Use the specified pan type and size. If you need to substitute a different pan, make sure both pans have a similar volume, which you can compare by measuring the amount of water each pan holds. (You'll read more about pan substitutions in Chapter 46.) Depth is another critical factor in pan substitution. A pan that's too deep or too shallow may cause the same problems as a temperature that's too high or low. Avoid any pan with warps and dents that will ruin the shape of the baked item.

You may recall that the material a pan is made from affects how it transfers heat. Most recipes assume the use of shiny metal pans. Pans made of glass or dark metal retain more heat and can create a thick crust. To compensate for this effect, lower the oven temperature by about 10 degrees to bake with dark metal pans and by 25 degrees for glass. If you're using cast iron or other materials, follow the manufacturer's directions.

Preparing the Pans

The recipe also tells you how to prepare the pan so the product can be easily removed after baking. Do this step before mixing ingredients.

Common directions for preparing pans include the following:

- **Grease and flour.** This means to coat a pan lightly with solid fat and then dust it with flour. See **Fig. 44-6.** Don't use salted butter or margarine. Salt creates a darkened crust that sticks to the pan. Use wax paper to spread the fat. Thoroughly grease the corners and the crease between the sides and bottom, where foods are most likely to stick. Sprinkle with a little all-purpose flour. Tilt and shake the pan to distribute the flour evenly. Turn the pan upside down over the sink and tap to remove any excess flour.
- **Spray with cooking spray.** This method is convenient but may leave a sticky film on pans. Since it may not work for all products, follow label or recipe directions for use.
- **Line with paper.** Use cooking parchment for this method. Ordinary brown paper contains

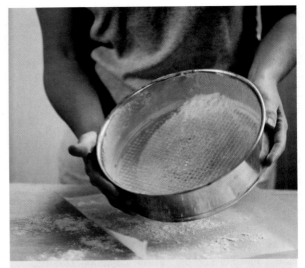

Fig. 44-6 To grease and flour a pan, apply the fat. Then add flour and shake the pan to distribute it. What happens to the extra flour?

chemicals that may be transferred to the food when heated. The wax in wax paper may melt and be absorbed by the crust. Cut a piece of parchment the same shape and size as the pan bottom. Grease the pan and line the bottom with the parchment. Remember to peel the paper off the product when you remove it from the pan.

Not all pans should be greased. Fats collapse air pockets in beaten egg white in foods like angel food cake, which also needs to cling to the sides of the pan to rise. Recipes that contain a high proportion of fat become oily. Also, greased or floured pans become sticky in a microwave oven.

Baking the Product

To bake evenly, items must be placed in the oven so the heated air can circulate around them freely. Allow at least 1 inch of space between pans and between pans and oven walls. Otherwise, they may create a **hot spot**, an area of concentrated heat that can cause uneven baking and browning.

If you're using one pan, place it in the center of the oven. Place two pans on separate racks in diagonally opposite corners. If you have three or four pans, stagger them so that one is not directly above another. See **Fig. 44-7.**

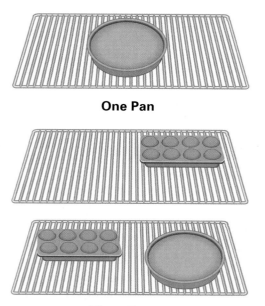

One Pan

Three Pans

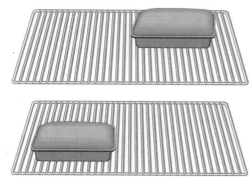

Two Pans

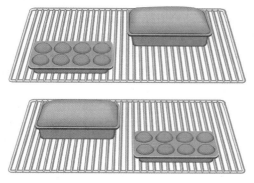

Four Pans

> **Fig. 44-7** When baking, pans need to be placed correctly in the oven. Correct placement for one, two, three, and four pans is shown here.

As soon as the pans are in the oven, set a timer. Start checking the product for doneness about 5 minutes before the time is up. To prevent heat loss, avoid opening the oven door until then.

Baking in a Convection Oven

Convection and conventional ovens bake foods using the same basic process, so the same rules about pan choice and placement apply. The continuous current of hot air created by the convection oven does speed some chemical reactions in foods, however. Products brown faster and lose less moisture. Some products also rise more quickly.

Most recipes for baked products are developed for conventional ovens but will likely adapt well to convection cooking. Baking temperature and time are the main differences. In general, you can reduce temperatures in recipes by 25 to 50 degrees, and baking time by one-third. The owner's manual might have more detailed conversions. You can also use a convection oven cookbook to find recipes similar to your own as a guide to making adjustments.

Baking in a Microwave Oven

Technically, microwave ovens don't bake; they cook with moist heat. As a result, baked products don't brown or develop a crust. They stay very tender and moist, however, because less evaporation occurs.

Adapted recipes for microwave ovens can be unpredictable. Factors like standing time, rapid cooking rates, and the pale appearance of baked goods can lead to overbaking. For best results, use a recipe developed for microwaving.

Removing Baked Products from Pans

Some baked goods should be removed from pans immediately. Otherwise, many cookies stick and muffins could overbake. Some cookies need to cool for just a minute to firm up before removal.

Most cakes and some breads need to cool partially in the pan to prevent cracking or tearing on removal. Cakes made without fat are cooled completely in the pans. Some items are served from the baking pan. Follow the directions for each recipe.

For any bakery item, use wire cooling racks to promote quick cooling. A countertop or other solid surface holds the heated air, which collects as moisture and makes a soggy product.

Remove cookies from baking sheets with a wide spatula and gentle handling. To remove yeast bread from a pan, turn the pan on its side on a wire rack. Ease the bread out with a clean pot holder or dish towel. Place the bread right side up on the wire rack. For cakes and quick breads, use this technique:

1. Run a spatula along the sides of the pan, if needed, to eliminate sticking points.
2. Place a wire cooling rack over the top of the cake or bread. See **Fig. 44-8A**.
3. Holding the pan and rack securely with pot holders, flip them upside down. Place the rack on a level surface. See **Fig. 44-8B**.
4. Lift the pan off the cake or bread, which is now upside down.
5. Quickly place another wire rack on the bottom of the baked item. See **Fig. 44-8C**.
6. Using both hands, grasp both racks without squeezing. Flip the racks so the baked product is right side up.
7. Remove the top rack and allow the item to cool completely. See **Fig. 44-8D**.

STORING BAKED PRODUCTS

Baked goods should be thoroughly cool before storing. Trapped heat in a container produces moisture that can make the food soggy and prone to spoilage.

Most cookies, cakes, and breads can be kept at room temperature in a sealed container or wrap for up to three days. They usually freeze well also. Perishable products, including those with custard, cream, or fruit fillings and frostings, must be refrigerated. Freezing is not advised, however; these fillings tend to separate when they thaw.

Career Prep

Anger Management

PEOPLE GET ANGRY WHEN THEY FEEL threatened. Anger is a burst of energy that prepared primitive humans for protective action—for fight or flight. Unfortunately, those options aren't very helpful today. The threat is emotional, not physical, so anger is often pent up until it swells into rage. Then it bursts through and wreaks havoc. Anger on the job can increase stress and reduce productivity. It also contributes to the growing problem of workplace violence.

You can learn to manage anger on the job and off. These steps can help:

- **Identify ideas, expectations, and attitudes that produce angry feelings.** You may be angry because a teacher or boss criticized something you did. Do you expect to be perfect all the time? Should people in charge ignore mistakes? Maybe you took the correction as a personal attack. On reflection, you see that none of these assumptions is true.

- **Learn constructive responses.** Channel the jolt of physical energy into mental energy. Think through your options and choose a useful one. If you made a mistake, learn how to correct it. If you think you were treated unfairly, explain your position. Remain assertive without becoming aggressive. To act assertively is to stand up for yourself calmly and firmly. To be aggressive is to intimidate through physical or verbal force. Aggression is threatening and provokes an angry response. If

Fig. 44-8

How to Remove a Cake from the Pan

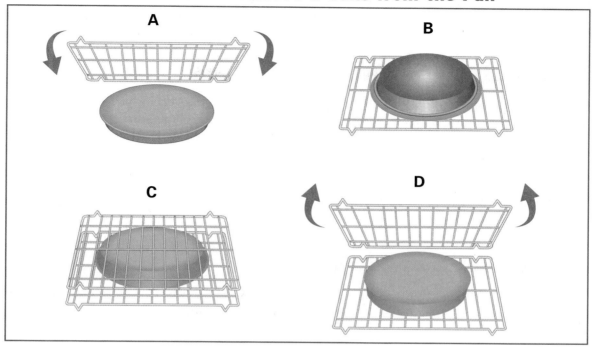

A

B

C

D

you must react physically, find a harmless outlet. Jog up and down stairs or take a walk.

Another useful tool for managing anger is conflict resolution, which settles disputes before they grow hostile. In conflict resolution, each person states the problem as he or she sees it and offers a solution. The parties discuss and debate each idea reasonably. They may agree to try one solution or to compromise, with all sides both giving in and getting part of what they want. They may ask an outside, objective party to mediate, or review both sides and suggest a resolution.

Some anger is chronic. It results not from any one situation, but from frustration with multiple problems that build over time. Such anger can be harmful to health. Defusing chronic anger may take the help of a professional counselor.

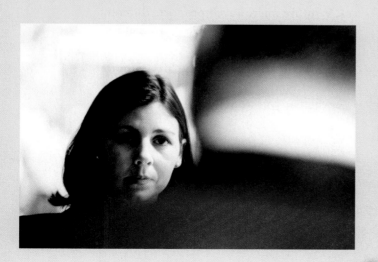

Career Connection

Practicing responses. With a partner, think of a conflict that could arise in a work setting. Then create and present a skit that demonstrates constructive responses to the situation. Have classmates evaluate your approach.

Summarize Your Reading

▶ Recipes for baked goods typically call for flour, liquid, one or more leavening agents, fat, sweetener, eggs, and flavoring.

▶ In baking, gluten must be produced from proteins in flour.

▶ Some baking ingredients need to be refrigerated, while others do not.

▶ The baking process includes choosing the correct oven temperature and pans. For successful results, methods also include correctly preparing the pans for baking and removing the baked products from pans.

▶ Although it is not possible to eliminate fat and sugar entirely, recipes can be adapted to limit fat and sugar in baked foods.

Check Your Knowledge

1. How is wheat made into flour?

2. Describe the action of **gluten** during mixing and baking.

3. What effect does mixing time have on gluten?

4. Compare hard, soft, and durum wheat.

5. How do **bleached** and **unbleached flours** differ?

6. Why do recipes with whole-wheat flour often contain all-purpose flour too?

7. Describe the kinds of flour used to make these flours: all-purpose, bread, cake and pastry, and gluten.

8. Describe the ratio of liquid to flour in pour batters, drop batters, soft doughs, and stiff doughs.

9. Why do baked goods need a **leavening agent**?

10. How do air and steam leaven products?

11. Why is baking soda mixed with dry ingredients before adding it to liquids in a recipe?

12. Compare **active dry**, **quick-rising**, and **compressed yeasts**.

13. What roles do fats play in baking?

14. Can you substitute oil for margarine in a baking recipe? Explain.

15. What contributions do **granulated sugar**, **confectioners' sugar**, and **brown sugar** make when baking?

16. How should flour, leavening agents, fats, and sugar be stored?

17. What is the role of eggs in baked goods?

18. What happens to biscuits when the oven temperature is not accurate?

19. Why is pan size important?

20. How can you avoid creating a **hot spot** when baking?

21. Why are microwaved products different from conventionally baked products?

22. **CRITICAL THINKING** A cook wrapped a loaf of banana bread in aluminum foil after removing it from the pan. Explain whether you would have done this.

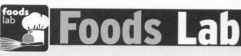
Apply Your Learning

1. **SCIENCE** **Gluten Balls.** Check the Internet to find information on how to make gluten balls. Conduct an experiment to make them. What do you learn about gluten from this activity?

2. **Flour Display.** Make a display of different kinds of flours. Label them with descriptions, protein levels, and storage hints. Include visuals that show how each flour type is used in baking.

3. **Sweeteners on Labels.** Read labels on baked goods to identify sweeteners used in them. Which sweeteners seem to be the most common? Why do you think these sweeteners were used?

4. **Pan Preparation.** Demonstrate how to prepare a pan for baking. Show the method for greasing and flouring a pan and also the method for lining a pan with paper.

5. **Removal from Pan.** Demonstrate how to remove a baked cake from the pans.

Foods Lab

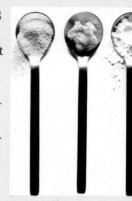

Testing Leaveners
Procedure: Using baking soda, baking powder, or yeast samples provided by your teacher, test each one for potency. First, mark the samples by type of leavener. If you are testing multiple samples of one type, mark them in this way: "Baking Soda A" and "Baking Soda B." The method for testing each leavener is different, so be sure to use the correct procedure. Record your observations.

Analyzing Results
❶ What leaveners did you test? What method did you use for each type of leavener?
❷ What did you observe when you tested each sample?
❸ Would you use any of the tested leaveners for baking? Why or why not?

Food Science Experiment

Leavening Actions

Objective: To identify conditions that promote chemical leavening.

Procedure:

1. Pour ½ cup of cold water into each of two microwave-safe containers. Dissolve ½ tsp. baking soda in one, and ½ tsp. double-acting baking powder in the other. Observe and record the results.

2. Add 1 tsp. vinegar to each container. Record the results.

3. Heat each solution in a microwave oven at full power for 30 seconds. Describe the results.

Analyzing Results
❶ Which factor seemed to have the greatest impact on the baking soda: water, acid, or heat? Which had the greatest impact on the baking powder?
❷ How might the results have been different with single-acting baking powder?
❸ Suppose you have a cake recipe that calls for baking soda and buttermilk, but all you have is low-fat milk. Would you try to prepare this recipe? Why or why not?

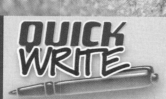

CHAPTER 45 Quick & Yeast Breads

QUICK WRITE

NARROWING A TOPIC. A specific topic is easier to write about than a general one. For example, what would you include in a paper with "inventions" as the theme? This broad topic could produce vague and rambling results. A more precise topic like "recent kitchen inventions" directs thoughts and research. Try narrowing the general topic, bread. List five specific topics for a written paper.

To Guide Your Reading:

Objectives

▶ Describe various types of bread.

▶ Explain the difference between quick and yeast breads.

▶ Compare methods for making quick and yeast breads.

▶ Describe and demonstrate how to make quick and yeast breads.

Terms

biscuit method

conventional method

cut in

drop biscuits

fermentation

kneading

muffin method

quick breads

quick-mix method

rolled biscuits

score

yeast breads

P

EOPLE HAVE BEEN MAKING BREAD FOR MORE than 10,000 years and seem to have come up with nearly that many variations. From pitas to tortillas, from pumpernickel to croissants (kraw-SAHNTS), there's bread for every occasion and every taste. You don't have to visit a bakery to enjoy nourishing, tasty, freshly baked breads. You can make them right at home.

MAKING QUICK BREADS

Quick breads are leavened by agents that allow immediate baking. Air, steam, baking soda, and baking powder are typically used. Most quick breads are made by one of two basic mixing methods: the muffin method or the biscuit method. Following each technique correctly helps ensure favorable results.

Muffin Method

In the **muffin method**, lightly mixing liquid ingredients into dry ingredients creates a product with a slightly coarse yet tender texture. The method makes a pour or drop batter for pancakes, muffins, some coffeecakes, fruit and nut loaves, and a soft cornbread casserole called spoon bread. See **Fig. 45-1**.

The challenge is to avoid overmixing. Because these recipes contain little fat as tenderizers, beat-ing the ingredients produces a chewy, heavy texture. Muffins end up with air spaces, or tunnels, on the inside and peaks on top. With that in mind, follow these steps, as shown in **Fig. 45-2** on page 624:

1. Measure all ingredients accurately.
2. Sift the dry ingredients together in a mixing bowl. If you're using whole-grain flour, blend

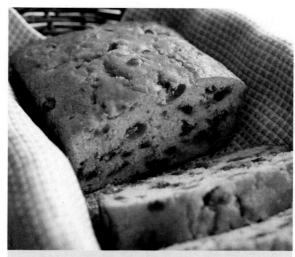

Fig. 45-1 Early bakers in history could only leaven with yeast or air and steam. In the 1800s, the use of baking soda and baking powder made the first quick breads possible.

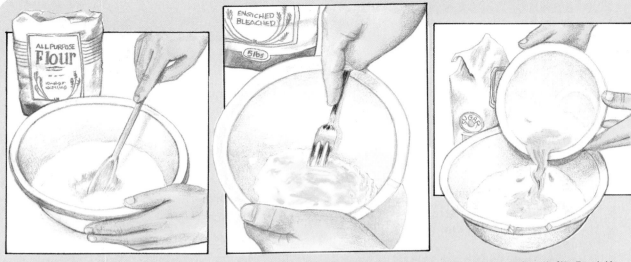

Fig. 45-2 For the muffin method, sift dry ingredients together and make a well in the center (left). Beat the liquid ingredients in a separate bowl (center). Pour the liquid mixture into the well all at once (right). Fold together without overmixing.

ingredients thoroughly with a spoon or whisk instead.

3. Using the back of a spoon, make a well in the center of the dry mixture.

4. In a small bowl, beat all liquid ingredients—eggs, milk or water, oil or melted fat, and flavorings—until well blended.

5. Pour the liquid all at once into the well in the dry ingredients. Fold in the dry ingredients just until they are moistened. Use as few strokes as possible. A few floury streaks can remain, and the batter should be lumpy.

For muffins or bread, gently spoon the batter into greased muffin tins or loaf pans. An alternative is to line muffin pans with paper baking cups. Fill cups no more than two-thirds full to avoid overflows. **Fig. 45-3** shows a muffin recipe.

For pancakes, pour small amounts of the batter onto a hot, greased skillet or griddle, making a few at a time. Waffles are baked in a waffle iron, according to the owner's manual.

Testing for Doneness

These signs indicate doneness in quick breads:

• **Muffins.** Muffins are lightly browned, with rounded, pebbly tops. Remove them from the tins immediately unless the recipe states otherwise. A well-made muffin has a symmetrical

shape and is fine, light, and tender on the inside.

• **Loaf breads.** Loaves are lightly browned and have pulled away slightly from the sides of the pan. The crust has a center crack and feels firm when tapped. Follow recipe directions for removing loaf breads.

• **Pancakes.** Pancakes are ready to turn when the edges look dry and the bubbles on top start to break. Cook until the underside is golden.

Muffins and pancakes are best served fresh and warm, although they may be reheated. Allow loaf breads to cool completely before serving. The flavors blend and the texture firms for easier slicing.

Biscuit Method

Unlike the muffin method, the **biscuit method** makes one basic type of bread—the biscuit plus its egg-enriched cousins, scones and shortcakes. This method also differs in that a solid fat is added to the dry ingredients before the liquids are lightly mixed in. The resulting bread has a delicate texture and a crisp but tender crust. The inside, slightly steamy and creamy white, peels apart in wafer-thin layers.

Biscuits also use a higher ratio of flour to liquid than muffins, making a dough rather than a batter. They are either rolled or dropped, depend-

Fig. 45-3

Cranberry Almond Muffins

Yield	Nutrition Analysis
12 muffins	***Per Serving:*** 300 calories, 15 g total fat, 8 g saturated fat, 0 g trans fat, 65 mg cholesterol, 10 mg sodium, 39 g total carbohydrate, 2 g dietary fiber, 26 g sugars, 4 g protein
	Percent Daily Value: vitamin A 8%, vitamin C 2%, calcium 2%, iron 6%

Ingredients

2 large eggs
1½ cups sugar
1½ tsp. almond extract
¾ cup (1½ sticks) unsalted butter, melted and cooled slightly, plus additional for greasing muffin pans

1½ cups all-purpose flour
1½ cups whole fresh cranberries, washed and sorted
¾ cup sliced almonds
confectioners' sugar

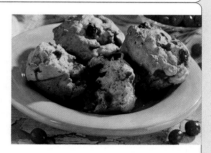

Directions

1. Place oven rack in middle position. Preheat oven to 350°F. Generously butter muffin pans.
2. In bowl of electric mixer, beat eggs and sugar together on medium speed until thick and light yellow in color, about 2½ minutes. Beat in almond extract and melted butter, about 30 seconds.
3. Add liquid ingredients to flour. Mix with spoon. Add cranberries and almond slices. Stir mixture briefly to combine. Mixture will be lumpy.
4. Spoon mixture into muffin cups, each two-thirds full. Bake until toothpick inserted in center comes out clean, about 45 minutes. Cool and sprinkle with confectioner's sugar.

ing on the amount of liquid in the recipe. Each type starts with these steps:

1. Measure all ingredients accurately.
2. Sift the dry ingredients together into a large mixing bowl.
3. Cut the fat into the flour until the particles are the size of peas or coarse bread crumbs. To **cut in** means to mix solid fat and flour using a pastry blender or two knives and a cutting motion. This technique disperses fine fat particles in the dough. During baking, the fat melts between layers of flour, and its liquid content turns to steam, giving rise to a flaky biscuit. Cold fat is cut in more quickly, making a lighter texture.
4. Make a well in the center of the dry ingredients, as in the muffin method.

5. Add the liquids all at once.
6. Using a fork, mix until the dry ingredients are just moistened.

Rolled Biscuits

Rolled biscuits are always mixed by the biscuit method. The dough is prepared, then rolled out to an even thickness and cut to biscuit size before baking. **Kneading** means working dough with the hands to combine ingredients and develop gluten. In order to create a light, flaky product, very little kneading is done with rolled biscuits.

When making rolled biscuits, the combined ingredients should make a dough that "cleans" the sides of the bowl—that is, it holds together in a ball and no longer sticks to the bowl. After the dough reaches this stage, follow these steps for rolling:

1. Turn the dough out on a board sprinkled with just enough flour to keep the dough from sticking. Too much flour toughens the texture.

2. Knead the dough lightly, but use only your fingertips to keep from melting the fat in the dough. If necessary, dust your hands with a little flour to keep the dough from sticking.

3. Gently fold the dough in half toward you and give it a quarter turn.

4. Continue to knead gently, fold, and turn as directed in the recipe, usually six turns or fewer. The dough should lose its stickiness. Overworking the dough creates tough, compact biscuits.

When the dough is ready, roll it out and cut the biscuits. See **Fig. 45-4** and the photo on page 632. This is how the biscuits are cut out:

1. On a clean, lightly floured surface and using a lightly floured rolling pin, roll the dough out gently to about ½-inch thickness. Keep the dough circular to avoid waste when cutting. Maintain an even thickness—lopsided biscuits bake unevenly. Dust the board and rolling pin with flour only as needed to prevent sticking.

2. Cut out the dough with a biscuit cutter lightly dipped in flour. You can also use the rim of a beverage glass. Cut straight down; a twisting or turning motion can pull the bis-

Fig. 45-4

Buttermilk Biscuits

Yield	Nutrition Analysis
18-20 biscuits	**Per Serving:** 100 calories, 5 g total fat, 2 g saturated fat, 0 g trans fat, 0 mg cholesterol, 160 mg sodium, 12 g total carbohydrate, 0 g dietary fiber, 2 g sugars, 2 g protein **Percent Daily Value:** vitamin A 0%, vitamin C 0%, calcium 4%, iron 4%

Ingredients

½ cup vegetable shortening
2¼ cups flour
2½ tsp. baking powder
½ tsp. baking soda

1 Tbsp. sugar
½ tsp. salt
1¼ cups buttermilk

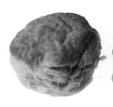

Directions

1. Preheat oven to 425°F. Grease a baking sheet. Wrap shortening with wax paper and place in freezer.

2. Tear off 2 pieces wax paper about 12 inches long. Sift flour, baking powder, baking soda, sugar, and salt onto one sheet of wax paper. Place empty sifter on other sheet. Sift mixture back and forth 4 more times and into a large mixing bowl at the end.

3. Cut shortening from freezer into small pieces, and scatter over dry ingredients. With fingertips, lightly rub shortening and flour together. Occasionally toss mixture so all particles of shortening are coated with flour. When mixture is flour-covered, begin adding buttermilk. Use a fork to lightly mix with dry ingredients.

4. Cover work surface with dusting of flour. Gather up sticky dough, and place on floured surface. Dust your hands with flour and knead the dough gently, adding only enough flour to make it manageable.

5. With a floured rolling pin, roll the dough into a disk ½ inch thick. Using a 2-inch biscuit cutter, cut out biscuits and place them on baking sheet. Bake for 12 minutes or until golden.

cuit out of shape. Square biscuits can be cut with a sharp knife dipped in flour. Work carefully to avoid tearing or pulling the dough. You can try cookie cutters, too, if they are deep enough to cut without flattening the dough. For a scone recipe, the circle is cut into wedges.

3. Pat leftover dough together, roll it again, and cut. Remember, however, that the more a dough is handled, the less tender and flaky the biscuits will be.

4. With a wide spatula, place the biscuits about 1 inch apart on an ungreased baking sheet. Bake as the recipe directs.

Drop Biscuits

Compared to rolled biscuits, **drop biscuits** have a little more liquid in proportion to flour. In fact, you can turn a rolled biscuit into a drop biscuit by increasing the liquid. The sticky dough holds its shape when mounded but doesn't clean the sides of the bowl. It is not kneaded or rolled. Oil sometimes replaces solid fat, and the muffin method may be used for mixing. These differences make drop biscuits more mealy than flaky.

To form drop biscuits, place large spoonfuls of dough about 1 inch apart on a greased cookie sheet, or use muffin tins for a more symmetrical shape. Bake according to recipe directions. You can also spoon drop biscuits onto a casserole as a topping or onto a fruit filling to make a cobbler.

Testing for Doneness

Both rolled and drop biscuits double in size. Rolled biscuits have golden brown tops and straight, cream-colored sides. Drop biscuits have golden brown, irregular contours.

THE MARVEL OF YEAST BREAD

 In contrast to quick breads, **yeast breads** are leavened with yeast. The dough must be well kneaded and allowed to rise before baking. Science has revealed the hidden workings in bread.

Yeast and the enzymes it contains produce alcohols and carbon dioxide gas by breaking down carbohydrates, a process called **fermentation**. As the gas leavens the bread, it also "pushes

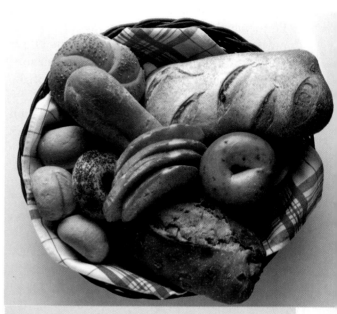

Fig. 45-5 Human ingenuity has produced yeast breads of countless types. Bread has been the mainstay of many meals for thousands of years.

around" protein and water molecules, enabling them to form more gluten. Meanwhile, the alcohols and other by-products of fermentation, including amino and fatty acids, mix into flavorful compounds.

The creativity of making yeast breads has kept pace with the science. Imaginative bakers harness yeast to make pizza crusts and pita bread, hard rolls and soft pretzels, puffy pastries and chewy bagels—with variations of added seeds, nuts, fruits, cheese, and seasonings. See **Fig. 45-5**.

Kinds of Yeast Breads

Despite the many variations, yeast breads fall into five basic categories:

- **Basic white bread.** Made only with all-purpose flour, yeast, salt, sugar, fat, and water or milk.
- **Batter bread.** Made like basic white bread, but with more liquid. The batter is beaten, so the texture is not as light as kneaded yeast bread.
- **Sweet white bread.** Uses basic white bread ingredients plus butter, eggs, extra sugar, and sometimes nuts and fruits. Pecan rolls and coffeecakes are examples.

- **Whole-grain bread.** Made with whole-grain flour, which replaces part or all of the all-purpose flour in basic white bread. Gluten flour may be added to lighten the loaf. You can substitute whole-grain flour for up to half of the flour in a recipe.
- **Sourdough bread.** Leavened with sourdough starter. This well-fermented mixture of yeast, water, and flour gives a tangy flavor and chewy texture.

MAKING YEAST BREAD

Making yeast bread is time-consuming yet flexible enough to fit into even a busy schedule. Some recipes can be started one day and finished the next. Kitchen appliances can help. A microwave oven heats liquids, brings cold ingredients to room temperature, and helps dough rise. A food processor or heavy-duty mixer with a dough hook saves a few minutes and some labor over hand kneading.

Making yeast bread involves several steps. "Hands-on" steps of kneading and shaping dough alternate with "hands-off" stages of letting dough rise.

$ Consumer FYI

Bread machines. If you have storage space and a yearning for fresh bread, a bread machine can be a handy appliance. These large metal boxes are easily programmed to produce one or two loaves of fresh-baked bread. You just put the ingredients in the compartment, set the machine, and come back when the bread is done.

To choose a machine, consider bread size and shape. Round, square, and rectangular loaves are all options. Check the cycles provided. You can adjust for crustiness as well as different flours. Other features to note are a removable bread pan, "keep warm" function that holds the bread until you get there, protection in the event of a power failure, and delayed start. Bread machines aren't for everyone, but sales have increased as people enjoy an easy way to fill the house with the aroma of fresh-baked bread.

Mixing the Dough

Mixing ingredients for yeast bread has two aims: making the dough and activating the yeast. Since bread flour is an excellent gluten producer, it is ideal for making yeast dough, but all-purpose flour is a less expensive, satisfying substitute. Have all ingredients at room temperature to promote yeast growth. Two common mixing methods used with yeast breads are the conventional method and the quick-mix method.

Conventional Method

In the **conventional method**, the yeast is first dissolved in warm water to activate growth. As you've learned, this is also a method of testing yeast, called proofing. Temperature is critical. Yeast won't grow if the water is too cool and will die if it's too hot. Check the water temperature with a candy thermometer if you have one. Otherwise, let a drop fall on the inside of your forearm. It should feel pleasantly warm.

1. Dissolve the yeast in water about 105°F to 115°F and let it stand for 5 to 10 minutes.
2. Heat the fat, sugar, and liquid to melt the fat. Cool the mixture to lukewarm.
3. Add the dissolved yeast to the liquid, along with any eggs in the recipe.
4. Add enough flour to make a soft or stiff dough, as the recipe indicates. Yeast recipes may give a range for the amount of flour, 4 to $4\frac{1}{2}$ cups, for example, rather than an exact figure. This is because flour varies in how much liquid it can absorb. On humid days, for instance, flour absorbs less liquid because it has already taken in some moisture from the air. You have added enough flour when the dough cleans the sides of the bowl.

Quick-Mix Method

The **quick-mix method** combines dry yeast with the dry ingredients. The liquids must be warmer because the dry ingredients absorb some of the heat. You can use a standard electric mixer until the dough thickens and becomes too heavy. Then switch to a sturdy spoon. Since the mixer develops gluten, kneading time is shorter.

1. Combine part of the flour with the undissolved yeast, sugar, and salt in a large bowl.
2. Heat the liquid and fat to between 120°F and 130°F.
3. Add the liquid to the dry ingredients and beat until well blended.
4. Add just enough of the remaining flour to make the kind of dough specified in the recipe.

Kneading the Dough

Except for batter breads, yeast dough must be kneaded to develop a strong gluten structure that holds up when the dough rises. Follow these steps:

1. Sprinkle a clean work surface and your hands with just enough flour to keep the dough from sticking—a very small amount. If the dough absorbs too much extra flour, the bread will be dry and tough.
2. Turn the ball of dough out on the surface and flatten it slightly.
3. With the heels of both hands, press the top of the dough and push away from you. See **Fig. 45-6**.
4. Pull the far side of the dough toward you, folding the dough in half. This traps air in the dough.
5. Rotate the dough one quarter turn.
6. Continue the push, fold, and turn technique for at least 8 to 10 minutes, using a steady rhythm. When the rough, sticky mass becomes a smooth, glossy, elastic ball, it is ready for the next step—rising.

Letting the Dough Rise

Letting the dough or batter rise allows yeast colonies to multiply and flavors to develop. With recipes that use quick-rise yeast, you can bake bread with only one rise. With the traditional method described here, the dough must rise twice—once after kneading and again after it is shaped.

For the first rising, place the ball-shaped dough in a large, lightly greased bowl. The bowl must be large enough to allow the dough to double in size. Turn the dough over so the greased surface is on top, and press plastic wrap lightly

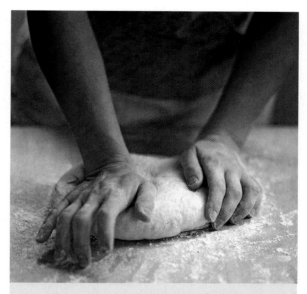

Fig. 45-6 Kneading develops yeast dough and builds muscles at the same time.

onto it. This helps keep the dough from forming a crust or drying out, both of which limit yeast growth. Cover the bowl with a clean, dry dish towel. Batter breads may be put directly into the baking pan to rise.

Choose a warm place for the dough to rise; 75°F to 85°F is ideal. Avoid drafts, which cool the dough, as well as radiators and furnace vents, which cook it. If you can't find a suitable spot, make one. Fill a large bowl two-thirds full of hot water. Set the dough on a wire rack over the water. Replace cooling water with hot water as needed. You can also use a microwave oven, but check the owner's manual for specific instructions, which vary with the oven's power and controls. The method usually involves warming the oven and then leaving it off for a time before additional warming.

Let the dough rise until double in bulk, usually about 1 to 1½ hours. Stiff doughs and those made with whole-grain flour or nuts and fruits take longest to rise. Allow extra time for refrigerated dough. If you're using quick-rising yeast, check the package to estimate rising time.

To test the dough, gently poke two fingers about ½ inch into the surface. If a dent remains, the dough is ready to shape. If the dent springs back, let the dough rise a little longer and test again.

Punching Down

Once the dough has risen, it must be punched down. Punching down lets excess gases escape, making the dough easier to shape. It gives the bread a fine texture by eliminating large air bubbles, which would leave large holes during baking. It also redistributes yeast cells, giving them fresh sugar and starch molecules to feed on as fuel for the second rising.

Punching down is just what it says: thrust your fist into the center of the dough with one quick punch. Then pull the dough away from the sides of the bowl and press it down toward the center to form a ball. Turn the dough out on a lightly floured surface. Many experts recommend letting the dough rest about 10 minutes after punching down to make it more flexible.

The dough is now ready to be shaped. If you can't go on to this step, simply let the dough rise again. You can cover and refrigerate it overnight, if needed. The dough will rise slowly and be ready when you are.

Batter breads are stirred down rather than punched down. Stir the batter with a sturdy spoon until it's close to its original size. Spread it in the baking pan for the second rising.

Shaping Dough and Second Rise

Basic bread dough is generally shaped into a loaf. Some breads are baked free-form on a baking sheet. Others are placed in pans. Usually the dough is cut in half. Use kitchen shears or a sharp knife for this task. Tearing the dough damages the strands of gluten. To shape a loaf:

1. Flour the work surface lightly. With a rolling pin, roll the dough into an 8 x 10 inch rectangle. Be sure it is the same thickness throughout. Roll out the bubbles in the edges.
2. Starting at one of the short ends, roll the dough up tightly. This helps press out air as you roll.
3. Turn the roll so the seam is on top. With your fingers, pinch the seam edge to the roll so it stays closed.

Career Prep

Problem Solving

ONE OF AN INTERVIEWER'S FAVORITE techniques is to have job hopefuls explain how they would solve a problem. Why do you think this is so? Problem solving is a process that involves varied thinking skills. Your response tells interviewers how well you recognize cause and effect, identify resources, predict consequences, weigh advantages and disadvantages, and use creativity. Problem-solving employees are an asset now and an investment in the future.

In practice, solving a problem can also test your people skills. To find solutions, especially at work, often means approaching and persuading diverse individuals to give the help you need.

How can you develop this ability that employers value and that can serve you well personally? Try working through your next problem using these steps:

- **Identify the problem.** Describe the situation as precisely as possible. Include the cause, since that can help you choose a solution. You may uncover several problems that need attention separately.

- **Identify your options.** List possible solutions. Indulge your creativity. Remember that even the most unlikely ideas can provide a kernel of usefulness.

- **Evaluate the options.** Now you can weed out the unworkable options. Consider each that

4. Turn the roll seam-side down. Hold your hands with palms pressed together. With the bottom edge of your hands, press down on both ends of the roll, about ¼ inch inside the edge, to pinch and seal them.

5. Tuck the flattened ends under the roll. Then turn the roll upside down and pinch the ends into it. Place the roll seam-side down in a greased loaf pan.

Yeast dough is very pliable and accepts many different shapes, limited only by your imagination. You can make a braid, a wreath, or a braided wreath. Twist rolls into figure-8s, cloverleaves, sailor's knots, or crescents. Stick smaller balls on larger ones for bunny heads or teddy bears.

Place the shaped dough in the baking pans. Cover with a dry dish towel and let rise again until double, which usually takes less time than the first.

Baking the Dough

Preheat the oven before the bread finishes rising. Loaves are sometimes scored just before baking. To **score** means to make slashes about ½ inch deep across the top of the bread. Scoring prevents the crust from cracking as the dough rises. Diagonal scoring adds a decorative touch.

The heat of the oven gives yeast one last burst of activity, resulting in a sudden rising called oven spring. This indicates a good start, and a nicely browned crust indicates the bread is nearly finished baking. Baking times vary considerably, however, so always bake as directed in the recipe. To check for doneness, remove the loaf from its pan and tap the bottom and sides. Well-baked bread sounds hollow. If you hear a dull thud, put the bread back in the pan and continue baking.

As soon as bread is done, remove it from the pan and place it on a wire cooling rack. Keep the bread away from drafts because rapid cooling can crack the crust top. Let loaves stand about 20 minutes for easier slicing. A quality product has risen well. The top is smooth, rounded, and nicely browned. Inside, the bread has a soft and springy texture that is consistently fine throughout.

remains in terms of available resources and effectiveness. Can it be done? How well would it solve the problem?

- **Choose the best option.** Carefully weigh the pros and cons and look at possible outcomes, including the unintended ones. Then decide.

- **Make a plan to carry out your decision.** Use your management skills to plan a course of action.

- **Carry out your plan.** This marks a turning point, from planning to acting. The more effort you put into earlier steps, the more confident you can feel about taking action.

- **Evaluate the results.** Did the option work as expected? If not, ask yourself why. Maybe hurrying through some steps led to the wrong choice. Perhaps your choice was good, but the plan was carried out poorly. As you go through the process again, aim to use it more effectively.

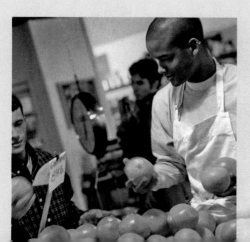

Career Connection

Finding solutions. Work with a team to identify a problem that could occur in a foods or nutrition work setting. Describe the situation on paper. Exchange papers with another team and suggest a solution to the problem described and a plan of action. Use the process outlined.

Summarize Your Reading

▶ Historically speaking, quick breads are a relatively new baked product. That's because the leavenings needed to make them weren't available for thousands of years.

▶ Quick breads are made using two different mixing methods that give distinctly different products.

▶ Yeast leavens bread through a chemical process. The bread must be kneaded and allowed to rise before being shaped and baked.

▶ Different methods can be used to mix the dough for yeast breads.

▶ Convenience breads include packaged mixes and ready-to-bake doughs.

Check Your Knowledge

1. How are **quick breads** leavened?

2. What basic methods are used to make quick breads?

3. Explain the **muffin method**.

4. How would you know when each of these quick breads is done: muffins, loaf breads, and pancakes?

5. What are signs of a well-made muffin?

6. How is the **biscuit method** different from the muffin method?

7. How do you **knead** rolled biscuits?

8. How do you cut out rolled biscuits?

9. How are **drop biscuits** different from **rolled biscuits**?

10. What are signs of a well-made biscuit?

11. How does **fermentation** cause yeast dough to rise?

12. What is the difference between basic white bread and whole-grain bread?

13. How can basic white bread become batter bread and sweet white bread?

14. Why should ingredients for making yeast bread be room temperature?

15. Why is the **quick-mix method** of making yeast dough faster than the **conventional method**?

16. How is kneading yeast dough different from kneading biscuit dough?

17. How do you prepare yeast dough for the first rise?

18. Why is yeast dough punched down after the first rise?

19. How do you shape yeast dough into a loaf?

20. How and why would you **score** a loaf before baking it?

21. **CRITICAL THINKING** If you were making bread from scratch, would you prefer to make quick bread or yeast bread? Why?

22. What are signs of well-made yeast bread?

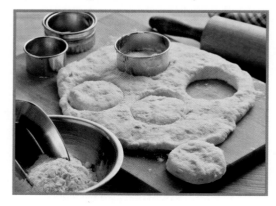

Apply Your Learning

1. **MATH** **Muffin Ingredients.** Assume you need six dozen assorted muffins for a brunch. Find the recipes and make a grocery list for all the supplies you'll need.

2. **MATH** **Quick Bread Comparison.** Compare the costs of quick breads made from scratch and from convenience mixes. Which is lower in cost? In what situations would each product be appropriate?

3. **Water Temperature.** Can you tell whether water is the right temperature to dissolve yeast? Pour a water sample that you believe is within the right range. Check it with a thermometer. How close were you? Practice until you can get three correct samples.

4. **Score Cards.** Develop score cards to use in evaluating quick and yeast breads. Include one each for muffins, rolled biscuits, drop biscuits, and basic yeast bread.

5. **Making Breads.** Demonstrate one of the following: a) the muffin method; b) making rolled biscuits; c) making drop biscuits; d) making yeast bread; e) making convenience bread.

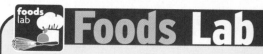 **Foods Lab**

Making Popovers

Procedure: Find and prepare a recipe for popovers or cream puffs, as assigned by your teacher. Copy the recipe you used, and display it with the baked goods for a class evaluation.

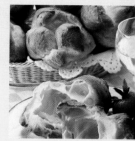

Analyzing Results

❶ Compare the recipes for popovers and cream puffs. How are they similar and how are they different?

❷ How does the interior of these products compare to that of other breads? What leavening agent created this effect?

❸ Compare the two recipes on taste, texture, and appearance. How are they similar and different in these qualities?

❹ Both of these foods are often served filled. What fillings would you choose for popovers? For cream puffs?

 Food Science Experiment

Leavening Action in Yeast

Objective: To compare stages of yeast development and leavening.

Procedure:

1. Preheat the oven to the lowest setting for five minutes. Then turn it off.

2. While the oven is preheating, dissolve one package of yeast and $\frac{1}{4}$ cup of sugar in 1 cup of warm water (about 110°F). Pour the mixture into a 1-gallon plastic freezer bag and seal securely, pressing out as much air as possible. Place the bag in the oven.

3. Repeat Step 2, replacing the sugar with an equal amount of flour.

4. Remove the bags after one hour. Observe and compare the results.

Analyzing Results

❶ How has the contents of each bag changed? In which bag is this change greater? What process caused this change in both bags?

❷ What type of carbohydrate is sugar? What type is flour? How might this difference relate to the rates of change you observed?

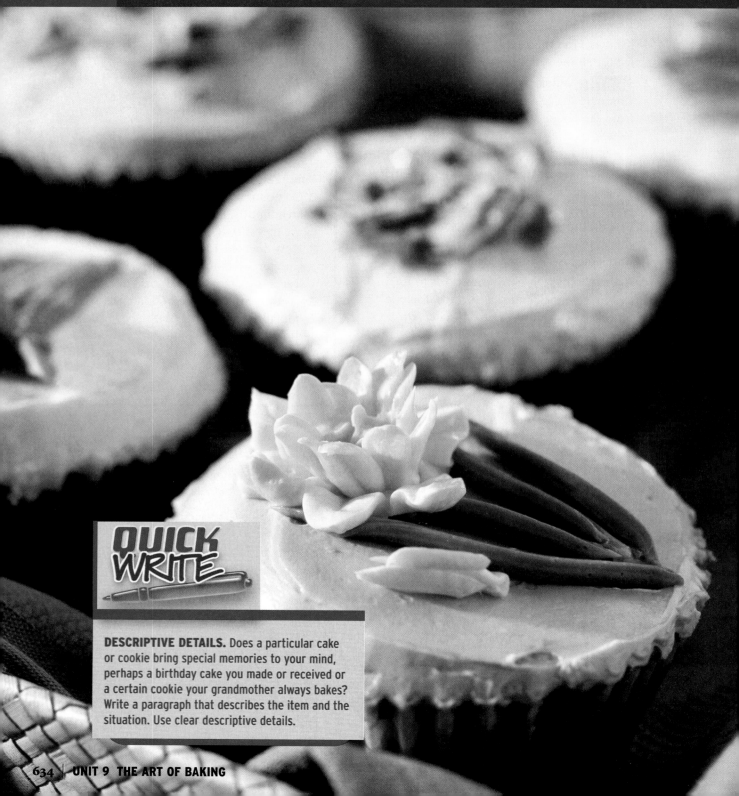

Cakes, Cookies & Candies

QUICK WRITE

DESCRIPTIVE DETAILS. Does a particular cake or cookie bring special memories to your mind, perhaps a birthday cake you made or received or a certain cookie your grandmother always bakes? Write a paragraph that describes the item and the situation. Use clear descriptive details.

I T'S NO SECRET WHY PEOPLE LIKE CAKES, cookies, and candies. They are rich with fat, sweetened with sugars, and often as appealing to look at as to eat. Due to those same ingredients, however, these treats should be enjoyed only on occasion—all the more reason to make them the highest quality possible. Learning the basic techniques behind cake, cookie, and candy creations helps you do just that. With the hundreds of varieties you'll be able to make, you can choose just the one to suit your craving and the occasion.

MAKING CAKES

You may have heard the advice before: for baking success, follow the recipe. Why is that so important? Ingredient amounts, mixing techniques, and baking times are all developed to work together with scientific precision. Mixing directions, for instance, are calculated to incorporate the right amount of air to give a cake batter the best volume and texture. Increasing the liquid changes the batter's consistency, but it can change the mixing time and method too. Check a reliable guide before making substitutions.

Generally, ingredients should be at room temperature when you begin. For example, this pre-

vents the possibility of curdling cold eggs that meet warm ingredients. Exceptions are common, however, so read and follow the recipe.

When you make a cake, you'll probably choose from two basic kinds. These are shortened and foam. See **Fig. 46-1**.

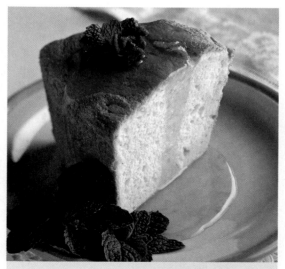

Fig. 46-1 Not all cakes are alike. A foam cake, like this angel food cake, is leavened by air.

Shortened Cakes

Shortened cakes are sometimes called butter cakes. They contain a solid fat—butter, margarine, or shortening—as well as flour, salt, sugar, eggs, and liquid. The main leavening agent is either baking powder or baking soda.

A quality shortened cake has good volume and moist, tender texture. Grain is fine and even, without tunnels. These qualities come in part from ingredients but also from skillful mixing. Ingredients are blended thoroughly but quickly to control the amount of gluten and air. Although mixing methods vary, the conventional mixing method is typical. Some recipes call for the faster one-bowl method.

Conventional Method

In the **conventional method**, fat and sugar are combined first. Sugar crystals "grate" against the fat, creating holes that fill with air. This builds volume into the batter. Alternately adding dry and liquid ingredients reduces the need for vigorous mixing, which contributes to a velvety texture. The recipe in **Fig. 46-2** uses the conventional method, which is described here:

1. Sift the dry ingredients together.

2. Cream the solid fat and sugar until the mixture has a light and fluffy consistency resembling whipped cream.

3. Beat the eggs into the creamed mixture according to recipe directions, typically one at a time.

Fig. 46-2　　　　　　　　　　　　　**Try This!** **Recipe**

Sunny Carrot Cake

Yield	Nutrition Analysis
9 servings	*Per Serving:* 220 calories, 8 g total fat, 1.5 g saturated fat, 0 g trans fat, 25 mg cholesterol, 340 mg sodium, 32 g total carbohydrate, 1 g dietary fiber, 19 g sugars, 4 g protein
	Percent Daily Value: vitamin A 50%, vitamin C 2%, calcium 6%, iron 6%

Ingredients

1¼ cups all-purpose flour
½ tsp. baking powder
½ tsp. baking soda
½ tsp. salt
⅓ cup margarine or butter
¾ cup sugar
1 tsp. grated lemon peel

1 tsp. vanilla
1 egg
2 egg whites
½ cup plain, vanilla, or lemon low-fat yogurt
1½ cups shredded carrots

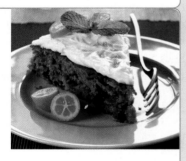

Directions

1. Preheat oven to 350°F. Grease and lightly flour a 9 x 9 inch baking pan.
2. Combine flour, baking powder, baking soda, and salt in small bowl. Set aside.
3. Beat margarine with electric mixer for 30 seconds in large bowl. Add sugar, lemon peel, and vanilla to margarine and beat well. Add egg and egg whites to margarine mixture, one at a time, beating after each addition.
4. Add flour mixture and yogurt alternately to margarine mixture, beating after each addition. Stir in carrots.
5. Pour batter into prepared pan. Spread evenly. Bake 30 minutes at 350°F or until toothpick inserted in center comes out clean. Cool in pan on wire rack.

4. Mix the liquid ingredients in a separate bowl.

5. Add the dry ingredients to the creamed mixture alternately with the liquids. Begin and end with the dry ingredients. This helps keep the fat from separating, which could allow air to escape. Add the dry ingredients in fourths and the liquids in thirds, beating just enough to mix the ingredients after each addition. Overbeating causes a coarse texture and poor volume. The batter should be thick and smooth.

One-Bowl Method

The **one-bowl method** is a quick way to mix ingredients for a shortened cake. The method combines dry ingredients first and then adds moist ingredients. Some cakes mixed with this method use oil instead of solid fat. Use this quick method only when specified in a recipe.

1. Combine the dry ingredients in a large mixing bowl.

2. Add the fat, flavoring, and part of the liquid. Mix to make batter.

3. Add the unbeaten eggs and the remaining liquid and beat until thick and smooth. Mixing can be done by hand or with an electric mixer. Scrape down the sides of the bowl several times to catch traces of unmixed ingredients.

Baking Shortened Cakes

Baking pans for shortened cakes range from muffin pans for cupcakes, to broad sheet pans, to elaborate pans that mold a cake into a work of art. Use the pan size specified in the recipe. If you must use a different size, be sure the batter fills no more than about one-half of the pan. Adjust the baking time accordingly. See **Fig. 46-3**.

Cakes continue to bake after reaching full volume. When done, the cake has a thin, shiny crust, nicely browned and slightly rounded. The sides start to pull away from the pan. The top feels firm but springy. To test for doneness, insert a wooden pick in the center. If it comes out free of moist batter, the cake is done.

Foam Cakes

Foam cakes are well named. They are leavened by air trapped in a protein foam of stiffly beaten egg whites, giving the cakes a light, spongy texture and high volume. Some call for baking powder as well. Other ingredients vary among the three types—angel food cake, sponge cake, and chiffon cake.

- **Angel food cakes.** In these fat-free cakes, egg whites are beaten with sugar until stiff and glossy. Flour is sifted over and gently folded in.
- **Sponge cakes.** These recipes include egg yolks, which are beaten until pale and thick and then mixed with the liquid ingredients. Flour is sifted and folded into the beaten egg whites, and the two mixtures are folded together.
- **Chiffon cakes.** Chiffon cakes combine three separate mixtures. Flour, sugar, and baking powder are sifted together. Egg yolks are beaten with oil and liquids. The liquid ingredients are stirred into the dry ingredients, and the beaten whites gradually folded into the batter.

Fig. 46-3

Baking Pan Equivalents	
Batter Amounts	**Pan Sizes to Use**
Four cups of batter	☐ 8 x 1½ inch, round cake or pie pan; ☐ 12-cup muffin pan
Six cups of batter	☐ 8 x 2 inch, round cake pan; ☐ 9 x 1½ inch, round cake pan; ☐ 8 x 8 x 1½ inch, square cake pan; ☐ 7½-inch Bundt® pan
Eight cups of batter	☐ 9 x 2 inch, round cake or pie pan; ☐ 8 x 8 x 2 inch, square cake pan; ☐ 9 x 5 x 3 inch loaf pan; ☐ 9-inch Bundt® pan

Baking Foam Cakes

A tube pan is not only traditional for foam cakes but also practical. The airy batter needs plenty of support in order to rise, which the ring shape provides. Two-piece pans have a separate bottom for removing the cake more easily. When using a one-piece pan, lining the bottom with parchment paper helps prevent sticking.

To test a foam cake for doneness, touch the top lightly. It should spring back. Cool the cake upside down in the pan to keep its fragile structure from falling. Some pans have legs on the rim for this purpose. You may also invert the cake on an empty glass bottle with a slender neck or on a large metal funnel turned upside down.

When the cake is cool, gently loosen it from the sides of the pan with a spatula. If the pan has a removable bottom, push it upward and use the spatula to free the cake. Invert the pan and the cake onto a serving plate.

Decorating Cakes

For many people, a cake isn't finished until it's frosted. Frosting, or icing, can complement a cake's flavor and appearance. It keeps the surface from drying out and "glues" layered and specially designed cakes together. See **Fig. 46-4**.

Frostings can be cooked or uncooked. Cooked frosting is cooked to a certain temperature on a candy thermometer, cooled slightly, and then beaten until creamy. A simpler version is cooked in a double boiler while beating with a mixer until the frosting stands in soft peaks.

Easier still are uncooked frostings. Confectioners' sugar is creamed with butter, margarine, or cream cheese. Milk is blended in to achieve a spreading consistency. Extracts add flavor. Thin glazes are also made this way.

Whatever frosting you use, cover the container as you work to keep the mixture from drying out and forming a crust. Dry frosting is difficult to use, and flakes of crust are unattractive.

To save the time of frosting a cake—and the fat, sugar, and calories that frosting supplies—you can drizzle on a glaze of confectioners' sugar and fruit juice. Another idea is to cut a stencil from a piece of paper—a snowflake, flower, stars,

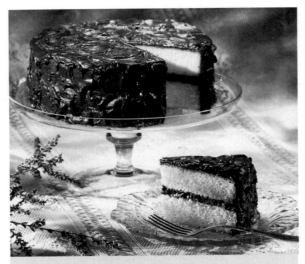

Fig. 46-4 To frost a layer cake, first brush off crumbs carefully. Frost the bottom layer first, but not the sides. Put the top layer in place. Frost the sides of the cake next and the top last.

or leaves—or use a decorative paper doily. See **Fig. 46-5**.

MAKING COOKIES

If you compare recipes for cakes and cookies, you'll notice a similarity in ingredients and proportions. The main difference is that cookies have relatively little liquid, giving them a more substantial texture.

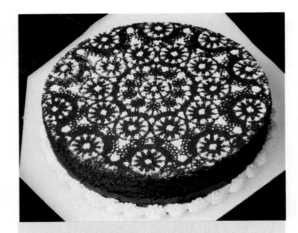

Fig. 46-5 To stencil a cake, place the design on top and sprinkle with confectioners' sugar, cocoa, ground cinnamon, grated chocolate, or finely ground nuts. Remove the stencil carefully.

Today cookies are a specialization in their own right. Choices range from crunchy butter wafers, to soft, jam-filled rings, to decorated cookie "pizzas." Despite the seemingly endless variety, cookies are conveniently grouped into six basic kinds based on how they are formed. These are bar, drop, rolled, molded, refrigerator, and pressed cookies.

Bar Cookies

Bar cookies are baked in a shallow pan and then cut into bars or squares. Some are soft doughs. Others are layered, with different bases, fillings, and toppings. Brownies, with their many variations, are the favorite of bar cookies.

Bar cookies are usually cut when cool. A sharp, thin-bladed knife makes clean, even cuts. Removing a corner piece first makes others easier to lift out.

Drop Cookies

The ever-popular chocolate chip cookie is an example of a drop cookie. **Drop cookies** are made from soft dough dropped onto a cookie sheet.

A small cookie scoop is handy for forming drop cookies. You can also scoop a rounded portion of the dough on a teaspoon and then push it onto the sheet with a rubber scraper or another teaspoon. Allow at least 2 inches between cookies since they spread and flatten a bit during baking.

Rolled Cookies

Beautifully decorated holiday cookies are often **rolled cookies**, which are made from stiff dough that is rolled out and cut into different shapes with cookie cutters. The cookies in **Fig. 46-6** are made this way.

Fig. 46-6

Try This! **Recipe**

Lemony Sugar Cookies

Yield	Nutrition Analysis
About 2 dozen cookies	*Per Serving:* 70 calories, 3 g total fat, 0 g saturated fat, 0 g trans fat, 10 mg cholesterol, 50 mg sodium, 9 g total carbohydrate, 1 g dietary fiber, 3 g sugars, 1 g protein
	Percent Daily Value: vitamin A 2%, vitamin C 0%, calcium 2%, iron 2%

Ingredients

1 cup all-purpose flour
3/4 cup whole-wheat flour
1 tsp. baking powder
1/3 cup margarine
1/3 cup sugar

1 egg
1 tsp. vanilla
1 Tbsp. lemon juice
1/2 tsp. lemon rind, grated

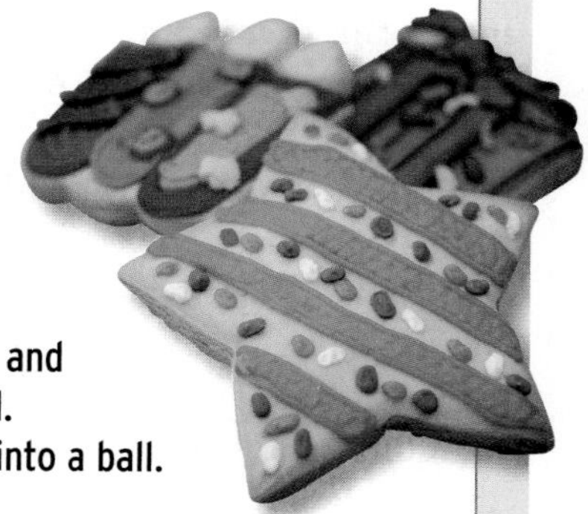

Directions

1. Preheat oven to 375°F. Lightly grease cookie sheet(s).
2. Combine both flours and baking powder and set aside.
3. Cream margarine in large bowl. Add sugar gradually, beating until light and fluffy. Add egg, beating well. Stir in vanilla, lemon juice, and lemon rind.
4. Add flour mixture to egg mixture, stirring until blended. Gather dough into a ball. Cover and chill dough thoroughly.
5. Place dough on lightly floured surface and roll to 1/4-inch thickness. Cut with cookie cutters into desired shapes and place on lightly greased cookie sheet.
6. Bake at 375°F for 8 minutes until golden brown. Remove from cookie sheet and cool on wire rack.

Rolled cookie dough is chilled for easier handling. Work with a small amount at a time, leaving the rest in the refrigerator. Roll the dough about ⅛ inch thick on a lightly floured surface. Use as little flour as possible to avoid drying out the cookies.

Before cutting, dip the cookie cutter in flour and shake off the excess. Try to cut efficiently by positioning cutters to minimize scraps of dough. These can be rolled and cut again, but they get a little tougher each time. Using a spatula, place the cookies on a baking sheet about 1 inch apart.

Molded Cookies

Molded cookies are shaped by hand. Balls of dough may be rolled in chopped nuts or other coatings before baking. Some are flattened with the bottom of a glass. Others are "engraved" with cookie stamps or tiles. Peanut butter cookies are pressed with a fork, creating their characteristic ridges. You might also make crescents, pretzels, logs, or twists.

Chilling the dough makes these cookies easier to shape. Pinch off walnut-size pieces of dough and form them quickly. Overworking makes cookies tough. Press the dough together so the cookies hold their shape.

Molded cookies are placed about 1 inch apart on a cookie sheet, or 3 inches apart if they are to be flattened. Dipping the glass or fork in flour or granulated sugar keeps it from sticking to the dough. Stamps are oiled lightly before being used and floured between cookies.

Refrigerator Cookies

To make **refrigerator cookies**, form the dough into long, even rolls about 1½ to 2 inches in diameter. Wrap the rolls well in wax paper, foil, or plastic wrap, and chill as the recipe directs. The dough can be prepared several days in advance.

To cut, slice the roll by encircling it with heavy thread and pulling the ends. Place slices about 1 inch apart on the cookie sheet.

Pressed Cookies

Pressed cookies are made by using a cookie press to force dough directly onto a baking sheet. Spritz cookies, made with a basic, versatile, butter dough, are probably the most familiar type. Cookie presses include disks for making an array of shapes, from clovers to camels. See **Fig. 46-7**.

The consistency of the dough is the key to these cookies. It must be soft enough to press but firm enough to hold its shape. Some doughs are chilled for this reason, and working quickly is essential. This stiff dough spreads very little, so you need only about half an inch between cookies on the sheet.

Baking and Storing Cookies

Cookies of uniform size bake more evenly. Let cookie sheets cool between batches. The dough softens and loses its shape on a hot baking sheet.

Cookies are delicately browned when done. To test drop and bar cookies, lightly press one with your finger. A slight imprint will remain. Unless the recipe states otherwise, remove cookies from the sheet as soon as they are done. Otherwise, the heat from the sheet continues baking the cookies.

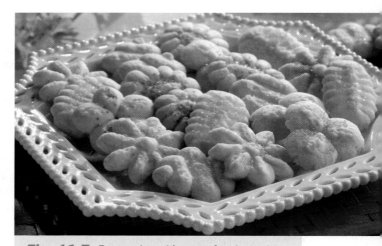

Fig. 46-7 Pressed cookies are fun to make. Once you learn how much dough to press out for each cookie and how to "let go" of the dough from the cookie press, you can make a large batch in a short time.

Cookies should be stored in a container after cooling. Cover crisp cookies with a lid that fits loosely and soft cookies with a tight-fitting lid, and store the two types separately. For longer storage, you can freeze cookies.

Convenience Cakes and Cookies

Cake mixes have come a long way, in quality and variety, since the first one-layer ginger cake was offered in 1947. Now, by adding water, oil, and eggs, you can have white, chocolate, butter pecan, or marble cake that rivals many homemade recipes. With a few extra steps and ingredients, you can try the variations that are often included on the box. For extra convenience, frostings are sold in mixes and ready-to-use form.

Cookies, too, are quickly and easily prepared from mixes. In fact, you can make cookies from cake mix by reducing the amount of liquid. You can also find ready-to-use cookie dough in the store's refrigerator case.

MAKING CANDIES

Compared to baking, making candy may seem simple. Candy making, however, is the more exacting art and science. You can't substitute ingredients in a candy recipe as you might in a cookie. Thirty seconds usually makes little difference in baking times. When you cook candy, however, thirty seconds can mean the difference between success and failure.

Given their sensitivity, increasing or decreasing candy recipes is tricky and not advised. If the yield is too small, make additional batches. If it's too large, remember that homemade candy makes a thoughtful gift.

Kinds of Candies

Someone who is overwhelmed with good choices might be likened to "a kid in a candy store." When you consider all the candy made, you appreciate the meaning of that expression.

Fig. 46-8 shows three types of candy, but a few other standards are described here. Nougat is a chewy or crunchy candy made by beating hot sugar syrup into beaten egg whites. Smooth, pliable fondant is usually a base for other candies, including mint patties and chocolate-covered cherries. Divinity is soft and puffy. It's made with stiffly beaten egg whites, sugar, corn syrup, and flavoring. While a batch of taffy cools, it is pulled and twisted into long strands to incorporate air and make a soft, chewy candy. Caramels brown as butter, milk or cream, and sugar cook.

New candy makers may want to build their skills by starting with easy-to-prepare candies that require little or no cooking. **Fig. 46-9** on page 642 is a simple recipe to try.

Principles of Candy Making

Before making candies, it helps to know something about the chemical processes involved. By knowing what is going on in that pan of bubbling syrup, you can better judge how well things are proceeding. Two main forces are of concern to candy makers: temperature and crystallization.

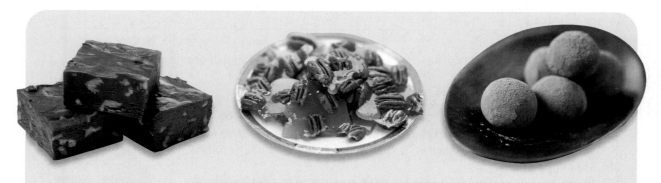

Fig. 46-8 Creamy, semisoft fudge (left) is made with sugar, corn syrup, butter, and cream. Crunchy brittle (center) is made with carmelized sugar and nuts. Rich, creamy truffles (right) are made with chocolate, sugar, butter or cream, and flavorings. They are rolled into balls and coated with chocolate.

The Role of Temperature

Why do candy recipes call for such unusual temperatures—248°F, for example? Imagine you're cooking a candy mixture. The mixture starts to boil. As the liquid evaporates, the mixture thickens. Its boiling point rises and continues to rise as more liquid escapes. Thus temperature is a measure of how much liquid is left in the mixture: the higher the temperature, the less liquid remains. This is one factor that decides whether a butter-and-sugar mixture becomes a chewy caramel or a crunchy toffee.

To monitor the mixture's temperature with the attention it needs, a candy thermometer should be placed in the pan so it can be read at any time. Make sure the bulb does not touch the pan bottom to ensure an accurate reading.

If you do not have a thermometer, you can use the **cold water test**, which estimates syrup temperature based on how it acts in cold water. Although it's often used in recipe directions, this test is less reliable than a thermometer. To use the cold water test, follow these steps:

1. With a clean wooden spoon, drop about ½ teaspoon of the hot syrup into a cup of cold, not icy, water.
2. Use your fingertips to form the drops of syrup into a ball in the water.
3. Remove the ball from the water and note its firmness. Hotter syrups form harder balls. If the syrup does not behave as the recipe directs, it has not reached the proper temperature. Cook it a few minutes longer and test again. **Fig. 46-10** describes the consistency of the cooked syrup for each temperature range.

The weather has an indirect impact on the temperature a candy mixture should reach. Sugar attracts moisture. On humid days, once the candy cools, it starts to reabsorb water vapor from the air. As a result, it stays softer than desired. That's why many people make candy only in dry

---

Fig. 46-9

Try This! **Recipe**

Chocolate Peanut Clusters

Yield	Nutrition Analysis
About 44 pieces	**Per Serving:** 110 calories, 8 g total fat, 2.5 g saturated fat, 0 g trans fat, 0 mg cholesterol, 90 mg sodium, 8 g total carbohydrate, 1 g dietary fiber, 5 g sugars, 3 g protein **Percent Daily Value:** vitamin A 0%, vitamin C 0%, calcium 2%, iron 2%

Ingredients
2, 7-oz. bars milk or dark chocolate

1, 16-oz. jar dry roasted, salted peanuts

Directions
1. Line two large cookie sheets with wax paper.
2. Break up chocolate into small pieces.
3. Put chocolate pieces in a microwavable bowl. Melt in microwave oven at 50 percent power for 3 to 4 minutes, stirring and checking every 90 seconds.
4. Stir in peanuts.
5. Drop by heaping teaspoonful onto the lined cookie sheets. Cool. Candy will set up in about an hour at room temperature. Refrigerate to speed set.

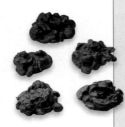

Fig. 46-10

Stages in Cold Water Test		
Stage	**Temperature**	**Consistency**
Thread stage	230–233°F	Forms a loose, sticky thread that won't form into a ball.
Soft-ball stage	234–240°F	Forms a soft ball that flattens.
Firm-ball stage	244–248°F	Forms a ball that holds its shape, is pliable, and doesn't flatten.
Hard-ball stage	250–266°F	Forms a hard, compact ball that holds its shape but flattens when pressed between the fingers.
Soft-crack stage	270–290°F	Forms firm threads that are pliable when removed from water.
Hard-crack stage	300–310°F	Forms brittle threads that break or snap easily when removed from water.
Caramel stage	320–338°F	Forms brittle threads, and liquid turns brown.

weather. You can compensate for the added moisture by cooking the syrup two degrees higher than the recipe states, which boils off more liquid.

Also recall that at higher altitudes, mixtures boil at lower temperatures. Use specially developed recipes to make candy at high altitudes.

Crystallization

Crystallization is the formation of sugar crystals in syrup. It occurs because the sugar molecules dissolved in the syrup, glucose and fructose, tend to reunite and return to their original form—granulated sugar. Crystallization can happen as a mixture boils, when less water is available to keep the molecules dissolved. Sometimes a solid sugar crystal or bit of lint falls into the mixture, starting a chain reaction of crystallization. Any sort of agitation can trigger the process as a mixture cools and it is less able to hold dissolved sugar.

Left alone, crystals grow slowly and get large. Large crystals feel gritty on the tongue. Small crystals create the smooth, silky texture that marks a superior candy.

Controlling crystallization, then, is the key to candy making. To keep sugar crystals small, recipes often include ingredients called **interfering agents**. Cream of tartar is an acid that breaks down sugar crystals, while fats literally get between the molecules to keep them apart. Corn syrup adds extra glucose to the syrup, disrupting the orderly crystalline formation.

Agitation is another way to manage crystal growth. You can induce crystallization by starting to beat the mixture when it has cooled to the right temperature. Continued beating speeds the process, producing more small crystals. If you keep beating until crystallization stops, you'll have a batch of creamy pralines or velvety truffles.

You can also use these principles to prevent crystallization entirely to make noncrystalline candies. Both toffee and caramels, for instance, contain a large amount of butter, an interfering agent. Both are cooled without stirring.

In addition to recipe directions, these steps can help prevent unwanted crystallization:

- Have all ingredients at room temperature.
- Use only clean pans, spoons, and thermometers. Wash and dry equipment before reusing it. Dip cold utensils in warm water to warm them.
- Rub pan sides with butter to prevent sugar from sticking.
- Put sugar in the pan first. Wash the sides with the liquid used in the recipe.
- While cooking, dissolve crystals on pan sides with a pastry brush dipped in hot water. Watch for crystals that start to slide into the syrup.
- When pouring out the mixture, work quickly. Be careful not to scrape the sides or the bottom of the pan.

Syrup that starts to crystallize can be saved by adding a small amount of water, but you will have to cook the mixture again.

Steps in Candy Making

Because candy making requires exact timing, pre-preparation is essential.

After reading the recipe, measure and arrange all ingredients so they are at hand when you need them. Also assemble the necessary equipment. In addition to cooling racks, baking sheets, and other standard items, you'll need the following:

- Candy thermometer.
- Heavy, deep pan with straight sides. Choose one that holds about three times the volume of the ingredients. If the pan is too small, the syrup can foam up and boil over, making a mess and possibly delivering a severe burn. If the pan is too large, the mixture may not be deep enough to cover the bulb of the thermometer.
- Wooden spoon with a long handle. Sugar syrups reach very high temperatures. Metal gets too hot to hold and plastic may even melt.

You'll need a mixer for some candies, such as nougat and divinity. Use a sturdy, free-standing model. Portable mixers don't have enough power. Some candies also require special equipment, such as candy molds and dipping forks. See **Fig. 46-11**.

Because candy recipes vary greatly, no single method makes them all. One common process is outlined here:

1. Clip the candy thermometer to the side of the pan.
2. Add sugars, liquids, and butter, if used.
3. Place the pan over low heat and stir until the sugar is completely dissolved. Stir constantly but carefully to minimize splashing. Avoid scraping the sides, which could trigger crystallization to occur.
4. Add other ingredients and bring the mixture to the desired temperature. Stir as the recipe instructs. You may be told to stir the boiling mixture occasionally or to stop stirring once the sugar dissolves.

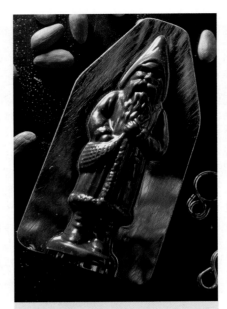

Fig. 46-11 Many candies can be made by pouring the mixture into molds.

5. Remove the pan from the heat. Stir in extracts, nuts, or other flavorings, as directed.
6. Let the mixture cool undisturbed to the temperature indicated. Some recipes advise placing the pan in water to speed cooling and encourage fine crystals to grow.
7. Beat the mixture according to the recipe. Pour or drop the candy onto baking sheets or pans, which are usually prepared by buttering or lining with wax paper.

Storing Candies

Allow candies to cool completely before storing them. Keep them in a cool place in a tightly covered container, layered between sheets of wax paper, plastic, or foil, or wrap them individually. Candies can keep in this way for up to three weeks, depending on type. Many candies can be frozen for up to one year.

Use separate containers for different kinds of candy, which otherwise may exchange moisture and flavors. Walnut toffee and peppermint fudge may be your favorite candies, but you probably don't want to taste them together.

Food Photographer

LOIS ELLEN FRANK: If a picture is worth a thousand words, Lois Ellen Frank's work could fill a library. Her photos tell of the wonder of food—not only as a commodity to be bought and sold but also as a core of culture that draws in a people's traditions, values, and history.

Focus on Food. Food and its many meanings were woven into Lois Ellen's childhood on Long Island, New York, including those passed on by her Jewish father and her mother, who is Kiowa and European. From both grandmothers, Lois Ellen inherited a love of cooking, and at age twelve she sold homemade bread to a nearby health food store. In high school, she helped grow and sell organic vegetables and met with friends to taste-test new recipes. She held a series of restaurant jobs. Another calling, however—photography—took her to the Brooks Institute of Photography in California.

A respect and reverence for food followed her. Lois recalls: "I worked in two restaurants to put myself through school and found myself preparing dishes for school assignments." Her understanding of how food behaves, paired with an artist's eye for color, balance, and drama, soon brought success. She has shot ads for many restaurants, food and culinary posters, magazine spreads, and cookbooks. Her work has won many awards.

The Wide-Angle View. With her career running full steam, Lois Ellen's quest for personal inspiration led her to explore her Native American roots and to Santa Fe, New Mexico, a region steeped in Native American lore. She was especially moved by the Indian reverence for food, which views food as a sacred life-giver and healer, connecting people to each other and to the earth, both physically and spiritually. Inspired, she found a mission: to help preserve this ancient philosophy, in which she found much wisdom.

Lois Ellen now lives in Santa Fe. After returning to school for a master's degree in cultural anthropology, she continues to research foods and is pursuing her Ph.D. in culinary anthropology. Working with culinary advisors, she produced a cookbook, *Foods of the Southwest Indian Nations*. The book won the 2003 James Beard Award in the Americana category. Part of the proceeds goes to a culinary arts scholarship to help young Native Americans carry on their food heritage and learn professional culinary techniques.

The Mission Continues. Besides traveling and arranging displays for photo shoots (she still makes much of the food herself), Lois Ellen teaches cooking classes on Native American foods, is a guest chef and lecturer, and works on museum exhibits related to native foods. She continues to be actively involved in her photographic and chef careers and looks forward to more publishing projects. She says: "No two days are ever the same. The challenges are always different and exciting. If you love what you do, you will love each day of your life that you do it."

On-line Connections

1. To learn more about topics in this article, search the Internet for these key words: Native American cooking; food photography.

2. To learn about related careers, search the Internet for these key words: artisanal baking; ecotour guide.

Summarize Your Reading

▶ Different kinds of cakes are mixed and baked in distinctive ways. Mixing techniques, ingredient amounts, and baking times are all developed to work together with scientific precision.

▶ Cakes can be frosted and decorated according to your originality and the occasion.

▶ Cookies differ in several ways from cakes, including texture. Cookie types determine the methods for making them.

▶ Convenience products make baking quick and easy when time is an issue.

▶ Making candy is an exact art and science that requires more than one sensitive chemical process.

Check Your Knowledge

1. Why should recipes for baked items be followed precisely?

2. What are signs of a quality **shortened cake**?

3. Compare the **conventional method** with the **one-bowl method** for mixing a shortened cake.

4. How can you tell that a shortened cake is done baking?

5. How does a **foam cake** differ from a shortened cake?

6. Describe how angel food, sponge, and chiffon cakes are made.

7. Why is a tube pan a good choice when baking a foam cake?

8. How do you test a foam cake for doneness?

9. Why is a foam cake cooled upside down?

10. How do you make cooked and uncooked cake frostings?

11. Describe two ways to decorate cakes without using frosting.

12. Compare cakes and cookies.

13. Describe **bar**, **drop**, **refrigerator**, and **pressed** cookies.

14. What is different about how **rolled** and **molded cookies** are made?

15. How can you tell when cookies are done baking?

16. Explain the role of temperature in candy making.

17. How do you take a **cold water test** to check a candy mixture for doneness?

18. How does weather impact the temperature a candy mixture should reach?

19. **CRITICAL THINKING** Why is controlling **crystallization** important when making candy?

20. How do **interfering agents** control the process of crystallization?

21. What techniques can a cook use to keep syrups from crystallizing?

22. Why is pan size important when making candies?

23. How should candies be stored?

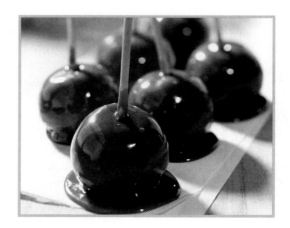

Apply Your Learning

1. **MATH Bake Sale.** Suppose you plan to donate a baked item for a school bake sale. What would you make and in what quantity? Will you use convenience products or bake from scratch? Why? What will your baked item cost and sell for?

2. **SOCIAL STUDIES Historical Cakes.** Research the history of cakes, learning about different types, such as "Lady Baltimore cake." Report your findings and make one of the historical cakes to share.

3. **Cake Decorating.** Try your hand at cake decorating. Study magazines and cookbooks to get ideas. Will you choose a theme for your cake?

4. **Skills Practice.** Make one of these in the foods lab and evaluate results: a) shortened cake; b) foam cake; c) one type of cookie; d) one type of candy. When and how would you serve the item you prepared?

5. **Making Fudge.** Find a recipe for fudge that calls for the cold water test. Research the principles of fudge making before preparing a batch. Evaluate results.

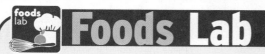

Foods Lab

Reduced-Fat Brownies

Procedure: Prepare the brownie recipe assigned by your teacher. You will either make a full-fat or a reduced-fat brownie recipe. What is the fat content per serving for your recipe? Serve samples of your recipe for a class taste test. Label your samples with a code, such as Team A. As you sample brownies, record the two samples you like best.

Analyzing Results

❶ Tally results to find out which brownies were preferred.

❷ What fat-reduction techniques were used in the reduced-fat brownies?

❸ Were reduced-fat or full-fat versions favored? Did any fat-reduction techniques produce better results?

❹ What do you conclude about full-fat versus reduced-fat recipes?

 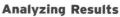

Food Science Experiment

Properties of Chocolate

Objective: To analyze reactions of ingredients in chocolate.

Procedure:

1. Place ¼ cup of chocolate baking morsels in a microwave-safe container. Heat the morsels in a microwave oven at 50 percent power for 10 seconds and stir. Repeat if needed until the morsels are almost melted. Stir the morsels to complete the melting.

2. Add 1 tsp. of water to the chocolate and stir in. Observe and record the results.

3. Add 2 more tsp. of water to the chocolate. Reheat for 5 seconds and stir. Observe and record the results.

Analyzing Results

❶ How did the chocolate react to the first addition of water?

❷ How did the chocolate react to the second addition of water?

❸ Chocolate is made of dry solids and fats. With this in mind, offer reasons for the reactions you observed.

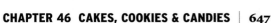

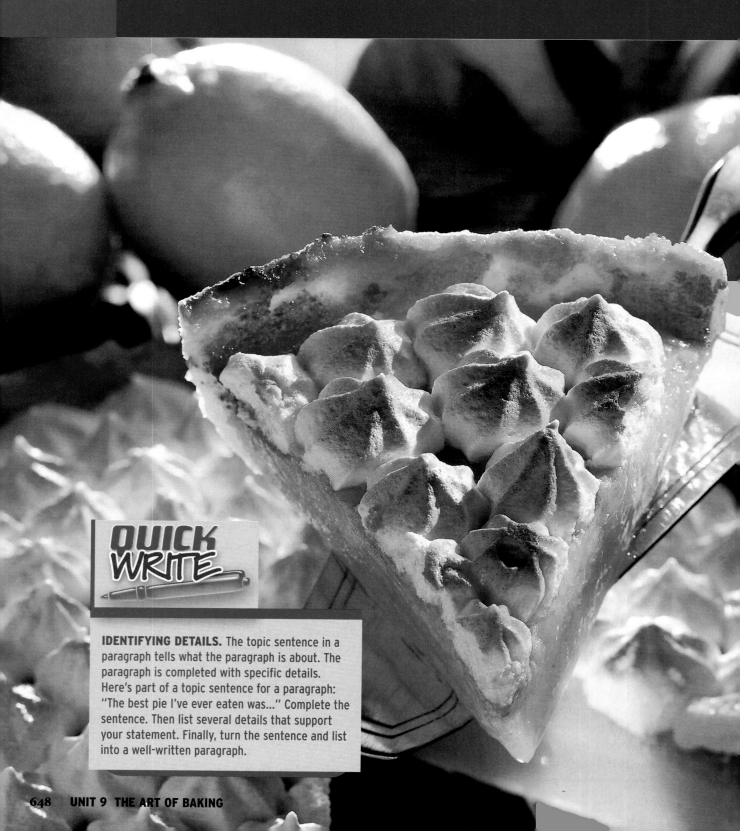

QUICK WRITE

IDENTIFYING DETAILS. The topic sentence in a paragraph tells what the paragraph is about. The paragraph is completed with specific details. Here's part of a topic sentence for a paragraph: "The best pie I've ever eaten was..." Complete the sentence. Then list several details that support your statement. Finally, turn the sentence and list into a well-written paragraph.

P IES ARE LITERALLY AS OLD AS CIVILIZATION. Over time, pies—and their cousins, tarts—have gone from simple to spectacular, from practical to delectable. Whether served as a main dish or a dessert, even ordinary foods seem dressed up when wrapped in a crust.

PIES

A **pie** is any dish consisting of a crust with a filling. See **Fig. 47-1**. What foods go into today's popular pies? Note their similarities and their differences.

- **Fruit pies.** Whole or sliced fruit is combined with sugar and a starch thickener. The ratio of sugar to thickener varies depending on the fruit. The sugar forms a syrup with the fruit juices. The thickener congeals the syrup to firm up the filling as it bakes. Common fruit pie thickeners include flour, cornstarch, and tapioca starch. Some pie makers blend thickeners to get the best qualities of each one, adding body and gloss but no color or flavor.
- **Cream pies.** The "cream" in these pies is closer to a pudding, consisting of eggs, milk, cornstarch, and flavoring. This mixture is cooked until thick, then cooled and poured into a baked, cooled crust. Flavors include lemon, banana, coconut, and butterscotch. **Fig. 47-2** on page 650 is a cream filling for another favorite flavor—chocolate.
- **Custard pies.** Similar in texture to cream pies, these pies start with uncooked custard, which is baked with the crust. Pumpkin and pecan pies belong to this category.
- **Savory pies.** In contrast to a dessert pie, a savory pie contains cooked meat, poultry, seafood, or vegetables in a thickened sauce. It's usually served as a main course. The first pies ever made were probably savory.

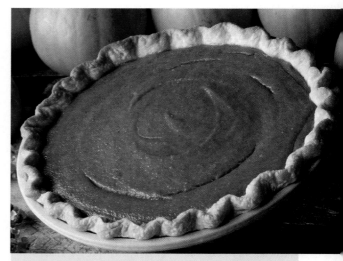

Fig. 47-1 The filling influences whether a pie is made with a single or double crust. Pumpkin and other custard pies have a single crust.

Fig. 47-2

Try This! **Recipe**

Chocolate Pie

Yield	Nutrition Analysis
8 servings	*Per Serving:* 220 calories, 7 g total fat, 2 g saturated fat, 0 g trans fat, 30 mg cholesterol, 85 mg sodium, 33 g total carbohydrate, 1 g dietary fiber, 13 g sugars, 5 g protein *Percent Daily Value:* vitamin A 4%, vitamin C 0%, calcium 8%, iron 8%

Ingredients

½ cup sugar
5 Tbsp. unsweetened cocoa
¼ cup cornstarch
2 cups fat-free milk

1 egg, lightly beaten
1 tsp. vanilla extract
9-inch, baked pie shell
nondairy whipped topping

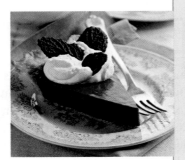

Directions

1. Combine sugar, cocoa, and cornstarch in medium saucepan.
2. Add milk gradually, stirring with wire whisk until well blended.
3. Bring to boil over medium heat. Cook 1 minute, stirring constantly.
4. Stir about ¼ of hot cocoa mixture into beaten egg. Add egg mixture to remaining hot cocoa mixture, stirring constantly.
5. Stir in vanilla.
6. Pour mixture into 9-inch, baked pie shell. Let cool 1 hour on wire rack.
7. Chill 3 hours or until set and serve with nondairy whipped topping.

Piecrust Basics

The foundation of any pie is its crust, not only in physical structure but in appeal as well. For many people, the crust "makes" the pie, especially a tender and flaky pastry crust. See **Fig. 47-3** for a recipe.

Pastry Dough Ingredients

A basic pastry dough relies on the interplay of four ingredients—flour, water, fat, and salt. Flour and water form the structure, balanced by the tenderizing qualities of the fat. Ice-cold water helps keep the fat from melting during mixing, which is needed for a flaky texture. The fat also adds flavor, which is enhanced by the salt. Recipes may include a little sugar and vinegar, which bind with flour proteins to limit gluten formation.

Most piecrust recipes call for all-purpose flour. For added lightness, some bakers use equal parts of all-purpose and cake flour. The resulting dough is softer and needs quick, skilled handling.

Because vegetable shortening and lard are pure fat, they make the flakiest crust. The water present in butter, margarine, and cream cheese creates a more crumbly texture, closer to a butter cookie. These flavorful crusts are often used for tarts.

Piecrust can also be made with oil instead of solid fat or hot water instead of cold. These changes require slightly different mixing methods, however, and produce crusts with a different texture. With oil, the texture is usually tender but more dry and grainy than flaky.

Preparing the Pastry Dough

Preparing piecrust is similar to preparing biscuits. Cut the fat into the flour with a pastry blender or two knives only until the mixture resembles coarse crumbs or small peas. Add water one tablespoon at a time, mixing lightly with a fork after each addition. Form a ball of dough that is neither crumbly nor sticky. You may need less water in humid weather.

Fig. 47-3

Pie Shell

Yield
9-inch diameter shell; 8 servings

Nutrition Analysis
Per Serving: 110 calories, 6 g total fat, 2 g saturated fat, 0 g trans fat, 0 mg cholesterol, 50 mg sodium, 12 g total carbohydrate, 1 g dietary fiber, 1 g sugars, 2 g protein

Percent Daily Value: vitamin A 0%, vitamin C 0%, calcium 0%, iron 4%

Ingredients
vegetable oil cooking spray
1 cup all-purpose flour
1/4 tsp. baking powder
1/8 tsp. salt

4 Tbsp. vegetable shortening
3 Tbsp. plus 1 tsp. ice water
1 tsp. lemon juice

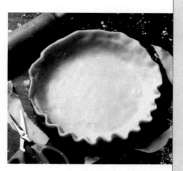

Directions
1. Preheat oven to 425°F and coat 9-inch pie pan with cooking spray.
2. Combine flour, baking powder, and salt in medium bowl. Cut in shortening with pastry blender until mixture resembles coarse meal.
3. Combine ice water and lemon juice in small bowl.
4. Sprinkle water mixture, 1 tablespoon at a time, over flour mixture. Toss with fork until dry ingredients are moistened and form dough.
5. Roll dough into an 11-inch circle. Fit dough into prepared pie pan. Trim to 1/2-inch overhang. Fold edges under and flute. Pierce bottom and sides of dough with fork.
6. Bake at 425°F for 14 minutes or until lightly browned.

Like biscuits, piecrust dough should be mixed and handled as little as possible to keep particles of fat separated by moistened flour. If the pastry is mixed too much, the particles break down. If handled too much, the particles melt from the heat in your hands. All of this work also overdevelops the gluten, transforming the texture from feathery to leathery.

Once mixed, the dough is rested to relax the gluten. This minimizes shrinkage during baking. You, on the other hand, might start working on the filling and perhaps on cleaning up. Cover the dough with wax paper and a towel so it doesn't dry out.

Rolling the Pastry Dough

Piecrust can be rolled on any clean, washable surface that is at a comfortable height.

1. Sprinkle the work surface and rolling pin with flour, or place the dough between two pieces of wax paper or plastic wrap. You won't need flour if you use the latter method.
2. Press the ball of dough to flatten it slightly. Gently roll the dough from the center out in all directions, giving it an occasional quarter-turn to maintain a circular shape. Roll out the dough evenly to a thickness of about 1/8 inch and a diameter 2 inches larger than the pie pan. Flour the rolling pin and surface only as needed to keep the dough from sticking.
3. Brush any excess flour off the dough. Place the pie pan nearby and transfer the dough to the pan by one of two methods. You can fold the dough in half or quarters. Lift it into the pan and gently unfold. You can also wind the dough loosely around the rolling pin, starting with the edge nearest you and rolling away. Hold the rolling pin over the far edge of the pie pan. Unwind the dough and let it settle into the pan.

4. Carefully center the dough in the pan. Push it gently onto the bottom and sides. Avoid stretching the dough, which increases its tendency to shrink.

Somewhere in the process the dough may crack or lose its shape. Patch or reshape it by cutting off a piece the size needed from an area where you have extra dough. With cold water, slightly moisten the area to be repaired. Place the patch on the dough and press firmly. Sprinkle with a little flour and roll with the pin to smooth and even out the patched spot.

Decorating the Edge

A piecrust should have a **fluted edge**, which creates an attractive, shaped finish. Examples are shown in **Fig. 47-4**. By pressing the dough gently with your thumbs and index fingers, you can make a rope- or V-shape. Make ridges with the tines of a fork.

Two-Crust Pie

Pies can be made with one or two crusts. Look for a recipe that makes the amount of dough you need.

To make a two-crust pie, divide the dough into two portions, one slightly larger than the other.

Roll out the larger portion and fit it into the pan. Then proceed as follows:

1. With scissors or a sharp knife, trim the bottom dough even with the edge of the pan.
2. Roll out the second ball of dough for the top crust. Cover to keep it from drying out.
3. Prepare the filling and pour it over the bottom dough.
4. Place the top dough over the filled pie.
5. Trim the top dough to about $\frac{1}{2}$ inch larger than the pie pan.
6. Slightly moisten the edge of the bottom dough. Tuck the overhanging top dough under the edge of the bottom dough. Press both together. This forms a seal to keep in juices. Flute the edge.
7. With a sharp knife, cut several slits in the top dough near the center to allow steam to escape during baking.

To add appeal, you can glaze the top dough before baking by brushing with milk and a light sprinkle of sugar or with beaten egg mixed with water. Cut shapes with a cookie cutter from rolled-out dough and place them on the filling.

Lattice Crust

A **lattice crust** makes an eye-catching woven top on a two-crust pie, especially one with a col-

Fig. 47-4 Piecrusts can be finished with different patterns on the edge. You can "rope" the edge by pinching the dough at an angle with your thumb and the knuckle of your index finger.

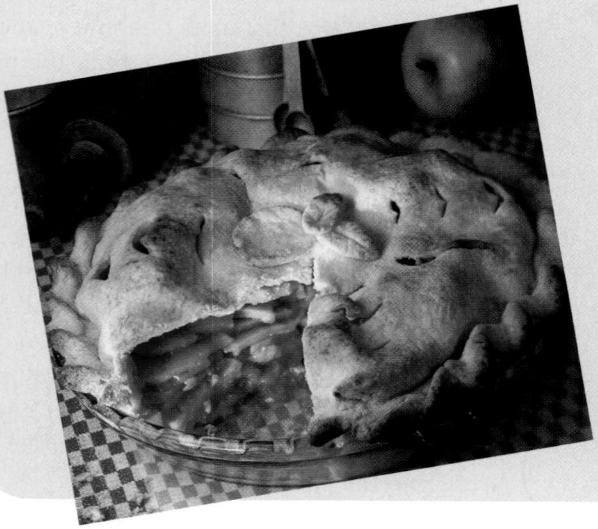

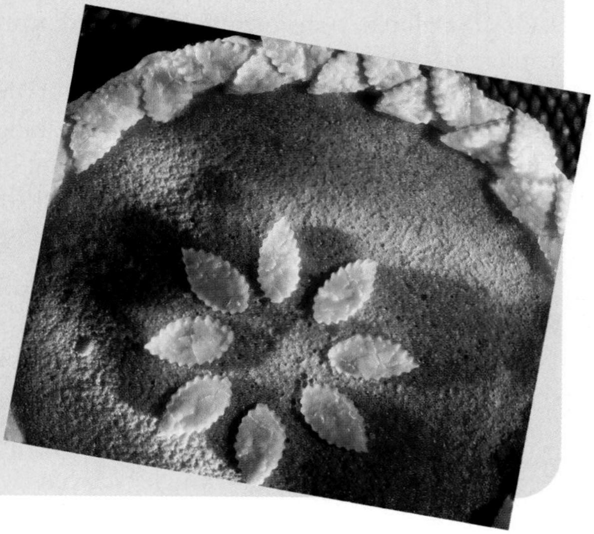

orful filling. To make a lattice crust, cut strips and weave them as shown in **Fig. 47-5**.

One-Crust Pie

For some one-crust pies, the crust and filling are baked together. For others, the crust is baked empty, or blind, and a prepared filling is added later. A bottom crust baked before filling is called a **pie shell**.

To make a one-crust pie:

1. Let the bottom dough rest in the pie pan for a few minutes.
2. Using scissors or a sharp knife, trim the dough ½ inch beyond the edge of the pan.
3. Tuck the overhanging dough under to form a double-thick edge.
4. Flute the edge.
5. Bake blind or fill as directed.

To keep a pie shell from puffing up when baking, use a fork to poke small holes all over the dough before putting it in the oven. This technique is called **docking**. You can also put a smaller pie pan on top of the dough in the pan. Another method is to line the dough with aluminum foil and then fill with dried beans or peas. Lift them out with the foil a few minutes before the crust is done.

Crumb Crusts

A **crumb crust**, made of crushed crackers or cookies, is a sweeter, simpler alternative to pastry dough for a one-crust pie. Graham cracker crusts are traditional for cheesecakes. Depending on the filling, you might try gingersnaps, sandwich cookies, vanilla wafers, or macaroons.

Use fine crumbs to make a crust. Coarse crumbs don't hold together as well. For variety, add chopped nuts, oats, coconut, or spices. Stir in melted butter or margarine and press the mixture into the pan. The crust may be baked or chilled for added firmness.

Fig. 47-5

How to Make a Lattice Piecrust

Lay half of the strips across the pie.

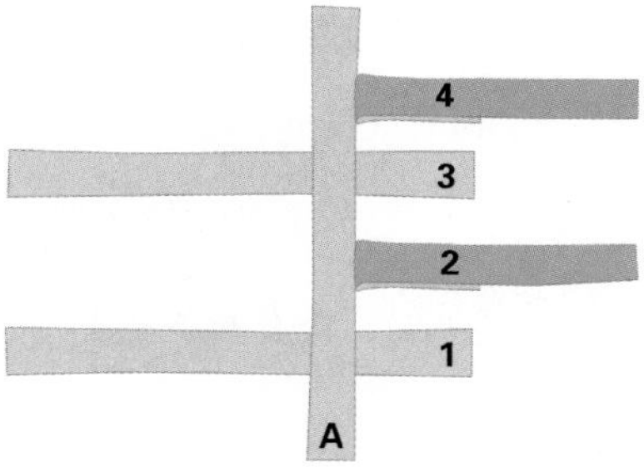

Fold back alternating strips (2 and 4) so folds are near pie edge. Add new strip (A) in opposite direction close to folds.

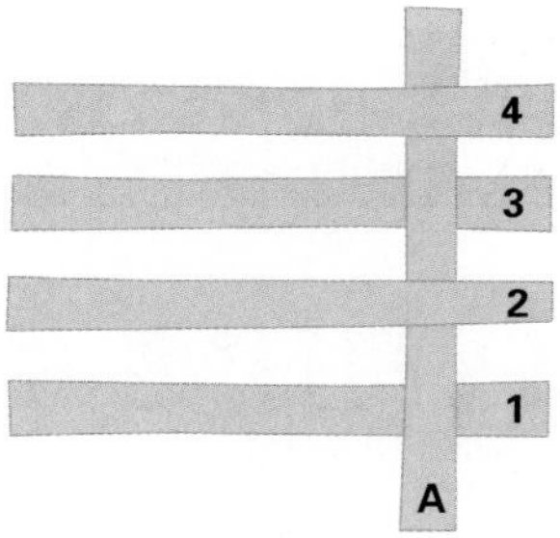

Unfold strips 2 and 4.

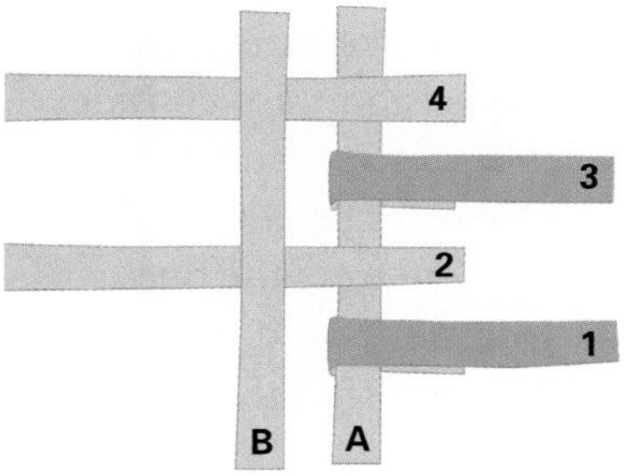

Fold back the other alternating strips (1 and 3) as far as they will go. Add strip B.

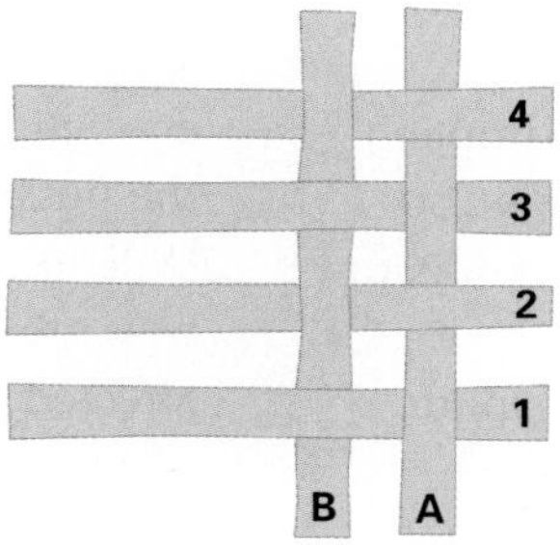

Unfold strips 1 and 3.

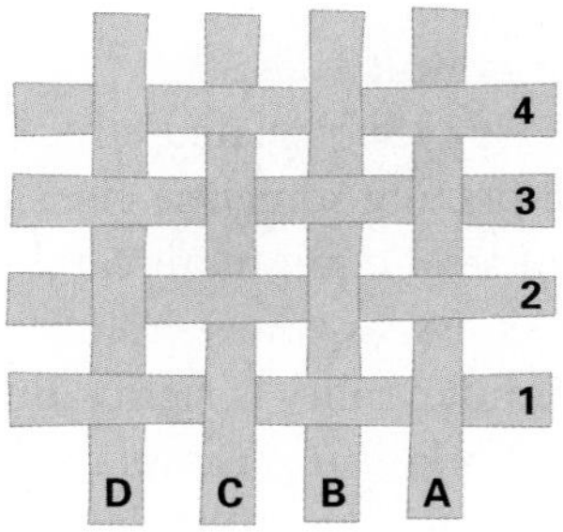

Continue this pattern until all strips are woven.

If a one-crust pie looks unfinished, scatter the top with crumbs from the crust mixture or with buttered breadcrumbs. For a sweet topping on a fruit pie, cover generously with a **streusel** (STROO-suhl), a crumbly mixture made by cutting butter into flour, sugar, and possibly spices.

Turnovers

A **turnover** is a square or circle of pastry dough folded over a sweet or savory filling. Bite-size turnovers may be served as appetizers or snacks. Large ones are a clever way to serve individual entrées or desserts. Turnovers may be baked or deep-fried.

To make a turnover, roll out the dough and cut it into squares or circles. Add the filling and brush a little water along the edge of the dough. Fold the dough over and press the edges together with the tines of a fork. Put one or two slits in the top.

TARTS

At first glance, you may see little difference between tarts and pies. Like some pies, a **tart** has a single crust; however, it is always removed from the pan before serving. See **Fig. 47-6**.

A full-size tart, also called a **flan**, is conveniently made in a two-piece flan pan. It has a removable bottom and a straight, fluted edge about 1 inch deep. Another option is a flan ring,

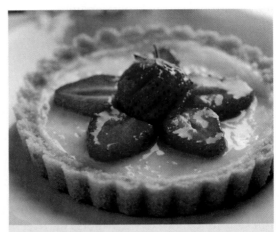

Fig. 47-6 Tarts can be appetizers, entrées, or desserts.

Career Prep

Ethics on the Job

ETHICS ARE PRINCIPLES OF RIGHT and wrong that govern actions and decisions. Many employers and professional groups have a written code of ethics based on universal ethics, including honesty, fairness, and supporting the community.

Many job-related ethical choices are simple. Respecting someone else's property is right, so you treat equipment carefully. You use it only for business, as your employer intends. Respecting confidentiality is right. You don't gossip about co-workers or discuss confidential company matters, even with friends. Giving fair value is right, so you give your best work in exchange for your wages.

Some workplace decisions, however, are ethical dilemmas. Right and wrong actions are not clear in these situations.

When faced with a difficult ethical choice, you can turn to your workplace, professional, and personal ethical code. Make sure you have enough facts to make a decision. Also consider the possible consequences for you and others. Will your decision and actions be fair to those who are affected by it? If you were the one affected, how would you feel? Could you comfortably explain your decision to family and friends?

Discovering dishonesty in others offers another challenge. Ignoring what you observe

a bottomless metal rim that is set on a cookie sheet to form a pan. You can also use a standard pie pan. A **galette** (gah-LEHT) is a hand-shaped tart made by folding and pleating the edge of the dough to form the sides.

Miniature tarts are made individually in deeper pans similar to small muffin or pie pans. You can buy inexpensive ones made of foil or you can use muffin pans and baking cups.

BAKING PIES AND TARTS

Baking times and temperatures vary among pie and tart recipes. Pie shells are usually baked at 425°F or 450°F for about 20 minutes. Filled pies are baked at a similar temperature for the first 10 minutes, and then at a lower temperature, around 350°F, to cook the filling.

If you suspect the filling might bubble over, put a shallow pan on the oven rack below the pie. Don't line the rack with foil. It prevents hot air from circulating evenly around the pan.

Soggy bottom crusts can be another problem. To keep crusts flaky, add the filling just before baking. You can also bake the shell blind and "moisture-proofed" with a light egg wash. Then fill and continue baking. In a baked and cooled shell, a coat of warm jelly or melted chocolate is a tasty, functional seal.

Color is the best indication of doneness in shells and two-crust pies. They should be golden brown and slightly blistered. If the edge browns too quickly, cover it with strips of aluminum foil. Test filled pies for doneness as the recipe directs.

CONVENIENCE PIES AND TARTS

If your desire for a pie exceeds the time available to make one, try a convenience form. Piecrust mixes are sold in the baking aisle, as are ready-made crumb crusts. Pastry crusts, some in their own foil pan, are sold in the refrigerator or freezer case. Refrigerated crescent roll dough also makes a flaky crust. For a dessert pie, line the pan with slices of refrigerated cookie dough.

For fillings, choose from canned fruit or cream fillings or pudding mixes. Garnish with fresh fruit, chocolate curls, or other creative touches.

may be easy, but standing up for what is right sets an example and encourages others to act ethically. A co-worker may only need to be reminded that an action is against company policy. On the other hand, if you suspect a supervisor of unethical behavior, it's wise to record your observations, including the date. Many companies offer a way to report unethical activities. If not, you can go to management, the human resources department, or an outside agency if necessary.

Ethical decisions, even minor ones, help shape personal growth. Whether people gossip, lie, or steal, such unethical behavior lowers them in the eyes of others. Most people also think less of themselves. Ethical principles are like good health habits: if practiced every day, they support you when it matters most.

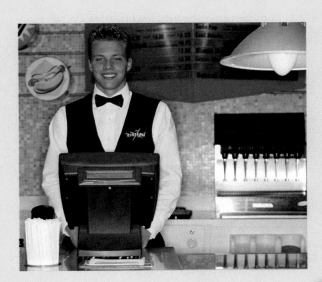

Career Connection

Codifying ethics. Suppose you're a restaurant owner. Write a one-page code of ethics that you think should be followed by all employees.

Summarize Your Reading

▶ Pies and tarts are commonly served as dessert, but they can also be a main dish.

▶ Pies and tarts can be simple or elaborate, depending on the crusts and fillings used to make them.

▶ Piecrusts can be challenging to make well, but knowledge of some basic principles helps the baker achieve successful results.

▶ Pastry dough is also used to make turnovers, flans, and galettes.

▶ Convenience forms are available for making both crusts and fillings for pies.

Check Your Knowledge

1. What is a **pie**?

2. Describe the following kinds of pies: fruit, cream, custard, and savory.

3. What are the four main ingredients in pastry dough?

4. Why should water be ice cold when making pastry dough?

5. Why do pastry dough recipes sometimes call for a little sugar and vinegar?

6. Compare crusts made with these fats: vegetable shortening or lard; butter, margarine, or cream cheese; and oil.

7. How do you mix pastry dough?

8. Why should pastry dough be handled as little as possible?

9. How do you roll pastry dough?

10. What are two ways to keep pastry dough from shrinking?

11. How can you repair a crust that is missing dough in one place on the edge?

12. What is a **fluted edge**?

13. How is the top crust for a two-crust pie made?

14. What is the basic procedure for making a **lattice crust**?

15. What is a **pie shell**?

16. What is the purpose of **docking**?

17. What ingredients are commonly used in a **crumb crust**?

18. **CRITICAL THINKING** What type of crust would you choose for these pies and why: a) banana cream; b) cherry; c) pumpkin; d) apple; e) chicken pot pie?

19. What is a **turnover**?

20. How do **tarts** differ from pies?

21. What can you do if you think a pie or tart might bubble over while baking?

22. How can you prevent a crust from becoming soggy on the bottom?

23. List convenience pies and fillings.

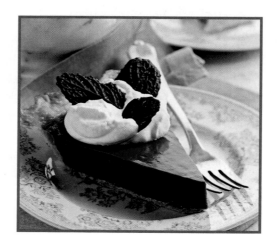

Apply Your Learning

1. **Crust Demonstrations.** Demonstrate one of the following: a) how to make a lattice crust (practice first with pieces of fabric until you master the weaving technique); b) how to make fluted edges on a pie (use dough for children's play, which can be re-formed to show various techniques).

2. **Crumb Crust.** Make a pie with a crumb crust on the bottom. What fillings work well with such a crust? Evaluate results and share samples.

3. **Chicken Pot Pie.** Prepare a chicken pot pie from scratch. Also bake a frozen chicken pot pie. Compare the two pies for taste, texture, and appearance.

4. **(MATH) Pie Costs.** Will you save money by making a pie at home or should you buy one ready-made? Choose one type of pie and compare costs from different sources. Make recommendations for consumers.

5. **(LANGUAGE ARTS) Advertisement.** Write an advertisement for a specialty bakery that sells homemade pies and tarts. What qualities will you emphasize?

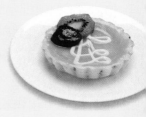

Foods Lab

Pies and Tarts

Procedure: Prepare one of the following pies: a) fruit pie; b) cream pie; c) custard pie; d) pie made with convenience products; e) fruit tarts. Serve samples for a class taste test.

Analyzing Results

❶ Evaluate your product on taste, texture, and appearance.

❷ How did your crust turn out? What would you do differently next time? Why?

❸ How did the convenience pie compare to similar pies made from scratch?

❹ Of the pie samples you tried, which type do you prefer? Why?

6. **Piecrust "Cookies."** Practice your crust-making skills by making piecrust "cookies." After rolling out the dough, cut it into shapes, sprinkle with sugar, and bake at 425°F for about 12 to 15 minutes or until lightly browned. Evaluate results.

 Food Science Experiment

Fats in Piecrusts

Objective: To compare how different fats affect qualities of piecrust.

Procedure:

1. Prepare the piecrust recipe provided by your teacher. You will make a crust using one of the following fats: lard, vegetable oil, or solid shortening.

2. Roll the dough into a rectangle about 6-by-10 inches. Place it on a cookie sheet. Poke holes in the crust with the tines of a fork and bake as directed.

3. Cut the cooled crust into equal-size servings for sampling, and mark them with the fat you used. Evaluate and compare the recipes made with different fats.

Analyzing Results

❶ Which crust had the lightest, flakiest texture?

❷ Which crust was most tender?

❸ Which crust do you think had the best flavor?

❹ How do the recipes compare nutritionally?

❺ What reasons can you give for the results?

UNIT 10

Global Foods

CHAPTER 48 **Foods of the United States & Canada**

CHAPTER 49 **Foods of Latin America & the Caribbean**

CHAPTER 50 **Foods of Western & Northern Europe**

CHAPTER 51 **Foods of Southern Europe**

CHAPTER 52 **Foods of Eastern Europe & Russia**

CHAPTER 53 **Foods of Southwest Asia & Africa**

CHAPTER 54 **Foods of South & Eastern Asia**

CHAPTER 55 **Foods of Australia & Oceania**

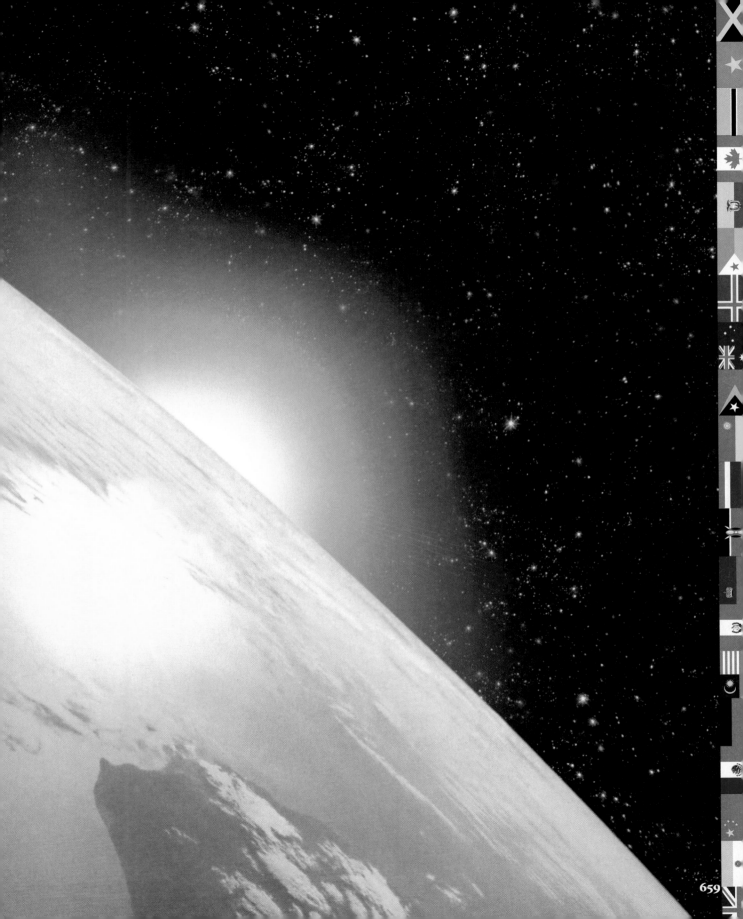

Foods of the United States & Canada

USING EXAMPLES. What foods are specialties in your region of the country? Choose a regional favorite that you would serve to a visitor who wants to experience the "local flavor." In writing, describe the example you've chosen. Explain how the food or dish represents your area's tastes and culture.

To Guide Your Reading:

Objectives

▶ Relate history and geographic location to cuisines in the United States and Canada.

▶ Identify typical ingredients used in dishes of the United States and Canada and explain their use.

▶ Describe and prepare dishes from the United States and Canada.

Terms

bannock	jambalaya
cioppino	poke
croquette	scrapple
étouffée	succotash
goulash	taro
gumbo	

W
HAT BETTER PLACE TO BEGIN EXPLORING global foods than right at home. Although you'll make your way around the world in this unit, the United States, by itself, offers glimpses into many ethnic cuisines. That's because the people who have made the United States their home over the years have a rich and varied heritage. Wherever people put down roots, their own unique foods and dishes became woven into the local food tapestry.

Out of this development came a land of unique regions, each with distinctive foodways—but times are changing. Quick travel and a growing interest in food are bringing foodways together as fusion cuisine. Although you'll read about regional foods in the U.S. and Canada, remember that food boundaries are less clear than they once were. See **Fig. 48-1**.

Fig. 48-1
Although the United States has fifty states, two are geographically separate. Alaska borders Canada's Yukon Territory. Hawaii is a group of islands in the Pacific Ocean. Canada is divided into ten provinces and three territories.

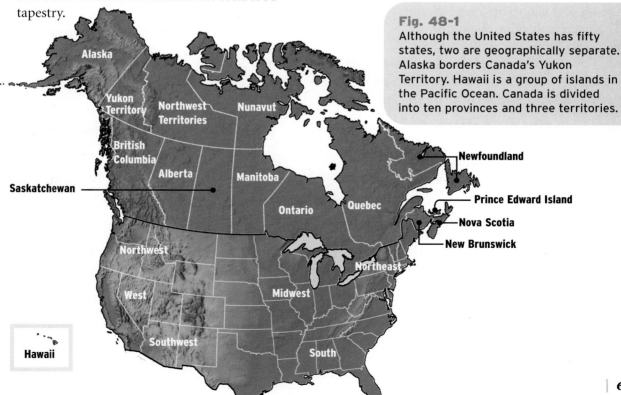

THE UNITED STATES

What is American food? Many foods might qualify, but where did they really come from? Many foods are not as "American" as you might think.

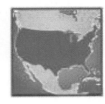

Northeast

Another name for the Northeast is New England. This region stretches from Maine to New Jersey along the northeastern seacoast of the U.S. Early settlers found corn, squash, beans, berries, maple syrup, wild turkeys, deer, and cranberries. Then and now, living along the coast means having a plentiful supply of lobster, clams, salmon, and many other fish. Codfish cakes and codfish balls, both mixed with mashed potatoes, are regional dishes in Rhode Island. Fish stews are common. See **Fig. 48-2**.

In New Jersey, blueberries, peaches, strawberries, and tomatoes are grown. Maple sugar and maple syrup are Vermont specialties.

The one-pot boiled dinner, or New England "potboiler," comes from British heritage. Cast iron pots filled with corned beef or brisket, mutton, or pork once hung over big fireplaces. The meat was cooked with carrots, onions, and squash. Red flannel hash is a New England classic. The name and color come from beets added to the finely chopped corned beef, potatoes, carrots, and onions. **Succotash**, originally a Native American dish of beans and corn, is one of the most well-known dishes from this region.

New York City and Boston

New York City is the ultimate melting pot, where hundreds of thousands of immigrants settled in neighborhoods with fellow countrymen. Ethnic markets, delis, and restaurants helped cooking styles survive. Chinatown and Little Italy are just two examples.

The city of Boston, where many Irish settled, contributes its name to some foods. Boston brown bread is dark, sweet, steamed bread made with rye and wheat flour, cornmeal, and molasses. Another dish is Boston cream pie. This dessert, with two layers of sponge cake, a custard filling, and a topping of chocolate or powdered sugar, isn't really a pie at all. Boston baked beans are sweetened with molasses. Molasses is also an ingredient in New England Indian pudding, which combines pumpkin with molasses, cornmeal, raisins, and spices. This might have been the first pumpkin pie.

Pennsylvania Dutch

The German people who settled in Pennsylvania are called "the Pennsylvania Dutch." They brought sauerkraut and other pickled vegetables. They also shared sausage-making skills. All kinds of "wursts" were made from pork and beef. Pretzels are a favorite of the Pennsylvania Dutch. See **Fig. 48-3**.

Like others of their generation, German immigrants were thrifty. They used everything, including pork scraps. **Scrapple** bakes pork scraps with cornmeal, flavored with thyme and sage. Then it's cut into slices and fried.

Shoofly pie, made with molasses, is also a Pennsylvania Dutch recipe. It's so sweet that you can guess how it got its name.

Midwest

In the eighteenth century, as large cities in the East grew crowded, adventurous pioneers set out to explore the wide-open spaces to the west. Settlers followed, establishing new homes in the Midwest.

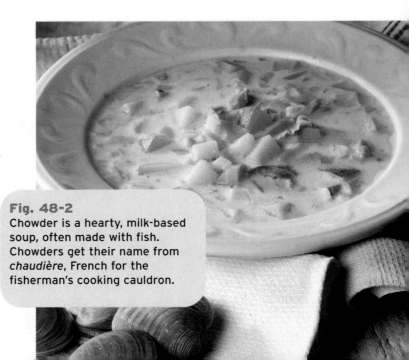

Fig. 48-2
Chowder is a hearty, milk-based soup, often made with fish. Chowders get their name from *chaudière*, French for the fisherman's cooking cauldron.

If you want meat and potatoes, America's Heartland is the place to find them. Steaks from the Midwest are renowned the world over. In Minnesota, beef is made into Swedish meatballs, which are cooked in sour cream. Acres of corn for livestock feed and cooking oil grow throughout the Midwest, especially in Iowa, Illinois, and Kansas. Corn-fed pork is prized.

In the mid-1800s, many Germans came to the Midwest. They were joined by Estonians, Ukrainians, Latvians, Scandinavians, and Hungarians. Of course, sausages like kielbasa came too. Many Swiss and Germans settled in Wisconsin to raise milk cows and produce the famed Wisconsin cheeses. See **Fig. 48-4**. Hungarian dishes include chicken paprika and stuffed bell peppers. **Goulash** is a Hungarian stew made with beef and vegetables and flavored with paprika. Sour cream is part of many Hungarian dishes.

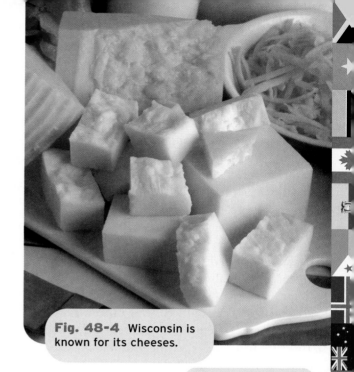

Fig. 48-4 Wisconsin is known for its cheeses.

Fig. 48-3

Try This! **Recipe**

Soft Pretzels

Yield
About 12 large pretzels

Nutrition Analysis
Per Serving: 190 calories, 0 g total fat, 0 g saturated fat, 0 trans fat, 0 mg cholesterol, 480 mg sodium, 43 g total carbohydrate, 1 g dietary fiber, 6 g sugars, 5 g protein
Percent Daily Value: vitamin A 0%, vitamin C 0%, calcium 0%, iron 15%

Ingredients
¼ oz. pkg. active dry yeast
¼ cup brown sugar
1½ cups warm water, about 85°F

5 cups all-purpose flour
4 cups water

1½ Tbsp. baking soda
coarse or kosher salt (optional)

Directions
1. Preheat oven to 475°F. Grease baking sheets. Combine yeast and brown sugar in large bowl. Gradually add 1½ cups warm water, stirring until yeast is dissolved. Let stand 5 minutes.
2. Stir in flour; blend well. Turn dough out onto lightly floured surface. Knead until smooth and elastic, 5 to 10 minutes.
3. Pinch or slice off enough dough to form a 1½-inch ball. On lightly floured surface, roll ball into a rope and shape into a pretzel.
4. Combine 4 cups water and baking soda in large saucepan or Dutch oven; bring to a boil. Lift pretzels with spatula and drop into boiling water, a few at a time. Boil until pretzels rise to the surface, about 1 minute.
5. Place pretzels on greased baking sheets. Sprinkle with salt, if desired. Bake at 475°F for 8 minutes. Serve warm.

South

To find Southern cooking, look to these states: Virginia, North Carolina, South Carolina, Georgia, Florida, Alabama, Mississippi, and Tennessee. Typical ingredients are rice, corn, peanuts, sesame seeds, sweet potatoes, and pork. African-American cooking has influenced many dishes.

Grits are a Southern specialty made from ground, dried corn called *hominy*. Grits are often served for breakfast. *Hushpuppies* are deep-fried corn fritters typically served with catfish. In the South, pork is a basic ingredient. Ham hocks, bacon, and salted pork flavor pots of beans and greens. Pork is also made into sausages and ham.

Dr. George Washington Carver brought acclaim to the peanut. He was born a slave but became an agricultural research professor at Tuskegee Institute, where he found many uses for this nutritious legume. In Florida, peanuts are boiled. South Carolinians call them goobers. North Carolinians add them to stuffing for roast chicken. Peanuts thicken soups in African-American kitchens in Alabama and Mississippi.

On the tables of typical Southern restaurants, you'll find chicken and dumplings, fried chicken, and fried catfish served with hot cornbread. Biscuits and gravy are a Southern specialty, often served for breakfast. *Brunswick stew*, originally made from squirrel and now usually with chicken, is a classic stew from Kentucky to Alabama.

Sweet Southern dishes include peanut brittle and sweet potato pie. Georgia is famous for peaches, which are often made into cobbler, a kind of upside-down pie with a biscuit-like crust on top. In the Florida Keys, where limes are grown, Key lime pies were a logical result.

Louisiana

Creole, or mixed heritage, cooking began in the 1700s when the French settled in New Orleans. Africans who worked in the kitchens of plantation owners blended African, French, Spanish, Caribbean, and Native American ingredients and techniques to create Louisiana Creole cuisine.

Jambalaya is the perfect example of Creole cooking. This rice dish cooks ham, seafood, chicken, and sausages with rice, vegetables, and seasonings. Another well-known Creole dish is **gumbo**, which combines the Spanish custom of mixing seafood and meat with French-style *andouille* sausages. See **Fig. 48-5**. Shrimp or crawfish, also called "mud bugs," are cooked **étouffée** (ay-too-FAY). This French word means "smothered," which is a typical Southern method of cooking food covered in liquid or sauce.

In 1755 the Acadians from Canada settled in Louisiana. Their descendents, the Cajuns, now live along the swampy bayous. Cajun cooking combines French cuisine with the American South. Cajun *maquechoux* is a relish of corn, onions, bell pepper, cayenne, and cream.

Southwest

The American Southwest includes New Mexico, Oklahoma, Texas, and parts of Arizona and Colorado. Cooking includes Spanish, Mexican, and Pueblo Indian influences. Spaniards introduced cattle to the area in the sixteenth century. The bison that roamed the region provided a ready meat source. By the 1800s, ranches dotted the Texas plains, with cowboys tending large herds of longhorn cattle.

Long before the Spaniards arrived, Pueblo Indians were raising such crops as corn, beans, pumpkins, chiles, and squash. Other tribes,

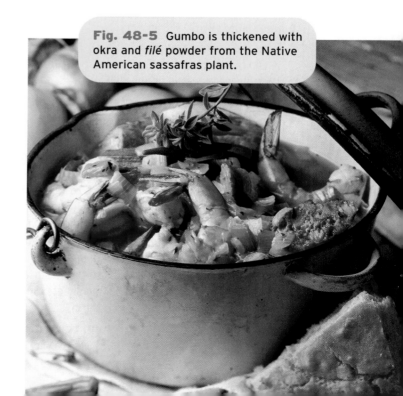

Fig. 48-5 Gumbo is thickened with okra and *filé* powder from the Native American sassafras plant.

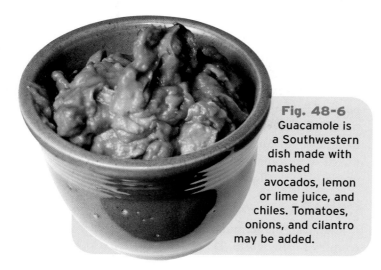

Fig. 48-6
Guacamole is a Southwestern dish made with mashed avocados, lemon or lime juice, and chiles. Tomatoes, onions, and cilantro may be added.

including Apaches, Comanches, and Navajos, cooked pumpkins and seasoned stews with the local juniper berries. Pine nuts, the nutritious seeds from pinecones, were staples. From European wheat, Native Americans made fry bread. Sopaipillas are sweet versions of fry bread topped with honey.

Corn, tomatoes, chiles, and beans are mainstays in New Mexico and Texas. See **Fig. 48-6**. As you know, the cuisine of Texas is often called Tex-Mex. The ultimate Tex-Mex dish is chili con carne. In honor of this "bowl of red," hundreds of annual competitions are held throughout the country. A Southwestern breakfast dish, huevos rancheros, is eggs topped with spicy tomato and pepper sauce. Another breakfast dish, called migas, has scrambled eggs with cheese, peppers, and tortillas.

Beef barbecue in Texas is legendary. Settlers built huge smokers to infuse beef with a smoky flavor. Like chili, barbecue recipes vary from cook to cook. Most agree that the meat in a true barbecue should be seasoned only with a "dry rub" of spices.

West

In the 1800s wagon trains trekked across the Great Plains and over the Rockies. They were loaded with people lured by the "golden life" promised in the West. During the dangerous and exhausting journey, they lived on meat jerky and biscuits.

Some, like the Basques from Spain, stopped when they got to Nevada. The Basque influence is still alive in restaurants and festivals in Nevada and the Sierra foothills in California. Grilled lamb chops and roasts are accompanied by pots of Basque beans and chewy sheepherder bread. Other settlers headed north and stopped in Wyoming and Montana, where there was plenty of wild elk, moose, bison, and bear.

California

In the 1700s, Spanish explorers settled in California and divided the land into ranchos, or small ranches. At one time, ranchos covered some of the most fertile land in California. Rancho cooking combined Spanish, Mexican, and Native American ingredients, influences, and techniques. It became a major culinary influence in California. Spanish stews, or pucheros, joined Mexican enchiladas, refried beans, carne con chile, and flour tortillas.

Plum, apple, and pear orchards grow in Northern California, and oranges in the southern part of the state. Olive trees and grapes thrive in this region. Avocados grow in the Santa Barbara area, and rice grows in the delta around Sacramento.

The great Central Valley, which runs through the middle of the state, is the market basket for everything from rice and quince (a tart-flavored fruit), to garlic and tomatoes, to wheat and corn. Artichokes, asparagus, and apples grow closer to the coast. The Pacific Ocean still provides a lucrative industry in crab, salmon, rockfish, shrimp, and tuna.

Cioppino (chuh-PEE-noh) is a San Francisco fish stew originally made at Fisherman's Wharf. This stew was invented when Italian vendors went from boat to boat asking fishermen to "chip in" a little of their fish. The Brown Derby Restaurant contributed the cobb salad. See **Fig. 48-7** on page 666.

Northwest

The Pacific Ocean is noted for its variety of seafood: clams, mussels, shrimp, giant halibut, salmon, and tiny Olympic oysters. Oregon, Washington, and Alaska are renowned for their seafood cuisines.

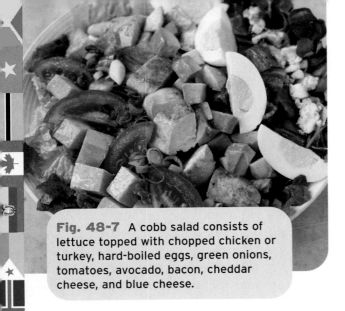

Fig. 48-7 A cobb salad consists of lettuce topped with chopped chicken or turkey, hard-boiled eggs, green onions, tomatoes, avocado, bacon, cheddar cheese, and blue cheese.

Sweet Walla Walla onions, plus apples, pears, hazelnuts, cherries, herbs, and vegetables are among the local crops of Washington State. *Aplets* and *cotlets* are Washington's famous candies made from apples and apricots, sugar, and walnuts. Washington grows wheat and potatoes and leads the country in apple production. Seattle is America's "gateway to Asia." The influences of Asian cuisines are found in restaurants and markets. Plenty of rainfall ensures continual sprouting of wild mushrooms in the forests of Washington and Oregon.

As the largest and coldest state of the American Northwest, Alaska has glaciers covering many areas. During the summer, sunlight lasts for 84 straight days in the northern part of the state. The nonstop sunlight creates giant-size vegetables. A good portion of the crop has to be canned, frozen, or otherwise preserved for the long cold winter.

Two foods synonymous with Alaska are king crab and salmon. See **Fig. 48-8**.

Hawaii

Hawaii has long been the stopping point for ships traveling between Asia and North America. The South Pacific islands of Hawaii are a paradise, with sandy beaches, palm trees, pineapples, coconuts, and perfect climate. Surrounding waters and inland streams provide flavorful fish. **Poke** is sliced raw fish mixed with seaweed, onions, chiles, and soy sauce.

Native Hawaiians share traditional Polynesian foodways at a *luau*. The luau is a celebratory meal cooked in a pit on the beach. Typically, a whole pig cooks for hours. An accompaniment might be *poi*, which is mashed, cooked **taro** root, the large tuber of the tropical taro plant. Other dishes include *lomi lomi*, salmon cut into pieces and mixed with tomatoes and onions, and *haupia*, a coconut-flavored pudding.

CANADA

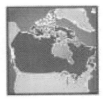

Canada is the second largest country in the world. Despite Canada's size, the population lives mainly on coasts and in cities that border the United States. As in the U.S., Canadian foods reflect the nation's natural resources and rich cultural diversity.

Only about five percent of Canada's land can be used for growing crops. Native ingredients include wild rice, maple syrup, Saskatoon berries, Jerusalem artichokes, wild mushrooms, reindeer, turkey, duck, trout, buffalo, fiddlehead ferns, and a wide range of freshwater fish and seafood. Two of Canada's most important crops are wheat and rapeseed, the seeds used to make canola oil.

Fig. 48-8 The Alaskans catch five kinds of salmon: chinook, sockeye, silver or coho, chum, and pink. Here you see salmon drying in Kodiak, Alaska.

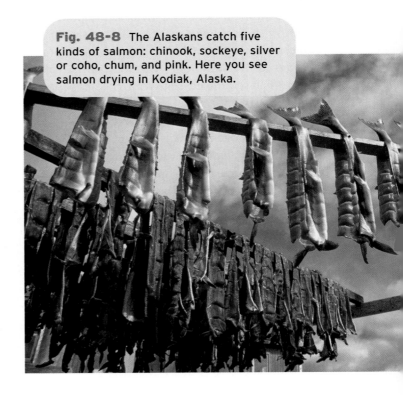

Canadian food reflects the nationalities of many immigrants from Eastern and Western Europe, Ukraine, Asia, and the Caribbean. Varied food traditions melded with local ingredients to form pockets of regional cuisine.

Traditional dishes are found throughout Canada. Scottish immigrants brought **bannock**, flat, biscuit-like bread made with flour or oats and cooked on cast iron over a hot grill. Classic Canadian desserts are raisin pie and butter tarts. A butter tart is a pie pastry filled with a mixture of brown sugar, corn syrup, butter, and vanilla. Date squares, known as "matrimonial cakes," are common in western Canada.

Canada is divided into provinces, each with distinctive foods and dishes.

Northeast

Newfoundland, Nova Scotia, New Brunswick, and Prince Edward Island make up northeastern Canada. Newfoundland is a land of startling beauty, with inland fjords and towering icebergs. The people have made their living from the sea for countless generations. Cod is the foundation of "Newfie" cuisine. Fishing supplies tables with tuna, herring, mackerel, squid, shrimp, snow crab, and lobster. See **Fig. 48-9**. The sweet flavors of blueberries and golden-colored cloudberries come naturally in Newfoundland.

In cold coastal Nova Scotia, farmed oysters and other fish are local businesses. Nearby Prince Edward Island is renowned for cultured (farmed) mussels. Seafood chowders are made with scallops, swordfish, cod, salmon, mussels, and clams.

New Brunswick is surrounded by the Atlantic Ocean. It is best known for farming and fishing. Potatoes are the most valuable crop, and the most valuable seafood catches are scallops and lobster.

East and Midwest

Quebec is a place of amazing scenic beauty and modern cities with old world charm. Visiting Montreal is like taking a trip to France. People speak French, and French culinary influences are everywhere. You'll find excellent fresh and aged cheeses from the milk of cows, goats, and sheep.

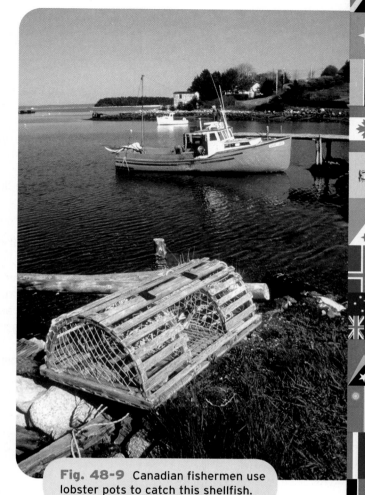

Fig. 48-9 Canadian fishermen use lobster pots to catch this shellfish.

Seafood is broiled, baked, and made into **croquettes** (kroh-kets). For this dish, the seafood is puréed and bound with a thick sauce and formed into small shapes. Then it's breaded and deep-fried. Quebec produces about 90 percent of Canada's maple syrup. See **Fig. 48-10** on page 668.

The other province in the East is Ontario. In the fertile southern region of Ontario, apple, peach, and plum orchards dot the landscape. Today, in addition to raising beef and pork, Ontario is home to game farms for quail, pheasant, and partridges. Cheddar cheese is a specialty.

The Midwestern provinces of Manitoba, Saskatchewan, and Alberta are known as Canada's "market basket." Vast fields of wheat, corn, rye, millet, and sunflowers cross this prairie land. Cattle and bison graze on the range.

Fig. 48-10

Maple Ice Cream Sandwiches

Yield	Nutrition Analysis
20 disks (10 sandwiches)	**Per Serving:** 360 calories, 18 g total fat, 5 g saturated fat, 0.2 trans fat, 30 mg cholesterol, 85 mg sodium, 47 g total carbohydrate, 1 g dietary fiber, 33 g sugars, 4 g protein
	Percent Daily Value: vitamin A 6%, vitamin C 0%, calcium 10%, iron 4%

Ingredients

1 cup pure maple syrup
½ cup light olive or canola oil

1 cup all-purpose flour
⅛ tsp. salt

5 cups vanilla ice cream

Directions

1. Generously spray baking sheets with vegetable oil spray. Place oven rack in middle position. Preheat oven to 350°F.
2. In heavy, medium-size saucepan, bring maple syrup and oil to boil, about 5 to 6 minutes. Boil for a few seconds and remove from heat.
3. Whisk flour into maple mixture. Mix until smooth, about 1 minute. Mix in salt. Drop maple batter by 1½ tablespoons onto baking sheets, allowing thin batter to spread (up to 6 circles per baking sheet).
4. Bake for 12 minutes or until batter is color of maple syrup, more brown than beige. Remove from oven and let sit for 2 minutes.
5. To make sandwiches, lay one maple disk on work surface. Gently add ½ cup ice cream and top with another disk.

Manitoba is known for excellent wild rice. Nearly five million pounds are harvested annually. From the many lakes in the province come a wide variety of fish, including Winnipeg gold eye, pickerel, northern pike, trout, carp, and Arctic char. Arctic char is similar to both salmon and trout.

Farms and farmers markets thrive in the fertile province of Saskatchewan. At many, you can pick your own tomatoes, berries, and herbs. The largest city, Saskatoon, is named for the local Saskatoon berry, which is made into pies and preserves. The local wild rice is often served as a stuffing in chicken or turkey.

In Alberta, the fertile prairies meet the Rocky Mountains. This is cattle country. Beans and potatoes grow here, as do Jerusalem artichokes, which are native to this part of the world. Also called sunchokes, these small tubers with bumpy skins have to be peeled and can be eaten raw in salads or sautéed as a vegetable.

West

In the province of British Columbia and the territories, the native Indian system of commerce was known as "potlatching." A potlatch is a feast with dancing and eating. Traditional potlatch foods included salmon, venison, moose, clams, huckleberries, blackberries, and oil made from the eulachon fish, a type of smelt.

The territories of Yukon, Northwest, and Nunavut are truly unspoiled land. Alaskan salmon, halibut, trout, Arctic Grayling, and Kokanee salmon are pulled from the abundant lakes and rivers. Popular wilderness dishes include caribou steak, venison, and buffalo burgers. The Northwest Territories and the territory of Nanavut are known as the "Land of the Midnight Sun." Seafood and the massive, shaggy, bison-like musk ox are harvested here. Musk ox meat is unique to Canada and found nowhere else in the world outside this extremely vast and beautiful land.

Career Pathways

Restaurant Owner

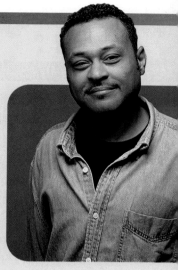

DERRICK ROBINSON: Derrick Robinson has fond memories of his grandfather barbecuing ribs, with "the crackle of the wood burning and the sizzle of the meat juices hitting the fire below, creating this indescribable smell." In this mouth-watering bit of nostalgia, he also sees the makings of a big-time franchise.

A Meaty Proposition. Being a cook was not Derrick's dream as a young man in Peoria, Illinois—being an entrepreneur was. He tried various jobs, from carpenter to stockbroker, all with the idea of starting his own business. Finally he found the opportunity right at home.

Derrick's grandfather, John Robinson, had been a meat packer, who barbecued for friends on weekends. His open-pit technique was so popular that friends started bringing him their meat for him to cook. He began selling barbecued meat at his wife's hamburger stand and opened his own restaurant in 1949. Over time, Big John's Barbecue became a Peoria legend. Peorians who moved away and tourists passing through remembered and returned to Big John's when they came back. "My grandfather gave me the perfect vehicle to drive my ambition for building a business."

Learning by Doing. Ambition alone does not build a business, of course. Derrick's contacts as a stockbroker helped him find financing, but "all of my experiences and education never prepared me for running my own business. I had to become a quick learner when it came to construction costs, contract negotiations, HR (human resources), and legal matters."

Derrick's on-the-job training continued when he opened Grandpa John's Rib Shack in 2002. Overseeing the kitchen, counting the day's receipts, evaluating employees, handling customer complaints, and even cleaning the toilets—it's all in a day's work. Then there are the typical challenges of equipment that breaks down and workers who don't show up. No wonder he calls customer relations and problem solving his greatest assets.

Ribs Across America. While he runs the daily operations, Derrick says, "I gain most of my enjoyment from the marketing and business development. I'm a big proponent of ideas and these areas allow me to utilize my creativity. My interest is not in owning a restaurant, but in creating a concept that incorporates what my grandfather taught me about barbecue and starting a national, if not international, chain of rib shacks."

That concept would include what his grandfather taught about dedication to quality. Grandpa John's Rib Shack uses the special spice blend and slow roasting and smoking that won the original "Big John" a loyal following. This culinary philosophy is good advice for growing a business as well: "It takes more time to produce our barbecue, but the end result is well worth it."

On-line Connections

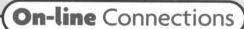

1. To learn more about topics in this article, search the Internet for these key words: franchising a business; business development; barbecuing meat.

2. To learn about related careers, search the Internet for these key words: customer service trainer; restaurant consultant.

CHAPTER 48 FOODS OF THE UNITED STATES & CANADA | 669

Summarize Your Reading

▶ Despite the number of states, the United States can be divided into regions when studying foodways. These regions, however, are less distinct than they once were as foods are shared and revised among cuisines.

▶ Many dishes in regions of the United States and Canada developed from the geography of the area.

▶ Hawaii and Alaska are physically separate from the rest of the United States, giving them unique heritage and cuisines.

▶ Although Canada is the second largest country in the world, it can use only about five percent of its land for growing crops. Nevertheless, the country has many distinctive foods and dishes.

Check Your Knowledge

1. **CRITICAL THINKING** The chapter states that food boundaries in the various regions of the United States are less clear than they once were. Do you think the same might be said about food boundaries around the world?

2. **CRITICAL THINKING** Are "American" foods truly American? Explain your thinking and give examples.

3. How did red flannel hash get its name?

4. What makes New York City a "melting pot"?

5. What is **scrapple**?

6. What contributions did the Germans make to Midwestern cuisine?

7. How have peanuts been incorporated in Southern cooking?

8. Why is **jambalaya** a good example of Creole cooking?

9. Describe these Southern foods: a) hominy; b) hushpuppies; c) Brunswick stew; and d) gumbo.

10. What is Cajun cooking?

11. How did Native Americans contribute to Southwestern cuisine?

12. How is typical Texas barbecue seasoned?

13. What people had a strong impact on foods in Nevada?

14. What is rancho cooking?

15. What is **cioppino** and how did it get its name?

16. What foods are commonly grown in the state of Washington?

17. What is *poi*?

18. **CRITICAL THINKING** Why do you think Canadians live mainly on coasts and along the border with the United States?

19. How do many people in Northeastern Canada make their living, and why?

20. What are **croquettes**?

21. Why are Canada's Midwestern provinces known as Canada's market basket?

22. What meats are typically eaten in the Canadian territories?

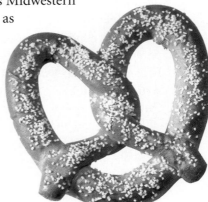

Apply Your Learning

1. SOCIAL STUDIES **Country Study.** Choose one region of the United States or Canada to study. Learn about the history, geography, foods, and dishes of the region. Using such visual aids as films and magazine photos, give a class presentation.

2. **Taste Test.** With your lab team, prepare a dish typical of one region in the United States or Canada. Present your dish with those of other teams for a class taste test.

3. MATH **Texas Barbecue.** Plan a Texas barbecue for your class. Use regional recipes, adjusting them for enough servings.

4. **Topic Exploration.** Report on one of the following topics: a) the history of African-American "soul food," including ingredients and dishes; b) Hawaiian luaus; c) the influence of Native Americans on food and cooking in America; d) the influence of Aboriginals on food and cooking in Canada.

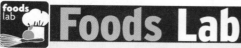

Foods Lab

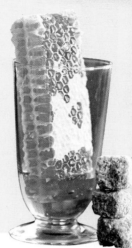

Comparing Sweeteners

Procedure: Do a taste test of sweeteners that are associated with different regions of Canada and the United States. Sample the sweeteners alone. Then pair each one in different combinations with available foods, such as squares of bread or fruit slices.

Analyze Results

❶ Describe the taste of each sweetener.

❷ How might you use each sweetener in cooking? In baking?

❸ How do you think the availability of a specific sweetener in a region influenced the cuisine that developed?

Food Science Experiment

Composition of Potatoes

Objective: To compare the composition of different varieties of potatoes.

Procedure:

1. Weigh one russet potato and one red potato. Record the weights.

2. Scrub and pare the potatoes. Boil each one in a separate saucepan until tender. Drain the potatoes well, reserving some water for comparison.

3. When cool enough to handle, weigh each potato again. Record the weights.

4. Slice the potatoes lengthwise. Evaluate and compare their appearance and texture. Note the qualities of the cooking water.

Analyze Results

❶ How did each potato's weight change after cooking? Which potato lost or gained a greater percentage of its weight?

❷ How did the cooking water from each potato look and feel?

❸ Which potato had a firmer texture? Which felt mealy? How might these qualities be related to the results you described in questions 1 and 2?

❹ Different varieties of potatoes are grown in different regions. Why would that interest consumers? Professional chefs?

Foods of Latin America & the Caribbean

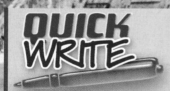

GRABBING INTEREST. In a written paper, the first paragraph, especially the first sentence, should grab the reader's interest. For example, which of these openers is more attention getting: "Habañeros are hot peppers" or "It will be a hot day at the North Pole before I ever eat a whole Habañero pepper again"? Try writing an interesting opener for a theme related to some aspect of Latin American foods.

To Guide Your Reading:

Objectives

▶ Explain the impact of European explorations and geography on Latin American cuisines.

▶ Identify typical ingredients used in dishes of Latin America and the Caribbean and explain how they are used.

▶ Describe and prepare dishes from Latin America and the Caribbean.

Terms

cassava	jerk
ceviche	masa
chorizo	mole
empanada	salsa
frijoles	sopas

WHEN CHRISTOPHER COLUMBUS SET FOOT on a Caribbean island in 1492, he couldn't have imagined how his discovery would shape world history and, in turn, food history. By opening a door between Old World Europe and New World America, he opened a floodgate of culinary exchange.

Over the next 300 years, Spain, Portugal, France, and Great Britain would lay claim to nearly all of Latin America and many of the Caribbean islands. The blend of European foods and food traditions with those of the native peoples would create some of the most exciting cuisines on any continent.

LATIN AMERICA

Latin America boasts dramatic contrasts in climate and geography, from rugged mountain ranges, to crystal blue bays, to lush tropical rainforests. See **Fig. 49-1**.

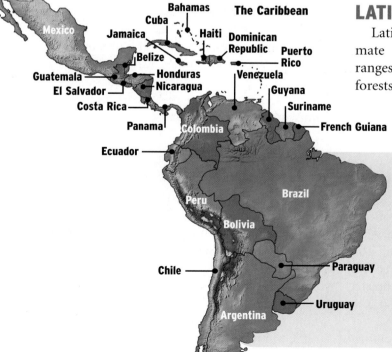

The Caribbean

Bahamas
Cuba
Jamaica · Haiti · Dominican Republic · Puerto Rico
Mexico
Belize
Guatemala · Honduras · Venezuela
El Salvador · Nicaragua · Guyana
Costa Rica · Suriname
Panama · French Guiana
Colombia
Ecuador
Brazil
Peru
Bolivia
Paraguay
Chile · Uruguay
Argentina

Fig. 49-1 Latin America lies below the United States, beginning with Mexico at the southwestern border. South of Mexico is Central America, which extends from Belize and Guatamala to Panama. Beyond Panama is Colombia, one of the many countries in South America. Look east of Central America and you'll see the islands in the Caribbean Sea. Among these island countries are the Bahamas, Dominican Republic, Haiti, Puerto Rico, Cuba, and Jamaica.

Three native cultures dominated the early history of Latin America: the Aztecs in Mexico; the Mayas in Central America; and the Incas in South America. All enjoyed a rich harvest of foods. They cultivated corn, beans, chiles, squash, potatoes, tomatoes, avocados, and a starchy root vegetable called **cassava** (kuh-SAH-vuh). See **Fig. 49-2**. The waters and land teemed with seafood and game.

As European colonists arrived, they brought their own staples with them. The Spanish and Portuguese brought wheat and hogs. Wheat flour made leavened baking possible. Pork became the most important meat in Latin America, except in Argentina and northern Mexico, where the grassy plains fed the Spaniards' beef cattle. The Spanish also introduced rice, goats, sheep, and chickens. The French brought herbs, including thyme and chives, and a sophisticated culinary tradition. The English planted coffee shrubs.

The native chile provides the most characteristic flavor of Latin American cuisine. Both red and green chiles lend a full range of hotness to dishes.

Besides their role in seasoning, chiles are the basis for another staple, the **salsa**, or sauce. Most recipes are chunky mixtures with added tomatoes, onions, garlic, and spices. Mexican, Brazilian, and Caribbean salsas, however, can be as simple as chopped chiles, salt, and lime juice. *Adobo* is a spicy vinegar salsa used as a rub or serving sauce for meats. *Escabèche*, originally a Spanish pickling sauce, is a marinade for cooked fish, chicken, and vegetables. The annatto seed is ground with chiles, onions, and herbs to make *achiote* sauce.

Latin American Dishes

The Latin American diet is based on corn, rice, and beans. Separately or together, these foods might appear in any part of *la comida*, the meal. As a main dish, for instance, rice is paired with chicken in *pollo con arroz*. As a side dish, rice helps cool a fiery salsa. Rice pudding is enjoyed for dessert. These foods also provide complete protein, a real concern in a land where meat is a luxury for many people.

When meat is served, barbecuing and grilling are popular preparations. Leftovers may be chopped with onions, garlic, and herbs and used

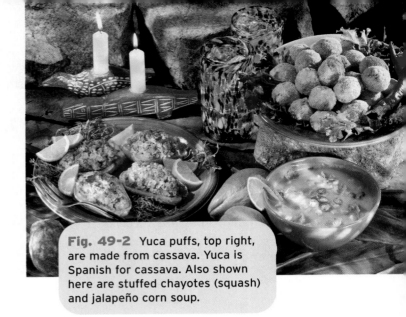

Fig. 49-2 Yuca puffs, top right, are made from cassava. Yuca is Spanish for cassava. Also shown here are stuffed chayotes (squash) and jalapeño corn soup.

in an **empanada** (em-puh-NAH-duh), a turnover filled with meat, vegetables, fruit, or all three. Empanadas were introduced by the Spanish, as were *albondigas*, meatballs that are sometimes made with rice. **Chorizo** (chuh-REE-zoh), a spicy sausage, flavors many stews.

Seafood is plentiful around coastal areas, from the Gulf of Mexico to Chile's Cape Horn. Each region has a recipe for **ceviche** (suh-VEE-chay), an appetizer of raw fish marinated in citrus juice until firm and opaque. The fish is drained and served with chiles, tomatoes, and onions.

Some soups, or **sopas**, feature meat as the main ingredient. Peanuts and squash are also used. Toasted cassava meal, cornmeal, ground nuts, and potatoes thicken soups.

Mexico

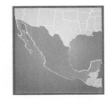

Although their land hasn't been the best for agriculture, the Mexican people have made good use of it. They grow corn, beans, wheat, and rice for food at home. Main food exports are coffee, vegetables, fruit, and livestock. Some crops are grown in the north, but the hilly landscape suits ranching better. With recent industrialization, much of Mexico's growing population has settled in the central part of the country. Besides farms, bustling cities thrive there. In the south, large plantations produce coffee and sugarcane amidst small farming villages where people struggle to raise food for their families.

Mexican Ingredients

Mexican cuisine has kept the Aztec influence. The Aztecs considered corn sacred, and even today corn is held in high regard. About 60 varieties are grown. Corn is enjoyed in soups and fresh on the cob. Mainly, however, corn is dried, cooked, soaked in limewater, and then ground into dough, or **masa** (MAH-suh). Dried, ground masa is sold as *masa harina*, a coarse-grained corn flour. People use masa to make tortillas, a flatbread that is part of nearly every Mexican meal. For convenience, people buy tortillas at bakeries in many Mexican cities.

Two other native foods found in pantries today are avocados and squash. Chilled soups and salads feature avocados. They are also mashed into guacamole, a spread seasoned with garlic, cilantro, and a little tomato. Squash and squash blossoms appear in soups, fritters, and empanada fillings.

Chocolate came to Mexico from trade with the Maya in Central America. The Aztecs used it in a hot, frothy beverage that they enriched with corn milk and seasoned with chiles, vanilla, and other spices. Hot chocolate, sometimes thickened with cornstarch or flavored with vanilla, is still a favorite. Chocolate even seasons sauces and main dishes.

Mexican Dishes

Tortillas filled with any combination of meat, poultry, beans, fish, and cheese is the basic recipe for many Mexican dishes. As tacos, tortillas are folded over filling and eaten out of hand. See **Fig. 49-3**. When tortillas are folded around cheese and grilled, they make quesadillas. For enchiladas, tortillas may be dipped in chile sauce before they are filled and baked. Flautas are deep-fried. Uncooked masa is spread on cornhusks and rolled into tamales.

Beans—**frijoles** (free-HOH-lees) in Spanish—are equally prominent in meals. They are in main dishes as tortilla fillings or as beans and rice.

Frijoles refritos is a side dish of red or pinto beans, mashed and fried in lard. Like other Latin American countries, Mexico has regional recipes for bean stew, or *cocido*, often made with pork and vegetables.

Soup also plays various roles. A first course might be a tortilla soup made with tomatoes, onions, garlic, and chiles. *Posole* is a main-course soup of pork or chicken and dried corn. *Menudo*, a popular morning "pick-me-up," combines tripe (the lining of a cow's stomach), hominy, and chiles. In the northern Mexican state of Sonora, a favorite dish is potato soup (*sopa de papas*) laced with melted cheese.

Salsas are an everyday condiment. In Guadalajara, a salsa is made with *chipotle* chiles (smoked jalapeños) and *tomatillos* (Mexican green tomatoes). A **mole** (MOH-lay) sauce may blend dozens of ingredients. It's based on chiles, ground pumpkin or sesame seeds, onions, unsweetened chocolate, and spices. Many variations may include tomatoes, bananas, sugar, or raisins. The best-known version, *mole poblano*, traditionally accompanies turkey.

Seafood recipes take advantage of local varieties. In the Gulf of Mexico, shrimp is plentiful. It's often prepared with puréed plantains (a starchy banana), onion, tomato, and salsa. On the Yucatan peninsula, shrimp is served chilled *en escabèche* or grilled in an achiote paste.

Fig. 49-3 These Mayan women are preparing pibil turkey tacos. Traditionally, pibil cooking was done in a pit, but modern methods wrap and steam foods.

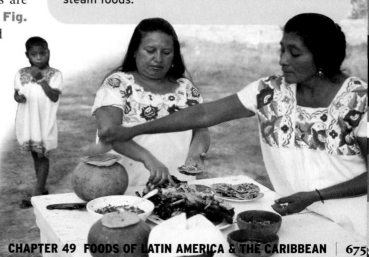

Central America

Joining the North and South American continents are the tropical countries of Central America. Rural living is common in these countries, with many people living in villages and on farms.

Central American countries share some food tastes. The native berry allspice flavors many sweet and savory dishes. Chicken is widely eaten, sometimes flavored with pineapple, tomatoes, or raisins. Chayotes are a squashlike fruit native to Central America. They are stuffed with cheese in the dish described in **Fig. 49-4**.

At the same time, each country has distinct specialties. Chicken in a spicy sauce with sesame and pumpkin seeds is Guatemala's *pollo pepian*. Oysters are a favorite there as well. In El Salvador the signature dish is *pupusa*, a corn cake filled with refried beans, cheese, and pork and served with a cabbage, onion, and carrot slaw.

A popular dish in Nicaragua is *nacatamal*, cabbage, plantain, and pork steamed in banana leaves. In Costa Rica you'll find *gallo pinto* (fried black beans and rice) and *arroz con tuna* (rice with tuna). A Panamanian breakfast tortilla is a thick corn pastry, deep-fried and topped with cheese and eggs.

South America

Thirteen countries make up South America in an area about three times the size of the United States. As you might imagine, in a land this vast, no single cooking style predominates.

Brazil

Regional Brazilian cuisines vary because so many cultural groups settled in the country. The overriding influence goes back to the 1500s when Portuguese colonists and African slaves worked the sugar plantations.

The national dish is an Afro-Brazilian specialty, an elaborate meal called *feijoada completa*. For the main course, black beans and various meats are simmered together in a well-seasoned stock. Meats include fresh and dried beef, chorizo, pig's feet, and other cuts of pork. Simple side dishes like orange slices and rice round out the meal. Other dishes might be greens sautéed in *dende* oil, a bright orange palm oil, or *farofa*, a crumbly mixture of sautéed cassava meal and nuts, raisins, or other ingredients. The dish in **Fig. 49-5** is traditional in the province of Bahia.

Brazil is also noted for seafood stews, another African contribution. *Moqueca* contains seafood, from swordfish to shrimp. The base is coconut milk and tomatoes. A popular soft drink, *guarana*, is made with fruit of the same name. It's also sold as a powder and syrup.

Argentina

More Western and Eastern Europeans immigrated to Argentina than to other South American countries. Their influence shows in Argentine kitchens. Seasonings include milder, Old World herbs as well as spicy chiles. Pastas are enjoyed, and yeast breads are as common as tortillas. Many Argentineans take afternoon tea with a South American beverage, *yerba mate*, which is brewed from holly leaves.

With the country's vast grasslands, or pampas, it's no surprise that beef is the major industry and national food. It's often grilled outdoors and served with Argentina's signature sauce, *chimichurri*. In the sauce, vinegar joins olive oil in a complex seasoning blend that typically includes garlic, parsley, onion, and oregano. Meats are also combined with local fruits or vegetables in various recipes for *carbonada criolla*, or mixed stew.

Andean Countries

In the Andean nations of Colombia, Ecuador, Peru, and Chile, the geography is dominated by mountain, seacoast, and tropical rainforest. These features also influence the cooking landscape.

Corn, beans, and potatoes grow in the cool, dry climate of the fertile Andean foothills. Potatoes, in fact, may have been "born" there. The Pacific Ocean provides seafood in enormous array, from sea bass to sea urchin. The tropical zone offers cassava and chiles, although dishes are less spicy than those of Mexico and Central America. With grazing land limited, meat comes

Fig. 49-4

Chayotes Rellenos con Queso

Yield
4 servings

Nutrition Analysis
Per Serving: 150 calories, 9 g total fat, 3 g saturated fat, 0 g trans fat, 60 mg cholesterol, 490 mg sodium, 13 g total carbohydrate, 2 g dietary fiber, 3 g sugars, 6 g protein

Percent Daily Value: vitamin A 8%, vitamin C 15%, calcium 10%, iron 6%

Ingredients
2 chayotes, halved and seeded
1 small onion, chopped
1½ Tbsp. margarine or butter
½ tsp. salt

¼ tsp. pepper
1 egg, slightly beaten
⅓ cup Monterey Jack cheese, shredded
⅓ cup fresh bread crumbs

Directions
1. Cook chayotes in boiling water until tender, about 45 minutes. Scoop out pulp without tearing shells. Mash pulp in bowl. Set shells and pulp aside.
2. Melt margarine or butter in medium saucepan. Add onion and sauté until translucent, about 3 minutes. Add chayote pulp, salt, and pepper. Cook and stir 2 to 3 minutes. Remove from heat. Stir in egg and cheese.
3. Fill chayote shells with pulp mixture and top with bread crumbs.
4. Place filled shells in greased baking pan. Bake at 350°F until crumbs are golden brown, 20 to 25 minutes.
5. Serve chayotes in the shell. Discard shell after filling has been eaten.

from easily kept animals, including chicken, llama, and guinea pig.

These shared ingredients lead to shared foods. One dish common to these countries is *arepa*, a small griddlecake made with cooked cracked corn. *Aji*, which is a local chile and a hot sauce made from it, is a favorite seasoning. In the Andes, llama meat is salted and dried to make *charqui* (jerky).

In addition, each nation puts its own stamp on popular combinations of food. For example, Colombia is known for *ajiaco*, a soup of chicken, potatoes, and corn. Boiled potatoes and corn on the cob are also traditional accompaniments to a Peruvian specialty, *anticucho*—cubes of beef heart in an aji marinade, skewered and grilled.

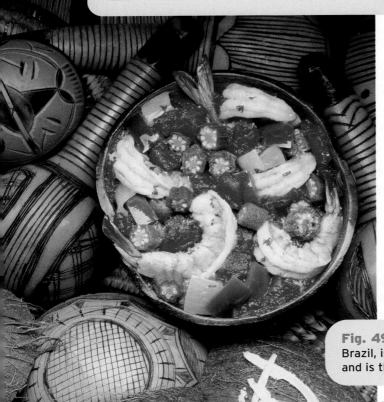

Fig. 49-5 This stew from Bahia, a province of Brazil, is called *shrimp caruru*. It contains okra and is thickened with manioc flour.

THE CARIBBEAN

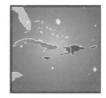

Hundreds of tropical islands lie in the Caribbean Sea. The earliest known inhabitants of these islands were the Caribs and the Arawaks. It is thought that these natives taught European colonists two important skills: to barbecue and to season with chiles. The result of this and other culinary criss-crossing is a lively fusion of cuisines—native, Spanish, French, African, British, and Dutch.

As you might guess, seafood is a sta   in the Caribbean. Conch, a prized shellfish, i   ed for special occasions. Chicken is just as like   o show up in main dishes—as are pork and goat on some islands. Rice and legumes are also central to meals, especially black and red beans, black-eyed peas, and pigeon peas. Black beans are an ingredient in the recipe in **Fig. 49-6**.

Tropical fruits are everywhere in Caribbean cooking. Mangoes, figs, pomegranates, and coconuts are tasty snacks. They also flavor meats and appear in side dishes.

Caribbean Dishes

Dishes in each Caribbean country show different cultural influences. African elements are prominent in Jamaica. The national dish combines two West African imports—saltfish, or dried cod, and ackee, a tropical fruit.

Escaped African slaves may have been the first who mingled sweet and hot flavors to create Jamaica's jerk recipes. **Jerk** is a blend of chiles, onions, garlic, allspice, and other herbs and spices. It seasons meat, poultry, and fish. Marinades are made by adding oil, citrus juice, and molasses.

Some of Haiti's dishes show a French influence in more subtle seasonings and cooking techniques. In a *griot*, cubes of meat marinate in citrus juice, salt, pepper, and thyme. They are then simmered and fried. Pork is used by those who can afford it, but chicken is more common.

Cuban cuisine leans toward Spanish cooking. Many main dishes start with a *sofrito*. This sauté of onion, garlic, and bell pepper in olive oil is similar to the Creole cooking of New Orleans.

Fig. 49-6

Try This! **Recipe**

Cuban Black Bean Soup

Yield	Nutrition Analysis
4 servings	*Per Serving:* 170 calories, 3.5 g total fat, 0 g saturated fat, 0 g trans fat, 0 mg cholesterol, 630 mg sodium, 34 g total carbohydrate, 11 g dietary fiber, 3 g sugars, 10 g protein *Percent Daily Value:* vitamin A 2%, vitamin C 15%, calcium 8%, iron 20%

Ingredients

1 medium onion, chopped
1 rib celery, chopped
1 garlic clove, minced
1 Tbsp. vegetable oil

1 cup chicken or vegetable broth
2 cans black beans, 1 lb. each, drained

dash cayenne pepper
1 Tbsp. lemon juice
salt and pepper, if desired

Directions

1. In stock pot or Dutch oven, sauté onion, celery, and garlic in oil until tender.
2. Add broth, beans, and cayenne pe   r. Simmer over medium heat, stirring occasionally, until heated throu   t 5 minutes.
3. Carefully purée mixture in sma   in blender or food processor. Return to stock pot.
4. Stir in lemon juice and simmer   Add salt and pepper to taste. Serve hot.

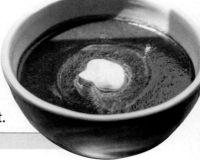

Career Pathways

Entrepreneur

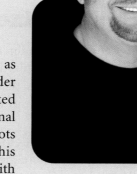

PARK KERR: The American West is known for adventurers, and Park Kerr is carrying on the tradition. Harnessing an independent spirit and an unconventional approach to business, he has created the El Paso Chile Company, the most successful seller of gourmet salsas in the country.

Life-Changing Chiles. In college, Park majored in marketing but preferred "cool school courses that I thought would affect the rest of my life, like graphic design, cooking, fashion merchandising, anything fun." His instincts would later prove right for him. "Everything I took set me up for success in some way or another. I learned trend scouting from fashion merchandising and how foods work in cooking class. Cultural anthropology showed me how to look at cultures."

Meanwhile, Park needed a job. Inspiration came in the form of a ristra, a decorative string of chile peppers often seen in the Southwest. Park found that ristras could be bought for $3 in New Mexico and sold for $15 back home in El Paso, Texas. His first ristra dealership was a homemade street-corner stand. With his mother's help, it grew into a successful booth at a large Dallas gift show. Within a few years, the El Paso Chile Company employed a dozen workers, and their ristras and wreaths appeared on the cover of the fashionable Neiman-Marcus catalog.

Chiles are in season for just a few months, however. Once the supply is gone, ristra making shuts down until the next harvest. The business needed another business.

Hot Foods, Hot Markets. For Park, a ninth-generation Texan in the heart of Tex-Mex country, the direction seemed obvious. With interest in ethnic food on the upswing, the company added a line of gourmet salsas and hot sauces. Park wrote a cookbook, a marketing move that gave him status as an "expert" in border cuisine. He promoted the book on a national tour, landing him spots on television and his own cooking show. With all this creative effort, it's no wonder the El Paso Chile Company has grown over the years.

Today the company's line includes salsas, barbecue sauces, bean dips, and Park's best-selling cookbooks. All the foods, including dog treats, are made from natural ingredients only, with no preservatives. Park's sister and her husband now oversee daily operations, freeing Park for new product development and promotion: "I get left alone to dream, design, and develop the next big thing. It is very progressive that, as the business has become huge, the entrepreneurial spirit is totally fostered throughout the organization."

While creativity and risk taking are the heart of the entrepreneurial spirit, Park offers this no-nonsense advice for budding business owners: "When offered free advice, shut your mouth, shelve your ego, and open your ears. People see your business differently than you do and will give you million-dollar ideas. Trust me on this one."

On-line Connections

1. To learn more about topics in this article, search the Internet for these key words: chile peppers; specialty food trade; border cuisine.

2. To learn about related careers, search the Internet for these key words: food product design; food business entrepreneurs.

Summarize Your Reading

▶ As people from Spain, Portugal, France, and Great Britain colonized in Latin America and the Caribbean, their culinary traditions blended with those of the people already living there.

▶ The earliest cultures to establish foods in Latin America were the Aztecs in Mexico, the Mayas in Central America, and the Incas in South America.

▶ Chiles play a major role in dishes throughout Latin America.

▶ The geography of Latin America has high impact on the foods eaten there.

▶ Hundreds of tropical islands can be found in the Caribbean Sea.

Check Your Knowledge

1. What parts of the world make up Latin America?

2. How would you describe the general geography of Latin America?

3. Why did beef become an important meat in Argentina and northern Mexico, yet pork was more common in other Latin American countries?

4. How are chiles commonly used in Latin American cuisine?

5. What three foods are basic in the Latin American diet?

6. Describe an **empanada**.

7. How are central Mexico and southern Mexico different?

8. What is **masa** and how is it made?

9. How did the Aztecs use chocolate in Mexico?

10. How might **frijoles** be used in Mexican dishes?

11. What kind of sauce uses unsweetened chocolate as an ingredient?

12. What are the seven countries in Central America?

13. How might a family in Nicaragua use banana leaves?

14. How does South America compare in size to the United States?

15. Why are Brazilian cuisines so varied?

16. What is *chimichurri*?

17. How does the geography of the Andean nations affect the foods available?

18. What did natives of the Caribbean likely teach to European colonists?

19. What tropical fruits are common in Caribbean cooking?

20. What is **jerk**?

21. **CRITICAL THINKING** Why do you think Mexican dishes are more known in the United States than dishes from South America?

22. **CRITICAL THINKING** If you could take a culinary journey to one part of Latin America, where would you go and why?

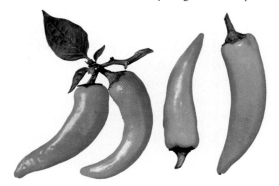

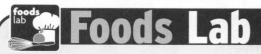
Apply Your Learning

1. **SOCIAL STUDIES** **Country Study.** Choose one country in the chapter to study. Learn about the area's history, geography, and culture. Using such visual aids as films and magazine photos, give a class presentation.

2. **Taste Test.** With your lab team, make one Latin American or Caribbean dish. Present your dish with those of other teams for a class taste test.

3. **Ethnic Meal.** Plan, prepare, and serve a Latin American meal.

4. **Chile Peppers.** Create a chile pepper display for the class, showing the various kinds and labeling their degree of hotness. Learn how to prepare very hot chile peppers for cooking and demonstrate the technique for the class.

5. **SOCIAL STUDIES** **Mexican Holiday.** Despite its name, the Mexican holiday, the Day of the Dead, is a festive occasion. Research and report on this holiday, including information about the foods that are part of the festivities.

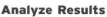 **Foods Lab**

Making Salsa

Procedure: Develop and prepare a recipe for tomato-based salsa. Refer to existing recipes for ideas about ingredients and techniques. Then experiment with your own seasonings and proportions. Serve samples with baked tortilla chips, along with a copy of your recipe.

Analyze Results

❶ What different ingredients did other lab teams use? How did the salsas compare in heat, sweetness, and other flavor factors?

❷ After tasting other salsas, would you alter your recipe in any way? If so, how?

❸ Calculate the cost of your salsa. How does the cost compare to ready-made salsas from the supermarket?

 # Food Science Experiment

Starches in Tortillas

Objective: To compare qualities of the grain products used in tortillas.

Procedure:

1. Measure ½ cup of wheat flour in a small bowl. Gradually stir in ½ cup of water.

2. Mix the water and flour with a fork for five minutes. Pause at one-minute intervals to observe the mixture's appearance and consistency. Record your observations.

3. Repeat Steps 1 and 2, replacing the wheat flour with an equal amount of *masa*, the ground corn product used in corn tortillas.

Analyze Results

❶ What changes, if any, occurred as you mixed the water and flour? The water and *masa*?

❷ Review Chapter 44's discussion of flour. Suggest an explanation for the results you noted in question 1.

❸ Recipes for flour tortillas include a leavening agent. Why do you think this ingredient is not used in corn tortillas?

CHAPTER 50

Foods of Western & Northern Europe

QUICK WRITE

THE MYSTERY OF WORDS. Despite their shared language, British and American people have unique names for some foods. Write what you think these British foods might be: crisps, chips, toad-in-the-hole, and bloater paste on toast. Then research what these foods actually are.

I MAGINE THIS MENU FOR A DAY TRIP IN EUROPE. You rise in Denmark to an early breakfast of Danish pastry and Dutch cocoa; munch on sausage and pumpernickel while motoring across Germany; and dine late on French onion soup with melted Swiss cheese just outside Paris.

Such is the diversity of European foods. Some countries are smaller than some American states. History and geography have combined, however, to create very different cultures and cuisines—as different as those of the Vikings who settled in Norway and the chefs in the royal courts of France. See **Fig. 50-1**.

WESTERN EUROPE

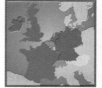

Western Europe has an ample food supply. Rolling green fields support sheep and cattle, with room for chicken and pigs. Dense forests are alive with fowl, deer, and hare. Hardy grains and root vegetables thrive in the temperate, wet climate. Fruits flourish in the south. Seafood is important in coastal areas, although even landlocked nations are not far from an ocean or sea.

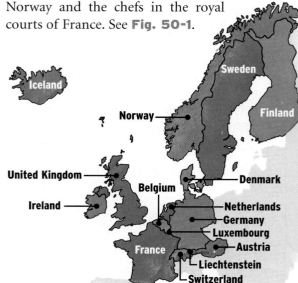

Fig. 50-1 The European continent is a great peninsula that breaks into smaller peninsulas and has bordering islands. Here you see Northern and Western Europe. The Scandinavian countries of Norway, Sweden, Denmark, Finland, and Iceland make up Northern Europe. The United Kingdom includes England, Scotland, and Wales, collectively called Great Britain. Northern Ireland is also part of the UK, but the Republic of Ireland is a separate country. What other countries make up Western Europe?

The United Kingdom and Ireland

Separated by the North Sea and the English Channel, the British have developed a cuisine that is unique in all of Europe. Dishes reflect a heritage of hard-working people closely bound to the land. Traditional British cooking is simple, substantial, and nourishing.

The nations in the United Kingdom—England, Scotland, Wales, and Northern Ireland—and the Republic of Ireland are proud of their individual identities, yet a love for tea unites them all. "Low" tea is just a light, mid-afternoon meal of small sandwiches, bread and jam, or scones and clotted (thickened) cream. Scones might also be topped with the spread shown in **Fig. 50-2**. Low tea is followed by a larger late dinner. "High" tea is itself an evening dinner. Menus include meats, fish, cheeses, bread and butter, and pastries.

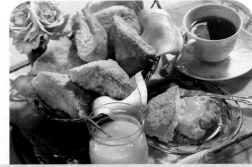

Fig. 50-2

Fish and chips are almost as universal. This favorite "street food" pairs deep-fried fillets, usually haddock, cod, or sole, with french-fried potatoes, sprinkled with salt and splashed with malt vinegar.

England

The English fondly call their standard dinner "meat and two veg," or meat and two vegetables. One vegetable is usually potatoes. A typical example is bangers and mash (sausage and mashed potatoes) served with peas.

Meat pies are a familiar main dish. Shepherd's pie features lamb or beef with diced carrots and peas under a mashed potato crust. Steak and kidney pie may include oysters or mushrooms. Cornish pasties are handheld turnovers filled with meat and root vegetables and shaped like a half moon. The classic Sunday dinner, however, is roast beef and **Yorkshire pudding**, a popover baked in the hot pan drippings from the roast beef.

Try This! Recipe

Lemon Curd

Yield	Nutrition Analysis
3 cups (2 Tbsp. per person)	**Per Serving:** 140 calories, 10 g total fat, 5 g saturated fat, 0 g trans fat, 110 mg cholesterol, 0 mg sodium, 14 g total carbohydrate, 0 g dietary fiber, 13 g sugars, 1 g protein **Percent Daily Value:** vitamin A 8%, vitamin C 15%, calcium 2%, iron 2%

Ingredients

juice and grated rind of 5 lemons
1½ cups sugar

1 cup butter, cut into small pieces
10 egg yolks, beaten

Directions

1. In double boiler, combine lemon juice, lemon rind, sugar, and butter. Over medium heat, stir continually until sugar and butter melt and are well mixed.
2. Add egg yolks and whisk briskly to combine.
3. Set aside whisk and continue to stir until mixture coats the back of spoon. Prevent curdling by not letting the mixture boil.
4. Strain mixture through a fine sieve to remove rind. Mixture will appear thick and creamy. Let cool and keep refrigerated. Serve on pound cake, bagels, toast, biscuits, or scones.

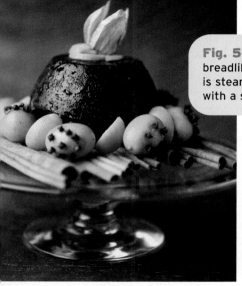

Fig. 50-3 Plum pudding is a breadlike British dessert that is steamed and often served with a sauce.

Everyday English desserts include fruit cobbler, shortbread biscuits (cookies to Americans), and bread-and-butter pudding. See **Fig. 50-3**. Special occasions might call for a trifle, with varied layers of sponge cake, jam, gelatin, custard, and whipped cream, or a **fool**, puréed fruit folded into whipped cream.

Recent immigration from India and Asia has contributed to the new cuisines developing in England. Indian curries are one of the most popular foods. Chinese "takeaways" (take-out restaurants) are as common as fish-and-chips shops.

Scotland

In Scotland, oats are a dietary staple. Oat porridge is eaten at breakfast. Sweet oatcakes are offered at tea. Toasted oats are folded into whipped cream and layered with fresh fruit in a dessert called *cranachan*.

Meat is supplied by two Scottish natives, Angus cattle and Blackface sheep. Steak and meat pies are common uses. Leftovers might end up in *stovies*, a hash of fried onion, chunks of potato, and beef or lamb. Chicken and leeks are found in *cock-a-leekie* soup.

The North Sea and Atlantic Ocean provide a bountiful catch, including swordfish and mackerel. Salmon from Scotland is considered the best in the world and is widely exported. Smoked herring, called kippers, and potted (pickled) herring are enjoyed at breakfast and tea. *Finnan haddie* is lightly smoked haddock. It's often poached and served with potatoes in seasoned milk or over toast in a white sauce.

Ironically, Scotland's most famous dish is probably more talked about than eaten. **Haggis** is an ancient recipe. A sheep stomach is stuffed with a mixture of oats, organ meats, onions, and beef or lamb suet and then boiled. See **Fig. 50-4**. Traditional side dishes are *bashed neeps* (mashed turnips) and *chappit tatties* (mashed potatoes).

Wales

Welsh cooking developed as thrifty meals to sustain miners and farmers. A typical breakfast is bacon, eggs, and a stack of *crempog* (buttermilk pancakes), layered with butter. Cawl is a lamb stew with assorted root vegetables, usually leeks, potatoes, and turnips, depending on what's on hand. Leftover meat and vegetables might be used to fill *oggies* (turnovers).

Simplicity prevails in baking too. Tea breads like *bara brith* ("speckled bread") are flavored with currants or cinnamon. Cakes may be sprinkled with fine-grained caster sugar. *Teisen sinamon* (cinnamon cake) is spread with meringue and jam. Lemon marmalade sweetens a steamed Snowdon pudding. Gooseberries and loganberries go into pies.

Herring, mackerel, and oysters are important ocean catches. Deep rivers teem with salmon and sea trout. Cockles, or heart clams, are dear to the Welsh. A classic scene is women harvesting cockles and packing them on donkeys. Now men with tractors do the job, but cockles remain a favorite in appetizers and savory pies, especially served with **laverbread**. This distinctively Welsh product

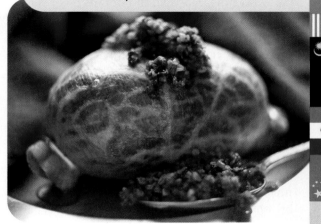

Fig. 50-4 For the Scots who grew up eating haggis, the dish is a revered tradition. Many consider it an acquired taste.

Fig. 50-5

Try This! Recipe

Ratatouille

Yield	Nutrition Analysis
4 servings	**Per Serving:** 170 calories, 14 g total fat, 2 g saturated fat, 0 g trans fat, 0 mg cholesterol, 160 mg sodium, 11 g total carbohydrate, 3 g dietary fiber, 5 g sugars, 2 g protein **Percent Daily Value:** vitamin A 15%, vitamin C 80%, calcium 4%, iron 6%

Ingredients

¼ cup olive oil
½ cup thinly sliced onion
1 clove minced garlic
1½ cups green pepper strips

2 cups cubed eggplant
2 cups sliced zucchini
1½ cups peeled, seeded, tomato chunks

1 tsp. basil
½ tsp. oregano
¼ tsp. salt
⅛ tsp. pepper

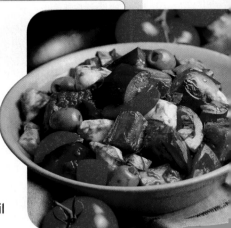

Directions

1. Heat oil in large skillet. Sauté onion and garlic in oil for about 3 minutes.
2. Add green pepper. Cook about 5 minutes longer, stirring occasionally.
3. Stir in eggplant and zucchini. Simmer, covered, about 20 minutes.
4. Add tomato, basil, oregano, salt, and pepper. Stir gently. Cover and continue simmering until mixture is thick and vegetables are soft, about 15 minutes. If mixture is too watery near the end of cooking, remove cover and simmer until excess liquid evaporates.

is processed seaweed. Griddlecakes of laverbread and oatmeal, called *bara lawr*, are a traditional breakfast food.

Ireland and Northern Ireland

The potato has been *the* staple in Ireland since the 1600s. The roots of Irish cuisine, however, are older. Sheep, pigs, cattle, and fish have long inhabited the land and coasts. The soil yields oats, barley, carrots, cabbage, and onions.

This variety shows in dishes like Irish stew, which combines lamb or mutton, potatoes, and onions. Other stews are a medley of root vegetables in a barley-thickened broth. Fish pies are filled with cod, scallops, and oysters in a thick white sauce. Corned beef is brined brisket and goes back to a time when beef was preserved with pellets of salt called corns. The Ulster Fry, named for Northern Ireland, is a skillet breakfast of bacon, black pudding (blood sausage), eggs, and mushrooms. Buttermilk is essential to Irish soda bread and oat bread for leavening as well as flavor.

The potato expanded food choices. It's mashed with leeks and mixed with chopped, cooked cabbage in **colcannon**. It's mashed and fried with cabbage in butter or bacon fat to make *bubble and squeak*.

France

France's location makes a remarkably varied cuisine possible. Mountains in the east and southwest, alternating with coastlines, create a range of climates across the country—warm summers and cool winters; hot summers and cold winters; light rains and heavy ones. Add the rich soil of the Alpine valley and the stage is set for the world's most famous cuisines.

Regional French Cooking

France's regional cooking is defined by local foods, including the fat. Olive oil is used in southeastern France, near the Mediterranean Sea. It's the first ingredient in the fish stew *bourride* and the base of an accompanying hot pepper and breadcrumb sauce, *rouille*. The recipe in **Fig. 50-5** is also from this region. In the southwest, duck or goose fat flavors such dishes as *cassoulet*, a casserole of white beans, duck, and sausage.

In the northwest, cooks use butter and cream from the area's many farms. Shellfish is sautéed in butter and served in a cream-based béchamel sauce. Caramelized sugar and cream are gently cooked into *crème caramel*. Apples from area orchards fill the buttery crust of a *galette des pommes* (apple tart).

Eastern France shares a "meaty" heritage with neighboring Germany. Lard seasons dishes like *choucroute garni*, a platter of sauerkraut cooked with sausage and various cuts of pork.

Types of French Cuisines

French home cooking is *cuisine paysanne*, or "country cooking." "Provincial" is another term for this cuisine. The main meal might include seafood stew or roast chicken, mixed greens, and seasonal vegetables. Recipes are simply prepared and seasoned with sage, tarragon, rosemary, and other common herbs. Bread is part of every meal. A long, crusty **baguette** (ba-GET) may be bought fresh daily. Leftovers are used for *pain perdu*, or "lost bread," called French toast by Americans.

Assorted cheeses and fruits end the meal. France produces more than 400 different kinds of cheese. *Brie*, *Camembert*, and *chèvre* (goat cheese) are among the best known, but many local varieties exist.

What many people think of as French cooking is **haute cuisine** (oht kwih-zeen). This classic French cuisine is known for high-quality ingredients, expertly prepared and artistically presented. Dishes are complicated and often rich, featuring Hollandaise and béchamel sauces. Stunning desserts are a treat for the eye as well as the taste buds, as you can see in **Fig. 50-6**.

In the 1970s, a new style of haute cuisine arose in reaction to traditional heavy dishes. *Nouvelle cuisine* emphasizes the food's natural flavor and uses smaller servings of fresh foods, lighter cooking, and less butter and cream. This made it easier to enjoy French foods while watching fat and calories.

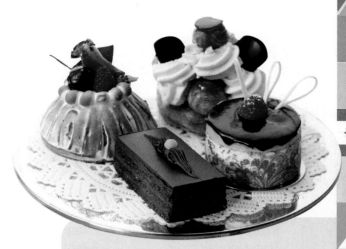

Fig. 50-6 French pastries are known for their beautiful and creative presentations.

Germany

German cooking is considered robust. Meats have long played a leading role, especially *wursts* (sausages), *schnitzels* (cutlets), and *bratens* (roasts). *Bratwurst* is a sausage of veal and pork seasoned with ginger and caraway seed, a common spice in German cuisine. *Wienerschnitzel* is a breaded, fried veal cutlet. A beef roast marinated in vinegar with cloves, bay leaves, and peppercorns becomes **sauerbraten**.

The need to preserve foods has made cured meats as common as fresh. *Braunschweiger* is a smoked, spreadable sausage made with pork liver. Acorn-fed pigs produce the famous Westphalian ham. Smoked eel and herring are popular in northern Germany.

Dishes made with root vegetables round out a meal. Examples are *linsensuppe*, lentil soup; *kartoffel klöbe*, potato dumplings; and *himmel und erde* ("heaven and earth"), potatoes and applesauce topped with fried onions and bacon. Another vegetable, red cabbage, is used for the dish in **Fig. 50-7** on page 688.

Wheat grown in southern Germany supports a great tradition of baking. Breads range from plain hard rolls to **stollen**, a yeast bread filled with dried fruit. Layers of chocolate cake, cherries, and whipped cream create *schwarzwälderkirschtorte*— the celebrated Black Forest cake.

Fig. 50-7

Blaukraut

Yield	Nutrition Analysis
4 servings	**Per Serving:** 120 calories, 3 g total fat, 1 g saturated fat, 0 g trans fat, 5 mg cholesterol, 570 mg sodium, 21 g total carbohydrate, 3 g dietary fiber, 15 g sugars, 4 g protein **Percent Daily Value:** vitamin A 25%, vitamin C 100%, calcium 6%, iron 6%

Ingredients

4 slices diced bacon
6 cups shredded red cabbage
1 cup apple slices
½ cup thinly sliced onion

½ cup chicken broth
2 Tbsp. apple cider
2 Tbsp. vinegar
2 Tbsp. brown sugar

½ tsp. salt
1 tsp. caraway seeds
(optional)

Directions

1. Fry bacon in 2½-qt. saucepan until crisp.
2. Add cabbage, apple, and onion. Cook uncovered over medium heat for 5 minutes.
3. Combine broth, apple cider, vinegar, brown sugar, and salt. Stir into cabbage. Sprinkle with caraway seeds, if desired.
4. Cover and cook just until cabbage is tender, 5 to 10 minutes longer.

Belgium

Various cultures, from Spanish to Scandinavian, contribute to Belgian cuisine. Consider the range between the three foods considered national dishes. *Carbonnade flamande* is beef stewed in a thickened broth that includes onions and brown sugar. It's rivaled by the native endive, a white lettuce. Called "white gold," endive is featured in cream soups or braised with a lemon juice and sugar sauce. Finally, potatoes are prepared in every manner. They may be stuffed and mashed, in pancakes and in croquettes. *Pommes frites* (french-fried potatoes) are dipped in béarnaise sauce.

Seafood is also popular, especially mussels. See **Fig. 50-8**. A thick stew, *waterzooi van tarbot*, combines monkfish, cod, or other whitefish in a broth enriched with egg yolks and cream. Belgian waffles, topped with fruit or jam and cream, are a favorite street food. Belgians are producers of—and great consumers of—some of the world's finest chocolate.

The Netherlands

The Netherlands borders the North Sea. Cool, damp weather and fishing are facts of life. Fish stalls do a thriving business in fresh mussels and oysters. Street vendors sell baked fish and seafood salads. Herring eaten raw and salted is a particular favorite.

Dishes that warm the body are appreciated. *Stamppot* combines mashed potatoes or leeks with kale or cabbage. Plate-size yeast pancakes are served with sausage or vegetables as a main dish or topped

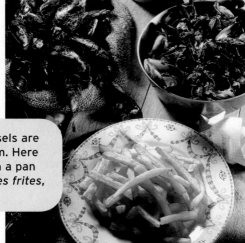

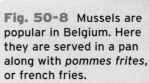

Fig. 50-8 Mussels are popular in Belgium. Here they are served in a pan along with *pommes frites*, or french fries.

with apples and whipped cream as dessert.

Dairy foods are a staple at most meals, especially such cheeses as Gouda, Edam, and quark, an unripened cheese similar to sour cream. *Vla*, a custard, is a common dessert.

Trade with the West Indies expanded Dutch tastes. They adapted an Indonesian custom, calling it *rijsttafel*, or "rice table." This is a buffet of rice and a variety of highly seasoned sauces, meats, and vegetables. They also added cinnamon, cloves, and ginger to cakes and cookies. It was the Dutch who found a way to process the cacao bean into cocoa powder, leading to the creation of chocolate candy.

Switzerland, Liechtenstein, and Luxembourg

The cuisines of Switzerland, Liechtenstein, and Luxembourg are influenced by their German and French neighbors. A specialty of Zurich, Switzerland, near Germany, is *Zürcher geschnetzeltes*, strips of veal in a mushroom cream sauce. Meats are often smoked and dried. Smoked pork and broad beans, or *judd mat gaardebou'nen*, is a national dish in Luxembourg.

People enjoy a small but varied crop of local produce: apples, berries, carrots, beans, and potatoes. *Roesti*, pan-fried, shredded potatoes and onions, is a common side dish. Asparagus is a favorite in Liechtenstein.

Swiss dairy cows give rich milk that makes superior cheeses, found in many dishes. A cheese fondue is traditionally made by melting Emmentaler and Gruyère and eaten by dipping chunks of bread into the hot mixture. *Râclette* is a dish of melted cheese smothered over individual potatoes and served with gherkin pickles. See **Fig. 50-9**. In Liechtenstein, *roesti* is a main dish, seasoned with bacon, topped with Gruyère, and served with a fried egg.

In the late 1800s, Swiss scientists powdered the milk and added it to chocolate, creating the milk

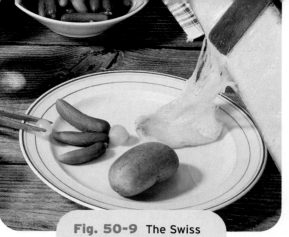

Fig. 50-9 The Swiss make a cheese called Râclette and serve it with potatoes and pickles.

chocolate for which the country is renowned.

Fruit pastries are well liked. Plum and pear tarts are a specialty of Luxembourg.

Austria

Austria draws culinary influences from all around the region, which it once controlled. *Tafelspitz*, beef brisket boiled with carrots and onions, is from the Eastern European tradition. Two "German" dishes are equally popular in Austria: sauerkraut and *weinerschnitzel*—literally, "Vienna cutlet," named for the Austrian capital.

Dumplings, or *knödel*, are used inventively. *Speckknödel* are bacon-filled potato dumplings. *Semmelknödel* are made from stale bread cubes soaked in beaten eggs and milk.

Austrian pastries are internationally known. In *strudel*, layers of paper-thin pastry are rolled with a sweet or savory filling. Fruit, cheese, and nut are well-liked varieties. A **torte** is a rich cake made with a small amount of flour and often with ground nuts or bread crumbs. *Sachertorte* is a dense chocolate layer cake, thinly spread with apricot jam and a glossy chocolate glaze. *Dobos torte* is a six-layer, vanilla sponge cake filled with chocolate cream. From the city of Linz comes *linzertorte*, a hazelnut crust filled with raspberry jam.

NORTHERN EUROPE

Europe's northernmost countries—Denmark, Sweden, Norway, Finland, and Iceland — are collectively called Scandinavia. The tip of this land mass extends into the Arctic Circle. Foods tend to be filling, yet creative. They are based on fish, cured meats, and dairy foods.

Creativity shows in the smorgasbord. Originating in Sweden, a **smorgasbord** is a buffet laden with cured fish, cold meats, cheeses, salads, and vegetables. A typical spread might offer smoked salmon, herring salad, cheese-stuffed eggs, spiced gooseberries, and pickled beets.

Denmark

Denmark is a squiggle of land separating the North and Baltic Seas. Salmon, cod, and herring are staples. Eel is baked, pickled, or stuffed. Balls of salted cod and mashed potatoes are fried as *torkesboller*.

Denmark has the greenest terrain in Scandinavia. Most farmland is used to raise cattle and hogs. Many meat dishes, such as *frickadeller* (meatballs), are sharpened with sour cream and horseradish. Roasts might be sweetened with apples, prunes, or plum-filled potato dumplings called *blommeboller*.

Carrots, cabbage, potatoes, and kale supply side dishes. They may be creamed or glazed in sugar and vinegar. Some are ladled out in soups.

Typically, at least one meal each day is a *smorrebrod*, or open-face sandwich. Whole-wheat and rye breads are preferred, often spread with herbed butter and simply but artistically filled. Anchovy paste is topped with slices of hard-cooked egg or a sweet pickle fan. Bacon, Danish blue cheese, and spinach are arranged in stripes.

Sweden

Swedish foods offer an intriguing mix of flavors. *Köttbullar* (Swedish meatballs) are spiced with nutmeg and served in sour cream gravy. Mustard mayonnaise traditionally accompanies *gravlax*, salt- and sugar-cured salmon.

Potatoes make popular side dishes, including pancakes and bacon-filled dumplings called *kroppkaker*. *Jannson's frestelse* (Jannson's temptation) is a casserole of potatoes, onions, anchovies, and cream.

Fruits also figure prominently. The chilled soup *fruktsoppa* features dried fruits. Lingonberry preserves, a favorite in Sweden, accompany small, thin pancakes called *plattar*.

Career Prep

Working with the Public

WHEN YOU DEAL WITH THE PUBLIC ON your job, some of your employer's success is in your hands. Satisfied customers are the best advertisement. Since customers have more options than ever, winning them through outstanding service is more important than ever. Bricks-and-mortar businesses compete with Web sites, TV shopping channels, and mail-order catalogs.

The formula for dealing with the public is a time-tested one: treat others as you want to be treated yourself. Offer the same service you appreciate when you shop or do business.

When you are your employer's "customer interface," other tips include the following:

- **Use personal contact to advantage.** Web sites and catalogs may be efficient, but they can't make a customer feel welcome like a human being can. Acknowledge people when they arrive, even if you can't wait on them. Make eye contact, smile, and greet them. It's been shown that smiling tends to make you feel more cheerful, and it's contagious.

- **Know your business.** In a diner, would you order a dish if the waiter couldn't tell you what was in it? A company's representative is expected to be familiar with products, services, and policies. This helps ensure that clients will be happy with their choice, which promotes good relations and return business.

- **Treat customers with respect.** Wait on customers in order, looking at them when they talk and thanking them. These aren't only good business practices. They are signs of respect that everyone deserves.

Norway

Small family farms are traditional in Norway. Farm products supplement such fish dishes as herring burgers and **lutefisk** (dried cod soaked in culinary ash and water). Ground beef and pork are often seasoned with ginger, nutmeg, and black pepper to make cabbage rolls and patties called boneless birds.

Dairy products are found throughout the meal. Cream enriches dishes ranging from fish pudding (*fiskepudding*) to *lefse*. *Lefse* is a soft potato flatbread made from kneaded rolled dough. Like the Mexican tortilla, it's used in a variety of ways.

Whipped cream is a standard filling for layer cakes and for *krumkaker*, wafer-thin waffle cookies that are rolled into a cone. Other bakery treats include tortes, fruit pastries, and decorative, cardamom-spiced cookies.

Finland and Iceland

Despite a short growing season, Finnish farmers raise almost all food eaten in the country. Karelian hot pot is a stew of beef, pork, and lamb. It's often served with potatoes or turnips. For *kalakukko* fish and meat are seasoned and encased together in pastry dough before baking. *Roselli* combines carrots, potatoes, and beets with a creamy sweet-and-sour dressing.

The range of foods found in Iceland, in the far North Atlantic, may be surprising: mutton and lamb; numerous fish, game, and dairy foods; and potatoes, rutabagas, cabbage, and rhubarb. Greenhouses warmed by the island's hot springs add tomatoes, peas, and even bananas to the menu.

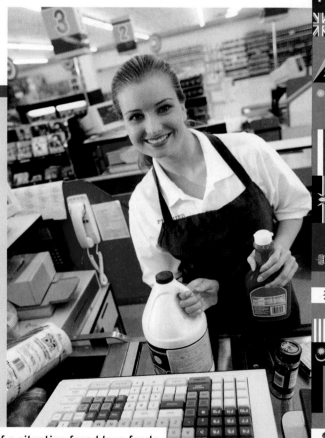

- **If you must disagree, stay agreeable.** Contrary to the popular saying, the customer is sometimes wrong. You can't always give them what they want. Keep a helpful tone and bring in your supervisor. This takes the burden off you. More important, it shows customers that they merit added attention.

- **Return rudeness with understanding.** Like you, customers can have bad moods and bad days. When you're on the receiving end of unjustified anger, don't take it personally. Instead, go out of your way to be extra polite and helpful. This at least stops the bad temper from spreading. It might even turn someone's day for the better—and maybe yours too.

Career Connection

Rehearse for the worst. With a classmate, think of a situation faced by a foods or nutrition worker and a challenging client. Briefly describe it on paper. With your teammate, draw a paper with a situation provided by another team. Improvise the situation for the class, using problem-solving skills to reach a positive outcome. Analyze approaches to the situations.

Summarize Your Reading

▶ Western Europe includes the United Kingdom of Great Britain and Northern Ireland, Ireland, France, Germany, Belgium, Netherlands, Luxembourg, Liechtenstein, Switzerland, and Austria. These countries have an ample food supply.

▶ The countries of Northern Europe are collectively called Scandinavia. They are Norway, Sweden, Denmark, Finland, and the island of Iceland.

▶ With different historical backgrounds, the countries in this chapter have developed distinctive cuisines.

▶ Seafood is a major part of the diet in these areas of the world. Even the countries that don't border the water are not far from it.

Check Your Knowledge

1. What countries make up the United Kingdom?

2. What is "low" tea in the United Kingdom?

3. What are fish and chips in the United Kingdom?

4. Describe these English foods: a) **Yorkshire pudding**; b) trifle; c) **fool**.

5. **CRITICAL THINKING** Why do you think haggis may be talked about more than it's eaten?

6. What classic scene is linked to a food in Wales? Why?

7. What is *bubble and squeak*?

8. How does the geography of France impact cuisines?

9. What fats are commonly used in different areas of France?

10. Describe three basic types of cuisine in France.

11. Why is German cooking considered robust?

12. **CRITICAL THINKING** Based on what you know about German foods, what nutrition concerns might be valid?

13. What three foods are national dishes in Belgium?

14. Why do people in the Netherlands appreciate foods that warm the body?

15. What two examples show how the Swiss make use of cheeses?

16. Describe these Austrian pastries: a) strudel; b) **torte**; c) linzertorte.

17. In general, what is a **smorgasbord**?

18. How is Denmark geographically different from the other Scandinavian countries?

19. What are *gravlax*?

20. What are *lefse* and *krumkaker*?

21. Why are people in Iceland able to have tomatoes and bananas on the menu?

Scandinavian marinated cod

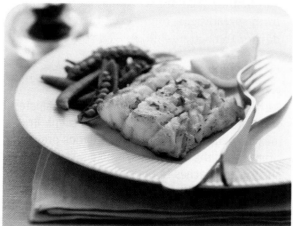

Apply Your Learning

1. **SOCIAL STUDIES** **Country Study.** Choose one country in the chapter to study. Learn about the area's history, geography, and culture. Using such visual aids as films and magazine photos, give a class presentation.

2. **Taste Test.** With your lab team, prepare a dish from one of the countries in the chapter. Present your dish for a class taste test.

3. **Ethnic Meal.** Plan, prepare, and serve a meal with dishes from one of the countries in the chapter.

4. **SOCIAL STUDIES** **Swedish Holiday.** Although Santa Lucia Day has been celebrated in Sweden only since the 1920s, the history of this holiday is much older. Research and report on the holiday and related foods.

5. **Exploration.** What is marmite? Find out and explain it to the class.

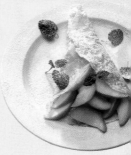

Foods Lab

Making Crepes

Procedure: Find and prepare a recipe for crepes. Fill them with your choice of fruits, meats, cheeses, vegetables, or other ingredients to create a dessert or main dish. Serve samples for a class taste test.

Analyzing Results

❶ How do crepes differ from pancakes?

❷ What was the effect of combining the taste of eggs with a sweet filling? With a savory filling?

❸ What special precautions did you take to prepare and serve this egg-rich dish?

❹ What challenges did you encounter in making or serving the crepes? How could these be managed?

Food Science Experiment

Root Vegetables

Objective: To compare qualities of different root vegetables.

Procedure:

1. Scrub and pare one of the following root vegetables assigned by your teacher: potatoes, parsnips, turnips, or rutabagas. Cut the vegetables into ½-inch slices. Measure 2 cups of the slices.

2. In a large bowl, combine 2 Tbsp. oil, 1 Tbsp. chopped parsley, ¼ tsp. salt, and ⅛ tsp. pepper

3. Toss the vegetables in the oil mixture until well coated. Place them in a single layer on a baking sheet and roast at 400°F until tender, about 20 minutes.

4. Serve samples of the vegetable in a blind taste test with other lab teams. Record each vegetable's appearance, texture, and taste. Try to identify each one. After testing, reveal the identity of your vegetable.

Analyzing Results

❶ What qualities did the vegetables you sampled share? How were they different?

❷ How well did the vegetables absorb the flavors of the seasonings?

❸ Which vegetables were you able to identify?

❹ Based on this experiment, why do you think root vegetables are staples of Western and Northern European cuisines? What other factors might play a role?

Foods of Southern Europe

QUICK WRITE

WRITING AN INVITATION. Suppose your class is going to prepare an Italian dinner to serve to school board members. Write an invitation to the dinner. What information must be included? How can you make the invitation unique or creative so that people are eager to accept?

M

ANY PEOPLE IN THE UNITED STATES today are following "the Mediterranean diet." This eating plan is based on whole grains, fresh fruits and vegetables, fish, and poultry, with lesser amounts of meat and dairy foods. Meals feature small servings of varied dishes. Other people have been following a Mediterranean diet all of their lives. It's the standard in many parts of Southern Europe. At a sunny Greek café overlooking the Aegean Sea, you won't see schnitzel on the menu.

MEDITERRANEAN CUISINES

Compared to typical foods in countries to the north, diets in Southern Europe are decidedly lighter. Fresh fish and poultry are at least as common as beef and sausage. Sauces are lighter, with olive oil the main cooking fat. Citrus fruits and warm weather vegetables may literally grow in your own backyard.

A look at a map explains many of these differences. See **Fig. 51-1.** The warm waters of the

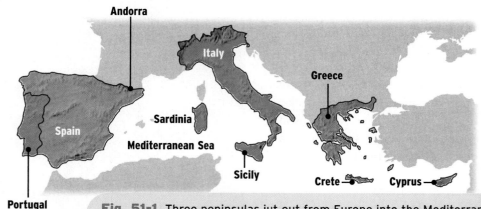

Fig. 51-1 Three peninsulas jut out from Europe into the Mediterranean Sea. Spain, Portugal, and the tiny nation of Andorra are on the Iberian Peninsula that nearly touches Africa. The familiar boot-shape peninsula is Italy, which includes the nearby islands of Sicily and Sardinia. The Balkan Peninsula lies between the Adriatic and Black Seas. Greece is at its southern tip. Many islands are scattered in the waters surrounding Greece, and not far away is the island nation of Cyprus. These countries are often collectively called the Mediterranean.

Mediterranean Sea keep summers mostly hot and dry and winters mild and wet. The Alps shield northern regions from the worst of the cold.

As in northern countries, the cuisines of Southern Europe often show pronounced regional differences. The Mediterranean was widely traveled and fought over throughout the long histories of these nations. The customs and culinary know-how of each dominant culture influence tastes today.

SPAIN

Spain covers most of the Iberian Peninsula of southwestern Europe, the gateway between the Mediterranean Sea and the Atlantic Ocean. In the days when ocean travel was a major means of transportation, this position made the country a center of commerce, drawing traders—and invaders—from all directions.

Spanish Ingredients

The Phoenicians arrived in Spain from the Middle East some 3,000 years ago. They found fish, shellfish, pigs, and sheep in abundance. They also supplied their colony with salt cod and garlic. A thousand years later, the Romans planted olive trees.

The main influence came with the Moors of North Africa, who ruled most of Spain from the seventh to the thirteenth century. They added eggplants, artichokes, tropical fruits, nuts, rice, and spices, most notably saffron. They also brought recipes for meats spiced with cinnamon and for rice cooked with dates. Pastries were sweetened with honey, enriched with egg yolks, and leavened by egg whites. The Moors also introduced **marzipan** (MAHRT-suh-pahn), a confection made of almond paste and sugar. Today the town of Toledo in central Spain is known for its marzipan creations.

Finally, European explorers returned with New World wonders like potatoes, tomatoes, peppers, beans, vanilla, and chocolate.

Spanish Dishes

Two broad statements apply to Spanish cuisine. First, garlic and olive oil are prominent in savory dishes, with pinches of saffron and sprinkles of parsley. Also, flan and custard-filled sponge cakes, part of the Moorish pastry tradition, are favorite desserts.

Within those guidelines, recipes are customized to fit local staples and influences. Consider **paella** (pah-EH-luh), a dish of rice seasoned with saffron and mixed with meat and seafood. Paella in Valencia, on the southeastern coast, may use only shellfish. Up north in Catalonia, food traditions from Germany and France filtered in over the Pyrenees Mountains. Paella here is likely to include sausage and chicken. See **Fig. 51-2**.

Another example is *cocido*, an elaborate stew of beans, mixed meats, vegetables, and a starch cooked in one pot and served separately. Madrid's well-known *cocido madrileño* includes garbanzo beans, bacon, beef, chicken, chorizo, and rice or fine noodles. A Catalan cocido may use pig's feet, lamb shank, a local sausage called *butifarra*, and potatoes.

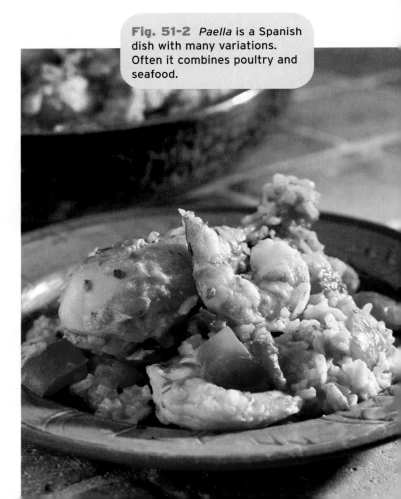

Fig. 51-2 *Paella* is a Spanish dish with many variations. Often it combines poultry and seafood.

Fig. 51-3

Gazpacho

Yield	Nutrition Analysis
4 servings	*Per Serving:* 80 calories, 4 g total fat, 0 g saturated fat, 0 g trans fat, 0 mg cholesterol, 380 mg sodium, 10 g total carbohydrate, 2 g dietary fiber, 4 g sugars, 2 g protein *Percent Daily Value:* vitamin A 15%, vitamin C 40%, calcium 4%, iron 6%

Ingredients

16-oz. can whole tomatoes, with liquid

½ cup finely chopped green peppers, divided

½ cup finely chopped cucumbers, divided

½ cup chopped onion, divided

1 Tbsp. vegetable oil

1½ tsp. ground cumin

1½ tsp. cider vinegar

¼ tsp. salt

¼ tsp. pepper

½ cup croutons, unseasoned

Directions

1. Put into a blender the tomatoes (with liquid), ¼ cup green pepper, ¼ cup cucumber, ¼ cup onion, vegetable oil, cumin, cider vinegar, salt, and pepper. (Save remaining ingredients.)
2. Cover and blend ingredients on medium speed until smooth.
3. Place blended mixture in covered container. Refrigerate for 1 hour or more. Serve soup cold. Garnish with croutons and remaining chopped ingredients.

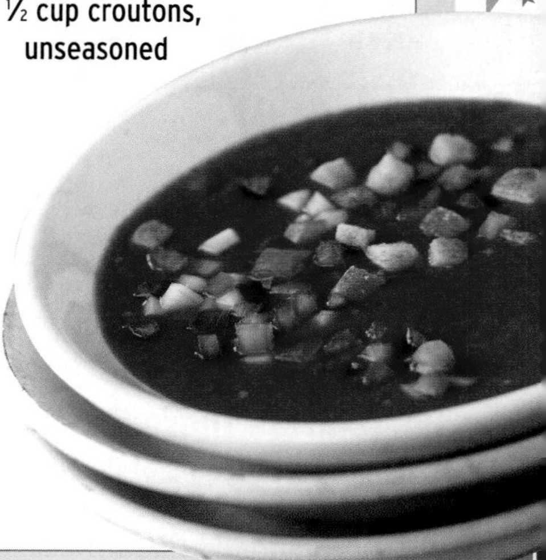

Small snacks or appetizers, called **tapas** (TAH-puhs), are immensely popular and greatly varied. You might find battered and fried olives in the southern region of Andalusia, where both the food and the technique are specialties. In Galicia, the northwestern corner of Spain, cooks are expert in preparing all types of seafood. A tapa might include grilled squid or octopus.

Local Dishes

Each region also has signature dishes. Catalonia's adventurous cooks make *zarzuelas*, stews of a half-dozen kinds of fish and shellfish plus almonds and hazelnuts. Andalusia is home to *gazpacho*, a cold soup based on dry bread soaked and puréed with tomatoes and garlic. A variation is shown in **Fig. 51-3**. Chopped tomatoes, cucumbers, sweet peppers, and onions may be passed at the table.

Lamb and suckling pig, which are roasted in wood-burning brick ovens, are the pride of the central Castile region. The area due north, Asturia, is known for *fabada*, a casserole of white beans, chorizo, ham, and blood sausage. It resembles the cassoulet found across the bay in France. In Galicia, the Celtic people of central Europe left their imprint. It shows in the form of fish and meat pies, including *empanadas*.

A unique place in regional cuisine belongs to the Basques, a cultural group living on both sides of the Spanish-French border. Sheepherders by tradition, their cooking takes in seafood, pork, and beans as well as lamb and mutton. Specialties include young eel and smoked cheese from sheep's milk. In *bacalao pil-pil*, salt cod is gently heated in olive oil and garlic, releasing the gelatin to thicken the sauce.

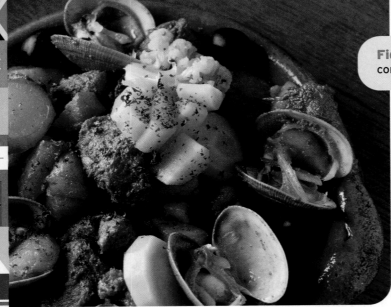

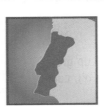

Fig. 51-4 Seafood and pork are combined in this Portuguese stew.

PORTUGAL

Although Portugal is overshadowed by Spain in size, its cuisine is not just a variation of Spain's. Portugal has a food history and tradition all its own.

Portuguese Ingredients

The culinary roots of Portugal parallel those of Spain. The Celts raised cattle and pigs in the north. The Romans added cilantro, parsley, and fava beans. The Moors cultivated rice in the marshy south. They also improved the technology. Their irrigation system turned dry land into groves of almonds, figs, lemons, and oranges. They simmered seafood or small pieces of meat in a *cataplana*, a copper vessel with rounded sides and a hinged, domed lid. The technique is called "*na cataplana*" even today.

In the 1500s, traders in Indian and Indonesian spices brought cinnamon, black pepper, and curry powder. New World colonies supplied green beans, tomatoes, and potatoes. From Africa came fiery *piri-piri* chiles, the base of numerous hot sauces. Portuguese sailors helped inspire the nation's love of salt cod. They caught and preserved the fish in great quantities on long voyages.

Portuguese Dishes

Traditional Portuguese recipes are thrifty, nourishing, original combinations. Salt cod, or *bacalhau*, is a good example. The Portuguese are said to have 365 ways to prepare cod, one for each day of the year. It may be simply grilled or fried in fish cakes. A more interesting recipe is *bacalhau à Gomes de Sá*, a layered casserole of salt cod, sliced potatoes, and sautéed onion and garlic, garnished with hard-cooked eggs and black olives.

Pork is a favorite meat. See **Fig. 51-4**. *Linguiça* is a smoked sausage seasoned with garlic, paprika, and pepper. It flavors stews, beans, and egg dishes. A smoked ham, *presunto*, is thinly sliced and served with figs as an appetizer. Pairing meat with seafood is distinctive of Portuguese cuisine. Marinated pork cubes and clams are browned and simmered to make *porco a alentejana*.

Chicken with piri-piri is a common poultry recipe. A fancier entrée is roasted chicken, marinated in paprika and garlic and stuffed with ground pork, onions, olives, and hard-cooked eggs. Grilled steaks are entrées in restaurants.

Soups are also prominent. A simple chicken soup, *canja*, is flavored with lemon and mint. The more elaborate *caldeirada de peixe* is a layered stew. A variety of fish—traditionally, whatever is available at the market—alternates with sliced tomatoes, onions, and peppers. "Dry" soups called *açordas* are thickened with bread, using a technique similar to making gazpacho.

The best-known vegetable soup is the deep green *caldo verde*, finely shredded kale and mashed potatoes in a broth seasoned with garlic and pepper. Another recipe combines pumpkin and onion.

Rice is the grain of choice, often served with seafood and chicken. In *paelha* (Portuguese paella), it's spiced up with linguiça and piri-piri sauce. Breads range from *pao doce*, a light, slightly sweet loaf, to *broa*, a "peasant" bread made heavy by stone-ground cornmeal.

ITALY

Italian is the leading ethnic cuisine in the United States, yet the Italian food served in American restaurants is often different from the meals served in a home in Italy. What's more, the menu varies depending on whether you're far up the "boot" in Venice or on the islands of Sicily and Sardinia.

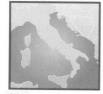

Italian Ingredients

In Italy, a harvest from land and sea is brought to market daily. Lengthy coastlines teem with seafood, from anchovies to tuna and from shrimp to squid. In the rich volcanic soil in the south grow olives, artichokes, fennel, lettuce, and chard from Greece; the Moors' spinach and eggplant; and New World squash and tomatoes. Goats and sheep are pastured in the foothills.

In northern river valleys grow staples like wheat, rice, corn, beans, peppers, and specially bred chicory called radicchio. Dairy cows produce the butter and cream used in regional dishes. From beef cattle and pigs come cured meats: Parma ham, Genoa salami, and sausages like pepperoni and **pancetta** (pan-CHEH-tuh).

Finally, the well-stocked Italian pantry includes garlic, onions, basil, oregano, rosemary, sage, and saffron.

Italian Dishes

The first course of a traditional Italian dinner is a light soup, such as vegetable *minestrone*, or appetizers called **antipasto** ("before the meal"). See **Fig. 51-5**.

Pasta is usually the second dish. It appears in hundreds of shapes and sizes, depending on region and recipe. North Italians favor meatier sauces and **pesto**, a sauce of ground fresh basil, pine nuts, garlic, Parmesan cheese, and olive oil. Sturdy ribbons of *fettucini* might be their choice. In the south, delicate *capelli d'angelo*, "angel hair," may be tossed with crushed tomatoes sautéed in olive oil and garlic.

In northern Italy, pasta is often replaced by rice, by **gnocchi** (NAW-kee), which are potato dumplings, or by a thick cornmeal porridge called **polenta** (poh-LEN-tuh). Gnocchi and polenta are served with meat and tomato sauce. See **Figs. 51-6** and **51-7** on pages 700 and 701. Polenta is the preferred accompaniment to rabbit stew. Rice may be cooked in chicken broth with saffron as *risotto alla milanese*. Other versions use chicken or spring vegetables. Parma ham or bacon seasons rice and peas in *risi e bisi*.

When served, meats vary with circumstances. Pork is frugally used in the far south, from stews to stuffed pork rinds. A festive occasion in central Italy and Sardinia might feature roast suckling lamb. In Milan it might call for *osso bucco* (braised veal shanks) garnished with *gremolata*, a mixture of parsley, garlic, and lemon peel.

Seafood is common on the coast. Sicilians bake swordfish with chopped tomatoes, olives, raisins, and pine nuts. Their northern neighbors in Tuscany prepare *cacciuco*, a soup of fish, shellfish, and squid.

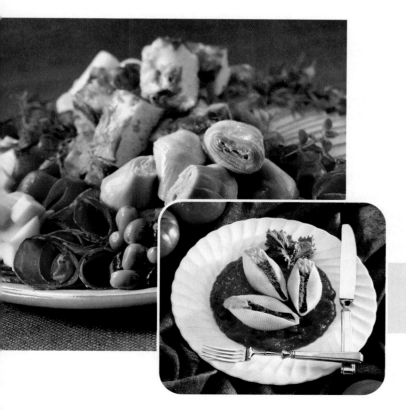

Fig. 51-5 A typical antipasto platter might include olives, pickled peppers, thin slices of salami, cheese, and marinated artichoke hearts. Pasta dishes are another Italian favorite.

Vegetables are found in numerous dishes besides soups and antipasto. Fresh green salads are common. Peppers, onions, and eggplant may be used in sauces or roasted in olive oil and tossed with basil. Raw vegetables and *bagna cauda*, a warm anchovy and garlic dip, are served as an appetizer.

In Italy, cheese is a course in a meal as well as an ingredient. Asiago and blue-veined Gorgonzola are made from cow's milk. Pecorino is made with sheep's milk. Mozzarella from the milk of water buffalo is traditional and thought superior, but cows are a more typical source.

Fresh fruits provide a sweet ending to a meal. Apricots, plums, and melons are seasonal summer fruits. Apples, pears, oranges, and grapes are more available in fall and winter.

Breads and Pastries

Breads are important to Italian tradition. Breakfast might be a small, loaf-shaped roll, or *panino*, with butter or jam, along with coffee or hot chocolate. Panino with a chunk of cheese or walnuts is an afternoon snack. A chewy Tuscan loaf complements soup.

Pizza began as focaccia, a yeast flatbread drizzled with olive oil and sprinkled with herbs. In 1889, a pizza chef in Naples topped his creation with red tomatoes, white mozzarella cheese, and green basil. The colors represented the Italian flag to impress an honored customer—Italian Queen Margherita. Pizza Margherita remains a specialty in Naples. Other regions have their own versions, using combinations of fresh herbs, olives, peppers, onions, mushrooms, sausage, and seafood. Crust thickness also varies with local tradition, but toppings are still light, and baking in a wood-fired brick oven is essential.

The Italians' well-known way with pastry borrows from the Moors. *Panforte*, a Christmas confection, is chewy, with honey and dried fruits.

Fig. 51-6

Try This! **Recipe**

Gnocchi

Yield	Nutrition Analysis
6 servings	*Per Serving:* 350 calories, 2.5 g total fat, 0.5 g saturated fat, 0 trans fat, 70 mg cholesterol, 420 mg sodium, 71 g total carbohydrate, 5 g dietary fiber, 3 g sugars, 10 g protein *Percent Daily Value:* vitamin A 4%, vitamin C 25%, calcium 4%, iron 15%

Ingredients

4 large baking potatoes
2 cups all-purpose flour
2 large eggs

½ cup chopped fresh sage
3 Tbsp. chopped fresh chives
1 tsp. salt
½ tsp. black pepper

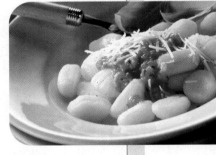

Directions

1. Put potatoes in large pot and cover with water. Bring to boil over high heat. Reduce heat to low, cover, and simmer about 25 minutes or until potatoes are fork-tender. Drain and cool potatoes completely.

2. In large bowl, mash the potatoes. Stir in flour, eggs, sage, chives, salt, and pepper. Knead mixture about 5 minutes, adding more flour if necessary. Dough should be a bit sticky inside. Do not overwork dough or it will require more flour, making the gnocchi heavy.

3. Cut dough into 12 pieces. On lightly floured surface and with floured hands, roll each piece of dough into ⅓-inch-thick rope. Cut rope into ½-inch pieces. Repeat with remaining dough; set aside.

4. In large pot, bring 3 quarts salted water to boil. Add gnocchi, stirring gently until they float. Drain and toss with the tomato sauce in **Fig. 51-6**. Sprinkle with Parmesan cheese if desired.

Fig. 51-7

Fresh Tomato Sauce

Yield	Nutrition Analysis
6 servings	**Per Serving:** 60 calories, 4.5 g total fat, 0.5 g saturated fat, 0 g trans fat, 0 mg cholesterol, 580 mg sodium, 4 g total carbohydrate, 1 g dietary fiber, 3 g sugars, 1 g protein
	Percent Daily Value: vitamin A 15%, vitamin C 15%, calcium 2%, iron 2%

Ingredients

2 Tbsp. olive oil
1 medium onion, peeled and diced

4 medium Roma tomatoes, diced
1 cup chopped fresh basil

1 large garlic clove, crushed
1½ tsp. salt
¼ tsp. freshly ground black pepper

Directions

1. In medium sauté pan over medium heat, add olive oil and onion and cook until transparent, about 6 minutes.
2. Add tomatoes, basil, and garlic. Cook on high heat for 2 minutes.
3. Reduce heat to low and simmer uncovered for 5 to 10 minutes or until most liquid is absorbed. Add salt and pepper. Serve over gnocchi or pasta.

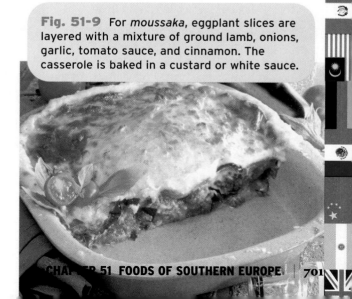

Deep-fried pastry tubes called **cannoli** and the sponge cake *cassata* brim with a mixture of sweetened ricotta cheese, citrus peel, pistachios, and shaved chocolate. Crunchy, anise-flavored **biscotti** ("twice-baked" cookies) are excellent for dunking in coffee.

GREECE

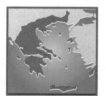

Since Greek history goes back 2,500 years, the cuisine is very old. Ancient Greek traditions have blended with those of Italy, Turkey, and the Middle East.

Greek Ingredients

In Greece, a little rich soil brings forth a wealth of foods. Farmers raise rice, wheat, beans, tomatoes, eggplant, onions, and garlic. Trees are laden with olives, nuts, figs, oranges, apricots, and lemons. The juice of lemons is a primary ingredient in **Fig. 51-8** on page 702. Oregano, rosemary, mint, and thyme grow wild in the hills. Sheep and pigs produce meat. Sheep and goats supply milk for the yogurt and the many cheeses

that are basic to Greek cuisine. Seafood is a staple, of course.

Greek Dishes

Greek main dishes are marked by zesty seasonings. In **moussaka**, sliced eggplant is featured. The casserole is baked in a custard or white sauce. See **Fig. 51-9**. *Souvlaki* is marinated, grilled meat served with *tzatziki*, a yogurt sauce flavored with

Fig. 51-9 For *moussaka*, eggplant slices are layered with a mixture of ground lamb, onions, garlic, tomato sauce, and cinnamon. The casserole is baked in a custard or white sauce.

Fig. 51-8

Try This! **Recipe**

Avgolemono (Egg-Lemon Soup)

Yield	Nutrition Analysis
4 servings	**Per Serving:** 140 calories, 5 g total fat, 2 g saturated fat, 0 g trans fat, 110 mg cholesterol, 200 mg sodium, 15 g total carbohydrate, 0 g dietary fiber, 2 g sugars, 9 g protein **Percent Daily Value:** vitamin A 2%, vitamin C 10%, calcium 4%, iron 6%

Ingredients

6 cups low-sodium chicken broth
⅓ cup long-grain rice

2 eggs
¼ cup lemon juice

salt (to taste)
white pepper (to taste)

Directions

1. Combine broth and rice in a 2-qt. saucepan. Bring to a boil. Reduce heat. Simmer until rice is cooked, about 15 minutes.
2. Beat eggs. Gradually add lemon juice, stirring constantly.
3. Gradually add ¼ cup hot broth to egg mixture, stirring constantly.
4. Gradually pour egg mixture into saucepan, stirring constantly.
5. Reduce heat. Cook until soup is heated through, about 3 minutes. Season to taste with salt and white pepper. Serve hot.

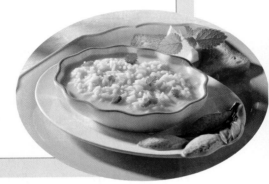

lemon, mint, and garlic. It's served on a skewer or in pita bread, garnished with tomatoes and onions. Whitefish is baked in a sauce of grated tomatoes, cayenne, and black pepper to make *bourtheto*, a specialty on the island of Corfu.

Vegetables are used in season, often in a variety of cooked and raw salads. Shredded cabbage and boiled beets are traditional in winter. *Horiatiki* is a summer classic—tomatoes, peppers, cucumbers, onions, and olives with oregano and olive oil, topped with feta cheese.

Stuffing vegetables is a Turkish technique. Onions are filled with *trahana*, an ancient crumbly pasta made of cooked bulgur and yogurt. Peppers, tomatoes, and eggplant may be stuffed with lamb, cheese, rice, or the rice-shaped pasta *orzo*. A Greek variation is **dolmas**, grape leaves folded and rolled with rice and ground meats and then steamed.

Layers of phyllo, a feathery pastry dough, add crispness to both sweet and savory dishes. See **Fig. 51-10.** Phyllo is filled with spinach and feta cheese to make *spanakopita*. Greece's famed **baklava** (bah-kluh-VAH) alternates tiers of phyllo with finely chopped walnuts or almonds mixed with sugar and cinnamon. The warm, baked pastry is cut into diamonds and steeped in warm honey syrup. Another dessert, *halva*, combines ground sesame seeds and honey.

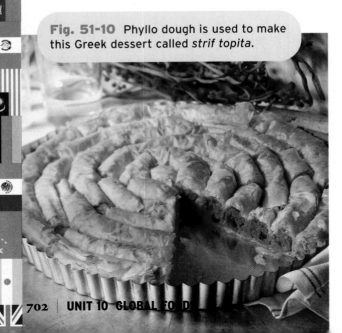

Fig. 51-10 Phyllo dough is used to make this Greek dessert called *strif topita*.

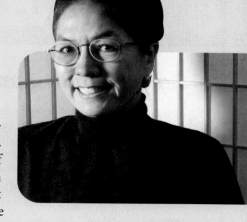

KATE HEYHOE: Kate Heyhoe remembers the day her husband Thomas, a computer consultant, returned from visiting a client, NASA's Jet Propulsion Laboratory. "He came home and said, 'Kate, I've seen the most amazing thing today.' This was in the early 1990s, and what he had seen was the World Wide Web." That discovery would change their lives and turn Kate into the editor of the first on-line food magazine.

From Food to Film. When it came to food, Kate already knew about "worldwide webs." Her mother served foods from her native Korea at dinner parties in their Dallas, Texas, home. As a student in Switzerland and in later travels, Kate explored world cultures and cuisines. Those experiences were invaluable in helping to discover her interests, yet she says, "I never really considered food as a career move." Her bachelor's degree was in journalism and her graduate studies in radio-television-film. She wrote a food column for a while, but with a love for cooking and sharing meals, "I kept finding my way back to the kitchen." Those kitchens included the restaurant she owned while living in Italy and the catering company she started after returning to Dallas.

Kate's interest in media was revived when a visiting film company hired her as a production coordinator. She moved to Hollywood and worked for several large studios as production manager. In this demanding position, she was responsible for everything from arranging auditions, to securing a location, to keeping track of the budget. It was good training for the diverse duties of editing a magazine.

The Global Gourmet. The electronic Gourmet Guide debuted on the Internet in 1994. The magazine's international flavor reflected Kate's fascination for exotic cuisines. Cooking experts were impressed by its range of recipes and depth of cultural notes. Famed chef Jacques Pepin made his first live, on-line appearance on the site; so did Julia Child. Meanwhile, Thomas's expertise ensured a flawless technical performance. Reviewers praised the site's ease of navigation and readability.

The success of the Gourmet Guide established Kate as a cooking authority. She built on that reputation with a string of cookbooks, including *Cooking with Kids for Dummies* and *Macho Nachos.*

In 1998, the magazine and the site combined under a new name, one that also describes its founder: the *Global Gourmet.* Today it is the longest-running "e-zine" on the Web.

While the Internet lets Kate juggle professional demands, including writing, research, and recipe development, it also helps her stay centered. Now back home in Texas, she can work at home, surrounded by other important things in life. "Being able to blend all the things I love—husband, pets, food, nature, and writing—is the most rewarding accomplishment."

On-line Connections

1. To learn more about topics in this article, search the Internet for these key words: creating a Web site; journalism degree; the Global Gourmet.

2. To learn about related careers, search the Internet for these key words: managing editor, television producer.

Summarize Your Reading

▶ The countries of Southern Europe lie on three peninsulas that jut into the Mediterranean Sea.

▶ Because this area was widely traveled and fought over throughout history, dominant cultures influenced cuisines in the many regions.

▶ Closeness to the Mediterranean Sea, or to the Atlantic Ocean for Portugal, means that fish and other seafood are common ingredients in cooking.

▶ The Moors of North Africa and the Basques helped shape Spanish cuisine. Traders brought spices and New World foods to Portugal.

▶ Italy and Greece share some ancient traditions, but they have distinctive cuisines.

Check Your Knowledge

1. What are the four main countries that make up Southern Europe?

2. **CRITICAL THINKING** Compare the diets of Mediterranean cuisines with typical foods in countries to the north. What geographical factors account for these differences?

3. Why was Spain's geographic location beneficial for the country?

4. What is **marzipan**, and which group of people introduced it to Spain?

5. What is **paella**?

6. What are **tapas**? Give examples.

7. Describe a local, or signature, dish from each of five regions in Spain.

8. Why is the Moorish technique of cooking seafood referred to as "*na cataplana*"?

9. What role does salt cod, or *bacalhau*, have in the Portuguese diet?

10. Describe Portuguese vegetable soups.

11. What vegetables are typical Italian ingredients?

12. What cured meats are included in the Italian cuisine?

13. Describe these Italian foods: a) **pesto**; b) **gnocchi**; and c) **polenta**.

14. How is cheese served in Italian cuisine, and what cheeses are typical?

15. Describe these Italian foods: a) *panino*; b) **cannoli**; and c) **biscotti**.

16. How did pizza originate?

17. What typical ingredients in Greek dishes are grown on trees?

18. What four ingredients basic to Greek cuisine do sheep, pigs, and goats supply?

19. Describe these Greek dishes: a) **moussaka**; b) souvlaki; and c) **dolmas**.

20. How is the feathery pastry dough, phyllo, used to make Greece's famed **baklava**?

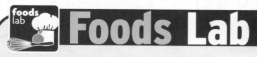
Apply Your Learning

1. **SOCIAL STUDIES** **Country Study.**
Choose one country in the chapter to study.
Learn about the area's history, geography, and
culture. Using such visual aids as films and
magazine photos, give a class presentation.

2. **Taste Test.** With your lab team, prepare a dish
from one of the countries in the chapter.
Present your dish with those of other teams for
a class taste test.

3. **Ethnic Meal.** Plan, prepare, and serve a meal
with dishes from one of the countries in the
chapter.

4. **SCIENCE** **Cheese Making.** Investigate the
science of cheese making. Demonstrate how to
make cheese for the class.

5. **LANGUAGE ARTS** **Meal Pattern.**
Research and report on the typical meal pattern
for a family in Greece. When and what is typically eaten throughout a day?

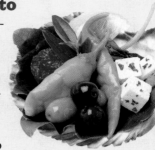

Foods Lab

Making Antipasto

Procedure: Find and prepare a recipe for
antipasto. Use authentic
ingredients if possible;
otherwise, substitute similar, more available foods.
Combine the antipastos
created by all lab teams to
make a buffet for sampling and evaluation.

Analyze Results

❶ Compare the appearance of some of the
antipastos. Which did you find most
attractive? Why?

❷ What tastes and textures did different
antipastos combine? Which were your
favorites? Why?

❸ Would a meal of these antipastos be
healthful? Explain.

Food Science Experiment

Roasting Peppers

Objective: To observe how roasting affects
taste and texture in peppers.

Procedure:

1. Adjust a broiler grid to about 4 inches from
the heat. Place green bell pepper halves, with
stem and seeds removed, on the grid. Broil
until the skin is blistered and scorched.

2. Carefully remove the peppers to a bowl and
cover with plastic wrap. Let them rest for 10
minutes, observing every few minutes.

3. When peppers are cool, peel off the skin.

4. Wash, slice, and seed one or more raw peppers. Compare the raw and roasted peppers
on taste and texture.

Analyze Results

❶ How did roasting affect the peppers' complex
carbohydrates, or fiber? How did it affect the
simple carbohydrates, or sugars?

❷ Which of the changes you noted in question 1
affected the peppers' taste more? Which
affected texture?

❸ What was the purpose of covering the bowl of
roasted peppers with plastic?

❹ Some people brush peppers with oil before
roasting. How might that affect the cooking
process and outcome?

Foods of Eastern Europe & Russia

QUICK WRITE

ABOUT TACT AND RESPECT. Suppose you're eating at the home of friends who have a Russian heritage. You've just tasted an unfamiliar Russian dish that they are proudly serving, but you don't like it. Write how you would handle this situation in a tactful and respectful manner.

To Guide Your Reading:

Objectives

▶ Relate history and geographic location to the cuisines of Eastern Europe, Russia, and the Independent Republics.

▶ Identify typical ingredients used in dishes of Eastern Europe, Russia, and the Independent Republics and explain how they are used.

▶ Describe and prepare dishes from the countries of Eastern Europe, Russia, and the Independent Republics.

Terms

bigos	kringel
blini	pelmeni
caviar	pierogis
kielbasa	pilaf
kolache	

MANY PEOPLE CAN NAME TYPICAL dishes of Russia or Poland, but what about Estonia or Moldova? The food traditions of many Eastern European nations, like their culture in general, stagnated through recent generations of closed societies and closed markets.

Today, people in these countries are renewing their culinary pride and sharing it with the world. Someday, you might take part by trying a piece of karask—an Estonian barley raisin bread. See **Fig. 52-1**.

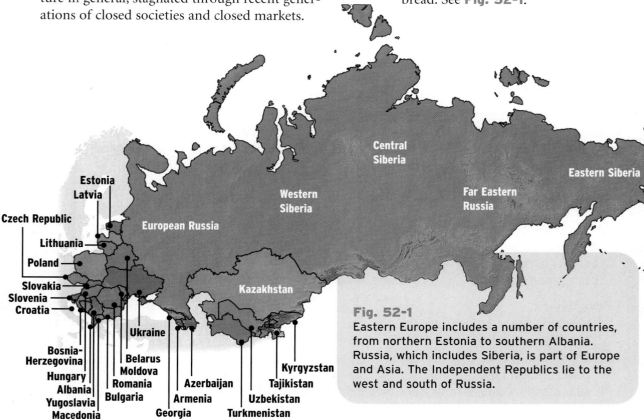

Estonia
Latvia
Czech Republic
Lithuania
Poland
Slovakia
Slovenia
Croatia
European Russia
Ukraine
Bosnia-Herzegovina
Belarus
Hungary
Moldova
Albania
Romania
Yugoslavia
Bulgaria
Macedonia
Georgia
Azerbaijan
Armenia
Kazakhstan
Western Siberia
Central Siberia
Far Eastern Russia
Eastern Siberia
Kyrgyzstan
Tajikistan
Uzbekistan
Turkmenistan

Fig. 52-1
Eastern Europe includes a number of countries, from northern Estonia to southern Albania. Russia, which includes Siberia, is part of Europe and Asia. The Independent Republics lie to the west and south of Russia.

EASTERN EUROPE

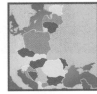

In terms of cooking, North and South meet in the republics of Eastern Europe. The Norse tradition of pickling and salting to stretch foods from a short growing season lives on in northern countries. Hearty meals sustain people through the long winter. Southern nations, on the other hand, share some customs with the Mediterranean. Still, as you trace cuisines down the continent, you find similarities in foods and techniques.

The Baltic Republics

Estonia, Latvia, and Lithuania are countries on the Baltic Sea. Cooking in these countries is real "meat and potatoes," or more accurately, "potatoes and meat." Potatoes are so basic that they're called "second bread." They're grated or mashed for puddings, pancakes, and dumplings and for small, savory tarts called *sklandu rausi*. Other sturdy vegetables, like fresh and pickled beets and cabbage, are tossed into pots for numerous soups and tossed with cooked eggs in salads.

Grains appear throughout the meal. The daily bread is a dark rye sourdough, dotted with caraway seeds, a common spice. Special occasions call for light breads. Lithuanians bake a "sausage" of barley groats (hulled kernels) and onions fried in bacon. Cooked farina leavened with beaten eggs is Latvia's chilled dessert, *buberts*. Sour milk thickened with cooked barley is a popular cold beverage.

Other dairy products are used in cooking. Sour cream dresses salads and garnishes soups, pancakes, and desserts. Farmer's cheese fills potato dumplings. It's cooked with beaten eggs in *Janu siers*, a cheese served in Latvia for the summer solstice. Butter is used in the region's many sweet and savory pastries.

Of meats, pork is most popular. An Estonian favorite, *sült*, is shredded pork and veal jellied in their drippings. *Pirags*, bacon-stuffed turnovers, often accompany soup in Latvia. Fish is plentiful. Perch, pike, and eel are taken from rivers, and herring and cod come from the Baltic Sea. Pheasant and other game may be found in the fall hunting season. A taste for smoked foods is traditional. Lithuanians enjoy a juniper-

Fig. 52-2

Try This! **Recipe**

Goulash

Yield	Nutrition Analysis
4 servings	***Per Serving:*** 540 calories, 31 g total fat, 10 g saturated fat, 0 g trans fat, 115 mg cholesterol, 370 mg sodium, 31 g total carbohydrate, 3 g dietary fiber, 4 g sugars, 34 g protein ***Percent Daily Value:*** vitamin A 20%, vitamin C 70%, calcium 4%, iron 25%

Ingredients

- 2 Tbsp. vegetable oil
- 1 lb. stew meat (beef, veal, pork, or lamb) cut in 1-inch cubes
- 1 cup chopped onion
- 1 cup diced green pepper
- 1 cup chicken broth or tomato juice
- 1 Tbsp. Hungarian sweet paprika
- ½ tsp. salt
- 4 small potatoes, peeled and cubed
- hot cooked noodles

Directions

1. Heat oil in heavy, 2-quart saucepan. Add meat and brown on all sides.
2. Add onion and green pepper. Sauté for about 3 minutes.
3. Stir in broth or juice, paprika, and salt. Bring to boil. Reduce heat. Simmer, covered, about 1 hour.
4. Add potatoes. Continue to simmer, covered, for 30 minutes. Serve over noodles.

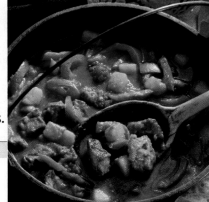

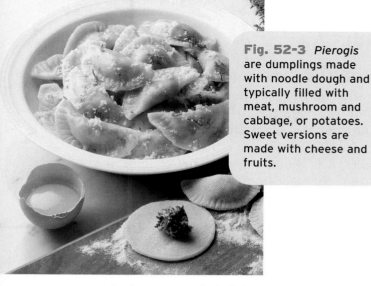

Fig. 52-3 *Pierogis* are dumplings made with noodle dough and typically filled with meat, mushroom and cabbage, or potatoes. Sweet versions are made with cheese and fruits.

smoked sausage called *skilandis*. Smoked lamprey eel is a delicacy throughout the Baltic area.

Many desserts feature fruits. A purée of cooked apples, plums, and rhubarb is thickened with potato starch to make Latvian *kîsêlis*. Blueberry dumplings served with sour cream are Lithuania's "cold noses." Birthdays in Latvia are celebrated with festively decorated **kringel**, a rich yeast oval or pretzel-shaped coffee cake. Some are made with nuts and others with fruit filling.

The Central Countries

A warmer climate and Western influences lighten menus somewhat in Poland, the Czech Republic, Slovakia, and Hungary. You'll still find smoked herring and pickled beets but also grilled trout and *paraszt-saláta*, a Hungarian "peasant salad" with fresh tomatoes, bell peppers, chopped parsley, and vinaigrette. Ground paprika, a red pepper, adds varying degrees of sweetness and heat to Hungarian and Slovakian cooking.

Wheat flour replaces rye in baking, so lighter breads are more common. Stews may be served with noodles, as in the Hungarian goulash recipe in **Fig. 52-2.** Dumplings, such as Polish **pierogis** (puh-ROH-gees), are made with noodle dough. See **Fig. 52-3.** Rice rivals potatoes as a side dish in Slovakia.

A German influence is seen in the popularity of breaded and fried pork cutlets, similar to *wienerschnitzel.* Likewise, the sweet-and-sour Polish stew **bigos** (BEE-gohs) includes fresh pork, apples, and sauerkraut as well as **kielbasa** (a Polish smoked sausage) and cabbage.

Pastries once made for Austrian royalty remain today. Poland's Easter specialty is the fruit- and nut-laden shortbread *mazurek.* A Czech **kolache** (koh-LAH-chee) is a sweet roll filled with fruit butter, nuts, or poppy seed paste. Hungary's *diós bukta* (walnut bread), a Christmas treat, can be a spiral of rich yeast dough filled with ground walnuts, dates, raisins, apples, apricot jam, and chocolate.

The Balkan Countries

Countries on the Balkan Peninsula between the Adriatic and Black Seas have a history of shifting borders and strong ethnic ties. The countries in this area are Slovenia, Croatia, Yugoslavia, Romania, Bosnia Herzegovina, Bulgaria, Macedonia, and Albania.

Like the Balkan people, cuisines of different cultures often live side by side in the same country. Slovenians and Croatians enjoy Austrian-style sausages, potato dumplings, and *jota*, a soup of sauerkraut, potatoes, and smoked pork. They also eat typical Italian dishes: minestrone, risotto, and meat dumplings (*zlinkrofi*) much like ravioli. **Fig. 52-4** shows a Bulgarian version of German strudel.

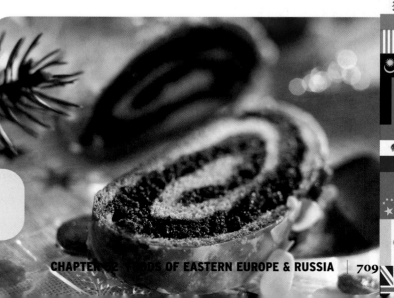

Fig. 52-4 Strudels are layers of dough rolled around sweet or savory fillings and then baked until golden. This Bulgarian version contains poppyseeds.

Republics farther south add Mediterranean elements. Lamb, eggplant, tomatoes, peppers, and yogurt are common ingredients. Yogurt, in fact, is a daily part of the Bulgarian diet. Lemon, garlic, and parsley are favored seasonings. Many recipes, like grilled meatballs and stuffed grape leaves, cross national borders. Phyllo dough layered with cheese or spinach is known as *banitsa* in Bulgaria and *byrek* in Albania. It's called *burek* in Yugoslavia, where a meat-filled version is preferred for breakfast. Potent Turkish coffee is brewed throughout the region.

In Romania, cuisines may blend in one dish. *Mamaliga*, a mainstay, is cornmeal porridge identical to Italian polenta. It's served with meat stew, sauerkraut, or sour cream and Greek feta cheese. *Samarle* can use any combination of grape or soured cabbage leaves, stuffed with a mixture of either ground pork and beef or lamb along with sour cream or yogurt. *Ciorba* (soup) is tart with sour cream, and may also include chicken, lemon, and parsley.

RUSSIA

Once the heart of the Soviet Union, Russia is the world's largest nation. The country stretches from European Russia, far across Siberia, and to Far Eastern Russia. With six and a half million square miles, it is almost twice the size of the United States. Farmland is limited, however, and the growing season short and cool. Traditional meals rely on grains, vegetables—especially potatoes, cabbage, and beets—beef, pork, and dairy foods. Mushrooms are gathered from field and forest. Fish are taken from inland waters and seas to the north and south.

Most dishes reflect the practical cooking of western Slavs, northern Vikings, and eastern Mongols. In striking contrast is the infusion of haute cuisine, a contribution of Russian Emperor Peter the Great. In the 1700s, he adopted Western ideas and technology to modernize his country—and introduced fine French food to the upper classes.

Fig. 52-5

Try This! **Recipe**

Kasha

Yield	Nutrition Analysis
4 servings	***Per Serving:*** 230 calories, 9 g total fat, 2 g saturated fat, 0 trans fat, 55 mg cholesterol, 430 mg sodium, 32 g total carbohydrate, 4 g dietary fiber, 0 g sugars, 8 g protein ***Percent Daily Value:*** vitamin A 6%, vitamin C 0%, calcium 2%, iron 6%

Ingredients
1 cup buckwheat groats (kasha)
1 egg, beaten
2 cups low-sodium chicken broth
2 Tbsp. margarine
½ tsp. salt
¼ tsp. pepper

Directions
1. Toast groats in skillet over low heat, stirring frequently.
2. Quickly stir in egg. Cook mixture, stirring and chopping, until egg is cooked and kernels have separated, about 3 minutes.
3. Combine broth, margarine, salt, and pepper in 1-quart saucepan. Bring to boil.
4. Stir broth mixture into groats. Simmer, covered, until kernels are fluffy and tender, about 15 minutes. Fluff with fork and serve.

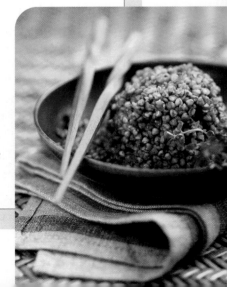

Russian Cuisine

Grains are basic to Russian cuisine. Bread is eaten at every meal—flatbread, wheat rolls, and especially Russian black bread. This moist rye loaf is flavored with chocolate, caraway, coffee, and molasses. A sweet, cold beverage, *kvas*, is even made by soaking black bread fermented with yeast.

Kasha is a versatile porridge usually made with buckwheat groats, but oats, barley, rice, or millet may be used. Kasha cooked with milk is eaten at breakfast. Adding cooked meat creates a main dish. Rice kasha with honey and raisins is a dessert. How would the recipe in **Fig. 52-5** be used?

Blini (BLEE-nee) are small, yeast-leavened, buckwheat pancakes. Most people enjoy them with jam or sour cream. They're also served as elegant *zakuski* (hors d'oeurves) with smoked salmon or sour cream and **caviar** (KAV-ee-ahr), the salted eggs of the sturgeon, a large fish. See **Fig. 52-6**. The *zakuska* table resembles the Scandinavian smorgasbord, from which it was adapted.

Salads and soups are varied mixtures of vegetables, mushrooms, and eggs. Both hot and cold soups are common. See **Fig. 52-7**. *Okroshka* is a cool summer soup of diced vegetables. *Shchi*, a soup made with cabbage, root vegetables, and broth, is served warm.

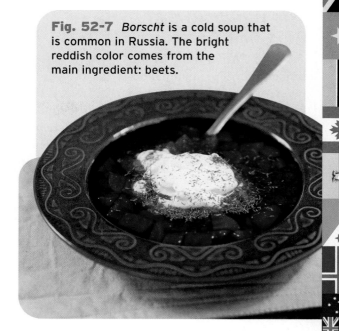

Fig. 52-7 *Borscht* is a cold soup that is common in Russia. The bright reddish color comes from the main ingredient: beets.

Main dishes often include ground meat. Pork and beef fill cabbage rolls and **pelmeni** (PELL-M'YE-NEE), dumplings. *Kulebiaka*, a large pie, may hold layers of meat, rice, and cooked eggs. French-inspired fare is fancier. Chicken Kiev is a breaded, fried chicken breast enfolding a square of seasoned butter. In beef stroganoff, beef strips are browned and simmered with mushrooms in a sour cream sauce.

Drinking tea is a time-honored tradition introduced from China in the 1600s. Russian tea (*zavarka*) is brewed strong and by tradition served in an urn called a samovar. It's poured into the cup, diluted with hot water, and sweetened with sugar, honey, or jam. At its most elaborate, two or three varieties are brewed separately and blended.

Simple Russian desserts include fruit dumplings, teacakes (butter cookies), and sweet cheese dishes. Easter brings two favorites filled with almonds and raisins. *Pashka* is a pyramid of cream, sugar, and eggs cooked and blended with cottage cheese. The yeast bread *kulich* is baked in a coffee can or other round mold. A typical cake alternates white and brown shortcake layers with caramel and cooked icing.

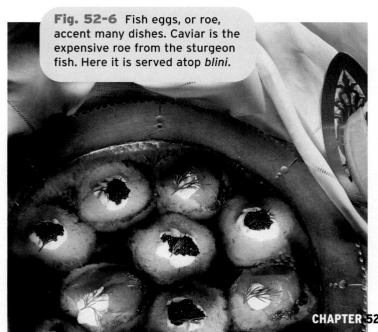

Fig. 52-6 Fish eggs, or roe, accent many dishes. Caviar is the expensive roe from the sturgeon fish. Here it is served atop *blini*.

THE INDEPENDENT REPUBLICS

When the Soviet Union broke up in 1991, many independent nations formed separate from Russia. Their cuisines are similar to one another and to Russia. Cultural differences, however, add variety to shared dishes. Influences from Eastern Europe and Turkey color the food landscape as well.

Ukraine, Belarus, and Moldova

A leading wheat producer, Ukraine has earned the name "the breadbasket of Europe." Bakers prepare a multitude of light breads in numerous shapes. Many are symbolic of holidays and other important events—doves and rosettes on wedding bread, for example. Another specialty is *kutia*, boiled wheat groats mixed with poppy seeds, honey, and nuts. It's served chilled on Christmas Eve.

In contrast, Ukrainian *borscht* is served hot, not cold as in Russia, and often includes meat.

Nakypliak is cabbage dressed up as a steamed soufflé.

Belarusian cooking has marked German and Polish accents. Potatoes are a staple. Grated potatoes are fried into *draniki* (pancakes) and folded with eggs in *babkas* (puffy casseroles). Pork is a favorite meat, and lightly smoked salt pork, a common flavoring. Both may be found in *machanka*, a stew of pork ribs and sausage. Native mushrooms add body to sauces and soups.

Moldovan meals include local versions of Romanian and Ukrainian foods. Poultry is more popular than pork. Some borscht recipes use chicken. A *ciorba* might combine chicken giblets and cabbage.

The Caucasus Republics

The Caucasus Mountain nations of Georgia, Armenia, and Azerbaijan lie just south of Russia, but their colorful cuisine puts them closer to their Mediterranean neighbors. An Armenian appetizer, *imom bayeldi*, is eggplant slices under a mound of sautéed onions, peppers, and toma-

---

Career Prep

Managing Life's Demands

ADULTS AREN'T ALONE IN TRYING to manage the demands of work, community, and personal life. If you've ever tried to study between customers at a car wash fund-raiser or postponed a birthday celebration, you already know about this "juggling act."

You also know that what happens in one area of your life directly affects other areas. If demands on your time and energy are increasing, how can you manage? The suggestions that follow can help you now and later:

- **Develop a sense of values and priorities.** When you decide what is most important to you, many of the pieces fall into place. If you value family ties, an afternoon might be spent with an older relative rather than with friends. On the other

toes, seasoned with garlic, mint, basil, and parsley. Azerbaijanis stay cool with *dovga*, a chilled yogurt and cucumber soup. Some versions include eggs and garbanzo beans. Others add raisins and walnuts. Plum and pomegranate sauces on meat and poultry are popular Georgian combinations. *Satvisi* is chicken with a walnut and garlic sauce, flavored with cinnamon and cilantro.

The region is also known for its way with grains. Western Georgians serve stews with *ghomi*, a millet porridge. Armenians might serve lahvosh, a thin, blistered flatbread. Rice and bulgur are stuffed into grape leaves or cooked in a **pilaf** (PIH-lahf), sautéed grains cooked in a seasoned liquid. Pilafs are often filled with dried fruit and nuts or strips of meat. An Azerbaijani pilaf may be cooked with milk.

Central Asian Republics

Five former Soviet states fall on the Asian side of the Eurasian divide: Kazakhstan, Uzbekistan, Turkmenistan, Kyrgyzstan, and Tajikistan. The climate is desert, the terrain largely rugged and desolate. Nevertheless, fertile valleys in Uzbekistan and irrigated land elsewhere produce an array of vegetables, fruits, and grains. Sheep, goats, camels, and horses graze on grassy flatlands.

Traditional foods reflect the age-old farming and herding life once common among the ethnic groups that call this region home. Flatbreads, called *nan* or *chorek*, are essential to meals. Some are yeast leavened; others use sour milk. Mutton fat may be added for tenderness, and sesame or poppy seeds scattered on top. In rural areas, they are still baked in the old way—on the inner wall of a brick oven.

Sheep provide meat for many main dishes. Cubes of lamb and onion are marinated in lemon juice or vinegar, skewered, and grilled as *shashlyk*. Mutton is ground to fill large, steamed meat dumplings called *manty*. It's also stewed with turnips, carrots, tomatoes, and garbanzo beans in *shurpa*.

hand, if you eat dinner with your family most nights, missing occasionally to meet with a study group might be reasonable. Put some thought into how you want to allocate your time.

- **Practice time management.** Time saved through planning can be spent where it's needed.

- **Practice stress management.** Like time, energy is a limited resource. You tackle responsibilities more enthusiastically if you avoid the wear of needless stress.

- **Practice saying no.** You might not be able to get involved with every cause you want to support or join in every activity you're invited to. Learn to say, "Let me think about it." After reflecting, if you feel you're stretching yourself too thin, simply say that you have other commitments. You might offer to help in some way that better fits your schedule.

- **Use technology to simplify life.** Take advantage of technology that will help you finish tasks more easily and quickly. Some business can be done via e-mail or the Internet. A microwave oven can simplify meal preparation. Remember to use extra time and energy according to your plans, not someone else's.

- **Build a support network.** No one person or family copes with all of life's demands unaided. Identify helpful resources and use them when needed. Employers are usually willing to meet workers halfway in resolving conflicts. Some companies have a human resources department to help with job-related problems.

Career Connection

Interviews. Interview an adult who works outside the home to learn how the person manages the varied responsibilities of work, community, and personal life. What resources and strategies are most helpful? What compromises or sacrifices have been made?

Summarize Your Reading

▶ Many countries make up Eastern Europe. Russia spans two continents and is bordered on the west and south by the Independent Republics.

▶ Many countries in this region of the world were formerly closed societies. Political change is now enabling them to share their culture and cuisines with other parts of the world.

▶ Farmland is limited in Russia, which includes the vast land of Siberia, a largely undeveloped area.

▶ Foods throughout the countries of Eastern Europe, Russia, and the Independent Republics vary partly due to geographic location.

Check Your Knowledge

1. **CRITICAL THINKING** How do you think cuisines were affected in countries that existed for many years under communist rule?

2. What geographic regions does Russia include?

3. How does the geography of the republics of Eastern Europe affect their cusines?

4. Why are potatoes referred to as "second bread" in the Baltic Republics?

5. How are dairy products used in cooking in the Baltic Republics?

6. What is a **kringel**, and how is this food used in Latvia?

7. Describe a Hungarian dish that contributes to lighter eating.

8. Describe these dishes: a) Polish **pierogis**; b) Polish **bigos**; and c) Czech **kolaches**.

9. Phyllo dough layered with cheese or spinach has three names in three countries. What are they?

10. Describe two foods commonly eaten in Romania.

11. Geographically, why is Russia the world's largest nation?

12. Why is Russian *kasha* so versatile?

13. What are **blini** and how are they served?

14. How is Russian tea, or *zavarka*, usually served?

15. What are the Russian desserts, *pashka* and *kulich*?

16. What happened in 1991 when the Soviet Union broke up?

17. Why is Ukraine called "the breadbasket of Europe?"

18. What are *draniki* from Belarus?

19. How do Armenians make **pilaf**?

20. Describe a traditional food that is still commonly eaten in the Central Asian Republics.

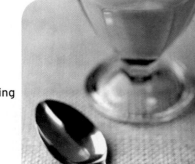

Rice pudding

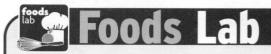

Apply Your Learning

1. **SOCIAL STUDIES** **Country Study.** Choose one country in the chapter to study. Learn about the area's history, geography, and culture. Using such visual aids as films and magazine photos, give a class presentation.

2. **Taste Test.** With your lab team, prepare a dish from one of the countries in the chapter. Present your dish with those of other teams for a class taste test.

3. **Ethnic Meal.** Plan, prepare, and serve a meal with dishes from one of the countries in the chapter.

4. **LANGUAGE ARTS** **First-Hand Experience.** Interview someone who has lived in or visited an area covered in this chapter. Prepare your questions in advance, including questions about foods. Deliver a speech to the class, explaining what you learn.

5. **SOCIAL STUDIES** **News Update.** Collect news clippings about the countries in this chapter. What current events are shaping this part of the world?

Foods Lab

Breads of Eastern Europe

Procedure: Sample different types of breads that are popular in Eastern Europe and Russia, such as black bread, potato bread, sesame seed, pumpernickel, and varieties of rye bread. Try them with different spreads, meats, or cheeses.

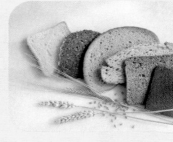

Analyzing Results

❶ What grains were used in the breads you sampled? What did they add to the breads' taste, texture, and appearance?

❷ How do these breads compare in sensory qualities to those that are commonly served in this country?

❸ What foods, textures, and flavors do you think go best with the breads you sampled, as spreads and accompaniments? How do you think the type of bread affects the rest of a culture's cuisine, and vice versa?

Food Science Experiment

About Sauerkraut

Objective: To explore how sauerkraut is made.

Procedure:

1. Research how sauerkraut is made.
2. Prepare and sample at least two brands of store-purchased sauerkraut. Include canned and bagged. You may wish to serve the sauerkraut with sausage.

Analyze Results

❶ From what food is sauerkraut made?

❷ What biological reaction produces sauerkraut? How does it work?

❸ Why is the vegetable typically washed when sauerkraut is made?

❹ What is the purpose of salt when making sauerkraut?

❺ Which sauerkraut sample did you prefer and why?

❻ Why do you think sauerkraut was routinely prepared in Eastern Europe and Russia?

CHAPTER 53

Foods of Southwest Asia & Africa

PARAGRAPH UNITY. In a rambling paragraph, sentences stray from the paragraph's point. In a unified paragraph, the sentences relate to the purpose of the paragraph, which is usually stated in a topic sentence. Write one or more unified paragraphs on this topic: an interesting experience you've had while studying global foods.

Objectives

▶ Relate history and geographic location to cuisines in Southwestern Asia and Africa.

▶ Identify typical ingredients used in dishes of Southwestern Asia and Africa and explain how they are used.

▶ Describe and prepare dishes from Southwestern Asia and Africa.

Terms

injera

mezza

saffron

sumac

tagine

tahini

I N THE REGION WHERE THE CONTINENTS OF Asia, Europe, and Africa meet, you'll find the countries of Southwest Asia and North Africa. Below North Africa stretches the vast African land below the Sahara Desert. See **Fig. 53-1**. Ways of life in these parts of the world might not be familiar to you, but the cultures have supplied many foods that you may recognize and already enjoy eating.

SOUTHWEST ASIA

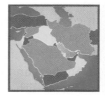

Southwest Asia is more commonly called the Middle East. This land mass lies across the Black Sea from Eastern Europe and across the Red Sea from Africa. Some of the countries may sound familiar, for example, Lebanon, Syria, Saudi Arabia, Israel, Iraq, and Turkey. The area also includes lesser-known states, like Qatar, Oman, and Yemen.

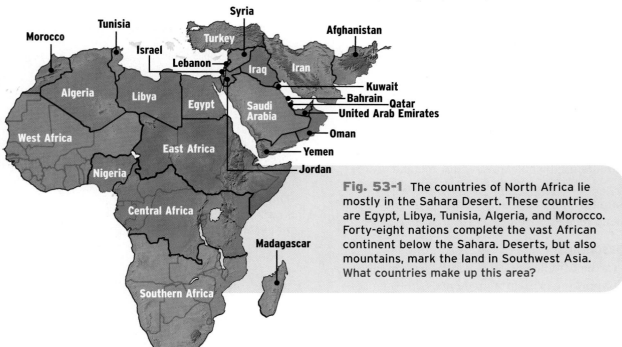

Fig. 53-1 The countries of North Africa lie mostly in the Sahara Desert. These countries are Egypt, Libya, Tunisia, Algeria, and Morocco. Forty-eight nations complete the vast African continent below the Sahara. Deserts, but also mountains, mark the land in Southwest Asia. What countries make up this area?

People have lived in the Middle East since at least 10,000 B.C. This is where farming began and continues along the great rivers—the Tigris, the Euphrates, the Nile, and the Jordan—as well as in Lebanon's Bekaa Valley. Wheat and barley were among the earliest crops. Rice, sugarcane, and olives were later additions. Today, irrigated fields and hothouses produce vegetables and fruits, from cabbage and potatoes to bananas and watermelon.

Southwest Asian Ingredients

Ingredients in Southwest Asian dishes draw from a bazaar of food traditions from around the Mediterranean and parts of Asia. Lamb and chicken are favored for main dishes. Goat is not uncommon. Seafood, fresh or preserved in olive oil, comes from the Mediterranean Sea and Persian Gulf: grouper, snapper, tuna, sea bream, shrimp, and prawns. Nile perch arrives frozen or dried from East Africa.

Yogurt (*laban*) is so necessary that some families make their own. It's eaten plain or with cucumbers and raisins. It's stirred into meat and vegetable dishes or served as a sauce. A diluted, lightly salted yogurt drink goes by various names and recipes. Iranians call it *abdug*. Afghanis like their *dugh* with mint.

Wheat is central to the region's impressive baking tradition. Rice and bulgur are essential to numerous main and side dishes. Arab cooks prefer basmati rice, a long-grain, aromatic variety from Pakistan and India.

Fruits and vegetables are too numerous to name. Favorite fruits include lemons, oranges, dates, figs, grapes, raisins, and quince. Eggplant, spinach, zucchini, artichokes, tomatoes, and okra are prominent vegetables. Garbanzo beans, fava beans, and lentils are popular legumes. Sesame seeds are used whole, pressed for oil, and ground into a thick paste called **tahini** (tuh-HEE-nee). Almonds, walnuts, and pistachios also play a big role in recipes.

Seasonings

In the Middle Eastern kitchen, seasonings are as important as main ingredients. Choosing seasonings from the wide store signifies a skillful cook. Vegetables, rice, beans, and meat might be spiced with coriander, cardamom, cinnamon, ginger, turmeric, and allspice. **Sumac**, a deep red native berry, usually ground, adds a fruity tartness. **Saffron**, the pungent, thread-like center of the crocus flower, turns rice a brilliant yellow. Pastries are aromatic with rose water, orange blossom water, or *mahleb*, the almond-flavored ground kernel of sour cherry pits.

Mint, parsley, dill, and cilantro are some of the most common herbs. Cooks may create their own combinations of *zatar*, a seasoning blend that includes marjoram, thyme, sumac, and salt. Olive oil flavors salads and cooked dishes. Honey, nuts, and fruits are also used as seasonings in dishes. See **Fig. 53-2**.

Southwest Asian Cuisine

Breakfast is a light meal in the Southwest Asian diet, often consisting of *labneh* (yogurt cheese) on a flatbread. *Marcook*, a dome-shaped flatbread, is baked on the surface of a rounded pan. *Taboun*, a thick Palestinian loaf, is traditionally baked on hot rocks in a round oven of the same name. A Lebanese favorite is the zatar-topped *manakeesh*.

The midday meal is the largest. It often starts with **mezza** (MEHZ-ZAH), or appetizers. Common choices include *hummus*, puréed garbanzo beans seasoned with tahini and sometimes garlic, and *baba ghannoush*, a similar purée of eggplant. Both

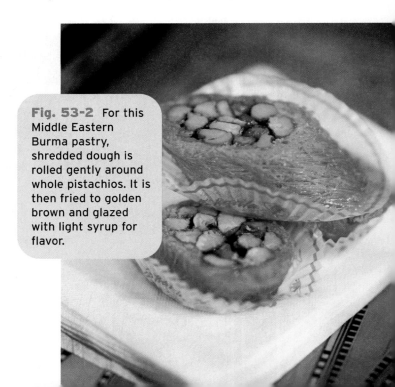

Fig. 53-2 For this Middle Eastern Burma pastry, shredded dough is rolled gently around whole pistachios. It is then fried to golden brown and glazed with light syrup for flavor.

Fig. 53-3

Hummus

Yield
5 servings; about ¼ cup each

Nutrition Analysis
Per Serving: 120 calories, 6 g total fat, 1 g saturated fat, 0 trans fat, 0 mg cholesterol, 70 mg sodium, 12 g total carbohydrate, 3 g dietary fiber, 0 g sugars, 5 g protein
Percent Daily Value: vitamin A 2%, vitamin C 6%, calcium 8%, iron 6%

Ingredients
1 cup canned garbanzo beans (chickpeas), drained and rinsed
¼ cup tahini (sesame paste)

2 Tbsp. lemon juice
1 clove garlic, minced
dash salt

1 Tbsp. minced parsley
pita bread

Directions
1. Puree beans in blender (or mash with fork). Add tahini, lemon juice, garlic, and salt. Blend until smooth.
2. Place mixture in serving bowl. Garnish with minced parsley. Serve as spread or dip with pita bread.

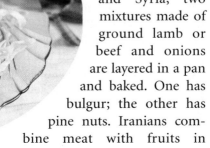

are served with strips of pita bread. See **Fig. 53-3**. You might find *falafel* (fuh-LAH-fuhl) served with a tahini sauce or yogurt dipping sauce. See **Fig. 53-4**. *Fatayer* is a turnover filled with meat, cheese, or spinach.

Vegetables and legumes appear in side dishes as well as mezza. A variety of fresh salads is built around cucumbers, tomatoes, and onions. *Tabbouleh* (tuh-BOO-luh) combines chopped parsley, tomatoes, onions, and bulgur with mint, lemon juice, and olive oil. Eggplant and zucchini lend themselves to stuffing with rice, nuts,

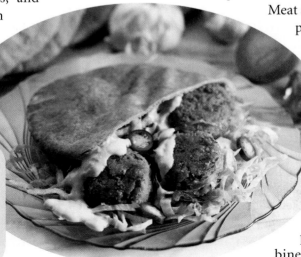

Fig. 53-4 These spiced patties of garbanzo or fava beans, onions, and garlic are called *falafel*. They are fried and often served inside pita bread.

and other vegetables. Slices may be breaded and fried. Lentils are added to soups and pilafs.

Many main dishes balance meats with grain and vegetables. Kebabs—small pieces or patties of meat, fish, or shellfish that are skewered and grilled—are usually served over rice. Meat and rice together stuff eggplant, zucchini, and cabbage or grape leaves to make *dolmas*. For *kibbeh*, the national dish of Lebanon and Syria, two mixtures made of ground lamb or beef and onions are layered in a pan and baked. One has bulgur; the other has pine nuts. Iranians combine meat with fruits in *zerkeshk polo*, rice with chicken, raisins, and bright red barberries.

Fish is readily found in coastal regions. Whitefish may be baked with tahini and pine nuts. Shrimp kebabs are basted with a garlic-seasoned yogurt marinade. *Chebeh rubyan* is balls of ground shrimp and rice, stuffed with onions, and simmered in a sauce of tomato and tamarind, a tart tropical fruit.

Coffee (*kahwah*) symbolizes hospitality throughout the Arab world. It's often made in the Turkish style—boiled three times, sweetened, and sometimes spiced with cardamom. Everyday desserts include fresh and dried fruit and *halvah*, bars of candy made with ground sesame seeds, honey, and sometimes nuts. The richer, syrup-drenched *katayef* contains sweetened cheese or cream custard between shredded pastry dough. *Mamoul*, nut-filled semolina cookies, are a tradition on the Islamic holiday Eid al-Fitr.

Israeli Cuisine

Some dishes from Israel are adopted in whole from Arab neighbors. Falafel, for example, is as common in Israel as in Jordan and Lebanon. Other foods show their immigrant roots. Eastern Europe is especially well represented. The Polish *pierogi* reappears as the *knish*, a turnover filled with potatoes, cheese, kasha, or chicken liver. *Bourekas*, a cheese-filled pastry similar to Serbia's *burek*, is a bestseller with street vendors. More recently, the Ethiopian influence has added curry powder and chiles.

Foods that can be prepared in advance are essential for the Jewish Sabbath (sundown Friday to sundown Saturday), when work is prohibited. *Cholent*, a stew of beans, potatoes, barley, and sometimes meat, is started Friday and cooked overnight. *Lokshen kugel* (noodle pudding) might be baked at the same time. Some foods take on special symbolism at holidays and holy days.

Fig. 53-5

Try This! **Recipe**

Moroccan Fruited Couscous

Yield	Nutrition Analysis
6 servings	**Per Serving:** 430 calories, 10 g total fat, 1 g saturated fat, 0 trans fat, 0 mg cholesterol, 170 mg sodium, 74 g total carbohydrate, 7 g dietary fiber, 24 g sugars, 11 g protein **Percent Daily Value:** vitamin A 2%, vitamin C 4%, calcium 8%, iron 15%

Ingredients

1 cup raisins
2 cups couscous, uncooked
1 medium onion, large dice (½ inch)
1 Tbsp. olive oil
⅛ tsp. turmeric

¾ cup slivered almonds, toasted
½ Tbsp. ground cumin
½ Tbsp. ground cinnamon
1 tsp. cayenne pepper

1 tsp. ground ginger
½ cup chicken stock
¼ tsp. salt (adjust to taste)
¼ tsp. pepper (adjust to taste)
1 Tbsp. honey (adjust to taste)

Directions

1. Place raisins in bowl. Cover with simmering water for a few minutes to plump. Drain and set aside.
2. Prepare couscous according to package directions. Set aside.
3. In large saucepan on medium-high heat, sauté onion in olive oil until onion is soft and translucent. Add turmeric and stir to release color. Add remaining ingredients except chicken stock, and sauté. Add chicken stock and bring to boil. Turn off heat.
4. Break up couscous into hot mixture and stir. Add honey, salt, and pepper to achieve a savory-sweet flavor.

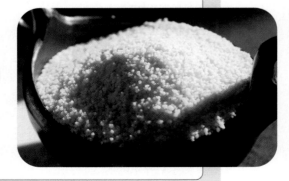

NORTH AFRICA

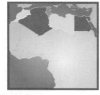

The daunting Sahara Desert sweeps across most of North Africa. Only a ribbon of land along the Mediterranean coast is hospitable to human, plant, and animal life. The Nile River waters crops, especially in Egypt—mostly wheat and barley, plus dates, nuts, olives, potatoes, and citrus fruits. Small farms are home to chickens, sheep, cattle, and goats. The Atlantic and Mediterranean supply seafood.

North African Dishes

North African foods show the influence of the Arab culture, with notable differences. The main grain is couscous, which is cooked by steaming. Traditionally, it's set over a simmering meat or vegetable stew, with which it is served, absorbing the moisture and the flavors. Couscous sweetened with sugar and dried fruit is a breakfast cereal.

North African cooks also use hotter spices. *Harissa*, a garlic-seasoned red pepper paste, is a common ingredient and condiment, especially in Morocco and Tunisia. It's sometimes found in *merguez*, a spicy Tunisian lamb sausage.

Likewise, each nation has specialties similar to, yet distinct from, those in the Middle East. Morocco has its **tagines**, well-seasoned stews made in a covered pot of the same name. Meat and fruit combinations, like lamb with prunes, are particularly popular. A dish with fruit and couscous is shown in **Fig. 53-5**. A *b'stilla* is an impressive pie filled with cooked, spiced chicken in a curdled egg sauce and topped with sugar- and cinnamon-coated almonds. Preserved lemons are the cuisine's characteristic flavoring.

Fava beans (*ful*) are favorites in Egypt. The Egyptian variety, small and brown, is preferred over garbanzo beans in falafels. *Ful medames*, a thick stew of lightly mashed beans garnished with cooked eggs, may be eaten any time of day.

Libyan cuisine stands out for its macaroni dishes, a reminder of Libya's days as an Italian colony in the early twentieth century. A Tunisian *brik* (turnover) has a filling that includes a whole egg, which is soft-cooked as the pastry fries. Algerians add raisins, almonds, and cinnamon to

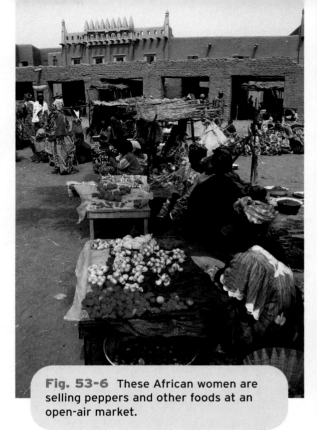

Fig. 53-6 These African women are selling peppers and other foods at an open-air market.

the sweet lamb stew *el ham lahlou*. Eggs are poached over sautéed tomatoes, peppers, and onions in *chakchouka*.

SUB-SAHARAN AFRICA

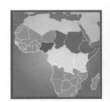

Sub-Saharan Africa is a land of dramatic contrast. In many cities, people have the same easy access to foods as you do. The food supply in rural areas, however, is a fragile chain, vulnerable to drought, poor transportation, and political instability. Many Africans rely on whatever food they can raise. Malnourishment is widespread. Famine is a constant threat.

Nevertheless, African cooking is bold in flavor and color. See **Fig. 53-6**. Only its starchy base—rice, corn, millet, plantains, cassava, and yams—is plain. Legumes and vegetables include black-eyed peas, groundnuts (peanuts), tomatoes, sweet peppers, squash, okra, and greens of all types, from beet leaves to spinach. Meatless meals are common, but so are chicken, guinea fowl, beef, fish, and goat. Chiles, red and black pepper, onions, garlic, cinnamon, nutmeg, ginger, peanut butter, and coconut milk add sweetness and heat. Tropical fruits, of course, are readily found.

Sub-Saharan Dishes

As in other parts of the world, foods and recipes vary among the regions of Sub-Saharan Africa. Customs and ingredients sometimes blend local crops and traditions with a long history of colonization by Europe.

Stew and a starch is the typical main meal. A common stew base is *moambé*, an oily broth made of palm nut pulp, seasoned with a diluted sauce. A Central African might use the peppery *egusi* sauce, a blend of ground, roasted squash seeds and tomato paste. Ethiopia's *berberé* paste includes varying amounts of red pepper, fenu-

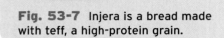

Fig. 53-7 Injera is a bread made with teff, a high-protein grain.

greek, allspice, cloves, cardamom, and turmeric.

Rice often accompanies stew. Mashed cassava is common in Central Africa, as are mashed yams in West Africa. Both foods are locally known as *fufu*. East Africa's *ugali* and Southern Africa's

Career Prep

Managing Stress

STRESS: IT CAN LEAVE YOU ANXIOUS, angry, sad, or depressed; it can lead to overeating or loss of appetite and to oversleeping or lack of sleep; it can cause stomachaches, headaches, and muscle aches; it can even cripple a relationship.

Despite all this, stress is not a disease. It's a normal response to life events and uncertainties. At work, stress may be caused by high expectations, repetitive tasks, and fatigue. People involved in international trade, for example, might work around the clock.

Not surprisingly, stress is also a leading cause of worker disability, through accident and "burn out." Certainly, coping with stress in positive ways is a valuable work skill. These suggestions can help:

- **Pinpoint the cause.** The cause of stress may be obvious, or it may be a combination of factors. Stress caused by positive events can be hardest to identify. You might be so excited about a vacation that you don't notice how the preparations are stressing you. Once you

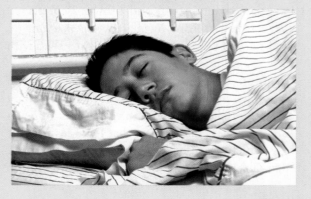

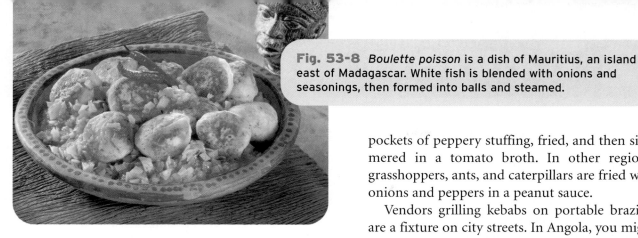

Fig. 53-8 *Boulette poisson* is a dish of Mauritius, an island east of Madagascar. White fish is blended with onions and seasonings, then formed into balls and steamed.

mealie meal both refer to a mound of fine cornmeal porridge, shaped and used as an edible scoop. Ethiopians use **injera**, a thin, spongy, sourdough flatbread, for the same purpose. See **Fig. 53-7**. Kenyans serve stew in a ring of *irio*, a mash of peas, potatoes, corn, and greens.

Other dishes also reflect local staples and traditions. **Fig. 53-8** shows a common fish dish on the island of Mauritius. Senegal's *thiebou dienn* (rice and rice) uses a technique typical on Africa's Atlantic coast. Fish steaks or fillets are filled with pockets of peppery stuffing, fried, and then simmered in a tomato broth. In other regions, grasshoppers, ants, and caterpillars are fried with onions and peppers in a peanut sauce.

Vendors grilling kebabs on portable braziers are a fixture on city streets. In Angola, you might find beef kebabs in *piri-piri* marinade, the fiery chiles brought by Portuguese colonists. On the east coast, it may be goat with garlic, ginger, and curry powder.

South African cuisine is uniquely stamped by the Dutch, German, and French settlers who blended to create the nation's Afrikaner ethnic group. It includes the sausage *boerewors* and *hoender pastei*, a pie of chicken, hard-cooked eggs, and ham, seasoned with pickling spices.

uncover the source, apply problem-solving skills to deal with it.

- **Don't procrastinate.** Avoiding an unpleasant job only prolongs the stress of having to do it.
- **Break down large tasks into short-term goals.** Achieving small goals builds a sense of confidence and control, which is essential for handling stress. Reward yourself along the way with breaks or small treats.
- **Eat right.** A nutritious diet is stress defense. It supplies physical strength to meet daily demands. Complex carbohydrates aid production of the brain chemical serotonin, which promotes a sense of well-being.
- **Get enough sleep.** Sleep is an often overlooked pillar of physical and emotional health. Cells grow and are repaired during rest. The mind is refreshed.
- **Exercise.** Physical activity offers a mental break that releases pent-up energy. Also, stressed breathing is shortened and shallow, depriving the body of oxygen. Deep breathing restores oxygen while relaxing muscles.
- **Laugh—and cry.** Shedding tears of joy, or sadness, relieves stress by lowering the level of some proteins and hormones.
- **Make time for yourself.** Try to do something each day just because you like it, whether or not it's "productive." Do a jigsaw puzzle. Feed squirrels in the park. Choose something that pleases you.
- **Stay connected.** Family, friends, co-workers, and other social groups offer a sense of support and comfort that helps you cope.

Career Connection

Expert advice. Research one of the areas discussed above. Share a list of tips or a demonstration on a related topic, such as getting a good night's sleep, low-cost fun, or relaxation.

Summarize Your Reading

▶ The cultures of Southwest Asia and Africa have provided many foods that people all over the world enjoy.

▶ People have lived in Southwest Asia since at least 10,000 B.C. Farming first began in this area of the world.

▶ Lamb, chicken, and seafood are common in Middle Eastern dishes, as are many fruits and vegetables. Seasonings are important to the cuisine.

▶ Africa is a huge continent with many countries below the Sahara Desert.

▶ North African cuisine has similarities to Middle Eastern foods, but distinct foods as well. Sub-Saharan foods blend local crops and traditions with historical influences.

Check Your Knowledge

1. Where, geographically, are the countries of Southwest Asia and North Africa?

2. What is a common name for Southwest Asia?

3. How do people in Southwest Asia make use of yogurt?

4. What is **tahini**?

5. What special knowledge might be needed by a Middle Eastern cook, and why?

6. What is **mezza**?

7. Describe these Middle Eastern dishes: a) *marcook*; b) *baba ghannoush*; c) falafel; d) tabbouleh; e) *dolmas*; f) *kibbeh*; g) *halvah*; and h) *mamoul*.

8. What is a *knish*?

9. What geographic feature exists throughout North Africa?

10. What is the main grain in North African dishes, and how is it typically used?

11. What is a **tagine**?

12. What might cooks in Egypt use in place of garbanzo beans to make *falafel*?

13. Compare food availability in cities and rural areas of Sub-Saharan Africa.

14. What foods add flavor and color to Sub-Saharan dishes?

15. What is *fufu*?

16. Name and describe a dish that a street vendor in Angola might sell.

17. **CRITICAL THINKING** What effect do you think nature has had on the food supply in Africa?

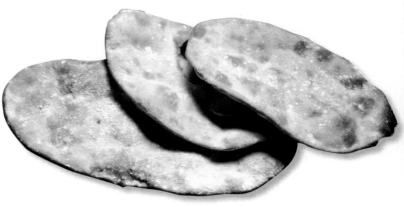

Apply Your Learning

1. **SOCIAL STUDIES** **Country Study.** Choose one country in the chapter to study. Learn about the area's history, geography, and culture. Using such visual aids as films and magazine photos, give a class presentation.

2. **Taste Test.** With your lab team, prepare a dish from one of the countries in the chapter. Present your dish with those of other teams for a class taste test.

3. **Ethnic Meal.** Plan, prepare, and serve a meal with dishes from one of the countries in the chapter.

4. **Middle Eastern Meal.** Suppose you are going to host a dinner party for eight people. The theme is Middle Eastern foods. Plan the menu and develop a work plan for preparing the meal, as you learned in Chapter 27.

5. **SOCIAL STUDIES** **Famine.** Write a news article about famine in East Africa. Research causes and potential solutions.

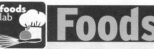 Foods Lab

Hummus Recipes

Procedure: Find and prepare a recipe for hummus. Experiment and create a dish using hummus as a spread, filling, or condiment. Share samples with the class.

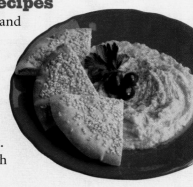

Analyzing Results

❶ How does hummus compare to popular American spreads or fillings in appearance, taste, and texture?

❷ What foods did the hummus best complement? In what ways?

❸ Describe hummus' nutrient profile. Would you suggest people include this food in their diet frequently or occasionally? Why?

 ## Food Science Experiment

Cooking Okra

Objective: To observe the properties of okra in cooking.

Procedure:

1. Cook ¼ cup of cut okra in a small amount of water over medium-low heat for five minutes. Observe the results.

2. Add one cup of beef, chicken, or vegetable broth to the saucepan. Simmer the broth for 15 minutes. Stir occasionally, noting any changes in the liquid.

3. Sample portions when the broth has cooled to serving temperature.

Analyzing Results

❶ What changes did you note after cooking the okra in water?

❷ Describe the taste, texture, and appearance of the broth after simmering. What do you think caused these results?

❸ What other vegetables have a similar effect in hot liquids? From what you observed while cooking the okra, do you think it works similarly to those vegetables, or differently? Explain.

❹ What other factors do you think make okra a common ingredient in many African soups and stews?

CHAPTER 54

Foods of South & Eastern Asia

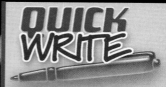

WRITING JAPANESE POETRY. Traditional Japanese foods are simply prepared, yet pleasing. The same is true of haiku, a form of traditional Japanese poetry. A haiku has three unrhymed lines of five, seven, and five syllables. Write a haiku about any aspect of Asian cuisine.

To Guide Your Reading:

Objectives

▶ Relate history and geographic location to cuisines in South and Eastern Asia.

▶ Identify typical ingredients used in dishes of South and Eastern Asia and explain how they are used.

▶ Describe and prepare dishes from South and Eastern Asia.

Terms

chutney	kimchee
curry	nori
daikon	sashimi
dal	sushi
dim sum	tandoor
hoisin	

CAN HUMAN HISTORY HINGE ON A cinnamon stick? The idea may sound extreme, yet think of the great world events that were spurred by the pursuit of the spices of South and Eastern Asia, including cinnamon. Explorations were launched. Nations were invaded. Entire cultures were changed—for both better and worse. See **Fig. 54-1**.

Meanwhile, Europeans overlooked another treasure—Asian cuisine, which had used these spices with such skill for some 3,000 years. The Dutch put cloves in their cookies and the British added ginger to their breads, but how many attempted an Indian curried rice or Chinese sweet and sour pork?

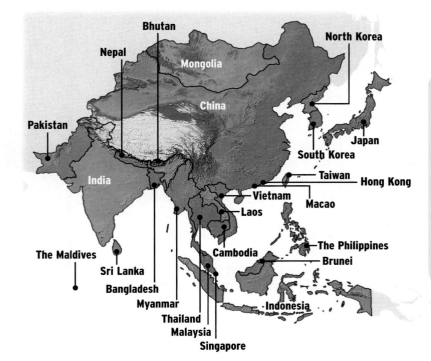

Fig. 54-1
The area of the world covered in this chapter is divided into three parts. South Asia includes India and several surrounding countries. East Asia includes China, Mongolia, Japan, the two Koreas, and nearby smaller countries. Below China and out into the Pacific Ocean are the countries of Southeast Asia. Among them are Thailand, Vietnam, and the islands of the Philippines.

SOUTH ASIA

South Asia is sometimes called the Indian subcontinent. That may lead you to forget that the region is home 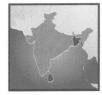 to smaller nations: Nepal, Bangladesh, and others. The term Indian, in this chapter, refers to the style of cooking that's common to all of these countries. Cooks in southern India and those in Sri Lanka may prepare different versions of the same dish.

Indian Ingredients

Farming is a major industry in South Asia. The Indus and Ganges Rivers deposit rich soil in the central plains of Pakistan and India as well as in Bangladesh's Ganges Delta. Southern India and Sri Lanka have tropical climates. These conditions are ideal for the staples that have come to define Indian cuisine: basmati rice, wheat, legumes, chiles, coconuts, mangoes, tamarinds, almonds, pistachios, and tea. Cattle, sheep, and goats are raised in hilly northern pastures. Oceans and rivers supply seafood ranging from shrimp to shark.

It's the spices that Indian cuisine is best known for, however. Cinnamon, cumin, cardamom, cloves, ginger, pepper, turmeric, garlic, cilantro, fenugreek, and mint—all these and more are expertly used. Indian cooks create personal recipes for *garam masala*. To make this mixture, they grind their favorite combinations of whole seeds, pods, and buds with a mortar and pestle. The aromatic and flavorful blends season foods and sauces. They can be tailored for each dish.

Indian Cuisine

The complexity of seasoning and variety of ingredients explain the great diversity in Indian recipes. Also, cooks may change a recipe to take advantage of seasonal foods and herbs. **Curries,** for instance, are dishes of vegetables and legumes in hot, highly seasoned sauces. Ingredients may include mung beans with pumpkin, or lentils with plantain. Seafood may be added in coastal curries. **Dal** (dahl) is a mixture or purée of legumes—mung beans, garbanzo beans, split

Fig. 54-2

Try This! **Recipe**

Dal

Yield	Nutrition Analysis
4 servings	*Per Serving:* 230 calories, 8 g total fat, 1 g saturated fat, 0 g trans fat, 0 mg cholesterol, 590 mg sodium, 30 g total carbohydrate, 15 g dietary fiber, 4 g sugars, 14 g protein *Percent Daily Value:* vitamin A 2%, vitamin C 25%, calcium 4%, iron 25%

Ingredients

1 cup split, hulled lentils or yellow split peas
2 cups water or vegetable broth
1 tsp. salt

2 Tbsp. vegetable oil
1 tsp. black mustard seed (optional)
⅓ cup chopped green pepper
⅓ cup chopped onion

½ tsp. turmeric
½ tsp. curry powder
2 tsp. lemon juice
hot, cooked rice

Directions

1. Combine lentils or split peas, water or broth, and salt in 1½-qt. saucepan. Bring to boil. Reduce heat. Simmer, covered, just until tender, about 30 minutes.
2. Heat vegetable oil in skillet. Add mustard seed. Cover and let seeds pop. Stir in green pepper, onion, turmeric, and curry powder. Sauté until vegetables are soft, about 5 minutes. Remove from heat. Stir in lemon juice.
3. Stir seasoned vegetable mixture into cooked lentils or split peas. Serve with hot, cooked rice.

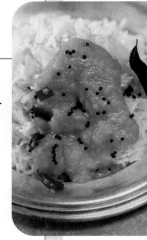

peas, and more—as well as onions, chiles, and tomatoes. See **Fig. 54-2**.

In addition, there is **chutney**, a zesty condiment made from fruit, sugar, spices, and vinegar. Chutneys, hot or mild, balance contrasting flavors—sweet and hot peppers, for instance, or mangoes and raisins with pepper and nutmeg. Cooler yogurt condiments, *raitas*, may include cucumber or onion and mint or garlic.

Nonetheless, due to different histories and geographies, some dishes and ingredients are more typical of northern or southern cuisine.

Northern Indian Cuisine

Both bread and rice are common in northern India. Both may be found in the same meal. *Nan*, the traditional flatbread, is usually yogurt leavened. Like other baked foods, it's cooked in a **tandoor**, a rounded, clay, charcoal-burning oven. See **Fig. 54-3**. A *chapati* is an unleavened disk of whole-wheat flour and water. Breads serve as a scoop for main dishes. Eating with the fingertips of the right hand is proper Indian etiquette.

Main dishes in the North often include meat. Chicken kebabs are marinated in seasoned yogurt in *murgh tikka masala*. Lamb simmered in a yogurt sauce, *rogan josh*, is served over rice. *Biryani* is a casserole of meat sautéed in *ghee* (clarified butter), then cooked with rice and flavored with fried onions.

Desserts often feature sweetened dairy foods. Northeastern India is known for "burned milk" dishes like *sandesh*. In this dish, condensed milk is cooked with *paneer*, a firm yogurt cheese similar to ricotta. *Gajar halwa*, a custard of grated carrots cooked with milk and sugar, is garnished with raisins and nuts. Shredded coconut is moistened with condensed milk and wrapped around a center of ground pistachios to make *coco pista pasand*.

Southern Indian Cuisine

Overall, Southern cuisine is more vegetarian, although some who follow Hindu practices eat

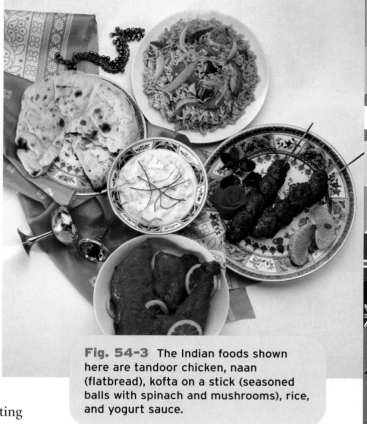

Fig. 54-3 The Indian foods shown here are tandoor chicken, naan (flatbread), kofta on a stick (seasoned balls with spinach and mushrooms), rice, and yogurt sauce.

animal products selectively—only fish, chicken, or eggs, for example. Religious beliefs and the tropical setting lead to greater use of legumes and vegetables. Sesame oil may be used instead of ghee.

Rice is the preferred grain in the South. Bowls of rice may be served plain. Parboiled rice and soaked beans are ground to make the batter for *dosa*. These large, crisp but flexible crepes may be filled with spiced potatoes, another staple starch. A special meal might include puffy, deep-fried rounds of bread called *poori*. The sauces in **Fig. 54-4** on page 730 often accompany dishes.

Southern foods tend to be more highly spiced than in the North. Chiles are used abundantly, often cooled by a coconut milk sauce. Shrimp simmered in coconut milk and curry powder, served over rice, is typical of southern coastal cuisine.

Northern tastes in desserts apply as well to the South. You may also find colorful fruit salads of pears, bananas, melons, and grapes, glistening with honey and orange juice and garnished with nuts.

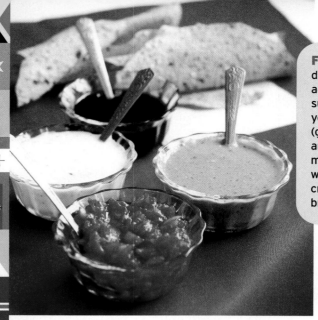

Fig. 54-4 Indian dishes are often accompanied by such sauces as yogurt (white), mint (green), onion (red), and tamarind. They may also be enjoyed with *papadum*, a crispy, crackerlike bread.

coli, spinach, cabbage, eggplant, peppers, green beans, bean sprouts, and mushrooms—all may fill the wok and steamer daily. Carrots, **daikon** (an Asian radish), and other root vegetables are also common. Pork, chicken, beef, and duck, much of it raised on family farms, have been favored meats since the second century B.C.

Wheat, rice flour, and bean starch are used to make noodles and dumplings. Soybeans are the base of soy sauce, a staple seasoning. The Chinese are credited with inventing tofu, the soy curds that they use in both savory and sweet dishes. With colorful names like cloud ears and tiger lily buds, mushrooms provide texture and flavor.

A variety of condiments add sweetness and spice. Besides soy sauce, cooks use plum sauce, oyster sauce, and **hoisin** sauce, which is thick, soy-sauce-based paste seasoned with chiles and garlic. See **Fig. 54-5**. Black and red beans and dried shrimp are mashed into pastes. For extra heat, Chinese mustard is used alone or mixed with other condiments. Sesame and peanut oil lend the flavor and aroma of lightly roasted nuts to fried foods.

EAST ASIA

Although many people tend to think of Chinese, Japanese, and Korean foods together, fans of East Asian cuisine know that no single description fits them all. The more you learn of these cuisines, the more you will see the similarities and differences.

One common thread in these cuisines is striving for balance in flavors, textures, and techniques. This balance is known as "yin and yang." The five basic flavors of sweet, salty, sour, bitter, and umami (savory) are incorporated in the balance.

China

Five thousand years ago, people were raising cattle and rice in northern China. The reverence for cooking and food may be just as old. A Chinese proverb says, "Govern the Empire as carefully as you would cook a small fish."

Chinese Ingredients

Although it's the world's third-largest nation, China has relatively little farmland. This lack is balanced by a wide range of climates and, in the south, a long growing season. In fact, farmers supply almost all the food needs of their one billion fellow citizens, and in great variety.

Long-grain rice and vegetables are the mainstays of Chinese cooking. Onions, scallions, broc-

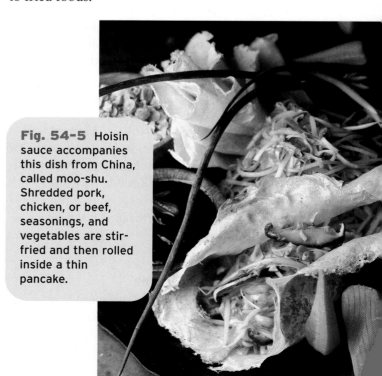

Fig. 54-5 Hoisin sauce accompanies this dish from China, called moo-shu. Shredded pork, chicken, or beef, seasonings, and vegetables are stir-fried and then rolled inside a thin pancake.

With fuel scarce in China, stir-frying became the cooking method of choice. Steaming is also common, and some foods are deep-fried. A food might even be deep-fried first to get a crispy crust before steaming to complete the dish.

Chinese Cuisine

Unlike other food customs you've read about, Chinese cuisine grew from within, with little outside influence. In a country so immense, it may come as no surprise that different styles developed in different regions, with people using the same basic ingredients.

South Coastal China

The southeastern seacoast near Canton is the heart of Cantonese cuisine. Tropical weather and an abundant supply of fresh food, especially seafood, are its inspiration. Cantonese foods are mildly seasoned and lightly cooked, often steamed or stir-fried. Bass steamed with ginger, onion, and soy sauce is a popular dish. So are fried rice and spring rolls, which are similar to egg rolls but smaller and more delicate. See **Fig. 54-6**. Buddha's delight, a stir-fried medley of carrots, mushrooms, snow peas, water chestnuts, and other vegetables, may be tossed with noodles or bean curd sticks.

Cantonese cuisine is also known for **dim sum**—bite-size dishes eaten at tea or between courses of a banquet. *Dim sum* morsels are meant to delight the eye as well as the tongue with their artistry and variety. A tray may include small plates of steamed meat- or vegetable-filled dumplings, deep-fried sesame balls, custard tarts, and fried chicken feet flavored with star anise and ginger.

Fig. 54-6

Try This! **Recipe**

Asian Fried Rice with Peas

Yield
8 servings, about ½ cup each

Nutrition Analysis
Per Serving: 140 calories, 2 g total fat, 0 g saturated fat, 0 g trans fat, 0 mg cholesterol, 135 mg sodium, 27 g total carbohydrate, 2 g dietary fiber, 3 g sugars, 4 g protein
Percent Daily Value: vitamin A 10%, vitamin C 15%, calcium 2%, iron 10%

Ingredients
1 Tbsp. canola oil
½ bunch green onions, divided, and cut into thin spirals
2 Tbsp. fresh chopped cilantro

4 cups cooked, long-grain white rice, chilled or room temperature
1 tsp. cumin

1 Tbsp. soy sauce
1½ Tbsp. seasoned rice vinegar
1 cup frozen peas
1 cup bean sprouts, washed and trimmed

Directions
1. In large, nonstick skillet or wok over medium-high heat, sauté half of the sliced green onions in oil until fragrant, about 1 minute. Add chopped cilantro and mix well.
2. Add rice, stirring to separate grains until heated, about 2 minutes.
3. Add cumin, soy sauce, and rice vinegar. Stir-fry until well mixed.
4. Sprinkle in frozen peas and bean sprouts and sauté until mixture is hot and peas are warmed. Transfer rice to serving plate and garnish with remaining chopped green onion spirals.

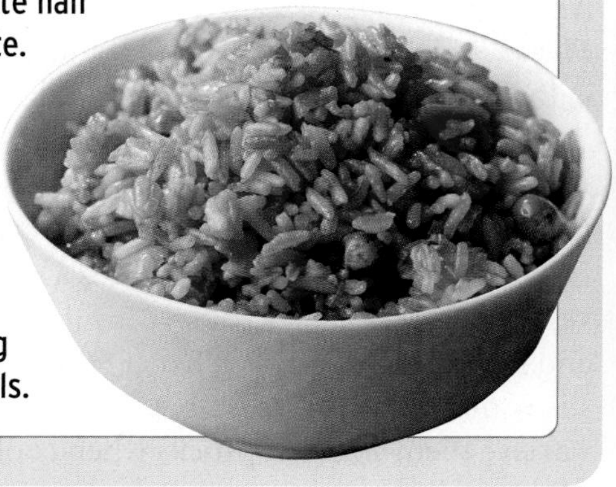

Fig. 54-7

Edamame Salad

Yield	Nutrition Analysis
4 servings	***Per Serving:*** 190 calories, 6 g total fat, 0 g saturated fat, 0 g trans fat, 0 mg cholesterol, 1000 mg sodium, 17 g total carbohydrate, 3 g dietary fiber, 5 g sugars, 17 g protein ***Percent Daily Value:*** vitamin A 15%, vitamin C 8%, calcium 15%, iron 15%

Ingredients

1 package (1 pound) edamame beans, cooked, shelled, and chilled

¾ cup chopped green onion

2 Tbsp. sesame seeds and dried sea vegetable seasoning (homemade or prepared)

2 Tbsp. ponzu sauce (or mix splash of lemon with 2 Tbsp. soy sauce)

1 Tbsp. seasoned rice vinegar

¼ tsp. salt

Directions

1. In medium-size bowl, toss together edamame beans, green onion, and sesame and sea vegetable seasoning.
2. Add ponzu sauce, rice vinegar, and salt. Mix thoroughly with rubber spatula.

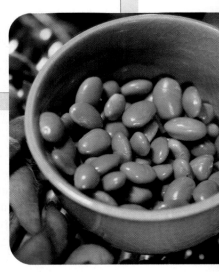

North China and Mongolia

Since natural resources are scarce in the northern region of China, much of the food is simply prepared. Wheat and millet grow in the region rather than rice. Cabbage is the main vegetable. Noodle soups with shreds of meat and vegetables, grilled lamb or mutton, and a minimum of seasoning characterize the cooking.

From China's capital of Beijing comes simple, but refined, cuisine. Peking Duck is the most famous dish of the north. (Peking is the old spelling for the city.) The two-day preparation yields a moist duck with crispy, golden skin. Another specialty is called *Lotus Buns* or *Beijing Flower Rolls*. These are steamed dumplings filled with minced green onion and ham.

Cooking on the dining table is a specialty in northern China as well as Mongolia, a neighbor to the north. One dish known around the world is the Mongolian Hot Pot that uses a special brass vessel set on the table. The pot is filled with broth and heated with charcoal. Diners drop wafer-thin slices of meat and vegetables into the pot and retrieve them with chopsticks when cooked. After cooking, diners drink the broth.

Central and Western China

Highly seasoned flavors typify the cooking of Szechuan, Hunan, and Yunnan provinces. Chiles season many dishes and sesame oil is commonly used. The aromatic Szechwan peppercorn is used liberally. *Su ch'un chuan* are crisply fried vegetarian spring rolls served with sweet and sour sauce. Carp from the Yellow River is served with bean sauce or sweet and sour sauce. Hot and sour soup is a specialty.

East Coastal China

In Hangchow, Soochow, and Shangai, you'll find dishes marked by a careful blend of sweet and sour flavors. Cooks prepare steamed dumplings and thick round noodles. Seafood and fish from the Yangtze River are mainstays. A rice dish called *juk* accompanies meals. Many dishes are braised, and the signature sauce is rich brown sauce. Bird's nest soup comes from this area.

Japan

Four main islands make up Japan. The islands are mountainous, with only twelve to fifteen percent of the land fertile enough to raise crops.

Japan adapted and refined ingredients and methods from China, Portugal, and America. Japanese cuisine evolved over the centuries into an orderly and aesthetic style. It reflects the industriousness of the people, who have created a remarkable industrialized society on a relatively limited land base.

Japanese Ingredients

Nowhere is the soybean more important than in Japan, where it was brought from China by Buddhist monks in the seventh century. Soy sauce is a primary seasoning ingredient. Tofu is sautéed, broiled, and deep-fried for dishes. *Miso*, a fermented bean paste, comes in a variety of flavors and colors. It flavors and thickens broths, marinades, sauces, and salad dressings. **Fig. 54-7** is a recipe that uses soybeans.

The Japanese harvest sea vegetables and cultivate mushrooms. As in the rest of Asia, rice is essential in Japan.

Japanese Dishes

The Japanese are famous for *Kobe* beef. Kobe beef comes from cattle raised on a special diet in Kobe, Japan. Prior to steak-size portions of Kobe beef, all meat was cut into small pieces for such dishes as *sukiyaki* and *teriyaki*. Sukiyaki is uniformly thin slices of seasoned beef and vegetables that are quickly grilled, sometimes at the table. Teriyaki refers to grilling or broiling small, marinated slices of chicken or fish until they have a shiny glaze.

The Japanese make good use of mushrooms. The matsutake mushroom, with steaklike texture and unusual aroma, is prized. Shiitake, oyster, and enoki mushrooms are cultivated.

The sea rules Japanese life. The Japanese bring in the world's largest fish catch annually. They cook fish whole with the skin on to keep the flesh moist. They dry tuna into bonito flakes to make *dashi*, a stock for soup or for flavoring other dishes. *Tempura* is a dish of crisp, batter-fried vegetable and fish morsels. The fish in Japan is so fresh that they serve it raw with condiments as **sashimi**. **Sushi** is the name of the vinegary rice that is rolled up in sashimi or **nori** (seaweed wrapper). See **Fig. 54-8**.

North and South Korea

Korea is situated on a peninsula between China and Japan. Korea is currently divided into North and South Korea. Korean cuisine is based largely on rice, vegetables, fish, seaweed, and tofu.

The nation is renowned for its traditional dish called **kimchee**. Kimchee is made by a unique process of preserving vegetables by fermentation. Made with cabbage, daikon radish, or cucumbers, the ingredients are seasoned with salt, pepper, garlic, and chiles and packed into stone jars. It's then left until the ingredients ferment. Kimchee is served as a very hot condiment.

Chiles and peppers season most dishes. Other seasonings include garlic, soy sauce, and ginger. Sesame seeds are used toasted, as oil, or as a paste. Abalone, crayfish, scallops, clams, shrimp, squid, and octopus are among the seafoods cooked with noodles or rice.

Bulgogi is Korean barbecue. Diners grill their own paper-thin slices of beef on a small grill in the middle of the dining table and then dip it in a hot pepper sauce.

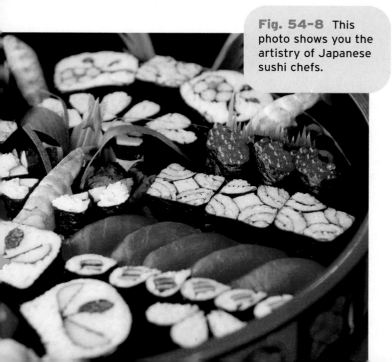

Fig. 54-8 This photo shows you the artistry of Japanese sushi chefs.

SOUTHEAST ASIA

The countries of Southeast Asia lie south of China and east of India. The area includes a peninsula and thousands of islands. Fresh flavors and a balance that leaves all the tastes satisfied describe the cooking of Laos, Thailand, Cambodia, and Vietnam. The most important seasoning in the region is fish sauce, called *nam pla* in Thailand and *nuoc nam* in Vietnam.

A specialty of Laos, Cambodia, and Vietnam is wrapping ingredients in leaves. One example is ground pork, seasoned with herbs and spices, and grilled and wrapped in lettuce leaves.

In Thailand you'll find colorful green, yellow, and red curries that use fish, pork, duck, and vegetables. Spring rolls are made with soft rice papers wrapped around crab, pork, mushrooms, bean threads, and bean sprouts. See **Fig. 54-9**. A favorite dessert in Thailand is *Kha Ya Khoo*, green rice cream.

Vietnam's national dish is *pho*, a beef and noodle soup. Another regional specialty is *chao tom*.

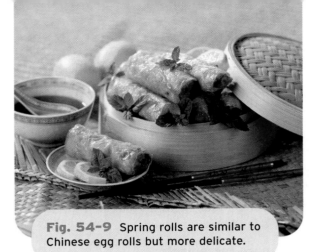

Fig. 54-9 Spring rolls are similar to Chinese egg rolls but more delicate.

For this, a length of sugarcane stalk is peeled, coated with a layer of pounded shrimp, and grilled. It's dipped in a fish-based sauce and served with fried shrimp wafers. Fried bananas on custard is a typical Vietnamese dessert.

Wild mushrooms grow in Laos, where the national dish is *o-lam*. This is a combination of cubed water buffalo meat cooked with local beans, eggplant, several types of wild mushrooms, and fennel.

Career Prep

Workplace Laws

THE SAFETY AND FAIRNESS PEOPLE have come to expect at work didn't always exist. Those features result from a body of federal law that covers almost all private and public employers, including employment agencies. Fair treatment is required in all areas of employment, from hiring and promotions, to use of company facilities, to the language used in want ads. Laws also ban retaliation against workers who pursue their rights under these statutes.

Some significant pieces of legislation are summarized here:

- **The Fair Labor Standards Act of 1938** establishes a national minimum wage and requires at least time and a half (regular wages plus 50 percent) for over 40 hours worked in a week. It also regulates child labor.

- **The Equal Pay Act of 1963** requires an employer to pay the same wage to men and women who perform substantially the same work.

- **The Civil Rights Act of 1964** bars discrimination, including harassment, based on race, national origin, religion, or gender. Pregnancy and childbirth must be treated like other temporary conditions. This act created the Equal Employment Opportunity Commission (EEOC), the independent federal agency that enforces antidiscrimination law.

Indonesia

The islands of Indonesia (Java, Bali, Borneo, Sumatra, and Celebes) are known as the "Spice Islands." They cover nearly 800,000 square miles on more than 15,000 islands in the Pacific Ocean. They straddle the equator between Australia and the Asian mainland. In this tropical zone, turmeric, cloves, nutmeg, mace, and cinnamon grow. Such fruits as oranges, mandarins, grapefruits, mangoes, bananas, pineapples, papayas, avocado, and coconut are plentiful. See **Fig. 54-10**.

One distinguishing condiment unique to Indonesia and other parts of Southeast Asia is the sweet soy sauce called *ketjap manis*. Other typical seasonings include coconut, lemon grass, shrimp paste, and chiles.

The Philippines

The traditional cooking of the Philippines is obvious in classic dishes. Next to rice, which is eaten three times a day, seafood is the most important ingredient. *Kinilaw* is fish preserved in a vinegar-and-salt mixture.

Filipino noodles, called *pansit*, are made with rice flour and are typically sautéed with garlic. *Lumpia* are spring rolls dipped in a soy sauce, vinegar, and garlic mixture. The main vegetables used are sweet potatoes, tomatoes, cabbage, and eggplant.

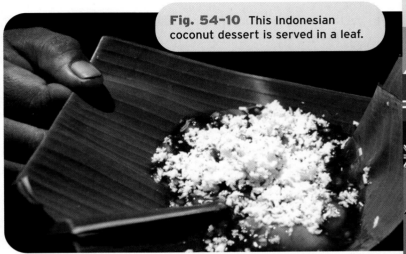

Fig. 54-10 This Indonesian coconut dessert is served in a leaf.

- **The Age Discrimination in Employment Act of 1967** protects workers and job applicants 40 years and older from unfair treatment based on age.

- **The Occupational Safety and Health Act of 1970** is a landmark in worker welfare. It created the Occupational Safety and Health Administration (OSHA) and empowered the agency to set and enforce standards to prevent workplace illness and injury.

- **The Americans with Disabilities Act of 1990** bars discrimination of qualified employees due to disability, an impairment that seriously limits a major life activity, such as breathing or learning. Employers must make "reasonable accommodation," such as shifting some duties, unless it would cause "undue hardship." "Accommodation" doesn't include lowering standards or goals.

- **The Family and Medical Leave Act of 1993** gives workers 12 weeks unpaid leave annually for childbirth or adoption or for their own or a family member's illness.

Career Connection

Teen rules. Visit the Teen Workers pages of the OSHA Web site and take the quiz on teens' legal rights and restrictions. Check your answers.

Summarize Your Reading

▶ In addition to part of Russia, many of the countries in this chapter make up the Asian continent.

▶ As the largest country in South Asia, India is the farthest south, stretching into the Indian Ocean.

▶ China is the world's third largest country. Japan is a chain of islands, with the Sea of Japan to the west and the Pacific Ocean to the east. These two countries, along with others, are in East Asia.

▶ Below China and out into the Pacific Ocean are the countries of Southeast Asia. They include Thailand, Vietnam, and the Philippines.

▶ While cuisines in all these countries have common characteristics, they also have many distinctions.

Check Your Knowledge

1. How did spices have an impact on Asian history?

2. What staples define Indian cuisine?

3. Describe these Indian dishes: a) **curries**; b) **dal**; and c) **chutney**.

4. What is a **tandoor** and how is it used?

5. How might rice be used in southern Indian cooking?

6. Since China has relatively little farmland, how is it able to raise enough food for the population?

7. How do Chinese foods get much of their sweetness and spiciness?

8. What cooking methods are commonly used in China?

9. What is **dim sum**? In what cuisine is it a specialty?

10. Why is food prepared simply in northern China?

11. What characteristic is common to both Szechuan and Hunan cuisines in central and western China?

12. What ingredient is particularly important in Japan?

13. Describe the Japanese dishes, *sukiyaki* and *teriyaki*.

14. Describe two ways the Japanese eat raw fish.

15. How is Korean **kimchee** made?

16. **CRITICAL THINKING** Why do you think foods like *kimchee* are made in Asia?

17. How is the Vietnamese dish *chao tom* made and served?

18. What seasonings grow in Indonesia?

19. In the Philippines, what are *pansit* and *lumpia*?

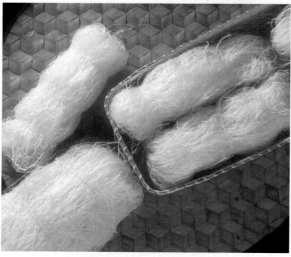

Korean cellophane noodles

Apply Your Learning

1. **SOCIAL STUDIES** **Country Study.** Choose one country in the chapter to study. Learn about the area's history, geography, and culture. Using such visual aids as films and magazine photos, give a class presentation.

2. **Taste Test.** With your lab team, prepare a dish from one of the countries in the chapter. Present your dish for a class taste test.

3. **Ethnic Meal.** Plan, prepare, and serve a meal with dishes from one of the countries in the chapter.

4. **Menu Interpretation.** Obtain a menu from a restaurant that serves Indian cuisine. Choose five terms related to dishes and learn what they mean. *Korma* and *vindaloo* are two examples.

5. **Mushroom Investigation.** Visit an Asian market to see the kinds of mushrooms available. What dried and fresh mushrooms can you find? Prepare an Asian recipe that uses a mushroom variety that you haven't eaten before.

 Foods Lab

Serving Traditional Meals

Procedure: Learn how a particular food is traditionally served in Japanese, Chinese, or other Asian culture. Demonstrate this technique for the class. If possible, use authentic foods, serving pieces, and table settings.

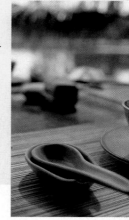

Analyzing Results

❶ How does this method of serving compare to that used in typical American meals?

❷ How do you think this way of serving reflects the culture's philosophy of cooking or sharing meals?

❸ What elements of this service would you like to adapt to American meals? How would you do this?

 Food Science Experiment

Cooking Rice

Objective: To evaluate different methods of cooking rice.

Procedure:

1. Prepare ¼ cup of dry, uncooked rice using one of the methods below, as assigned by your teacher:

   Method 1: Stir together the rice, ½ cup of water, and 1 tsp. oil in a saucepan. Bring the mixture to a boil. Immediately reduce the heat and simmer, covered, for 15 minutes.

   Method 2: Combine the ingredients as for method 1. Simmer uncovered for 15 minutes.

   Method 3: Combine ingredients as for method 1. Simmer, covered, for 15 minutes. Stir well every three minutes.

2. Set the saucepan of cooked rice on a counter for class evaluation and comparison.

Analyzing Results

❶ Compare the appearance and texture of rice produced by each method. Which method produced the best rice?

❷ Why do you think each result occurred?

❸ Some recipes, such as risotto, call for sautéing raw rice in hot oil and then gradually adding liquid while stirring continuously. Why do you think those recipes are successful?

CHAPTER 55
Foods of Australia & Oceania

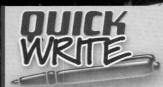

WRITING AN OPINION. Many people are intrigued by the idea of visiting Australia or an island in the South Pacific. Does that sound appealing to you? Write your opinion, giving reasons that explain your thinking.

To Guide Your Reading:

Objectives

▶ Relate history and geographic location to cuisines in Australia and Oceania.

▶ Identify typical ingredients used in dishes of Australia and Oceania and explain how they are used.

▶ Describe and prepare dishes from Australia and Oceania.

Terms
breadfruit
flummery
guava
rissoles

THIS CHAPTER MARKS YOUR LAST GLOBAL foods exploration. Until now, much of your study has been above the equator, in the Northern Hemisphere, or top half, of the world. Now it's time to travel "down under," that is, below the equator to Australia and the many islands of the South Pacific. See **Fig. 55-1**.

Papua New Guinea

Australia

Fiji

New Zealand

Fig. 55-1 Australia is the world's sixth largest country. It is mostly deserts and dry grasslands. East of Australia are thousands of islands known as Oceania. The largest of these is New Zealand. You may be familiar with other South Pacific islands, such as Fiji, New Guinea, Tahiti, Guam, Samoa, Bora Bora, and Tonga.

AUSTRALIA

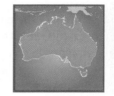

Do you know what country is surrounded by water although it's not an island? Because of Australia's size, geographers consider it to be a continent rather than an island. It's the smallest continent in the world, with a size slightly smaller than the United States.

Look to the southeastern corner of Australia and you'll see where much of the population lives. Besides the largest cities, this area also has a narrow plain with fertile farmland. More farmland is along the southern coast of the country.

If you're familiar with Australia, you've probably heard of the vast inland area called the "outback." There, dry grasslands are home to such unusual animals as kangaroos, koalas, dingoes, wombats, kookaburras, emus, dugongs, and bandicoots. Pastureland supports sheep and cattle ranches, or stations, as well as mining towns. Australians call remote rural regions the "bush."

Like the United States, Australia is a "melting pot" of ethnic influences. Since it wasn't on major trade routes, Australia has a history all its own.

TRENDS in TECHNOLOGY

BUSH TUCKER

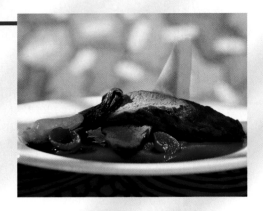

Americans might call it "down home" or "country" cooking. In Australia, it's "bush tucker," the foods and preparation methods of the Aborigines, and it's a recognized cuisine today. The bush is the outback, the rugged, remote land of Australia's Northern Territory. "Tucker" is Australian slang for food. Eating bush tucker is literally living off the land. Staples include a bounty of native game and seafood, nuts and seeds, grubs (immature worms), and wild greens, herbs, fruits, and vegetables.

Preparation technology is basic but effective. Cooking might be done in a *kup-murri*, or ground oven, a kind of outdoor grill. Coals are placed in the bottom of the pit, allowed to burn down, and then covered with stones. Meats or root vegetables, wrapped in palm leaves or paperbark (from the Mellaluca tree) are set on top. Leaves and dirt line the oven sides and cover the food.

Utensils also show Aboriginal resourcefulness. A root vegetable might be shredded with a piece of bark, then tied in a small bag and hung in a stream to rinse away any bitterness. It would be drained through a bundle of grass and roasted over coals.

Lately, food processors have applied modern technology to take advantage of bush tucker's current appeal. You can now buy everything from jars of *quandong* (wild peach) preserves to *witchetty* grubs in cans.

THINK BEYOND>> How might commercially prepared bush tucker compare to the original recipes in taste?

Culinary History

The first people to live in Australia were the Aborigines, who came from Southeast Asia around 40,000 years ago. Most Aborigines were hunter-gatherers. While they didn't grow crops, they still preserved foods. They gathered palm nuts, which they sliced and dried in the sun. Then they wrapped the kernels in bark and stored them in an earthen trench. After pounding the dried kernels into flour, the Aborigines made a primitive bread or biscuit that was cooked on hot rocks over a fire. To preserve meat, they shredded it into strips and placed it in the sun to dry. The original meat was from snakes, crocodiles, emus, wallaby, and kangaroo.

In the late 1770s, the voyages of Captain James Cook provided the British with a claim to Australia. The British king, George III, established a colony for prisoners there. Gradually, British settlers followed, bringing their love of meat and potatoes with them.

In 1792, the settlers began farming huge tracts of land and growing food for the colony. Sugarcane became a major crop. Raising sheep became a major industry.

Since these early days, immigrants from many countries have brought their own culinary specialties to Australia.

Australian Ingredients

Australians have come a long way from the first foods of the colonists. With a range of climates and advanced farming techniques, ingredients are now grown for just about any cuisine in the world.

An Australian cook can use traditional European foods, such as potatoes, cabbage, onions, carrots, and barley. American peppers, chiles, sweet potatoes, pumpkins, and corn are grown. In the tropical areas, mangos, pineapples, papayas, lemons, limes, and oranges flourish. Other available fruits include grapes, figs, nectarines, peaches, apricots, apples, plums, pears, and bananas. Leeks, broad beans, artichokes, almonds, and olives also thrive in Australia.

Australia's favorite meats are lamb, beef, and pork; however, duck, turkey, chicken, and kangaroo are also eaten. A huge variety of cheeses are made from the milk of cows, sheep, and goats. *Cheedam*, for example, is a golden yellow cheese similar to cheddar.

Australian Dishes

At one time, Australians depended on mutton stew, potatoes, peas, and tinned foods from England. British meat pies that contained oysters, lamb, beef, and such local ingredients as candied lemon and lime peel were a favorite. Leftover corned beef with onions was made into deep-fried pastries called **rissoles** (rih-SOHLS).

Some dishes have survived from the past. Flour dough is made into *johnnycakes*, which are like scones. Called "dampers," these were a staple to the Australian cowboys, or "drovers." See **Fig. 55-2**. Breakfast is oatmeal with brown sugar, muesli (cereal) and fruit, or eggs, bacon, and sausages, which the Australians call "snags." Cooking on the "barbie," or barbecuing, is a favorite cooking method for simple as well as

elaborate meals. A classic dessert is **flummery**, a sweet pudding thickened with gelatin or cornstarch and flavored with oranges or passion fruit.

In recent years, many changes have occurred in Australian cuisine. If you walk down the street in Sidney, Melbourne, or Brisbane, you'll find restaurants and foods similar to those in the United States.

OCEANIA

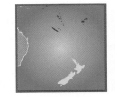

Although Australia is not an island, there are many islands in this area of the world: in fact, about 25,000 of them. Collectively called Oceania (oh-shee-A-nee-uh), these islands all lie in the southern part of the Pacific Ocean. The two largest islands are New Zealand and New Guinea.

Due to the climate and geography, the islanders cook with similar ingredients. The main crops on the islands include sugarcane, cocoa, and tropical fruits. **Breadfruit** is native to the region. This large tropical fruit is related to the fig family. It may be served baked, grilled, fried, or boiled. Seafood is also a major source of food and income.

New Zealand

Although it looks close on the map, New Zealand is a thousand miles from Australia. It is one of the most geographically isolated countries in the world. The first settlers in New Zealand were the Maori, who came from Polynesia around the ninth century.

The most famous culinary contribution of the Maori is *hangi*. This is the name for the traditional Maori feast, which is cooked in a rock-lined earth oven. It's similar to a Hawaiian luau, the Mexican *barbacoa*, Peruvian *pachamanca*, and the Australian Aborigines' earth oven.

The hangi is a feast of vegetables, meats, poultry, and fish. Peeled potatoes, sweet potatoes, and pumpkin are wrapped in taro or cabbage leaves. A leg of lamb or pork, whole chickens, and fish are placed in baskets made from flax or chicken wire.

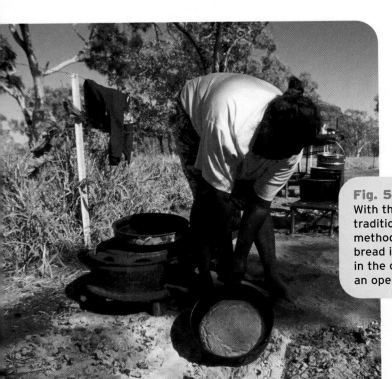

Fig. 55-2
With the traditional method, damper bread is baked in the coals of an open fire.

Once the fire burns to embers, the food baskets are placed on top. The meat goes in first, then the poultry, and lastly, the vegetables and fish. Wet sacks are placed over the top of the food, and dirt is shoveled on to cover it. After three to five hours of cooking time, the dirt is scraped away, the food is removed, and it is ready for serving.

All over New Zealand, people enjoy seafood. Cockles, oysters, lobsters, scallops, cod, flounder, king fish, snapper, squid, and salmon from the sea and rainbow trout from local streams are abundant. A classic New Zealand dish is *whitebait*. These tiny transparent fish are served as omelet-like patties.

Cows are raised in most parts of New Zealand. The beef is cut into thick juicy steaks. Cows' creamy milk makes excellent ice cream and cheese.

Veal, duck, and venison are favorite meats. Coconuts, citrus fruits, pineapples, papayas, bananas, tomatoes, yams, beans, and coffee beans are used in everyday New Zealand cuisines. Taro root is also a regular at meals.

New Zealand has been described as a "land of plenty." It is known throughout the world for lamb. The favorite way to prepare lamb is roasted

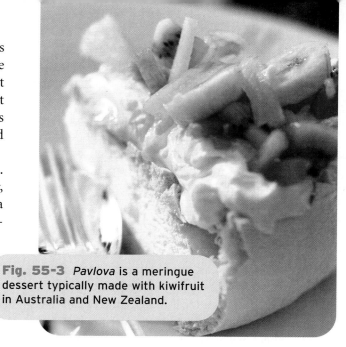

Fig. 55-3 *Pavlova* is a meringue dessert typically made with kiwifruit in Australia and New Zealand.

with garlic and served with a vinegary mint sauce.

The country is also known for kiwifruit. See **Fig. 55-3**. Kiwifruit was brought to New Zealand by the Chinese a hundred years ago. Kiwi is the Maori name for a chicken-like bird similar to an ostrich or emu. New Zealanders are nicknamed "kiwis" throughout the world.

Career Prep

Career Advancement

WILL YOU HAVE ONE JOB FOR LIFE?
Probably not. Whether you change jobs or move to different positions within a company, career advancement is likely. For many, it's a goal. To make career advancement part of your career path, take advantage of these resources:

• **Mentors.** Mentors are more experienced workers who advise and support you in career decisions. Some experts say good mentors are the most valuable asset in career advancement. Some companies pair older and younger workers in formal programs, but mentors exist in

every workplace. Look for those who share your career area as well as your work philosophy. If you value spending time with family, someone who enjoys 60-hour work weeks might not steer you in the path you desire.

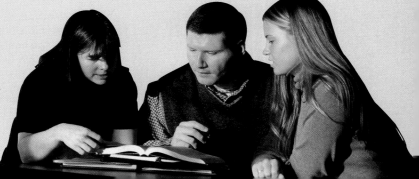

French Polynesia

The islands of the South Pacific are scattered over 70 million square miles. French Polynesia has steep mountains, beautiful waterfalls, and dense tropical foliage. Coconut palms, banana trees, and banyan trees grow everywhere. The people grow vanilla beans of high quality and raise poultry, pigs, and cattle.

Tahiti is the largest island found in French Polynesia. Restaurants and ingredients show the French influence. The tropical staples, including grapefruit, limes, bananas, and coconuts are the backbone of the local cuisine. See **Fig. 55-4**. **Guava** is a sweet tropical fruit eaten raw or used for preserves. Such seafood as swordfish, *mahi mahi* (dolphin fish), and tuna is plentiful.

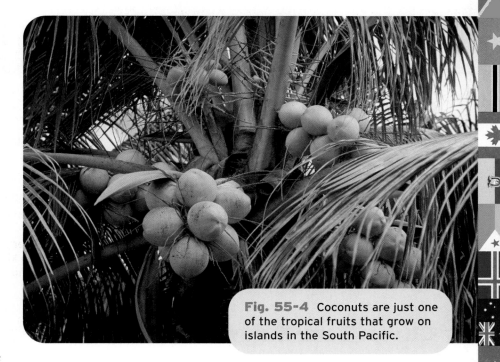

Fig. 55-4 Coconuts are just one of the tropical fruits that grow on islands in the South Pacific.

The traditional pit cooking is *hima'a* and the feast is called *tamaaraa*. Ingredients that go into a Tahitian hima'a include chunks of peeled breadfruit, peeled taro, suckling pig studded with garlic, and a whole fish or two. The food is wrapped in banana leaves and cooked in a fire pit.

- **Networking.** The same skills that help you find a job can help you advance in one. As you settle into the field, add new connections. Introduce yourself at trade shows, and get involved with professional groups. Don't forget family and friends. They may have valuable ties in other areas, plus a desire to help. Networks are a two-way street. Just as others support you, you can help others.

- **Continuing education.** An advanced degree is useful, and sometimes required, to move ahead in some fields. Extra training also looks good on a resumé. It gives employers more confidence in your abilities and shows that you take your job and career seriously. Opportunities to continue formal education are growing. More schools offer classes online, on weekends, at night, and during the summer. Weekend or one-day seminars may sharpen skills. Employers often help with schedules or tuition. Some companies offer training programs for aspiring managers.

Ideally, you choose to leave a job for one you like more. As you look for a new job, arrange interviews around your current work. Give at least two weeks notice and offer to help train your replacement. If you're pressured to quit a job or are fired, strive to leave on the same positive terms.

Career Connection

Interview. Interview a human resources representative from a local company. Ask what qualities and experiences are most useful for getting promoted. Report what you learn.

Summarize Your Reading

▶ Australia is the smallest continent in the world. It's slightly smaller than the United States.

▶ Australia is a "melting pot" of ethnic influences even though it wasn't on major trade routes.

▶ Australians have interesting names for some foods, such as "dampers" and "snags."

▶ About 25,000 islands make up Oceania. The country of New Zealand is a thousand miles from Australia.

▶ Seafood and tropical fruits are obvious staples in Oceania.

Check Your Knowledge

1. Why isn't Australia considered an island?

2. How is the southeastern corner of Australia different from the "outback"?

3. What is "bush tucker"?

4. **CRITICAL THINKING** Why do you think interest in "bush tucker" has grown in recent times?

5. What are two methods the Aborigines used to preserve food?

6. How did the British make use of Australia in the late 1770s?

7. What two factors give Australians the ability to grow ingredients for almost any cuisine in the world?

8. What are Australia's favorite meats?

9. Describe the following Australian foods: a) **rissoles**; b) "dampers"; c) "snags"; and d) **flummery**.

10. What is the geographic location of the islands collectively called Oceania? What two islands are the largest?

11. What is **breadfruit**, and how might it be served?

12. Who were the Maori?

13. Describe the Maori *hangi*.

14. How do cows contribute to the ingredients that make up the New Zealand cuisine?

15. Why have natives of New Zealand been nicknamed "kiwis"?

16. What is **guava**?

17. What ingredients go into the Tahitian *hima'a*?

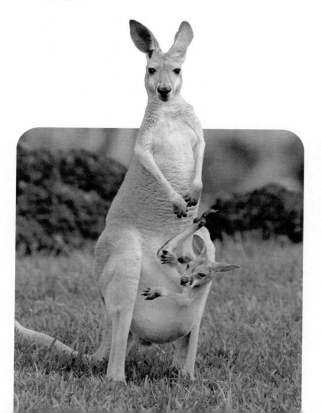

Apply Your Learning

1. **SOCIAL STUDIES** **Country Study.** Choose one country in the chapter to study. Learn about the area's history, geography, and culture. Using such visual aids as films and magazine photos, give a class presentation.

2. **Taste Test.** With your lab team, prepare a dish from one of the countries in the chapter. Present your dish for a class taste test.

3. **Ethnic Meal.** Plan, prepare, and serve a meal with dishes from one of the countries in the chapter.

4. **LANGUAGE ARTS** **Pavlova History.** Research the history of "Pavlova." Write a short feature for a culinary magazine, titled "The True Story of Pavlova."

5. **Coconut Exploration.** Find information about coconuts, including how and where they grow, their use, and their nutritional value. Bring a coconut to sample in class.

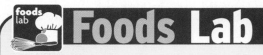

Foods Lab

Anzac Biscuits

Procedure: Find and prepare a recipe for Anzac biscuits, a traditional Australian cookie. Serve the cookies as part of a class taste test.

Analyzing Results

❶ Describe the cookie's texture. How do you think it was produced?

❷ How do the techniques for preparing these cookies compare to methods used for other cookies you've made?

❸ How do Anzac biscuits compare nutritionally to other cookies? What changes could you make to improve the nutrient profile?

Food Science Experiment

Enzymes in Tropical Fruits

Objective: To observe how tropical fruit enzymes affect other foods.

Procedure:

1. In a large bowl, combine a small package of gelatin dessert powder and ¾ cup of boiling water. Stir to dissolve completely.

2. Combine cold water and ice to equal 1¼ cups and add to the gelatin mixture. Stir until slightly thickened. Remove any remaining ice.

3. To the partially set gelatin, stir in ½ cup of just *one* of the following fruits, as instructed by your teacher: fresh pineapple, fresh papaya, or fresh kiwifruit, all cut into chunks.

4. Refrigerate the gelatin overnight. The next day, set the bowl on the counter for a class evaluation and comparison.

Analyzing Results

❶ Describe the consistency and appearance of each product.

❷ These fruits contain an enzyme called papain. Review earlier discussions of enzymes and protein and explain the results you observed here.

❸ These fruits, in any processed form, would not have the same effect. Why do you think this is true?

Glossary

A

absorption Movement of nutrients into blood stream. (5)

active dry yeast Partially dormant yeast contained in flour granules. (44)

added sugars Sugars extracted from plants and used to sweeten foods. (6)

adequate intake (AI) Dietary reference intake used when dietary allowance for a nutrient can't be scientifically established. (5)

adipose cells Cells that store fat from foods and grow larger as they store additional fat. (7)

aerobic exercise Vigorous activity that increases heart and breathing rate for at least twenty minutes. (11)

agroforestry Ancient practice of raising shade-loving crops under shelter of trees. (3)

air cell Pocket of air between membranes of egg at wide, round end. (35)

à la carte Items listed and priced individually on restaurant menu. (19)

albumen Thick fluid commonly known as egg white. (35)

al dente Doneness stage meaning firm to the bite. (32)

amino acids Chemical building blocks of proteins that link together in many arrangements. (7)

anaerobic exercise Exercise that involves short, intense bursts of activity. (11)

analogs Foods made to imitate actual foods in appearance but containing different ingredients. (4)

anemia Blood disorder characterized by lack of energy, weakness, shortness of breath, and cold hands and feet; caused by lack of iron. (5)

annual percentage rate (APR) Yearly interest rate charged when buying item. (22)

anorexia nervosa Eating disorder in which an extremely thin person sees self as fat and has intense fear of gaining weight. (12)

antioxidants Substances that protect body cells and immune system from damage by harmful chemicals in air and foods. (8)

antipasto Appetizers that might include olives, pickled peppers, thin slices of salami, cheese, and marinated beans and artichoke hearts. (51)

appetizer Small portion of food served at beginning of meal to whet the appetite. (18)

aquaculture Raising seafood in enclosed areas of water. (3)

arcing Electrical sparks caused by placing anything metallic in microwave oven. (26)

aromatic vegetables Such vegetables as onions, garlic, celery, and bell peppers, which add aroma and flavor when sautéed. (31)

B

aseptic packages Packages made for shelf-stable food storage. (4)

au gratin Casserole topped with buttered breadcrumbs or grated cheese. (42)

au jus To serve roast with natural meat juices. (43)

baguette Long, crusty French bread. (50)

bakeware Equipment for cooking food in oven. (22)

baklava Greek dish that alternates layers of phyllo with finely chopped walnuts or almonds mixed with sugar and cinnamon. (51)

bannock Flat, biscuit-like bread made with flour or oats and cooked on cast iron over hot grill. (48)

bar cookies Cookies baked in shallow pan and cut into bars or squares. (46)

basal metabolism Minimum amount of energy needed to maintain basic body processes. (5)

basic sandwich Two slices of bread with filling in between. (40)

beading Brown droplets on surface of meringue. (35)

behavior modification Process of making gradual, permanent changes in eating and activity habits. (11)

beta-carotene Phytochemical used by body to make vitamin A. (9)

bigos Sweet and sour Polish stew that includes fresh pork, apples, and sauerkraut. (52)

binder Liquid that helps hold mixture together. (42)

binge eating disorder Disorder in which person eats abnormally large amounts of food in short time. (12)

biodegradable Describes materials that break down in soil over time. (23)

biodiversity Wide variety of plant and animal species. (3)

bioterrorism Intentional use of biological agents—bacteria, viruses, and toxins—to harm people, animals, or plants. (20)

biscotti Crunchy, anise-flavored, twice-baked Italian cookies. (51)

biscuit method Making quick breads by adding solid fat to dry ingredients before mixing in liquids. (45)

bisque. Rich cream soup that uses shellfish as base. (43)

blanching Cooking vegetables briefly in boiling water to neutralize enzymes. (29)

bleached flour Flour chemically treated to neutralize yellow pigment. (42)

blini Small, Russian, yeast-leavened buckwheat pancakes eaten with jam or cream cheese or served as hors d'oeurve with salmon or sour cream. (52)

bloom Patches of white on chocolate; occur as cocoa butter surfaces when stored in warm area. (39)

body fat percentage Amount of body fat person has in relation to muscle. (11)

body mass index (BMI) Ratio of weight to height. (11)

boiling-water bath Used to process high-acid foods, such as fruits, by covering with boiling water in water-bath canner. (29)

bouillon Another name for broth. (41)

bouquet garni Bundled herb blend that flavors foods while cooking and is later removed. (28)

bran Edible, outer layer of grain kernel. (32)

breadfruit Large, tropical fruit related to fig family. (55)

broth Flavorful liquid, or stock, made by simmering meat, poultry, fish, or vegetables in water. (43)

brown sugar Granulated sugar coated with molasses, which adds moisture and caramel flavor. (44)

budget Plan for managing money. (16)

buffet Serving style in which people help themselves to food prepared and set out on a table. (18)

bulimia nervosa Eating disorder; binge eating is followed by purging to rid body of food and calories and prevent weight gain. (12)

bulk foods Shelf-stable foods sold loose in covered bins or barrels. (16)

C

caffeine Stimulant in coffee, tea, chocolate, cocoa, and cola drinks; affects nervous system, heart, and kidneys; produces unwanted side effects in some people. (39)

calorie Amount of energy needed to raise temperature of 1 kilogram of water 1 degree Celsius. (5)

calzone Double-crust, semicircular pizza with pizza fillings. (40)

canapés Small pieces of bread cut in decorative shapes; have flavorful toppings. (18)

cannoli Deep-fried Italian pastry tubes. (51)

carbohydrates Nutrient that is a person's main source of energy; found mostly in plant foods. (6)

carbonated Describes beverages that are bubbly due to added carbon dioxide. (39)

carbon monoxide Odorless, highly poisonous gas. (21)

cardiopulmonary resuscitation (CPR) Technique used to revive someone whose breathing and heartbeat have stopped. (21)

carnivores Group of organisms that feed mostly upon animals and convert this food into usable energy. (3)

carrageen Sea vegetable that helps produce consistency of such products as ice cream, salad dressings, soups, and puddings. (31)

cassava Starchy root vegetable. (49)

casserole Flavorful combination of precooked or quick-cooking foods in one-dish meal. (42)

caviar Salted eggs of sturgeon fish. (52)

ceviche Appetizer of raw fish marinated in citrus juice until firm and opaque, drained, and served with chilies, tomatoes, and onions. (49)

chalazae Two thick, twisted strands of albumen that anchor yolk in egg's center. (35)

chlorophyll Green pigment in plants; must be present for photosynthesis to occur. (6)

cholesterol Fat-like substance in all body cells; needed for many essential body processes. (7)

chorizo Spicy Spanish sausage that flavors many stews. (49)

chronic Long-term or recurring, as in health problems. (12)

chutney Zesty condiment made from fruit, sugar, spices, and vinegar. (54)

chyme Thick liquid resulting as stomach breaks down food mechanically through peristalsis. (5)

cioppino San Francisco fish stew originally made at Fisherman's Wharf. (48)

clone Genetic copy of an organism. (4)

club sandwich Made with three slices of toasted bread and two layers of different fillings. (40)

coagulate For an egg, to become firm, changing from liquid to semisolid or solid state when heated. (35)

coating Applying thin layer of one food onto another food for flavor and texture. (25)

cocoa Product of cocoa powder, combined with warm milk or water to make hot cocoa. (39)

cocoa butter Fat from chocolate liquid used in making many chocolate products. (39)

cocoa powder Solids left behind when fat, or cocoa butter, is extracted from chocolate liquid. (39)

code dating Series of numbers and letters that indicate where and when product was packaged. (17)

coffee bean Twin seeds of deep-red fruit produced by tropical coffee plant. (39)

colcannon Popular Irish dish made when potato is mashed with leeks and mixed with chopped, cooked cabbage. (50)

cold cuts Processed slices of cold meat and poultry. (36)

cold water test Estimates temperature of syrup based on how it acts in cold water. (46)

collagen Thin, white, transparent tissue found in tendons, between muscle cells, and between muscles. (36)

colostrum Thick, yellowish fluid in breast milk; rich in nutrients and antibodies, proteins that protect baby from infection. (13)

comfort foods Familiar foods, usually creamy, soft, and rich, that make people feel good when stressed, troubled, bored, or unhappy. (1)

commodities Surplus food purchased from farmers and distributed to those in need of food assistance. (16)

comparison shopping Process of matching prices and characteristics of similar items to determine which offers best value. (17)

complete proteins Proteins that contain all essential amino acids. (7)

complex carbohydrates Carbohydrates with complicated structures; starches. (6)

compressed yeast Combination of yeast and starch; moist and comes in small, individually wrapped cakes. (44)

condiments Accompaniments to food. (28)

conduction Method of transferring heat by direct contact. (26)

confectioners' sugar Pulverized, granulated sugar with trace of added cornstarch; also known as powdered sugar. (44)

connective tissue Thin sheets of protein material that bind muscle fiber into bundles. (36)

conservation Concern for environment and its future, shown by managing resources wisely. (23)

consommé Clarified broth, completely strained of all particles and sediment; may be served warm as appetizer. (43)

contaminants Substances that make food unfit for use. (20)

convection Movement of molecules through air or liquid. (26)

convection oven Uses convection currents created by air rising as it warms; fan circulates heated air to equalize temperatures throughout oven. (22)

convenience foods Commercially processed foods that are easy and quick to use. (16)

conventional method Bread-baking method in which yeast is dissolved in warm water to activate growth. (45)

cooked dressing Salad dressing thickened with starch paste instead of eggs. (41)

cooking greens Greens typically cooked before being seasoned and eaten, including collards, dandelion greens, kale, mustard greens, and chard. (31)

cooking power Amount of energy microwave oven uses to generate microwaves. (26)

cookware Equipment for cooking food on top of range. (22)

cornstarch Fine, white powder that is pure starch made from endosperm of corn kernel. (43)

cover Arrangement of a table place setting. (18)

credit Financial arrangement that delays payment. (22)

critical thinking Process of analyzing and evaluating what you hear and read for better understanding and interpretation. (1)

croquettes Seafood that is puréed, bound with thick sauce, formed into small shapes, breaded, and deep-fried. (48)

cross-contamination Spread of harmful bacteria from one food to another. (20)

croutons Small pieces of bread made crisp by baking or sautéing. (41)

cruciferous vegetables All vegetables from cabbage family. (9)

crumb crust Made of crushed crackers or cookies. (47)

crustaceans Shellfish with long bodies and jointed limbs; includes crabs, crayfish, lobsters, and shrimp. (38)

crystal Glassware made with lead, giving it clarity and sparkle. (18)

crystallization Formation of sugar crystals in syrup. (46)

cuisine A culture's representative foods and specific styles for preparing them. (2)

culture Set of customs, traditions, and beliefs shared by large group of people. (2)

curdling When milk separates into solids and liquids. (34)

curds Solid clusters formed when milk separates into solids and liquids. (34)

curries Indian dishes of vegetables and legumes in hot, highly seasoned sauces. (54)

custard Thickened blend of milk, eggs, and sugar used as base for many main dishes. (35)

custom Established practice repeated over time. (2)

customary system Measuring system in U.S. based on such units as inches and ounces. (24)

cut Specific, edible part of meat, such as steak, chop, or roast. (36)

cut in To mix solid fat and flour with pastry blender or two knives and cutting motion. (45)

cutting Dividing food into smaller parts using sharp-bladed tool. (25)

D

daikon Asian radish common as Chinese ingredient. (54)

Daily Value Current recommendation for a nutrient based on 2,000-calorie diet, expressed as percentage, set by federal government. (10)

dairy dressings Dressings based on buttermilk, yogurt, sour cream, or cottage cheese, with added seasonings. (41)

dal Mixture or purée of legumes, onions, chiles, and tomatoes. (54)

decaffeinated coffee Coffee with caffeine removed. (39)

dehydrated Lack of water in the body; signs include dark-colored urine, dry lips and skin, and constipation. (9)

developing nations Countries not yet industrialized or just beginning to industrialize. (3)

diabetes Condition in which the body can't control blood sugar levels. (12)

dietary fiber Plant materials that are eaten but can't be digested by human enzymes. (6)

Dietary Guidelines for Americans General USDA recommendations on food and fitness. (10)

dietary reference intakes (DRIs) Standards for assessing nutrient needs among people of different age and gender groups. (5)

dietary supplements Such substances as vitamins, minerals, amino acids, and herbals taken in addition to foods. (10)

digestion Mechanical and chemical process that breaks food down to release nutrients in forms the body can absorb for use. (4)

dim sum Bite-size dishes, such as dumplings and tarts, eaten at tea or between banquet courses in Asia. (54)

disaccharides Formed when two monosaccharides (single sugars) combine chemically. (6)

docking Poking small holes all over pie shell before baking to prevent puffing. (47)

dolmas Greek dish of grape leaves rolled around rice and ground meats and then steamed. (51)

dovetail Fitting different tasks together when cooking to make good use of time. (27)

down payment Portion of purchase price paid right away when buying on credit. (22)

drawn fish Whole fish with scales, gills, and internal organs removed. (38)

dressed Drawn fish with head, tail, and fins removed; also called pan-dressed. (38)

drop biscuits Biscuits made with more liquid in proportion to flour, as compared to rolled biscuits. (45)

drop cookies Cookies made from soft dough dropped onto cookie sheet. (46)

drupes Fruits with single hard seed (pit or stone), soft inner flesh, and tender, edible skin, such as cherries. (30)

dry-heat cooking Cooking food uncovered without added liquid or fat. (26)

dry legumes Seeds of mature plants left in field to dry; includes dry beans, peas, and lentils. (33)

dry-pack method Freezing unsweetened fruit by packing small whole fruits directly into freezer containers. (29)

E

eating disorders Conditions marked by extreme emotions, attitudes, and behaviors related to food, eating, and weight. (12)

eating pattern Mix of food customs and habits that include when, what, and how much people eat. (14)

ecosystem Environment containing community of organisms that interact and depend upon each other. (3)

elastin Tough, elastic, yellowish connective tissue found in ligaments and blood vessel walls. (36)

electrolyte minerals Sodium, chloride, and potassium, which control and balance fluid flow in and out of cells. (8)

empanada Spanish turnover filled with meat, vegetables, fruit, or all three. (49)

emulsifiers Substances such as egg yolks that hold together two liquids that normally won't stay mixed, such as water and oil. (35)

emulsion Mixture of two liquids that normally don't combine. (41)

endosperm Largest part of grain kernel; made of proteins and starches and contains plant's food supply (32).

EnergyGuide label Tool for estimating appliance's energy costs. (22)

enrichment Food production method that restores nutrients lost in processing to near original levels. (4)

entrée Main dish at meal. (14)

enzymatic browning Occurs when oxygen reacts with an enzyme, causing some fruits to turn brown. (30)

enzymes Special proteins that help chemical reactions take place. (5)

equivalents Different units of equal measure. (24)

ergonomics Study of ways to make space and equipment easier and more comfortable to use. (4)

esophagus Tube that connects mouth and stomach. (5)

essential amino acids Amino acids that the body needs but cannot provide; obtained from foods. (7)

ethnic Anything related to a culture, as in ethnic foods. (2)

étouffée Southern U.S. method of cooking food, such as shrimp, covered in liquid or sauce. (48)

F

fad diet Popular weight-loss method that ignores sound nutrition principles. (11)

fajitas Sandwiches made with grilled meat or poultry rolled in warm tortilla; served with foods to mix in, such as refried beans, salsa, and guacamole. (40)

falafel Small, deep-fried patties made with highly seasoned, ground garbanzo beans; Middle-Eastern filling for pita. (40)

family service Serving food by passing it around table in serving dishes. (18)

famine Most severe form of food shortage, which can last for months or years and cause thousands of deaths. (3)

fasting Abstaining from all or certain foods for period of time; practiced in some religions. (2)

fat-soluble vitamins Vitamins absorbed and transported by fat. (8)

fatty acids Chemical structures that make up fats. (7)

fatty fish Fish with more than 5 grams of fat in $3\frac{1}{2}$ ounces, such as herring and salmon. (38)

fermentation When yeast and enzymes it contains break down carbohydrates to produce alcohols and carbon dioxide gas for leavening. (45)

fetus Unborn baby. (13)

fillets Sides of fish cut lengthwise away from bones and backbone. (38)

finance charge Total amount paid for borrowing, expressed as dollar figure. (22)

fish Aquatic creatures with fins and center spine with bones. (38)

flan Full-size tart made in two-piece pan with removable bottom and straight, fluted edge. (47)

flatbread Unleavened bread made without yeast or baking powder. (32)

flatware Knives, forks, and spoons plus larger utensils, such as gravy ladles and cake servers. (18)

flummery Sweet Australian pudding thickened with gelatin or cornstarch and flavored with oranges or passion fruit. (55)

fluted edge Attractive, shaped finish on piecrust edge. (47)

foam Structure of air and protein that forms when cream or egg white is whipped. (34)

foam cakes Tall, spongy cakes leavened by air trapped in protein foam of stiffly beaten egg whites. (46)

focaccia Round, herbed, Italian bread brushed with olive oil. (40)

food additive Natural or chemical substance added to food for specific reason during processing. (3)

food allergy Abnormal response to certain foods by body's immune system. (12)

foodborne illness Sickness caused by eating food that contains harmful substance. (20)

food chain Cycle in which organisms obtain food from other organisms and environment; consists of sun, producers, consumers, and decomposers. (3)

food cooperative Food distribution business mutually owned and operated by members. (17)

food intolerance Adverse physical reaction to food, not involving immune system. (12)

food safety Keeping food safe to eat by following proper food handling and cooking practices. (20)

food science Scientific study of food and its preparation. (4)

food waste Any edible food that is discarded, such as uneaten servings on plate. (23)

fool Puréed fruit folded into whipped cream. (50)

formal service Most elaborate food service style, requiring hired help; often used for banquets. (18)

formed products Foods made from inexpensive sources and processed to imitate more expensive foods. (4)

fortification Process of adding a nutrient not normally found in a food. (4)

fraud Occurs when people gain something of value, often money, by deceiving others. (10)

free radicals Harmful by-product excreted when cells burn oxygen to produce energy. (8)

freezer burn Moisture loss caused when frozen food is improperly packaged or stored too long. (20)

fresh cheese Mild-flavored cheese made from pasteurized milk and not ripened or aged. (34)

fresh legumes Legumes from young plants, including green beans and green peas; picked ripe and sold as vegetables. (33)

frijoles Spanish word for beans. (49)

frittata Similar to omelet, but egg mixture isn't folded after cooking. (35)

fritters Cut-up fruit dipped in batter and deep-fried until golden brown. (30)

fruit Part of plant that holds seeds. (30)

fruit-flavored drinks Drinks that contain no juice; usually have water, sweeteners, flavorings, and other additives. (30)

functional foods Foods that provide health benefits beyond basic nutrition; many aim at disease prevention. (4)

fusion cuisine Cooking that creates new recipes by blending different ethnic food traditions. (2)

G

galette Hand-shaped tart made by folding and pleating dough edge to form sides. (47)

garnish Food added to dish as decorative or savory touch. (28)

gelatinization Thickening of a starch mixture; heat causes starch granules to absorb water, swell, burst, and run out to thicken liquid quickly. (43)

genetic engineering Process by which genes are removed from one organism, such as a plant, animal, or microorganism, and transferred to another. (4)

germ Seed of grain kernel that grows into new plant. (32)

giblets Edible internal organs of poultry. (37)

glucose Blood sugar formed when carbohydrates are fully broken down chemically. (5)

gluten Elastic substance formed when certain proteins in wheat flour combine with liquid. (44)

glycogen Storage form of glucose. (5)

gnocchi Potato dumplings. (51)

goulash Hungarian stew made with beef and vegetables and flavored with paprika. (48)

grain Lengthwise direction of muscle. (36)

grains All plants in grass family, such as wheat, corn, rice, oats, rye, barley, buckwheat, and millet. (32)

granulated sugar Highly refined sucrose crystals derived by boiling juice of sugarcane or sugar beets. (44)

GRAS list Additives classified by FDA as "Generally Recognized as Safe" due to long history of safe use. (20)

gratuity Extra money, or tip, given to restaurant server for good service. (19)

grazing Eating five or more small meals throughout the day instead of three large ones. (14)

grounding Minimizes risk of electric shock by providing path for current to travel back through electrical system, rather than through person's body. (22)

groundwater Water beneath earth's surface; fills cracks between rocks and sediment and is brought to surface by digging wells. (3)

guacamole Mexican dish made with mashed avocados, lemon or lime juice, and seasonings. (40)

guava Sweet tropical fruit eaten raw or used for preserves. (55)

gumbo Creole dish that combines Spanish custom of mixing seafood and meat with andouille sausages. (48)

gyro Greek specialty made with minced, roasted lamb, grilled onions, sweet peppers, and cucumber-yogurt sauce, wrapped in pita. (40)

H

haggis Sheep's stomach stuffed with mixture of oats, organ meats, onions, and beef or lamb suet and boiled; ancient Scottish recipe. (50)

haute cuisine Classic French cuisine known for high-quality ingredients, expertly prepared and artistically presented. (50)

HDL Lipoprotein that picks up cholesterol and takes it back to liver for excretion; "good" cholesterol. (7)

headspace One-inch space left between food and container lid when foods are preserved. (29)

heating units Energy sources in a range. (22)

Heimlich maneuver Procedure for dislodging an object from throat of choking person. (21)

hemoglobin Protein with globular shape; transports oxygen in blood to all body cells. (7)

herbals Plants used for medicinal purposes. (10)

herbivores Group of organisms that feed entirely on plants and convert this food into usable energy. (3)

herbs Flavorful leaves and stems of soft, succulent plants that grow in temperate climate. (28)

herb tea Caffeine-free tea made from flowers, leaves, seeds, and roots of herbs and plants, not tea leaves. (39)

hero Large sandwich with layered meats and cheeses on loaf of Italian or French bread or hard roll. (40)

high-altitude cooking Correcting recipes to prepare foods successfully in high altitudes. (24)

hilum Place where bean was attached to stem in pod; appears as scar on bean. (33)

HIV/AIDS Disorder that weakens immune system; infected people experience wide variety of nutrition-related problems. (12)

hoisin Thick, soy-sauce-based paste seasoned with chiles and garlic; used in Chinese cooking. (54)

holloware Serving containers made of silver, silver plate, or stainless steel. (18)

homogenized Process that breaks down fat and distributes it evenly and permanently in milk. (33)

hors d'oeuvres Small morsels of hot or cold food featured at formal receptions and usually eaten in one or two bites. (18)

hot-pack method Food preservation method that simmers food briefly before placing into jars with liquid. (29)

hot spot Area of concentrated heat in oven; can cause uneven baking and browning. (44)

hull Inedible outer coat of grain; removed after grain is harvested. (32)

hydration Receiving enough water to meet all the body's needs. (9)

hydrogenation Chemical process that turns vegetable oils into solids. (7)

hydroponic farming Growing plants without soil; plants are held in water, gravel, or sand and fed with nutrient-enriched water. (3)

hypertension High blood pressure linked to high salt intake. (8)

I

immature fruits Fruits picked before ripe; usually small for size and have poor color and texture. (30)

impulse buying Buying items, often unneeded, without planning; can harm budget. (17)

incomplete proteins Plant proteins that lack at least one essential amino acid. (7)

industrialized nations Developed countries in which organized food industry provides people with varied and nutritious diet. (3)

injera Thin, spongy, sourdough flatbread made with teff, high-protein grain native to North Africa. (53)

interest Fee paid for borrowed money. (22)

interfering agents Ingredients that control crystallization by keeping sugar crystals small; aid in candy making. (46)

internal temperature Temperature at center of thickest part of food; must be high enough to kill harmful bacteria. (20)

iron-deficiency anemia Lack of enough iron in body, resulting in fatigue, weakness, and shortness of breath. (8)

irradiation Process of exposing food to high-intensity energy waves to increase shelf life and kill harmful microorganisms. (20)

island Freestanding counter, open on all sides and often in center of kitchen. (22)

J K L

jambalaya Creole dish of ham, seafood, chicken, sausages, rice, vegetables, and seasonings. (48)

jerk Jamaican blend of chiles, onions, garlic, allspice, and other herbs and spices; seasons meat, poultry, and fish. (49)

juice Product that contains 100 percent fruit or vegetable juice. (39)

juice drinks Contain about 10 to 50 percent juice; rest is water, sweeteners, flavorings, and other additives. (39)

kielbasa Polish smoked sausage. (52)

kernels Small, separate, dry fruits produced by grains; harvested and processed for food. (32)

kimchee Very hot, fermented Korean condiment made with cabbage, daikon radish, or cucumbers and seasoned with salt, pepper, garlic, and chiles. (54)

kneading Working dough to combine ingredients and develop gluten. (45)

kolache Sweet roll filled with fruit butter, nuts, or poppy seed paste. (52)

kringel Latvian coffee cake made with yeast and sometimes nuts or fruit filling in oval or pretzel shape. (52)

lactation Production of breast milk. (13)

lacto-ovo-vegetarians People who eat foods from plant sources, dairy products, and eggs. (15)

lacto-vegetarians People who eat foods from plant sources and dairy products. (15)

lahvosh Armenian flatbread; larger and thinner than pita; available crisp or soft and in various flavors. (40)

lattice crust Woven strips of dough for top crust of pie. (47)

laverbread Processed seaweed. (50)

LDL Lipoprotein that takes cholesterol from liver to where needed in the body; can accumulate too much; considered "bad" cholesterol. (7)

leadership Ability to guide or direct people. (1)

leavened bread Bread that has risen due to use of yeast or baking powder. (32)

leavening agent Triggers chemical reaction that makes baked product rise. (44)

legumes Plants with seed pods that split along both sides when ripe. (33)

life span Stages of human development from birth through maturity. (13)

lipoproteins Chemical "packages" that transport fatty acids through bloodstream. (7)

low-fat fish Fish with less than 5 grams of fat in $3\frac{1}{2}$ ounces; includes bass, catfish, and halibut. (38)

lutefisk Norwegian dried cod soaked in culinary ash and water. (50)

M

macaroni Pasta made from durum wheat flour and water. (32)

Maillard reaction Browning on baked and fried foods and cooked roasts caused by chemical reactions between certain sugars and proteins in the food. (26)

major minerals Macrominerals with special duties in the body; calcium, phosphorus, magnesium, sodium, chloride, and potassium. (8)

malnutrition Deficiency or severe shortage of nutrient, caused by faulty or inadequate nutrition. (5)

management Using specific techniques to handle resources wisely in reaching for goals. (1)

manufactured food Product developed as substitute for another food. (4)

MAP packaging Modified atmosphere packaging in which mix of carbon dioxide, oxygen, and nitrogen is inserted into package before sealing to slow bacterial growth. (4)

marbling Small white flecks of fat in meat; may appear within muscle tissue. (36)

marzipan Confection made of almond paste and sugar; used to sweeten pastries. (51)

masa Dried, cooked corn, soaked in limewater and ground into dough. (49)

mature fruits Fruits that have reached full size and color. (30)

mayonnaise Thick, creamy dressing that is emulsion of oil, vinegar or lemon juice, egg yolks, and seasonings. (41)

meat Edible muscle of animals, typically cattle, sheep, and pigs. (36)

megadose Very large amount of a supplement that people believe will prevent or cure a disease. (10)

meringue Soft or hard foam made from beaten egg whites and sugar; used for baked desserts. (35)

metabolism Process through which living cells use nutrients in chemical reactions in order to provide energy for vital processes and activities. (5)

metric system Measuring system based on multiples of ten. (24)

mezza Southwest Asian term for appetizers. (53)

microorganisms Living creatures visible only through microscope. (20)

microwave time Actual time food cooks with microwave energy. (26)

microwaving Cooking foods from energy in the form of electrical waves. (26)

miscarriage Spontaneous expulsion of unborn child. (13)

mise en place French for "put in place"; all ingredients are arranged ahead in cooking order. (42)

mixing Combining two or more ingredients thoroughly so they blend. (25)

modified English service Formal way of serving meal at table; plates are placed in front of host, who puts food on plates and passes them. (18)

moist-heat cooking Cooking food in hot liquid, steam, or combination of the two. (26)

molded cookies Cookies shaped by hand. (46)

molded salads Gelatin salads that thicken and conform to a mold's shape. (41)

mole Sauce blending many ingredients; based on chiles, ground pumpkin or sesame seeds, onions, unsweetened chocolate, and spices. (49)

mollusks Creatures with soft bodies covered by rigid shell; includes clams, mussels, and oysters. (38)

monosaccharides Sugars with single-unit chemical structure. (6)

monounsaturated fatty acids Unsaturated fatty acids with one hydrogen unit missing. (7)

moussaka Greek dish of sliced eggplant layered with mixture of ground lamb, onions, garlic, tomato sauce, and cinnamon. (51)

muffin method Technique for making quick breads by lightly mixing liquid ingredients into dry. (45)

mulled Describes punch served hot and flavored with spices. (39)

multiple roles Specific responsibilities people have based on their different relationships to others. (16)

muscle Tissue made of long, thin cells, sometimes called muscle fibers, that are bound into bundles with thin sheets of protein material. (36)

myoglobin Reddish protein pigment where oxygen is stored in meat. (37)

MyPyramid USDA food grouping system that guides nutrition and health. (10)

NO

natural foods Foods that have been minimally processed and contain no artificial ingredients or added color. (17)

nonfat milk solids Solids in fresh milk that contain most proteins, vitamins, minerals, and lactose (milk sugar) in milk. (34)

nonrenewable resources Resources continually produced in nature, such as natural gas and oil, but at rate too slow to keep up with demand. (23)

nonverbal communication Messages sent using facial expressions or body language, not words. (1)

noodles Products made from durum wheat flour, with egg solids added for tenderness. (32)

nori Japanese seaweed wrapper that holds sushi. (54)

nutrient density Relationship between nutrients and calories in food. (10)

nutrients Life-sustaining chemical compounds in food; released as food breaks down. (1)

nutrition Study of nutrients and how the body uses them. (1)

Nutrition Facts panel Panel on food labels; has easy-to-read data about food's nutritional value. (10)

nuts Edible kernels surrounded by hard shell. (33)

obstetrician Physician who specializes in care of women during pregnancy and childbirth. (13)

omega-3 fatty acid Fatty acid in fish oils, especially fatty fish; may lower risk of heart disease. (7)

omelet Egg mixture in form of large, thick pancake filled with ingredients and folded. (35)

omnivores Organisms that eat both plants and animals. (3)

one-bowl method Quick way to mix ingredients for shortened cake; combines dry ingredients and then adds moist ingredients. (46)

open dating Calendar dates that indicate freshness of perishable foods, such as meat and dairy products. (17)

open-face sandwich Sandwich made with one slice of bread and topping. (40)

open stock When each piece in a tableware set can be purchased separately. (18)

organic farming Farming without pesticides and artificial fertilizers; stresses resource conservation. (3)

organic foods Foods produced without pesticides, artificial fertilizers, growth hormones, and antibiotics; not generally modified or irradiated. (17)

osteomalacia Disease caused by lack of vitamin D in adults. (8)

osteoporosis Condition caused by calcium deficiency; bones become porous, weak, and fragile. (8)

ovo-vegetarians People who eat foods from plant sources and eggs. (15)

oxidation Chemical reactions that combine elements with oxygen. (5)

P Q

paella Spanish dish of rice, seasoned with saffron, and mixed with meat and seafood. (51)

pancetta Italian cured sausage from beef cattle and pigs. (51)

pancreas Gland connected to small intestine; produces pancreatic juice that breaks down carbohydrates, proteins, and fats. (5)

pasta Italian word for "paste," or dough made from flour and water. (32)

pasteurization Heat-treatment that kills enzymes and harmful bacteria in foods. (34)

pediatrician Physician who cares for infants and children. (13)

peer pressure Influence of people in same age group. (13)

pelmeni Russian dumplings. (52)

peninsula Countertop extension open on two sides and one end. (22)

perishable foods Foods that spoil or decay, especially without proper storage. (17)

peristalsis Muscle action of esophagus (contracting and relaxing) that forces food into stomach. (5)

permanent emulsion Formed by different liquids that don't separate after they're mixed. (41)

personal hygiene Practice of keeping clean; helps avoid transferring harmful bacteria to work surfaces, utensils, and food. (20)

pesto Northern Italian sauce of ground, fresh basil, pine nuts, garlic, Parmesan cheese, and olive oil. (51)

photosynthesis Chemical process by which plants make carbohydrates. (6)

phytochemicals Naturally occurring chemical compounds in plant-based foods. (9)

pica Condition linked to iron deficiency; causes unusual appetite for ice, clay, and other nonfood items. (8)

pie Any dish with crust and filling. (47)

pie shell Single crust baked before filling. (47)

pierogis Polish dumplings made with noodle dough or potatoes. (52)

pilaf Sautéed grains cooked in seasoned liquid. (52)

pita Round, leavened flatbread. (40)

pizza Oversized, baked sandwich with yeast-bread base, usually served open-face with toppings. (40)

place setting Tableware for one person, including plate, glass, and typically knife, fork, and spoon. (18)

plankton Minute animal and plant life in water; absorbs mercury that settles at waterway bottoms. (38)

plate service Serving food by plating food in the kitchen and carrying plates to the table. (18)

poke Sliced, raw fish mixed with seaweed, onions, chiles, and soy sauce. (48)

polarized plugs Appliance plugs with one blade wider than the other; designed to fit matching outlet and reduce risk of shock. (21)

polenta Thick, cornmeal porridge of northern Italy. (51)

polysaccharides Complicated chemical arrangements that plants form by combining single glucose units to build starches. (6)

polyunsaturated fatty acid Unsaturated fatty acid with two or more hydrogen units missing. (7)

pomes Fruits with central core containing several small seeds, such as apples and pears. (30)

poultry Any bird raised for food. (37)

preheat To turn oven on early to have desired temperature when food is placed inside. (44)

pre-preparation Tasks to do before putting recipes together. (27)

preserve To prepare food so it can be safely stored for later use. (29)

pressed cookies Cookies made with cookie press that forces dough directly onto baking sheet. (46)

pressure canning Processing low-acid foods by placing jars of food in pressure canner in steam with temperatures above 212°F. (29)

principal Amount of money borrowed after deducting down payment from total purchase price. (22)

processed meats Meats changed by various methods to add flavor and help preserve them. (36)

produce Fresh fruits and vegetables. (30)

proofing Process for testing whether yeast is alive. (44)

punch Mixture of fruit juices and tea or carbonated beverage, such as ginger ale or seltzer water. (39)

quiche Pie with custard filling; may contain chopped vegetables, cheese, and chopped, cooked meat. (35)

quick breads Breads leavened by agents that allow for immediate baking. (45)

quick-mix method Combines dry yeast with dry ingredients to make yeast bread. (45)

quick-rising yeast Yeast that causes bread to rise in about half as much time as regular yeast. (44)

quorn™ Meat substitute made from fungal protein that is fermented and mixed with egg whites and vegetable oils. (15)

R

radiation Heat transfer as waves of energy. (26)

rancidity Spoilage caused by breakdown of fats. (20)

raw milk Milk that is not pasteurized. (33)

raw-pack method Method for preserving raw food; food is placed in jars of hot liquid, such as syrup, water, or juice. (29)

rebate Partial refund from maker of purchased item. (17)

recall Immediate removal of product from store shelves; occurs if manufacturer or FDA learns food is unsafe. (20)

reception Social gathering usually held to honor person or celebrate event. (18)

recipe Set of directions for making food or beverage. (24)

recommended dietary allowances (RDAs) Amount of a nutrient needed by 98 percent of the people in given age and gender group. (5)

reconstituting Process of restoring dried food to its former condition by adding water. (30)

recycle Reprocessing discarded products so they can be used again. (23)

reduction Simmering uncovered mixture until some of the liquid evaporates. (43)

refrigerator cookies Cookies made by forming dough into long, even rolls that are wrapped, chilled, and later cut to size. (46)

regreening The return of green chlorophyll to skin of ripe oranges; can be caused by bright lights in produce department. (30)

rehydrate To return water to foods that have been dried, often before use in recipes. (29)

renewable resources Resources that replace themselves rather quickly, sometimes immediately. (23)

reservation Arrangement made ahead for table at a restaurant. (19)

resources Things and qualities that can help in reaching goals. (14)

retail cuts Cuts of meat for sale. (36)

retort pouches Flexible pouches made of aluminum foil and plastic film; food is heat-processed in pouch; can store food after opening. (4)

rice Starchy seed of plants grown in flooded fields in warm climates. (32)

ripe fruits Mature fruit that has reached its peak of flavor and is ready to eat. (30)

ripened cheese Made by adding ripening agents, such as bacteria, mold, or yeast, to milk curds; cheese is then aged under carefully controlled conditions. (34)

rissoles Australian dish of leftover corned beef with onions made into deep-fried pastry. (55)

rolled biscuits Biscuits mixed by biscuit method; dough is rolled out to even thickness and cut before baking. (45)

rolled cookies Cookies made from stiff dough rolled out and cut into shapes with cookie cutters. (46)

roux Mixture of equal parts flour and fat used to thicken liquid. (43)

S

saffron Pungent, thread-like center of crocus flower for seasoning; turns rice bright yellow. (53)

salad Mixture of raw or cooked vegetables and other ready-to-eat foods, often served with dressing. (40)

salad dressing Seasoned mixture of oil and vinegar used to season salad. (41)

salad greens Leafy vegetables eaten raw. (31)

salsa Chunky sauce of tomatoes, onions, garlic, and spices. (49)

sandwich Filling of meats, vegetables, jams, or spreads between slices of bread. (40).

sanitary landfill System for burying trash in layers of soil. (23)

sanitation Prevention of illness through cleanliness and food safety. (20)

sashimi Fish served raw with condiments. (54)

saturated fatty acid Fatty acid that contains all the hydrogen it can chemically hold. (7)

sauce Flavored liquid often thickened and served to enhance food's flavor. (43)

sauerbraten German beef roast marinated in vinegar with cloves, bay leaves, and peppercorns. (50)

savory Describes dishes that are not sweet. (30)

scalded milk Milk heated to just below boiling. (34)

science Study of physical world at all levels. (4)

scorching Occurs when milk overheats and lactose rapidly caramelizes and burns. (34)

score To make slashes across top of bread; decorative and prevents cracks. (45)

scrapple Baked pork scraps with cornmeal flavored with thyme and sage. (48)

scratch cooking Preparing a dish from basic ingredients, or home cooking. (16)

seafood Saltwater fish and shellfish. (38)

sear To brown meat quickly over high heat. (26)

seasoning blends Combinations of herbs and spices. (28)

sea vegetables Seaweeds that grow in waters with filtered sunlight; classified as algae, not plants. (31)

seeds Edible, dried kernels of certain plants, such as the sunflower. (33)

seitan Meat substitute made by simmering flour in broth flavored with ginger, garlic, soy sauce, and seaweed to produce firm, chewy texture and brown color. (15)

self-esteem Perception you have of yourself. (1)

self-rising flour Flour with added baking powder and salt. (44)

sell-by date Indicates last day product should remain on shelf; allows time for home storage and use after the date. (17)

semi-vegetarians People who eat no red meat but who do eat poultry and fish. (15)

service contract Repair and maintenance insurance purchased to cover product for specific length of time. (22)

service plate Large, beautifully decorated plate used only for appetizer in formal service. (18)

shelf life Length of time food holds original flavor and quality. (3)

shelf-stable Can be stored at room temperature in original, unopened container without spoiling. (3)

shellfish Aquatic creatures with shell but no spine or bones. (38)

shirred eggs Eggs baked in greased, shallow dish and topped with small amount of milk. (35)

shortened cakes Cakes made with solid fat, flour, salt, sugar, eggs, liquid, and either baking powder or baking soda. (46)

simple carbohydrates Sugars formed from simple one- and two-unit structures. (6)

smoking point Temperature at which fat begins to break down. (26)

smoothie Beverage blend of milk or yogurt and fresh fruit. (39)

smorgasbord Swedish buffet of cured fish, cold meats, cheeses, salads, and vegetables. (50)

soft peaks Beaten egg whites that gently bend over like waves. (35)

solanine Bitter, toxic compound that forms green patches on potatoes with exposure to light. (31)

sopas Latin American soups. (49)

soufflé Puffy casserole made by folding stiffly beaten egg whites into sauce or puréed food and baking. (35)

soups Dishes of solid foods cooked in liquid. (43)

speed-scratch cooking Uses convenience foods along with basic ingredients for easier preparation. (16)

spices Dried buds, bark, fruits, seeds, stems, and roots of plants and trees in tropical or subtropical regions. (28)

spores Protected cells that develop into bacteria under the right conditions. (20)

standing time Time needed to complete cooking after microwaving. (26)

staple foods Most widely produced and eaten foods in particular area. (2)

staples Basic food items used on regular basis, such as milk, cereal, eggs, and bread. (16)

starches Formed when plants combine single glucose units into more complicated chemical structures. (6)

steaks Cross sections cut from large, dressed fish; may contain bones from backbone and ribs. (38)

steep To brew by pouring boiling water over tea and allowing it to sit for a few minutes. (39)

stew Any dish prepared by simmering small pieces of food in tightly covered pan. (41)

stiff peaks Beaten egg whites that stand up straight when beaters are lifted from the mixture. (35)

stir-fry Combination dish of bite-size pieces of food, stirred constantly while frying in small amount of oil over high heat. (42)

stollen German cardamom-spiced fruitcake. (50)

store brands Items produced and packaged for store, sometimes by name-brand producers. (17)

stress Physical or mental tension caused by reaction to a situation. (12)

streusel Crumbly, sweet topping for pie, made by cutting butter into flour, sugar, and possibly spices. (47)

subsistence farming When families raise their own food but have barely enough to live on. (3)

succotash Dish of beans and corn. (48)

sugar-pack method Coating fruit in sugar and freezing in containers to preserve it. (29)

sugars Simple carbohydrates chemically formed from plants; made of carbon, hydrogen, and oxygen. (6)

sugar substitutes Substances used in place of sugar to sweeten foods yet add few or no calories. (6)

sumac Deep red berry native to Middle East; adds fruity tartness when ground into spices. (53)

sushi Japanese vinegary rice rolled up in sashimi or nori. (54)

sustainable living Achieving economic growth while protecting environment and promoting human well-being. (3)

syrup-pack method Packing fruit in sugar syrup and freezing in containers to preserve it. (29)

T

tabbouleh Middle Eastern salad of cooked bulgur, chopped tomatoes, onions, parsley, mint, olive oil, and lemon juice. (41)

table etiquette Courtesy shown by good manners when eating. (19)

tableware Any item for serving and eating food. (18)

tagines Well-seasoned stews made in covered pot with same name. (53)

tahini Paste made from ground sesame seeds. (53)

tapas Small snacks or appetizers popular in Spanish regions. (51)

tandoor Rounded, clay, charcoal-burning oven. (54)

taring Adjusting food scale by subtracting container's weight so food can be weighed. (25)

taro Large tuber of tropical taro plant. (48)

tart Filled pastry with single bottom crust; always removed from pan before serving. (47)

task lighting Bright, shadow-free light over specific work areas. (22)

tea Leaves of shrub grown in tropical areas. (39)

teamwork Working well together to achieve goal. (27)

tea sandwiches Small, attractive, cold sandwiches often served at receptions and parties. (40)

technology Practical application of scientific knowledge. (4)

tempeh Pressed cake of fermented, cooked soybeans mixed with grain, usually rice. (15)

tempering Preventing curdling by bringing one food to the right temperature or consistency before mixing it completely with another. (34)

temporary emulsion Two combined liquids that begin to separate after mixing. (41)

timetable Table showing time needed to complete preparation tasks and when to begin each one. (27)

tofu Custard-like product made from soybeans. (33)

tolerance Maximum safe level for certain chemical in the human body. (20)

torte Rich Austrian cake made with small amount of flour and often with ground nuts or bread crumbs. (50)

tortilla Thin, round, unleavened flatbread made with either corn or wheat flour and baked on griddle. (40)

tossed salad Mixture of greens and other vegetables. (41)

toxicity Excessive amount of substance that reacts as poison in the body. (8)

toxins Poisons found in harmful bacteria. (20)

trace minerals Minerals needed in only small amounts but serving vital body functions. (8)

trans fats Fats produced when oils are turned into solids in food production; they increase LDL cholesterol levels and may lower HDL. (7)

tray-pack method Freezing whole fruits covered on tray without sugar, then packing in containers. (29)

trifle Layered dessert often made with cake, jam or jelly, fruit, custard, and whipped cream. (30)

triglycerides Type of lipid, commonly called fats. (7)

trussing To close cavity and bind legs and wings of bird before roasting. (37)

tuber Large, underground stem, the plant part that stores nutrients. (31)

turnover Pastry dough folded over sweet or savory filling and baked or deep-fried. (47)

twenty-second scrub Scrubbing hands with soap and warm water for twenty seconds to remove harmful bacteria. (20)

U V

unbleached flour Flour not chemically treated to neutralize yellow pigment; has slight beige tone. (42)

unit price Item's price per ounce, quart, pound, or other unit. (17)

universal product code (UPC) Series of black bars on food packages; scanner reads price and other information in code during checkout. (17)

underripe fruits Very firm fruits lacking flavor and top eating quality. (30)

universal design Home design that makes space usable for everyone, regardless of age or physical disability. (22)

use-by date Last date product can be used with high quality. (17)

vacuum bottle Bottle with structure and materials that prevent heat loss from hot foods inside. (18)

values Beliefs and concepts held as important. (14)

variety meats Edible organs and extremities of beef, veal, lamb, and pork. (36)

vegans People who eat only foods from plant sources. (15)

vegetarians People who eat plant-based diet but not meat, poultry, or fish. (15)

verbal communication Sending and receiving messages through speaking, listening, writing, and reading. (1)

villi Billions of tiny fingerlike projections that line folds of small intestine. (5)

vinaigrettes Mixtures of vegetable oil, vinegar or lemon juice, and seasonings. (41)

volume Amount of space something takes up. (24)

W X Y Z

warranty Manufacturer's guarantee that product will perform as advertised. (22)

water-soluble vitamins Vitamins that dissolve in water and pass easily into bloodstream during digestion. (8)

weep When liquid accumulates between meringue and pie filling because meringue was spread on cool filling. (35)

weight Measures heaviness of ingredient, as in "1 lb. ground beef" or "50 g chopped walnuts." (24)

wellness Person's total health, including physical, mental, and emotional well-being. (1)

wheat Grain that is one of the oldest plant foods. (32)

whey Thin, bluish liquid formed when rennin is added to milk. (34)

whole fish Fish sold as caught and the most perishable form. (38)

whole grain Describes grain products made with entire kernel and containing most of the original nutrients. (32)

wholesale cuts Large cuts of meat sold to retail stores. (36)

whole wheat Describes wheat products made with whole grain. (32)

wok Special bowl-shape pan traditional for stir-frying. (26)

work center Area designed and equipped for specific kitchen tasks, such as cooking. (22)

work flow Activity that starts with removing food from storage and continues to preparation and serving. (22)

work plan List of all tasks needed to prepare meal. (27)

work triangle Arrangement that connects the three main work centers. (22)

wrap Sandwich made by rolling filling in flatbread. (40)

yeast breads Breads leavened with yeast. (45)

yield Number of servings or amount recipe makes. (24)

yogurt Thick, creamy, custard-like product with tangy flavor made by adding harmless bacteria to milk. (34)

yolk Round, yellow portion of egg; encased in thin membrane and floats within albumen. (35)

Yorkshire pudding Popover baked in hot pan drippings of roast beef as part of classic English dinner. (50)

Credits

SW Productions, 216, 224(B)
SW Productions/Photodisc, 166(L)
Taxi, 660
Thinkstock, 150
Arthur Tilley/Taxi, 164
Rob Van Petten/Image Bank, 382
Yellow Dog Productions/The Image Bank, 187
John Waterman/Stone, 10, 176
Ed White/Taxi, 279
Frank Whitney/The Image Bank, 291(BR)
Angela Wyant/Stone, 271
Alden J. Ho, 87
Index Stock
    Annie Dowie, 520
    Susan Jaekel, 325
    Craig "Skip" Julius, 71
Brian Leatart, 99
Lonely Planet Images
    Doug McKinlay, 682
    Stephen Saks, 694
Joe Mallon, 6, 107(B), 117, 128, 153(B), 167, 201(L), 242, 243, 299(B), 300, 303, 315(TL), 323, 336, 357(TL), 357(B), 407, 501(B), 547(T), 550, 553
Map Resources/Bill Smith Studio, 661, 662, 667, 673, 674, 676, 678, 683, 689, 695, 696, 698, 699, 701, 707, 708, 710, 712, 717, 721, 727, 728, 730, 734, 739, 741
Kevin May, 302
Ted Mishima, 65(B), 455, 612
Mary Moye-Rowley, 357(R), 358(L), 359, 360, 361(L), 526, 575, 624
Morgan-Cain & Assoc., 289, 309, 311, 367, 368, 369, 509(B), 511
Steven Needham, 284
North Wind Picture Archives, 39(B), 153(T)
Olivia, 283
PhotoDisc, 47, 61, 88, 101, 110, 115, 127, 129, 139, 209, 237, 270, 273, 513(B), 657
    C Squared Studio, 295, 329
    Siede Preis, 235
PhotoEdit
    Dennis MacDonald, 245
Photo Researchers, Inc.
    P. Motta, 123
Paul Rico, 59, 197, 206, 282, 309, 351, 371(L), 466(T), 503(B), 513(T), 521, 535, 610, 722
Christopher Scalise, 169
Marty Snortum, 679
StockFood
    Arras, 38, 46, 470
    Iain Bagwell, 692
    Banderob, 432
    Bayside, 354
    Beery, 424
    Damir Begovic, 605

Leigh Beisch Photography, 213
Uwe Bender, 705
Benelux Press, 12(R), 37, 41, 161(B), 259(T), 363(T), 425(T), 438
Bischof, 417, 516
Bohle, 97
Bonisolli, 497(R)
Jean-Paul Boyer, 734
Michael Brauner, 432, 471, 554, 736
Cynthia Brown Studio, 342, 710
Buntrock, 414
Shelby C. Burt Fraser, 714
Angelo Caggiano, 635
Alan Campbell, 70
Christopher Campbell Photography, 646
Caspar Carlott, 699
James Carrier Photography, 392, 393, 464, 586
Cazals, 256(B)
Cephas Picture Gallery, 79
Cimbal, 485
Michael Cogliantry, 442, 641(C)
Renee Comet, 258, 393, 450, 641(L), 651
Conrad & Company Photography, 233
da Costa, 434
Achim Daimling-Ostrinsky, 395(C), 697
Thom DeSanto Photography, 104, 114, 589(T)
Duncan, 366
Eising Food Photography, 212, 257, 261, 267, 305, 340-341, 392, 414, 415, 418, 421, 425(B), 433, 436, 471, 529(T), 535, 546, 576, 606-607, 627, 611(R), 668, 688(T), 708
Susie M. Eising Food, 372
Element Photo, 345, 647
Colin Ericson, 561(B)
Douglas Evans, 23
Fairchild, 457
Thomas Firak Photography, 12(L), 401, 494, 563(T)
Foodcollection, 68, 74-75, 390, 434, 465, 471, 561(T)
Gabula Art-Foto, 702(B)
Dennis Gottlieb, 52, 137, 259(B), 684
Michael Grand, 252, 393
Grosskopf, 667
Rusty Hill, 14(C), 556-557, 699(L)
Holsten/Koops, 497(L)
Hunter, 125, 417
K. Iden, 417, 702(T)
Sian Irvine, 495(R), 685(T)
Douglas Johns Studio Inc., 262, 395(R), 398
Kob, 214, 218, 414, 415, 534
LaCroix, 473
Joerg Lehmann, 742

Louise Lister, 565
Geoff Lung, 28(R)
Rick Mariani Photography, 102, 131, 681
Maximilian Stock Ltd., 161(T), 194-195, 715
Meier, 535, 615
Chris Meier, 276-277, 677
Karl Newedel, 722, 724
Okolicsanyi, 56
O'Neill, 470
Paul Poplis Photography, 524, 640, 649, 663
Rees, 470
Z. Sandmann, 269(T)
Z. Sandmann/Cimbal, 693
Scherer, 452, 487(T)
Schieren, 339, 395(L), 414
Shaffer/Smith Photography, 551, 654
Shipes Shooter, 639
Slater Company Inc., 119
Smith, 600
Snowflake Studios, 623
Solzberg Studio, 66, 434
Studio Adna, 35
Studio Lipov, 709(B)
Sucre Sale, 410-411
Urban, 436
Frederic Vasseur, 644
Zabert Sandman Verlag, 621, 723
Volk, 495(L)
Westerman, 415
Wieder, 503(T), 538, 636
Frank Wieder, 28(L)
James Worrell Photography, Ltd., 252
Zila Photography, 362
Jeff Stoecker, 162, 324, 334, 466(B), 514
SuperStock, 48, 62, 172, 532, 544
    age fotostock, 742
    Mike Agliolo, 658-659
    Raphael Auvray, 142, 143
    Christopher Campbell, 168, 170
    Francisco Cruz, 234, 250, 691
    Digital Vision Ltd., 330
    Greer & Assoc., Inc., 130
    James May, 672
    Raoul Minsart, 196
    David Papzian, 558
    Pixtal, 448
    Stock Image, 158
    Stockbyte, 735
    Sucre Sale, 34, 648
    Thinkstock, 220, 712
Taylor Precision Products, 70, 326
Lee Tompkins, 397
USDA, 145, 241(L), 510
USDA/FSIA, 291(TR)
USDA/FSIS, 244
Vote Photography, 159, 226, 241(R), 244, 355, 376
Mel Waters, 669
Thomas Way, 703
Dana White, 65(B), 480
Ian Worpole, 92, 93, 163

Index

Page references for graphics and features are in *italics*.

A

Á la carte, 271
Absorption, 84
Accidents, 297-303, *298-303*
Active dry yeast, 612
Added sugars, 93-94, 95-96, *96*, 97
Additives. *See* Food additives
Adequate Intakes (AIs), *80*, 81
Adipose cells, 107
Adolescents (teens), 188-189, 202, 257, 258
Adulthood nutrition, 189-191
Advertising, 153, *153*, 159, 160, 167, 198, 223, 239, *244*, 244, 550
Aerobic exercise, 165-166
Agriculture, 25, 51
Agroforestry, 57, 58
Air cell, 491
Al dente, 456
Albumen, 491, *491*, 492
Alcohol, 24, 78, 124, 175, 257
Allergies, 67, 176, 214, *470*, 550
All-purpose flour, 610
Allyl sulfides, 136
Altitude, 349, 643
American Dietetic Association, 154
American Gas Association (AGA) seal, 312, *312*
American Red Cross, 303
American Standard Code for Information Interchange (ASCII), *337*
Amino acids, 84, 85, 103, 104, *105*, 120, 149
Anaerobic exercise, 166
Analogs, 64
Anemia, 78, 121, 125-126
Annual percentage rate (APR), 313
Anorexia nervosa, 177
Anthocyanins, 135
Antibiotics, 292
Antibodies, 105
Antioxidants, 118, 122, 134, 135, 431, *549*
Antipasto, *699*
Appetizers, 256-257
Appliances, 69, 70, 200, 311, 312, 312-313, 314-317, 332-333, *333*, 628, *628*
Aquaculture, 57-58
Arcing, 376
Aromatic vegetables, 442
Artificial sweeteners, 97
Aseptic packages, 66
Au gratin, 588
Au jus, 602

B

Baby vegetables, 439
Bacteria, 280, *280*
  bioterrorism using, 292
  bottled water and, 546
  in cheese, 481
  choice of materials in kitchen and, 309
  cleanliness to prevent spread of, 281-282
  cross-contamination, 282
  eggs and, 481, 492, *493*, 496, *496*, 497
  fish and shellfish and, 535, 538
  food temperature's effect on, 283-284, *332*
  juices and, 547
  in mayonnaise, 578
  in meat, *514*
  in meat grinding process, 290
  in milk, 483
  plastics as carrier of, *335*
  poultry and, 525, 526, 527
  in processed food, 407
  in raw milk, 478
  refrigeration and, 284
  in salad greens, 575
  in spoiled food, 285
  thawing food and, 284
  trash and, 333, 334
  on vegetables, 440
  in yogurt, 479
Baguette, 687
Bakeware and cookware, 313, *318-319*, 318-322, *320*, *321*, *322*, 616
Baking, 324-325, *325*, 348, 349, 373-374, 609-618
Baking powder/soda, 612, 613
Baklava, 702
Bannock, 667
Bar codes, 242, *242*
Bar cookies, 639
Basal metabolic rate (BMR)/basal metabolism, 86
Batters, 611
Beading, 502
Beans, 466-467, 573, 586-587
Behavior modification, 163
Berries, 413
Beta-carotene, 134-135, 136, 413
Better Business Bureau, 312
Beverages, 545-553
Bigos, 709
Bile, 84
Binders, 588
Binge eating disorder, 177
Biodegradable materials, 333-334
Biodiversity, 50, 57, 59, 67
Bioengineered foods, 66
Bioplastics, *335*
Biotechnology, 68
Bioterrorism, 292

Biscotti, 701
Biscuit method, 624-625
Bisque, 597
Blanching, 403
Bleached flour, 610
Blini, 711
Blood, 132
Blood sugar (glucose), 84, 85, 176
Bloom, 552
Body fat percentage, 162-163
Body image, 160
Body mass index (BMI), 161-162, *162*
Boiling, 370
Boiling-water bath, 405
Bottled water, 546
Bouillon, 594
Bouquet garni, 391
Braising, 371, *371*
Bran, 449, *449*, 450, 452
Bread flour, 610
Bread machines, *628*
Breadfruit, 741
Breads, 454-456, 617, 618, 623-631
Breakfast, 201, *201*, *227*, 227-228, *587*, 597
Breast-/bottle-feeding, 185-186
Broiling, 374
Broth, 593-594, 596, 597, 599
Brown sugar, 614
Brunch, 201
Budget, *222*, 222-223
Buffets, 255, 269
Bulimia nervosa, 177-178
Bulk foods, 230, 238, *238*, 245
Burgoo, 599
Burns and fires, 298-299, *299*
Burrito, 562
Butter, 479, 613
Buying (purchasing), 246-247

C

Cabinets, 320
Caffeine, 174, 185, 189, 545, *545*, 553
Cakes, 617, 618, *619*, 635-638
Calories, 26, *85*, 85, 86, *86*, 95, 96, 97, *105*, 145, 146, 160-161, 163, *163*, 165, *165*, 168, 175, 190, 226, *577*
Calzone, 566, *566*
Canapés, 256
Candies, 635, *641*, 641-644
Canned food, 242, 286
Canning, 39, 51, 52, 66, 225
Cannoli, 701
Carambola, *414*, 414-419
Carbohydrates, 78, *80*, 83-84, 85, *85*, *86*, 91-98, *92*, *93*, 112, 119, 120, 121, 185, 186, 188-189, 201, 228, 290
Carbon dioxide (CO2), 92, *485*
Carbon monoxide, 301, *314*

Carbonation, 545, 553
Careers, 28-29, 30-31
    anger management, 618-619
    attitude, 552-553
    business etiquette, 578-579
    communication, 426-427,
        458-459, 472-473
    dressing for work, 386-387
    education and training, 230-231
    ethics, 502-503, 654-655
    Family, Career and Community
        Leaders of America, Inc.
        (FCCLA), 178-179, 217, 529
    goal setting, 216-217
    industry aspects, 112-113
    information sources for, 58-59
    interests and aptitudes, 190-191
    jobs, 272-273, 350-351, 362-363
    leadership, 528-529
    learning and skills as aid to,
        126-127
    managing resources, 246-247
    positive work relationships,
        588-589
    preparing for, 136-137
    priorities, 540-541
    problem solving, 630-631
    resumé preparation, 336-337
    SPECIFIC, 45, 71, 87, 99, 155,
        169, 207, 263, 293, 302-303,
        327, 379, 397, 445, 517, 567,
        603, 645. See also list of spe-
        cific careers, 18
    technology in the workplace,
        486-487
    wages and benefits, 406-407
Carnivores, 50
Carotenoids, 134-135
Carrageen, 438
Cassava, 674, 674
Casseroles, 583, 586-589, 587
Caviar, 711
Celebrations, 26, 41, 42-43
Cells, 77, 77, 78, 103, 105, 106, 107,
    118, 132, 184
Centers for Disease Control and
    Prevention (CDC), 160, 292
Cereals, 454, 459
Certifications, 71
Ceviche, 674
Chalazae, 491, 492
Character, 528
Checkouts, 245, 245
Cheese, 480-481, 482-483, 485-486
Chemicals, 23, 24, 25, 56, 300-301,
    333
Cherimoya, 414, 419
Chicken, 522, 523, 524, 525, 526-
    529
Children, 187-188, 200, 224, 533.
    See also Adolescents (teens)
Chlorophyll, 92, 135
Choices of food, 24, 40, 64-66
Choking, 303, 303

Cholesterol, 80, 81, 107, 108-110,
    109, 111, 112, 175, 212
Chorizo, 674
Chowder, 597
Chutney, 729
Chyme, 83
Cioppino, 665
Citrus fruits, 413, 422
Clay-pot cooking, 321
Cleanliness, 281-282, 309, 311, 326
Cloning, 67
Coagulation, 494
Coating foods, 361, 361
Cocoa and hot chocolate, 551-553
Cocoa butter/powder, 552
Code dating, 242
Coffee/coffee beans, 547, 547-548
Colcannon, 686
Cold cuts, 512
Cold water test, 642
Collagen, 508
Color of food, 228-229
Colostrum, 185-186
Comfort foods, 26, 38, 174
Commodities, 223
Communication, 31, 44, 386, 528
Comparison shopping, 243, 246,
    313
Complete proteins, 104, 107
Complex carbohydrates, 93, 93, 95,
    97, 189, 571
Composting, 335, 337
Compressed yeast, 612, 613
Computers, 69-70
Condiments, 395, 560, 560, 563
Conduction, 367, 367-368
Confectioners' sugar, 614
Conflict resolution, 619
Connective tissue, 507, 507-508,
    513, 537
Conservation, 331, 332-337, 333
Consommé, 597
Consumers, 50, 225, 312-313. See
    also listing of Consumer FYI
    features, 19
Contaminants/contamination, 56,
    279, 292
Controlled atmosphere storage, 52
Convection cooking/ovens, 315,
    315-316, 368, 368, 374, 617
Convenience/convenience foods,
    225-228, 587, 594, 598-599,
    641, 655
Convenience stores, 236
Conventional method, 628, 636-637
Conversion, 346-347, 347, 348
Cookbooks, 27, 45, 350
Cooked dressings, 578
Cookie cutters, 396
Cookies, 613, 618, 635, 638-641
Cooking center, 308
Cooking classes, 370
Cooking greens, 437
Cooking methods, 367-378

Cooking oils, 613
Cooking power, 375-376
Cooking spray, 616
Cooktops, 314-315, 315, 332
Cookware and bakeware, 313, 318-
    319, 318-322, 320, 321, 322
Cooperation, 386
Corn, 452
Corn syrup, 614
Cornstarch, 594
Corridor kitchen plan, 308
Cost per serving, 244
Cotyledon, 466
Countertops, 310
Coupons, 244, 244-245
Cover, 253, 253
CPR (cardiopulmonary resuscita-
    tion), 303
Cream, 479, 484, 484-485, 618, 649
Creativity, 28, 126, 391
Credit, 313, 313
Critical thinking, 30-31
Croquettes, 667
Cross-contamination, 282-283
Croutons, 572
Cruciferous vegetables, 136
Crumb crusts, 653-654
Crustaceans, 534
Crystal, 252
Crystallization, 52, 614, 641, 643-
    644
Cuisine, 36
Culture, 35-36, 40, 197, 268-269,
    269
Curdling, 484
Curds, 480, 480, 481, 484, 485
Curing, 51-52, 53, 512
Curry, 728
Custards, 500-501, 501, 618, 649
Customary system, 344, 345
Customs, 36, 41-44, 42-43, 198, 198
Cuts (of meat), 508, 509
Cutting boards, 283, 358
Cutting foods, 358-360, 523, 523
Cutting in, 625
Cutting tools, 323, 323-324

D

Daikon, 730
Daily Values (DVs), 81, 81, 149, 152
Dairy dressings, 579
Dairy foods, 477-486, 478
Dairy substitutes, 214, 481-482
Dal, 728, 728, 728-729
Dating of products, 241-242
Decaffeinated coffee/tea, 548, 549
Decision making, 206, 206, 528
Decomposers, 50
Decorating cakes/piecrust, 638, 638,
    652, 652
Deep-fat frying, 372-373
Dehydration (lack of water), 133
Dehydration (of food), 406-407

Designer foods, 68
Developing countries/nations, 54, 55, 67
Dextrose, 92, *96*
Dietary fiber (fiber), *80, 81,* 84, 93, 95, 97, 98, *98,* 133, 149, 212, 369
Dietary Guidelines for Americans, 143, *144*
Dietary Reference Intakes (DRIs), 79-81, *80*
Dietary supplements, 149-152
Diet/diets, 36-37, 163-165, 167-168, 695
Digestion, 81-84, *82,* 104, 108, 189
Dim sum, 731
Dinnerware, 252
Disaccharides, 92, *92,* 93
Diseases, 24, 64, 68, 118-123, 134-136, 174, 189-190, 212, 241, 431, *549. See also* Centers for Disease Control and Prevention (CDC)
   beriberi, 119
   cancer, 160, 189, 212, 291, 431
   Crohn's disease, *169*
   diabetes, 24, 160, 176, 212
   heart disease, 24, 68, 149, 160, 189, 212, 431
   high blood pressure, 160, 175
   HIV/AIDS, 176
   hypertension, 124
   osteomalacia, 122
   osteoporosis, 123
   pellagra, 119-120
   rickets, 122
Dishwashers, *301,* 317, 333
Dish washing, 282, 298, 333
Distributors/distribution, 53, 55
Diversity, 34-44
DNA, 103, *103,* 120
Docking, 653
Dolmas, 702
Doneness, *514,* 514-515, *515,* 526, 537-538, 624, 627
Dough, 611, 628-631, 650-652
Dovetailing, 384
Dovi, 599
Down payment, 313
Drawn/dressed fish, 535, *536*
Dressings. *See* Salad dressings
Drop batters, 611
Drop biscuits, 627
Drop cookies, 639
Drugs, 24, 78, 106, 175, 257, 292
Drupes, 413, *414*
Dry ingredients, 356-358, *357*
Dry-heat cooking, *373*-375
Drying food, 52, 406-407
Dry-measure method, 358
Dry-pack method, 403
Duck, 523, 527
Dumplings, *599*

E

Eating disorders, 106, 176-179
Eating habits, 164-165, 205
Eating out, 202-205, 215-216, *216,* 270-273
Eating patterns, 199-200
Economics, 37-38, 54, 212, 222-223, 226, 243-245, 258, 331, *343,* 512-513, 523, 587
Ecosystem, 49, 50, 57, 67, 212, 292
Eggs, 65, 491-503, 573, 596, 600, 614, *640*
Elastin, 508
Elderly Nutrition Program (ENP), 224
Electric ranges, 315, *315*
Electricity, 300, *300,* 311, *311,* 316, 333
Electrolytes, 124, 125, 189
Electronic Benefits Transfer (EBT) card, 224
Emotions, 199
Empanadas, 674, 697
Employment/Age Certificate, *351*
Emulsifiers, 494, *495,* 578
Emulsions, 577-578
En papillote, 538, *539*
Endosperm, 449, *449,* 450, 452, 594
Energy, 85, 86, 91, 92, *93,* 95, 105, 118, 119, 120, 121, 201
Energy efficiency, 332-333
EnergyGuide/ENERGY STAR® labels, 312, *312,* 332, 333
Enhanced foods, 68
Enrichment of food, 68, 450, 452, 454
Entertaining, 260-262
Entertainment aspect of food, 26-27
Entrées, 204, 271
Entrepreneurship, 302-303, 679
Enzymatic browning, 422
Enzymes, 83, 93, 104, 105, 285, 404, 422, 480
Equipment for food preparation, 225. *See also* specific names of
Equivalents, 346, 347, *637*
Ergonomics, *69*
Esophagus, *82, 83, 83*
Essential amino acids, 104
Ethics, 67, *502-503, 654-655*
Ethnic food, 26-28, 29, 36, 44, 45, *99,* 215, *343,* 464, *567,* 599, *603*
Etiquette, 267-275, 578-579
Étouffée, 664
European Article Numbers (EAN), 242
European Union, 67
Exercise. *See* Physical activity (exercise)

F

Fad diets, 167-168
Fajitas, 562
Falafel, 562
Falls, 297
Families and food, 198, *198,* 199-200, 222, 227, 254, 257, 308, 586
Famine, 54, 55
Farmers Market Nutrition Program, *236*
Farmers markets, *236,* 236-237
Farms/farming, 51, 54, 55, 57-58, 59, 64, 67, 199, *573*
Fast food, 203, *203,* 225, 272, 559
Fasting, 39
Fat (in body), 85, 106, 107-108, 160
Fats (in food), 107-113
   absence of carbohydrates and, 95
   in baked goods, 613, *613*
   at breakfast, 201
   in breast milk, 185
   calories in, 85, *85,* 97
   in comfort foods, 26
   condiments, *560*
   in convenience foods, 226
   cooking in, 371-373, *372*
   dairy products, 477, *477*
   digestion of, 108, 174
   egg substitutes, 494
   fat replacers, 290
   and fatty acids, 84, 108
   fish, 534
   function of, 78
   legumes, 464
   limiting, *373*
   in low nutrient density foods, 144
   measuring, 357-358
   meat, 464, 507, 508, 510, 513
   poultry, 521, *521,* 522, 523
   recommendations about, *80, 81, 86, 86,* 110-111
   in roux, 596
   salad dressings, 577, 578
   salads, 571
   in sauces, 601
   structure of, 108
   in vegetables, 431
   in vegetarian diets, 212
   vitamins as aid to, 119, 120, 121
Fat-soluble vitamins, *121,* 121-123
Fatty acids, 84, 85, 108, 186, *213*
Fatty fish, 534, *535*
FCCLA, 178, 529
Federal Meat Inspection Act, 509
Feelings and emotions, 24, 26, 31, 41
Feijoa, *414,* 419
Fermentation, 627
Festivals for food, 27, 35, 41

Fetus, 184, *184*
Fiber. *See* Dietary fiber (fiber)
Fillets (of fish), 535, *536*
Fillings, 563-564, 565, 566, 618, 649, *649*, 655
Finance charge, 314
Fires and burns, 298-299, *299*
First aid, 303
Fish and shellfish, 37, 57-58, 533-541, 573, 574
Flans, 654-655
Flatbreads, 455
Flatware, 252, 253
Flavonoids, 135
Flavor of food, 83, 108, 228, 291, 484
Flavorings, 52, 479, 594, 614-615
Floors and walls, 310-311
Flour, 594-596, 609-611, *610*
Flouring pans, 616, *616*
Fluid consumption, 133, 174, 175, 189, 190, 205
Flummery, 741
Fluted edges, 652, *652*
Foam/foams, 484, 494-495, *495*
Focaccia, 564
Food additives, 52-53, *289*, 289-290
Food allergies, 67, 176, 214, *470*, 550
Food and Nutrition Board of the National Research Council, 200
Food budget, *222*, 222-223
Food chain, 49-50
Food choices, 197-199, 203-206, 213-216
Food contamination, 184
Food cooperatives, 236
Food gifts, *396*
Food groups, 144-145
Food Guide Pyramid, 143
Food intolerances, 176
Food labels, 239-242, *240*
Food myths, 152-153, *153*
Food poisoning, 279, 292
Food programs, 223-224, *236*
Food record, *205*, 205-206
Food Safety and Inspection Service (FSIS), 292
Food science, 63, 71, 369, 422, 424, 440, 456, 466, 485, 486, 494, 507, 510, 521, 526, 537, 574, 576, 578, 594, 609, 611, 615, 627, 642, 643
Food shortages, 199-200
Food Stamp Act, 223-224
Food terms, *204*, 240
Food waste, 230, 254, 335
Foodborne illness, 279-280, *280*, 284, 285, *290*, 291, 292, 404, 514, 538, *640*
Fool, 685
Formal service, 256-257
Formed products, 65

Fortification of food, 68, 477
Fraud, 154
Free radicals, 118
Freeze-drying, 52
Freezer burn, 288
Freezers, *301*, 316-317
Freezing food, 51, 225, 286-288, *287*, 348
Fricassee, 599
Friends and food, 198
Frijoles, 675
Frittatas, 499, *500*
Fritters, 425, *425*
Frosting/frosting cakes, 618, 638, *638*
Frozen food, 284, *288*, 288-289
Fructose, 92, *92*, 93, *96*
Fruits, 413
    beta-carotene in, 122, 135
    commercially processed, 423
    cooking, 423-427
    descriptions and uses, 415-418
    dietary fiber from, 98
    freezing, 403
    identifying, 413-419
    minerals in, 123
    nutrients in, 413, 420, 421, 424
    phytochemicals in, 135-136, 137
    in pies, 649
    preparing, 421, 421-422
    in salads, 574, 585
    selecting, 419-421
    serving, 422-423
    in soups, 597-598
    spreads made from, 406
    square, 420
    in stir-fries, 572
    sugars in, 93, 96
    vitamin C in, *118*, 118-119
    vs. juices, 546
    water in, 133
Frying and sautéing, 372
Fuel shortages/supplies, 55, 58
Functional foods, 68
Fusion cuisine, 44, 661

G

Galactose, 92, *92*, 93
Galettes, 655
Garnishes, *395*, 395-396, 598, *598*, 655
Gas ranges, 314-315
Gazpacho, 598
Gelatin, 574, 593
Gelatinization, 595
Genetic engineering, 66-67, 68
Genetically modified foods (GMFs)/organisms (GMOs), 66, 67
Germ, 449, *449*, 450, 452
Giblets, 524
Gifts of food, 396

Glassware, 252, *252*, 253
Global foods, 25-26, 29-30
    Africa, 717, 721-723
    Australia, *739*, 739-741
    Canada, 661, *661*, 666-668
    Caribbean, 673, 678
    East Asia, 730-733
    Eastern Asia, 727, *727*
    Eastern Europe, *707*, 707-710
    Latin America, *673*, 673-677
    Northern Europe, 683, *683*, 689-691
    Oceania, *739*, 741-743
    Russia, 707, *707*, 710-713
    South Asia, 727, *727*, 728-729
    Southeast Asia, *727*, 734-735
    Southern Europe, *695*, 695-702
    Southwest Asia, *717*, 717-720
    United States, *661*, 661-666
    Western Europe, *683*, 683-689
Global problems, 54-56, 59
Glucose (blood sugar), 84, 85, 95, *95*, 105, 188
Glucose (in plants), 92, *92*, 93, 94, *96*, 132
Gluten, 609, *610*
Gluten flour, 610
Glycerol, 108
Glycogen, 85, 95, 188, 189
Gnocchi, 699
Goose, 523, 525, 527
Goulash, 599, 663
Government food programs, 223-224, *236*, 243
Grain (of meat), 508
Grains, 37, 449-459, *450*, 573, 584, 586, 594
Granulated sugar, 614
GRAS (Generally Recognized as Safe) list, *289*, 289-290, 421
Gratuity, 271
Grazing, 202, 215
Greasing pans, 616, *616*
Green shopping, 59
Grilling, 259-260, 301, 326, *374*, 374-375
Ground meat, 510
Ground poultry, 524
Grounding, 311, *311*
Groundwater, 56
Guacamole, 562
Guava, 743
Gumbo, 664, *664*
Gyro, 562

H

Haggis, 685, *685*
Hand washing, 281, *281*
Haute cuisine, 687
Hazard Analysis and Critical Control Point (HACCP), 290, *291*, 534

Hazardous household chemicals, 300-301, 333
HDL (high-density lipoprotein), 109
Headspace, 403
Health
   antioxidants to protect, 118
   busy lifestyle and, *225*
   as career aid, *137*
   chronic problems with, 175-176
   claims on labels and, 241
   convenience foods and, 226
   eating out and, 203-205
   fast food and, *203*
   fats' effect on, 110
   fatty acids' role in, 108
   food budget related to, *223*
   food choices affecting, 24, 78-79, 205, 206
   illness and, 175
   lipids' effect on, 107
   minerals' effect on, 123-127
   phytochemicals' effect on, 134-137
   during pregnancy, 184
   proteins' effect on, 104, 105
   science and technology's effect on, 68-70
   snacks and, 202, *202*
   stress and, 26, 173-175, *174*
   tea and, *549*
   of teeth and gums, 95
   vegetarianism's effect on, 212
   vitamins' effect on, 118-123
   water's role in, 132
   weight's effect on, 160, 189
   wellness, 24
Health food stores, 236
Healthy Meals for Americans Act, 224
Heat exhaustion/stroke, 189
Heating units, 314
Heimlich maneuver, 303
Hemoglobin, 104
Herb teas, 550
Herbals, 149-152
Herbivores, 50
Herbs and spices, 391-395, *392-393, 394*
Heroes, 560-562
High-altitude cooking, 349, 643
Hilum, 466, *466*
Hoisin, 730, *730*
Hollandaise, 600
Holloware, 252
Homogenization, 478
Honesty, 502
Honey, 614, *614*
Hormones, 105, 160, 292
Hors d'oeuvres, 256
Hot chocolate and cocoa, 551-553
Hot spots, 616
Hot-pack method, 404

Hull, 449, 452, 473, *473*
Hunger and starvation, 30, 54, 55, 67
Hydration, 132
Hydrogen, 108, 110
Hydrogenated foods, 110, 481, 613
Hydroponic farming, 57
Hygiene, 281

I

Immature fruit, 420
Immigration/immigrants, 38, 199
Impulse buying, 238, 245
Incomplete proteins, 104
Independent grocers, 236
Indoles, 136
Industrial Revolution, 199
Industrialized nations, 54
Infants, 185-186, 224
Injera, 723
Insecticides, 282
Integrated pest management (IPM), 57
Interest, 313
Interfering agents, 643
Internal temperature, 283
Internet, 44, 54, 69-70, *70*, 154, 167, 237, 350
Intestinal juice, 84
Invitations, 261
Iodine, 126
Irish stew, 599
Irradiation, 290-291, *291*
Island, 308
Isoflavones, 135
Israeli wheat berry stew, 599

J

Jambalaya, 664
Jams/jellies, 406
Jerk, 678
Juice drinks, 546
Juices, 546-547

K

Kielbasa, 709
Kernels, 449, *449*, 470, 472, 473
Kilocalories, 85
Kimchee, 733
Kitchens, 281-282, 307-326
Kneading, 629, *629*
Knives, *323*, 323-324, *324*
Kolache, 709
Kringel, 709

L

Labels, 148, 239-242, 245
Lactase, 93

Lactation, 186
Lactose, 92, *92*, 93, *96*, 176, 186, 478, 479
Lahvosh, 562
Lard, 613
Lattice crusts, 652-653, *653*
Laverbread, 685
LDL (low-density lipoprotein), 109
Lead, *252*
Leadership, 31, *136*, 528-529
Leavened bread, 455
Leavening agents, 611-613, *612*
Leftovers, 284, 444, 512, 574, 584, 586, 587, 602
Legislation for food assistance, 223-224
Legumes, 463-469, *465*, 596, 597
Lettuce, 571, 574-575, *575*
Life span, 183
Lighting, 311, 333
Linolenic acid, 108, *213*
Lipids, 107-112
Lipoproteins, 108
Liquid ingredients, 356, *356*, 593-594, 611
Liver, *82*, 84
Low-fat fish, 534, *534*
Loyalty, 502
L-shaped kitchen plan, 308
Lunches from home, 257-259, *258*
Lutefisk, 691
Lutein, 135
Lychee, *414*, 419
Lycopene, 135, 431

M

Macaroni, 454
Maillard reaction, 369
Major minerals, *123*, 123-125
Malnutrition, 78, 106
Maltose, 93, *96*
Management, 31, 217, 246, 528, 712
Manners, 267-273, 578-579
Manufactured food, 64
Marbling, 508, 510
Margarine, 613, *613*
Marinating, 514, 602
Marzipan, 696
Masa, 675
Mature fruit, 419
Mayonnaise, 578
Meal patterns, 201-202
Meal replacement bars, *587*
Meals/meal planning, 69-70, 221-231, 332, 335
Measures and weights, 344-347, *346, 347*
Measuring ingredients, 355-358
Measuring tools, 322, *323*, *355*, 355-356
Meat, 37, 507-516, 573, 574
Meat alternatives, *463*, 464

Meat substitutes, 213-214
Media, influences, 198
Megadoses, 149
Melons, 413, *417*
Menu planning, 221-231, 335
Mercury, 533
Meringues, *501*, 501-503, *503*
Metabolism, 85-86, 132
Metric system, 79, 85, 344-345
Mezza, 718
Microorganisms, *279*, 279-280, 404, *405*, 421, *593*
Microwave ovens, 284, 316, *316*, 375-376, *376*, 378, *378*
Microwave time, 378
Microwaving, 375-378, *377*, 617
Milk and milk products, 37, 477-480, 484-485
Minerals, 78, 79, *80*, *81*, 85, 95, 97, 123-127, 132, 144, 149, 213, 369, 431, 441, 444, 450, 460, 464, 478, 492, 533, 545, 546, 571
    SPECIFIC, 122, 123, 123-127, *125*, 160, 175, 184, 213
Minestrone, 597
Miscarriage, 184
Mise en place, 584-585
Mixing, 324, *325*, 360-361
Modified atmosphere packaging (MAP), 65-66
Modified English service, 254-255
Moist-heat cooking, 369-371
Molasses, 614
Molded cookies, 640
Molded salads, 574
Mole, 675
Mollusks, 534
Monosaccharides, 92, *92*
Monounsaturated fatty acids, 108
Moussaka, *701*
Mouth, 83, *83*
Muffin method, 623, *624*
Mulled punch, 553
Mulligatawny, 597
Multiple roles, 221
Muscle, 507, 510, 521-522, 537
Mustard, 395
Myoglobin, 522
MyPyramid, 143
Myths about food, 152-153, *153*

N

Nanofiltration, *52*
Napkins, 253
National Electric Code, 311, *311*
National Marine Fisheries Service, 534
National School Lunch Act, 223
Natural disasters, 55
Natural foods/natural food stores, 236, 241
Natural resources, 50
Nonfat milk solids, 478

Nonrenewable resources, 331
Nonstick finishes, *322*
Nonverbal communication, 31, 458
Noodles, 454
Nori, 733
Nutraceuticals, 68, 136
Nutrient density, 145
Nutrients, 23. *See also* Nutrition
    absorption of, 25, 84
    as additive, 52
    analyzing intake of, *151*
    body's use of, 77, 78, 86
    chart for, *150-151*
    cooking's effect on, 368-369
    in dietary supplements vs. foods, 149
    in digestive process, 81-84
    as enrichment, 68
    excess of, 68
    in foods, 77-78
    as fortification, 68
    health affected by, 78-79
    listed, on Nutrition Facts panel, 148-149
    megadoses of, 149
    metabolism of, 85-86
    required, 79-81, *80*
    responsibility about, 86
    in soil, 50
    storage of, 85
    teamwork of, 79
    technology for saving, *52*
    transportation of, 84-85
    weight loss's effect on, 160
Nutrition, 23-24
    in adolescence, 188-189
    during adulthood, 189-191
    analysis, *152*, 344
    in childhood, 187-188
    convenience foods, 226
    dietary supplements, 149-152
    government's role in, 200
    illness affected by, 175
    improving, 68
    in infancy, 185-187
    during life span, 183
    limiting fat, *373*
    listed on food labels, 240-241
    lunches from home, 258-259
    meal times and, 201
    during pregnancy, 184-185
    research about, 69
    resources for, 143-149
    salad dressings, *577*
    salad greens, 575
    sandwiches, *559*
    at school, *203*
    soups, 596
    for special needs children, 188
    truth evaluation, 152-154
    vegetarian, 212-213, *213*
Nutrition Facts panel, 143, 148-149, *148*, *150*, 226, 239, 454

Nutrition Labeling and Education Act of 1990, 148
Nutritive Value of Foods chart, 150-151
Nuts, 469-472, *470-471*

O

Oats, 452, 453
Obesity (overweight), 78, 160-161
Obstetrician, 184
Oil-and-vinegar sauces, 602
Older Americans Act, 224
Omega-3 fatty acid, 108, *213*
Omelets, 499, *499*
One-bowl method, 637
One-wall kitchen plan, 308
Open dating, 241
Open stock, 252
Organic farming, 57
Organic foods, 236
Organic seal, 241, *241*
Organization, 386
Outdoor meals/cooking, 259-260, 326
Ovens, *301*, 314-316, 332
Ovo-vegetarians, 212
Oxidation, 85

P

Packaging, 53, 65-66, 288, 334
Paella, 696, *696*
Pan broiling, 372, *372*, 516
Pancetta, 699
Pancreas/pancreatic juice, *82*, 84
Parchment, 616
Parliamentary procedure, 579
Pasta, 454, *455*, 456-458, *457*, 574
Pasteurization, 477, 481, 547
Peanuts, *470*, *471*
Pectin, 402, 409
Pediatrician, 186
Peer pressure, 188
Pelmeni, 711
Peninsula, 308
Perishable foods, 238, 242
Peristalsis, 83, *83*
Permanent emulsion, 578
Pesticides, 51, 64, 66, 67, *291*, 291-292
Pesto, 699
Pests, 282, *282*, 291, 309, 333
Photosynthesis, 92, *92*, 456
Physical activity (exercise), 24, 86, 124, 133, 134, 161, 165-167, 175, 188-189, 190
Physically challenged people, 308-309
Phytochemicals, 78, 85, 97, 131, 134-137, 149
Phytosterols, 136
Pica, 126

Pickled foods, 406
Picnics, 260
Pie shells, 653
Piecrust, 650-654
Pierogis, 709, *709*
Pies, 649-654
Pilaf, 713
Pilot lights, *314*
Pita, 562
Pizza, 566
Place mats, 253
Place setting, 251, *251*
Placing pans, 616, *617*
Plankton, 533
Plants, 91, 92, *92*, 106
Plate service, 254
Poaching, 370
Poke, 666
Polarized plugs, 300
Polenta, 699
Politics and conflict, 55
Pollution, 333, 336
Polysaccharides, 93, *93*
Polyunsaturated fatty acids, 108
Pomes, 414, *414*
Population, 55, 56
Portal vein, 84
Portions, 147, 203, 223, 254
Posole, 599
Pots and pans. *See* Cookware and bakeware
Poultry, 521-529, 573, 574
Pour batters, 611
Poverty, 54
Power outages, 288-289
Precycling, 334
Pregnancy, 120, 133, 184-185, 533
Preheating, 615
Preparation of food, 37, 40, 69-70, 355-363
Pre-preparation, 384, 584
Presentation of food, 28, 396
Preserves, 406
Preserving food, 401-407
Pressed cookies, 640, *640*
Pressure canning, 405, *405*
Pressure-cooking, 371
Prickly pear, *414*, 419
Principal, 313
Problem solving, 126, 528, 630-631
Processing/processors of food, 25, 51-52, 53, 64-66, 67, 122
Produce, 419
Producers/production of food, 49-50, 51, 54, 56-57, 58, 64
Product dating, 241-242
Professionalism, 502, 654
Proofing, 613
Protein-energy malnutrition (PEM), 106
Protein/proteins, 78, 79, *80*, *81*, 84, 85, *85*, *86*, 95, 97, 103-107, 112, 119, 120, 121, 122, 160, 185-186, 201, 228, 290, 369, 571

Ptyalin, 83
Punch, 553
Punching down (dough), 630
Purchasing (buying), 246-247

Q

Quality of food, 242-243
Quercetin, 135
Quiche, 501, *501*
Quick breads, *623*, 623-627
Quick sauces, 602
Quick-mix method, 628-629
Quick-rising yeast, 612
Quorn™, 214

R

Radiation, 368, *369*, 374
Ragòut, 599
Rancidity, 286
Ranges, 314-316
Raw milk, 477-478
Raw-pack method, 404
Rebates, 244
Recalls, 291, 292
Receptions, 255-256, *256*
Recipes, 343
    changing, 347-349
    collecting, 349-350
    downsizing, 231
    files for, 351
    reading beforehand, 383
    SPECIFIC, 225, 226-227, 262, *262*, 344, 345, 402, 424, 442, 451, 457, 468, 487, 500, 512, 524, 539, 551, 561, 565, 572, 585, 595, 601, 625, 626, 636, 639, 642, 650, 651. *See also* list of specific recipes, 17
    trends in, 343
    weights and measures for, 344-347, 346, 347, 348
    well-written, 343-344
Recommended Daily/Dietary Allowances (RDAs), *80*, 81, 200
Reconstituting foods, 423, 444
Recycling, *336*, 336-337
Reduction, 594
Refrigerating food, 284, 286, *287*, 288, 289, *332*
Refrigerator cookies, 640
Refrigerator-freezers, 316-317, *332*
Regreening, 420
Reheating food, 284
Rehydration, 407
Religion, 39, 67, 212, 224
Renewable resources, 331, 332
Reservations, 270
Resources, 197-198, 224-225, 246-247, 330-336
Restaurants, 202, 270-273
Resveratrol, 135

Retail cuts, 508, *509*
Retailers of food, 53-54
Retinol/retinal/retinoic acid, 121
Retort pouches, 66
Rice, 37, 451-452, 458
Ripened cheeses, 481, *482-483*, 486
Ripeness, 419, 439
Rising, 629
Rissoles, 741
Roasting (and baking), *373*, 373-374
Rolled biscuits, 625-627
Rolled cookies, 639-640
Roux, 596, 601
R.S.V.P., 261
Runners, 253

S

Safety. *See also* Bacteria; Temperature, of food
    accidents, 297-303, *298-303*
    appliances, 300
    buffets, 255, 269
    canning/canned foods, 404, 405, *405*, 407
    children, *301*, 302
    choice of kitchen materials, 309
    choking, *303*
    cleanliness, 281-282
    contaminants/contamination, 56, 279, 282-283, 292
    cooktops, 298-299
    cutting, 358-359, *359*
    doneness, *514*, 514-515, *515*, 526, 537-538
    eating out, *281*
    eggs, *496*, *497*, 500, 572
    electrical system, 311, *311*
    families and food, 301-303
    family service, 254
    food, 280
    food allergies, 67, 176, 214, *470*, 550
    food label instructions, 240
    food supply, 289-292
    foodborne illness, 279-280, *280*, 284, 285, *290*, 291, 292, 404, 514, 538
    genetic engineering, 67
    hazardous household chemicals, 300-301, 333
    kitchens, 297-301, *301*
    knives, 298, 358-359, *359*
    lunches from home, 258
    marinades, 602
    mercury, 533
    microwaving/microwave ovens, *375*, 486, 500, 553
    milk, *485*
    mold, *481*
    odor of food, 289
    outdoor grilling, 60
    outdoor meals/cook⌐

ovens, 299, *299*, 301
physically challenged people, *302*, 302-303
picnics, 260, *260*
pilot lights, *314*
preserving/preserved foods, *405*, 407
raw dough, *640*
refrigeration, 284
science's role in, 25
seals of approval, 312, *312*
shopping, 246
stock, *593*
storing food, 284-289
takeout food, 203
washing foods, 421, *421*, 439-440
water, 300
Saffron, 718
Salad dressings, 572, 573-574, 575-579
Salad greens, 437, 574-575, *576-577*
Salads, *571*, 571-574
Saliva, 83, 93
Salsa, 674
Sandwiches, 559-565
Sanitary landfill, 333
Sanitation, 281, 290, 292, 317
Saponins, 136
Sapote, *414*, 419
Sashimi, 733
Saturated fatty acids, 108
Sauces, 395, 584, 585, 593, *600*, 600-602
Sauerbraten, 687
Sautéing and frying, 372
Savory, 414, 649
Scalded milk, 484
Scales, 358, *358*
School Breakfast Program, 224
Science, 24-25, 27, 28, 63, 69. *See also* Food science
Scorching, 484
Scoring, 631
Scrapple, 662
Scratch cooking, 225, *225*
Sea vegetables, 437-438, *438*
Seafood, 534, 565, 566, 583, 596
Seals of approval, 312, *312*
Searing, 372
Seasonings/seasoning blends, 391-395, 585, 588, 598, 602
Seeds, 472-473
Seitan, 214
Self-esteem, 30
Self-rising flour, 610
Sell-by date, 241, *241*, 286, 575
Senses and food, 83
Service contracts, 313
Service plate, 256
Serving food, 251-262, 284, 422-423, 439-440, 485-487, 568, 579, *579*
Servings of food, *145*, 146, 146-147, 148, *148*, 149, 244, *244*

Shaping dough, 630-631
Sharing food, 26, 28, 41, 203, 231
Sharp edges, 298, *298*
Shelf life, 51, 52, 286
Shelf-stable, 51
Shellfish. *See* Fish and shellfish
Shirred eggs, 498-499
Shopping for food, 235-247
Shopping lists, 238-239, *239*, 245
Shortened cakes, 636
Simmering, 370
Simple carbohydrates, *92*, 92-93
Sink center, 308
Sit-down restaurants, 270-272
Small intestine, *82*, 84, *84*
Smart appliances, 69, 70, 317, *317*
Smell, 83, 190
Smoking (tobacco), 257
Smoking point, 372
Smoothies, 551, *551*
Smorgasbord, 689
Snacking, 202, *202*, 230
Social aspect of food, 26, 40-41
Soft doughs, 611
Soft drinks, 96, 553
Soft peaks, 496, *497*
Solanine, 439
Solar energy, 58-59
Sopas, 674
Soufflés, 495, *495*
Soups, 593, *596*, 596-599
Source reduction, 334
Soy/soybeans, 106, 213, *213*, 214, *214*, *215*, *469*, 481, *573*, 597
Special needs, 188, 308-309
Specialty stores, 236
Speed-scratch cooking, 226-227, 262
Spices and herbs, 391-395, *392-393*, *394*
Spoiled food, 285, *285*, 575, *593*
Sponge cakes, 637
Spores, 280
Standing time, 378
Staple foods (staples), 37, 223, 239
Starches, 93, *93*, 94, 97, 456, 578, 587, 594, *595*, 597, *597*
Starvation and hunger, 30, 54, 55, 67
State governments, 223
Steaks (fish), 535, *536*
Steam, 612
Steaming, 370, *371*
Steeping, 550
Sterols, 107
Stewing, 371
Stews, 593, *599*, 599-600
Stiff doughs, 611
Stiff peaks, 496, *497*
Stir-fries/stir-frying, 373, *583*, 583-586, 731
Stock, 593, 601
Stocking food, 39
Stollen, 687

Stomach, *82*, 83, 83-84, *84*
Storage/storing of food, 55, 122, 240, 284-289, 308, 335
Store brands, 245
Store layouts, 238, 239
Stress, 26, 173-175, 205, 722
Streusel, 654
Subsistence farming, 54
Substitutions, 348, *349*
Succotash, 662
Sucrose, 93, *96*
Sugar, 614
Sugar alcohols, 97
Sugar substitutes, 97
Sugar-pack method, 403
Sugars (in plants), *92*, 92-94
Sumac, 718
Sun, 49, 122
Supercenters, 235
Supermarkets, 235-236
Supplements. *See* Dietary supplements
Supply of food, 30, 50, 51-54, 57, 64-67
Sushi, 733
Sustainable living, 59
Sweeteners, 613-614
Syrup-pack method, 403

T

Tabbouleh, 573
Table etiquette, 268-270
Table linens, 253
Table setting, 253-254
Tablecloths, 253
Tableware, 251-253
Taco, 562
Tagines, 721
Tahini, 718
Takeout food, 203
Tamarillo, *414*, 419
Tandoor, 729, *729*
Tapas, 697
Taring, 358, *358*
Taro, 666
Tarts, 649, *654*, 654-655
Task lighting, 311
Taste buds, 83, 190
Tea, 548-550, *549*, 550
Tea sandwiches, 564-565, *565*
Teamwork, 385-387, *387*, 503
Technology. *See also* listing of Trends in Technology features, 19
  appliances, 69, 200
  biotechnology, 68
  convenience foods, 200
  cooking, 39-40
  definition of, 63
  electronic communication, *472-473*
  farms/farming, 64

food supply and water problems, 57
health affected by, 68-70
influence on cuisines/customs, 39-40, 44
kitchen, *70*
military, 200
nutrients, *52*
processing/processors of food, 64, 66
for snacks, *202*
solar energy, 58-59
trade-offs, 70
wind power, 59
workplace, 486
Teens (adolescents), 188-189, 202, 257, 258
Tempeh, 214
Temperature
  in baking, 615, *615*
  for cake ingredients, 635
  in candy making, 641, 642-643
  in cooking methods, 370-371, 372, 373, 374
  in dough rising, 629
  of food, 203, 229, 283-284
    bacteria affected by, *283*, 283-284
    buffets, 255
    eating out, *281*
    family service, 254
    in freezer, 286, *287*
    lunches from home, 258
    picnics, 260
    in refrigerators/refrigerator-freezers, 286, *287*, 316, *332*
    room temperature, 286
  in recipes, 344, 346-347
  in yeast mixing methods, 628-629
Tempering, 484
Temporary emulsion, 577-578
Tenderness/tenderizing, 510, 511, 514, 516, *516*
Texture (and shape) of food, 52, 66, 108, 229, 291, 368, 424, 440, 481, 483
Thawing food, 284, *284*, 514, 525
Thermometers, 325-326, 514, *514*, 516
Thickening, 594-596, *595*, 597, *597*, 600, 601, 602
Time management, 540-541
Time-saving techniques, 227-228
Timetables, 384, 384-385
Tipping, *271*, 271-272
Tofu, 214, 468-469, 585, 587
Tolerance, 292
Tomato sauces, 601-602
Tomato-based sauces, *602*
Tools for food preparation, 322-326, *323*, 324, *325*, *326*, 355-356

Toppings, 588, *589*, 598
Torte, 689
Tortillas, 562, *563*
Tossed salad, 579
Toxicity, 122
Toxins, 280, 292
Trace minerals, 125-127
Trans fats, 110, 111
Transportation, 66
Trash, 333-337, *334*
Tray-pack method, 403
Trifle, 423
Triglycerides, 107, 108
Tropical fruits, 414
Trussing, 527, *527*
Tryptophan, 120
Tubers, 437
Turkey, 522, *522*, 524, 525, 526, 527
Turnovers, 654
20-second scrub, 281
Two-crust pies, 652-653

U

Ugli fruit, *414*, 419
Unbleached flour, 610
Underripe fruit, 419
Underwriters Laboratories (UL), 312, *312*
Unit price, 243, *243*
Universal design, 308-309
Universal product code (UPC), 242, *242*
U.S. Department of Agriculture (USDA)
  added sugars recommendation, *96*
  calorie recommendation, 86, *86*
  cutting board recommendations, 283
  Dietary Guidelines for Americans, 143, *144*
  Economic Research Service, 222
  food grading/inspection, 479, 509, *510*, 525, *525*
  Food Guide, 143, 144, 145
  food regulation by, *290*
  food standards, 478, 492
  FSIS as branch of, 292
  meat handling, 513
  Nutrition Facts panel, 143, 147-149, *148*, *150*
  organic seal, 241, *241*
  safe handling instructions, on food labels, 240
U.S. Department of Commerce, 57, 534-535
U.S. Department of Health and Human Services, 143, 160, 289

U.S. Environmental Protection Agency (EPA), 291-292, 333, *334*, 533, 546
U.S. Federal Trade Commission (FTC), 154
U.S. Food and Drug Administration (FDA), 289
  bioterrorism, 292
  bottled water standards, 546
  Daily Value (DV) guidelines, 81, *81*
  fat replacers, 290
  food additives, 52, 289–290
  food complaints, 247
  food labels, 239, *240*, 240–241
  food supply registration, *290*
  fraud, 154
  functional foods, 68
  Generally Recognized as Safe (GRAS) list, 289–290
  Hazard Analysis and Critical Control Point (HACCP), 290, *291*, 534
  irradiation, 290–291, *291*
  mercury guidelines, 533
  quorn™ approval, 214
  recalls, 291
Use-by date, 241, 286
U-shaped kitchen plan, 308
Utensils, *307*

V

Vacuum bottle, 258
Vacuum insulation panels (VIP), 66
Values, 199, 712
Variety meats, 511
Vegetable shortening, 613
Vegetables, 431
  baby, *439*
  beta-carotene in, 122, 135
  in casseroles, 587
  convenience forms of, 444
  cruciferous, 136
  descriptions and uses, *432-436*
  dietary fiber from, 98
  freezing, 403
  fresh, 438-444
  legumes as, 464
  minerals in, *123*, 124, 125, 444
  nutrients in, 431, *431*, 440, 441, 442, 444
  phytochemicals in, 135-136, 137
  plant parts, 431-437, *437*
  in salads, 572, 574
  spreads, 406
  starches in, 94
  in stir-fries, 583, 584, 585
  in thickening, 596
  types of, 431-438, *432-436*
  using leftover, 444
  vitamins in, *118*, 123, 444
  vs. juices, 546
  water in, 133